Contributors

JOSE AGUSTI, MD, specialist in preventive medicine and weight loss, St. Mary Medical Center, Hobart, IN

ADOLPHUS ANEKWE, MD, Clinical Assistant Professor of Medicine, Indiana University Northwest Center for Medical Education; Health Commissioner of the City of Gary; and Consultant, Internal Medicine, IN

STEVE BAILEY, MD, FACC, FSCAI, Chief of Cardiology, University of Texas Health Center at San Antonio, San Antonio, TX; President of the Society of Cardiac Angiography and Interventions, Washington, D.C.

TAM D BUI, MD, President, Cu Chi University of Health Sciences, Ho Chi Minh City, Vietnam, and San Francisco CA

THOMAS BUMP, MD, Electrophysiologist, Christ Hospital, Oak Lawn, IL

PAOLO CARDAIOLI, MD, Head Chief, Cardiovascular Diagnosis and Endoluminal Interventions Unit, Rovigo General Hospital, Rovigo, Italy

SHAO LIANG CHEN, MD, Vice-President of Nanjing First Hospital and Nanjing Cardiovascular Disease Hospital, Nanjing, China

GIM HOI CHOO, MD, KPJ Selangor Specialist Hospital, Shah Alam, Malaysia

ZHANG SHUANG CHUAN, MD, Key Member of Chinese Pediatric Association of Cardiology, Professor of Pediatrics, Director of Pediatrics, Department of Peking University; Shenzhen Hospital Guest Professor of Shenzhen Children's Hospital, Shenzhen, China

NGUYEN DUC CONG, MD, PhD, President, Thong Nhat Hospital, Ho Chi Minh City, Vietnam

ALEXANDER DOGANOV, MD, Director, Cardiac Catheterization Laboratories, National Heart Hospital, Sofia, Bulgaria

VIJAY DAVE, MD Director of Medical Education, Department of Medicine, Community Healthcare System, St. Mary Medical Center, Hobart, IN

HUAN QUANG DO, MD, PhD, Chief of Cardiology, Ho Chi Minh City Heart Institute, Ho Chi Minh City, Vietnam

HO THUONG DUNG, MD, PhD, Vice-Director, Thong Nhat Hospital, Chief Interventional Cardiology, Thong Nhat Hospital, Ho Chi Minh City, Vietnam

STILIANOS EFSTRATIADIS, MD, Interventional Cardiology, Quincy, IL

KRISHNA K GADDAM, MD, Cardiology fellow, Ochsner Clinics, New Orleans, LA

NGUYEN LAN HIEU, MD, PhD, Vice-Director, Cardiac Catheterization Laboratories, Vietnam Heart Institute, Hanoi, Vietnam

BAO VAN HO, MD, MSC., San Diego, CA

PHAM MANH HUNG, MD, PhD, Associate Director, Cardiac Catheterization Laboratories, Vietnam Heart Institute, Bach Mai Hospital, Hanoi Medical University, Hanoi, Vietnam

DONGMING HOU, MD, PHD, FACC, FAHA, Senior Scientist, Adjunct Assistant Professor of Indiana University School of Medicine (Cardiology), Indianapolis, IN; Adjunct Clinical Research Associate Professor of Mercer University (Pharmacy Practice), Atlanta , GA; Visiting Professor of Harbin Medical University, Harbin, China; Visiting Professor of Tongji University, Shanghai, China

HUNG D. HUYNH, Informatics Consultant, Riverside, CA

JOHN HUYNH, St. Louis University, St. Louis, MO

ANDREW M. KATES, MD, FACC, Associate Professor of Medicine; Director, Cardiovascular Fellowship Program, Washington University School of Medicine, St. Louis, MO

PHAM GIA KHAI, MD, FACC, Professor of Medicine, President of the Vietnam Heart Association, Hanoi, Vietnam

PHAM QUOC KHANH, MD, PhD, Director of Electrophysiology Laboratories, Vice-Director, Vietnam Heart Institute; Vice President, Vietnamese Interventional Cardiology Society, Hanoi, Vietnam

MOO-HYUN KIM, MD, Professor of Medicine, Director of Cardiology, Dong A Medical School, Director of Clinical Trials Center, Dong A University Hospital, Busan, Korea

XIANKAI LI, MD, Tongji University School of Medicine, Cardiology Department, Shanghai Tenth People's Hospital affiliated with Tongji University, Shanghai, China

DO DOAN LOI, MD, PhD, Vice-President, Bach Mai Hospital, Director, Echocardiography Laboratories, Vietnam Heart Institute, Hanoi, Vietnam

CHANGSHENG MA, MD, Professor of Medicine, Director of Atrial Fibrillation Center, Beijing An Zhen Hospital, Beijing, China

TUNG DINH MAI, BS, Department of Chemistry and Biochemistry, San Diego State University, San Diego, CA

PETER MCCULLOUGH, MD, Department of Medicine, Divisions of Cardiology, Nutrition and Preventive Medicine, William Beaumont Hospital, Royal Oak, MI

MARIO MARANHAO, MD, Professor of Medicine, Evangelic Hospitals and School of Medicine, Curitibo, Brazil

ANDREW D. MICHAELS, MD, MAS, FACC, FAHA, Associate Professor of Medicine, Department of Medicine, Division of Cardiology, University of Utah, Salt Lake City, Utah

HUYNH VAN MINH, MD, PHD, Chairman of the Department of Medicine, Hue Medical School, Hue, Vietnam

JOEL MULUNGU, MD, XiangYa School of Medicine, Central South University Third XiangYa Hospital, Division of Internal Medicine, Cardiology Department, Changsha City, Hunan, China

NAVIN NANDA, MD, Professor of Medicine, Director of UAB Heart Station/Echocardiography Laboratories, and Senior Scientist, the UAB Center for Aging, University of Alabama at Birmingham, Birmingham, AL

ARAVINDA NANJUNDAPPA, MD, FACC, FSCAI, RVT, Associate Professor of Medicine and Surgery, West Virginia University, Charleston, WV

NGUYEN THUONG NGHIA, MD, FSCAI, Vice-Chief, Interventional Cardiology Unit, Cho Ray Hospital, Ho Chi Minh City, Vietnam

JAMES NGUYEN, MD, Chief Resident, Internal Medicine, University of Arizona, Tucson, Arizona

THACH NGUYEN, MD, FACC, FSCAI, Co-Editor, the Journal of Geriatric Cardiology; Editorial Consultant, the Journal of Interventional Cardiology; Honorary Professor of Medicine, Capital University of Medical Sciences, Beijing, China; The Institute of Geriatric Cardiology, Chinese People's Liberation Army Hospital 301, Beijing, China; The Friendship Hospital, Beijing, China; The Vietnam Heart Institute, Hanoi, Vietnam; Clinical Assistant Professor of Medicine, Indiana University; Director of Cardiology, Community Healthcare System, St. Mary Medical Center, Hobart, IN; Visiting Professor of Medicine (cardiac physiology), Trinity School of Medicine, St. Vincent, West Indies

TUAN D. NGUYEN, MD, Anaheim, CA

MARKO NOC, MD, PhD, Professor of Medicine, Medical School, Ljubljana; Director, Center for Intensive Internal Medicine, University Medical Center, Ljubljana, Slovenia

JOHN B. O'CONNELL, MD, Executive Director, Heart Failure Program, Heart and Vascular Institute, St. Joseph's Hospital, Atlanta, GA

OLABODE OLADEINDE, MD, FACP, Consultant, Department of Medicine, St. Mary Medical Center, Hobart, IN; Assistant Professor of Medicine, Indiana University School of Medicine-North West, Gary, IN

BRIAN OLSHANSKY, MD, Professor of Medicine, Cardiac Electrophysiology, University of Iowa Hospitals, Iowa City, IA

LOAN T PHAM, MD, Hospitalist and Internal Medicine Consultant, Kaiser Permanente Hospital, Fontana, CA

HUNG CANH PHAN, MD, Norwalk, CA

HUNG NAM PHAN, MD, General Secretary, the Internal Medicine Society of Vietnam; Vice-Chief, Cardiovascular Section, Binh Dinh General Hospital, Qui Nhon, Vietnam.

TUONGMAN PHAN, BS, University of California San Diego, San Diego, CA

PHAN DINH PHONG, MD, Electrophysiology, Vietnam Heart Institute, Hanoi, Vietnam

TA TIEN PHUOC, MD, PhD, Cardiology Consultant, Vietnam Heart Institute, Hanoi, Vietnam

TOM PLOJ, MD, PhD, Center for Intensive Internal Medicine, University Medical Center, Zaloska Ljubljana, Slovenia

NGUYEN NGOC QUANG, MD, PhD, Interventional Cardiology, Vietnam Heart Institute, Hanoi, Vietnam

PETER RADSEL, MD, Center for Intensive Internal Medicine, University Medical Center, Ljubljana, Slovenia

JOHN REILLY, MD, Associate Director, Cardiac Catheterization Laboratory; Associate Director Cardiology Fellowship, Director Cardiovascular CT, Oschner Clinic, New Orleans, LA

GIANLUCA RIGATELLI, MD, PhD, Director, Section of Congenital and Structural Heart Disease Interventions, Cardiovascular Diagnosis and Endoluminal Interventions Unit, Rovigo General Hospital, Rovigo, Italy

AINOL SAHAR, MD, Director of Invasive Cardiac Catheterisation Laboratory, Department of Cardiology Serdang Hospital, Selangor, Malaysia

SHIGERU SAITO, MD, FACC, FSCAI, FJCC, Chief, Division of Cardiology and Catheterization Laboratories, Heart Center, Shonan Kamakura General Hospital, Kanagawa, Japan, Heart and Great Vessel Center of Beijing, You-Yi Friendship Hospital, Beijing, China

SIM KUI HIAN, MD, MBBS (HONS) (MONASH), FRACP, FACC, FCSANZ , FSCAI, FESC, FAPSIC, FNHAM, FASCC, FAHA, Head, Department of Cardiology; Head, Clinical Research Centre (CRC), Sarawak General Hospital, Malaysia, Adjunct Professor, Faculty of Medicine and Health Sciences, University of Malaysia Sarawak (UNIMAS)

CHITTUR A. SIVARAM, MD, FACC, Professor of Medicine and Vice Chief of Cardiovascular Section; Director, Cardiology Fellowship Training Program, University of Oklahoma, Oklahoma City, OK

THEODORE CONRAD TAN, MD, Resident, Department of Internal Medicine, West Virginia University; Charleston Area Medical Center, Charleston, WV

HUY VAN TRAN, MD, PhD, FACC, FESC, Deputy Chief, Department of Cardiology, Khanh Hoa Hospital, Khanh Hoa, Vietman; President, Khanh Hoa Heart Association; Vice-president, Vietnam Heart Association, Hanoi, Vietman

HOANG TRONG MINH TUAN, PhD CANDIDATE, Bioinformatics and Computational Biology, George Mason University, Fairfax, VA

NGUYEN QUANG TUAN, MD, PhD, Associate Professor of Medicine, Director of Interventional Cardiology, Vietnam National Heart Institute, Hanoi, Vietnam

DOBRIN VASSILEV, MD, PhD, Invasive Cardiology Department, National Heart Hospital, Sofia, Bulgaria

HECTOR VENTURA, MD, Section Head of Heart Failure Heart Transplant at Ochsner Clinic and Clinical Professor of Medicine at Tulane Medical School, New Orleans, LA

NGUYEN LAN VIET, MD, FACC, Professor of Medicine, Director of Vietnam Heart Institute, Hanoi, Vietnam

PHAM NGUYEN VINH, MD, PhD, FACC, Associate Professor of Medicine, Pham Ngoc Thach University of Medicine; Medical Director, Tam Duc Heart Hospital, Ho Chi Minh City, Vietnam

TIMOTHY YEE, Undergraduate Program, Notre Dame University, South Bend, IN

PRIDHVI YELAMANCHILI, MD, Fellow in Cardiology, Oschner Clinic, New Orleans, LA

RONG LIN ZHANG, MD, Vice President, Chief Cardiologist, Suqian People's Hospital of Nanjing, Nanjing University School of Medicine, China

LEFENG WANG, MD, PhD, Deputy Director of the Cardiology Center, Director of the Catheterization Laboratories, and Associate Professor, Chao Yang Red Cross Hospital, Beijing, China

SHIWEN WANG, MD, MCAE, Professor and Director, Institute of Geriatric Cardiology, General Hospital of Chinese People's Liberation Army, Beijing, China

WILLIAM H. WEHRMACHER, MD, Clinical Professor of Medicine, Loyola University Medical Center, Oak Lawn, Chicago, IL

YIDONG WEI, MD, Chief of Department of Cardiology, Shanghai Tenth People's Hospital of Tongji University, Shanghai, China

HAI YUN WU, MD, Institute of Geriatric Cardiology, General Hospital of Chinese People's Liberation Army, Beijing, China

Contents

Foreword

CHALLENGING TODAY'S AND FUTURE CARDIOLOGISTS, PHYSICIANS, AND HEALTH CARE PROVIDERS

Cardiovascular disease is a major health, social, and economic problem. On an individual basis, it limits the full development of a productive career, decreases earning potential, dampens the prospect of a challenging lifestyle, and shortens life expectancy. In the macroeconomic sphere, cardiovascular disease contributes directly to work absenteeism, lower production output, and incurs a large and disproportionate share of health care expenses.

With tremendous advances in the understanding of disease mechanisms and concurrent technology development, the management of cardiovascular disease has succeeded in decreasing mortality and improving morbidity. However, the question of today's cardiologists or of all health care providers is whether they are providing the best medical care at the lowest cost within the shortest time frame. Are we providing health care of the 21st century or do we still practice medicine invented in the 19th century? (N.B.: the majority of cardiac examination practices were discovered or invented before 1900.)

NEW CHANGES IN 21ST CENTURY SOCIETY

At the end of the first decade of the 21st century, we live in a world that has been changed forever with instant inter-human access (cell phones), instant information at the stroke of the fingertips (the Internet), wider 24/7 social communication (Twitter), and new ways of self-introduction and networking (Facebook). This is the normal way of life of many young and middle-aged people today. What are the social characteristics in regard to seeking and receiving medical care at the beginning of the 21st century?

Plenty of Information

The health care consumers coming to our offices are more informed than ever before. They access many resources from the Internet and do research on their health questions. At the same time, health care providers (cardiologists, physicians or nurses, allied health professionals) are bombarded by a never ending barrage of print or electronic media. The publications range from the "must-read" weekly editions of the Journal of the American College of Cardiology, Circulation, and the New England Journal of Medicine to the free, throw-away print-ings from scientific or business sources. For the lay readers as well as for the well-trained health care professionals, the problem is how to quickly distinguish between correct and false or relevant and irrelevant infor-mation in order to spend the time to read, memorize them, or throw them away.

Plenty of Options

In the diagnosis or treatment of a single medical problem, there are many options. Which tests among many will give the diagnosis with the least number of false positives? Which treatment among many can solve the problem with the fewest side effects?

Open Access and Transparent Process

Before coming to the office, health care consumers access the Internet, research their own health problems, and prepare questions for discus-sion during the meeting with the physicians. The patients want to play an active part in the planning and decision-making process of their own medical or surgical investigative and management plan. This process re-quires meaningful communication between the physicians, patients, and their families, thereby providing better results and greater compliance.

Cost- and Time-Effective Approach

Even though there are many options for treatment, which one is the best at an affordable price? The management should be cost- and time-effective because the time lost from patients, doctors, and nurses also costs money, especially in this era of hotly debated health care reform.

NEW SCIENTIFIC PERSPECTIVE ON THE CARDIOVASCULAR SYSTEM OF THE 21ST CENTURY

Standing a few feet away from a human being, an observer globally scans the human body with a bird's eye view. The results show that the cardiovascular system (CVS) looks like a closed-circuit irrigation net-work. The left ventricle is a main pump station receiving the blood from the lungs and propelling it to the aorta, distal peripheral arteries, and then the surrounding tissue. The blood returns to the right side of the heart and the pulmonary arteries against the earth's gravity thanks to the negative pressure of the thoracic cage during inspiration. The pul-monary venous system serves as a retention reservoir in a similar way that the abdominal cavity, wall, venous system and the deep and super-ficial venous system of the legs function for the right side of the heart (see Figure 2-1 in Chapter 2).[1]

From an information technology (IT) perspective, the CVS functions like a local area network (LAN) connecting various hardware devices together within a building by means of a continuous cable or an in-house voice-data telephone system. The anatomical structure of the heart and the CVS is the hardware. The mechanism running the heart and the CVS is the software. There is tight coupling between organs/compartments in the CVS, e.g., load balancing and congestion control, similarly seen in the interactions between components of a LAN.[2]

NEW SCIENTIFIC APPLICATIONS IN THE MANAGEMENT OF CARDIOVASCULAR DISEASE IN THE 21ST CENTURY

So when a cardiologist, physician, or allied health professional, wearing the hat of a hydraulics engineer, a physicist, or an IT consultant, investigates a cardiovascular (CV) problem, there are seven areas in the CVS on which to focus. The first area is that of the index problem (zone A), which causes the cardiac condition. Proximal to the index problem is the upstream area with hyperdynamic-producing activities in order to overcome the index problem (zone B). Distal to the index lesion is the downstream area with hyperdynamic-receiving capacity (compensatory state) (zone C). When this compensatory mechanism is overwhelmed, then a state of disease occurs. Another mechanism to overcome the index problem is the bypass (or work-around) system (zone D), which tries to maintain the usual cardiac function at lower capacity without correcting the index (or root cause) problem or while the root cause problem is being fixed. In addition to these four areas, the set-up (configuration) of the CVS (zone E) needs to be checked. The other systems (pulmonary, renal, cerebral, peripheral venous return) (zone F) are also involved in the production of symptoms and signs of a cardiac condition (see Figure 2-2 in Chapter 2).[1]

Applying the trouble-shooting and debugging techniques when correcting a problem in IT to the medical or surgical management of a CV problem, the majority of cardiovascular treatments fall into one of four strategies:

1. Reversing the index abnormality (e.g., unblocking a coronary lesion by stenting).
2. Enhancing a compensatory mechanism (e.g., giving tissue-plasminogen activator (tPA) for acute myocardial infarction).
3. Bypassing the index abnormality and connecting two healthy areas (e.g., coronary bypass graft surgery), and
4. Correcting the excesses of the compensatory mechanisms (e.g., angiotensin converting enzyme inhibition in heart failure).

Therefore the treatment could be to fix the hardware (e.g., replace the aortic valve in aortic stenosis) or the software (e.g., use beta blockade in acute myocardial infarction or in atrial fibrillation caused by hyperthyroidism). The above new concepts become the compass guiding the cardiologists, physicians, or allied health professionals in the investigative or management trail of a CV abnormality.[2]

The *Evidence-Based Cardiology Practice: A 21ˢᵗ Century Approach*, in its first edition by the People's Medical Publishing House-USA, Shelton, CT, brings together clinical consultants from different areas of expertise to address the day-to-day implications of conventional and frontline investigation and treatment for major CV problems. In a frank and honest review and evaluation of data from randomized trials or meta-analysis, we present a wide range of solutions, incorporating evidence-based medical information, from conventional to investigational, into daily practice. The strategic programming of the investigations and management is planned under the perspective of hydraulics and IT with the CVS as an irrigation network and run by a supercomputer.

Each major option is supported by the abstract of a clinical trial or two from opposing views that have been well received or hotly debated by the cardiology community. The cardiologists, physicians, or allied health professionals may use these data in the investigation or management trail of a CV problem.

THE HEART OF THE MATTER

However, data and facts alone do not necessarily lead to solutions. It is the critical analysis of the facts that delivers the correct answers. Medical decisions are made on the basis of *critical thinking,* and *clinical judgments* are based on the relevancy of the collected data. The medical decisions and clinical judgments are the results of the long thought processes generated from formal learning, data from guidelines and practice standards, experience, an understanding of the incidence of disease in the population that the patient represents, and the likelihood of a disease being present in a specific patient. Even so, at the end of a bedside encounter with a patient, it is the cardiologist or physician *alone* who makes a decision about what is relevant and what is helpful to patients. These decisions come from wisdom and compassion, which can only occur through *experience and introspection*, which are unique human traits.[2]

This small and humble book (or any medical or cardiology book) does not have all the answers, nor can we offer a perfect solution to every question, because clinical questions will always arise as long as the human body evolves and new technologies are invented. As many theories and hypotheses are being elegantly discussed in many quarters, we present just a few principles and applications that are the most likely treatments of the future. Following this principle, we channel our limited time, our limited number of brain cells and their connections, and our overflowing intellectual interest and emotional enthusiasm into these few promising investigations and treatments.

As editors and authors of this book, we hope that we achieve our role as effective communicators to our readers, who are all friends and colleagues. We have tried to make the messages simple and easy to understand, so they can be easily remembered and applied in all of our daily rounds. This is the one simple goal we have for ourselves and our readers.

SHORTCOMINGS

In this book, especially in the first two chapters, there are a lot of discussions about the cardiovascular system from the physics, hydraulics, or information technology point of views. These ideas are still very primitive and very controversial and provocative. In our writings and thinkings, the lead author and senior authors can explain the problems of heart failure or coronary artery disease by these new concepts; however, how to explain arrhythmia under this new technology? How about cancer? If any colleagues and friends have any ideas to suggest or to discuss, kindly e-mail them to *thach@jgcard.com*. Your ideas will be warmly welcomed and treasured.

CREDITS

While in medical school, in training programs, or in daily practice, I (TN) rely on writings (and teachings) from many sources, including the text Heart Disease: A Textbook of Cardiovascular Medicine, by Dr. Eugene Braunwald, published by W. Saunders; the Physical Examination of the Heart and Circulation, by Dr. Joseph K. Perloff (5th edition by People's Medical Publishing House-USA, Shelton, CT); the Cardiac Pearls by Dr. Williams P. Harvey, by Leannec Publishing; and lately the wonderful Handbook of Patient Care in Vascular Diseases by Rasmussen T.E. et al., published by Lippincott Williams & Wilkins. Since my interest has focused on the cost-effectiveness of treatment, I daily access the website www.clinicalevidence.com of the British Medical Journal group. As lead author of many chapters, I quote clinical pearls extensively from these books and websites. I credit the success of my patient care to the information I use from these books and websites. I would like to offer my heartfelt thanks to the authors of these giant pillars of medicine.

Autumn 2009, Beijing, China, Laporte, IN, New York, NY, Busan, Korea, Kanagawa, Japan and Royal Oak, MI

References

1. Nguyen, T., Yee, T., Hoang, M.T. T., et al.: Futuristic Applications to Today's Management of Cardiovascular Problems. In Hu, D.Y., Nguyen, T., Kim, M.H. et al., eds. Evidence-Based Cardiology Practice: A 21st Century Approach, by PMPH-USA, Shelton, CT.
2. Nguyen, T., Hoang, M.T. T., Yee, T., et al.: Practicing Cardiology of the 21st Century. In Hu, D.Y., Nguyen, T., Kim, M.H. et al., eds. Evidence-Based Cardiology Practice: A 21st Century Approach, by PMPH-USA, Shelton, CT.

Section I

Clinical
Evaluation

Practicing Cardiology of the 21st Century

CHAPTER

1

Thach Nguyen, Hoang Trong Minh Tuan, Timothy Yee, Cindy Grines, Dayi Hu, and John Reilly

Chapter Outline

INTRODUCTION

Practicing medicine is a time-honored profession. The clinical approach of investigating and treating disease is well documented, tested, and practiced. How can a physician provide better cardiac care with the help of modern information technology (IT)?

In this chapter, the first section is reserved for the usual merits of a clinical approach so dear to the hearts of all physicians and health care providers. The second section will discuss the useful application of artificial intelligence (AI) in medicine. New terms and definitions are clarified for the medical and professional readers. The third section discusses how to apply the principles of works and the methodologies of AI in the investigation and management of cardiovascular (CV) disease. Their clinical applications for two CV conditions, the simple coarctation of the aorta (CoA) and the complex acute myocardial infarction (AMI), complicated by heart failure (HF), are presented in detail. In the last section, the pros and the cons of the new approach are discussed and principles of how to apply AI and IT methodologies in daily practice are suggested.

CONVENTIONAL CLINICAL APPROACH

Diagnostic imaging has made enormous advances in the past 20 years and has significantly improved the accuracy with which a diagnosis of cardiac disease can be assured. At the same time, the availability of non-invasive imaging has reduced the need for a detailed physical examination that was the hallmark and pride of clinical cardiology. This section will discuss the continuing need for an accurate and thorough history, physical examination (H and P), and comprehensive management plan in the evaluation and management of patients with known or suspected cardiac disease. All of these are done through the lens of (1) a physician, (2) a Computer Automated Decision Support System (DSS), or (3) a physician equipped with an Automated DSS.

Investigative Plan

In all patient encounters, it is essential to understand the reason for the patient's need for a cardiac consultation. Failing to understand the chief complaint will impair the physician's ability to focus on solutions to both the diagnosis and therapy. At the same time, the physician should approach the patient with an open mind, without prejudice, and without using racial, age, or gender profiling.

Within the first five minutes of a conventional history interview, the large area of investigation of a cardiac symptom or disease should be narrowed gradually to a few major leads. The typical method used is a deductive analysis based on initial symptoms, with the "if...then" process—a core programming construct, widely used in information technology (IT) language—and now being reapplied in the medical diagnostic investigation.[1] Following such a hierarchical approach, the questions from a broad spectrum narrow down to be more specific in time, place, location, and characteristics. The ultimate goal is to try to establish a plan to lead the investigative trail for a subsequent comprehensive H and P to support diagnoses considered in the differential diagnosis. However, the guiding plan should be flexible and modifiable, according to the details that keep emerging from the ongoing history interview and physical examination. The diagnosis to be identified and the differential diagnoses to be ruled out are moving targets.

Other Information

In all patients for whom a diagnosis can or cannot be made based on the initial history, a complete review of systems is still indicated in order to uncover any additional potential information. The social and family history should be asked about in detail. Patients' medications should be reviewed, including all over–the-counter drugs and supplements. Recent changes in medications should be addressed to rule out drug-to-drug interactions or a new side effect. Allergy information should be gathered, and the specifics of the reaction should be documented.

Preliminary Diagnosis and Differential Diagnoses

Once the H and P is done, the physicians would look at all sources of data for decision-making, including the results of previous studies, hospital records, physician's notes, and information from family members. From there, the physicians can deduct a preliminary working diagnosis and a short list of differential diagnoses. In essence, for a physician specializing in cardiovascular disease, it is vital not to misdiagnose or miss some major and important diagnoses (Table 1-1).

TABLE 1-1: Diagnoses That Physicians Should Not Miss	
Acute myocardial infarction	Acute mitral regurgitation
Acute surgical abdomen	Acute aortic regurgitation
Rupture of aortic aneurysm	Subacute bacterial endocarditis
Cardiac tamponade	Aortic dissection
Pulmonary embolism	Acute limb ischemia
Transient ischemic attack and stroke	Acute mesenteric ischemia
	Pulmonary edema

TABLE 1-2: Concerns Before Ordering Tests

Pretest probability
Sensitivity and specificity
What is the least risky strategy for the patient?
  False-negative diagnosis
  False-positive diagnosis
Are there guidelines for appropriate use of tests?
Should cost be considered in the evaluation?
Are you chasing a red herring?
Are there urgent or emergency situations?
Is the availability of facilities limited?

Selection of the Right Tests

With the preliminary working diagnosis and a short list of differential diagnoses, it is necessary to confirm the diagnosis and rule out the differential diagnoses with objective tests. To make a diagnosis is to evaluate the results of the tests and then to use this information to confirm the probability that a patient has a given disease is greater than the other possible diagnoses. The results of the test also help to determine whether one therapy would be a better choice over another. The selection of a test depends on several factors, including the availability of technology, local experience and expertise on a given modality, patient-specific factors, and pretest and post-test probability within a context of time and a cost-effective approach (Table 1-2).

Should all the tests be done selectively or is there a place for the "do everything at once" shotgun approach? How should cost-and time-effective testing be done on an individual and societal basis? A continued provision of excellent cost-effective care is due to reduced overuse of imaging and procedures. However, the diagnostic accuracy of the tests has to be confirmed first before their cost-effectiveness can be estimated.

Art or Science?

Discussion of clinical diagnosis that employ probabilities and odds ratios are akin to statistics and science. Clinical diagnosis is an art that depends on creating likelihoods for a list of diagnoses based upon human interactions. It is also a science based on many years of learning and experience. What else can help the physician to provide better care for cardiovascular disease patients?[1]

ARTIFICIAL INTELLIGENCE METHODOLOGY

Scientists and physicians have been "manually" extracting information from data for centuries, but the overwhelming volume of data after the explosion of the Internet requires more automatic approaches. As data sets and the information extracted from them have grown dramatically in size and complexity, direct hands-on data analysis has become obsolete.[2]

With the proliferation, ubiquity, and increasing power of computer technology aiding data collection, processing, management, and storage, the captured data need to be converted into information, and once the information is verified, it becomes clinically useful knowledge. Even so, medical knowledge has become so vast and complicated that no one human brain can memorize everything. Computers are designed exactly for that—to sift through huge databases and match known questions and answers. It is crucial to know what kind of data and what types of tools, functions, and methods can help physicians in culling these to arrive at only essential information.[2] The ultimate goal is to provide a faster solution to patient problems, improve delivery of care, and reduce errors during treatment.

Clinical Investigation (Data Collecting)

The physician can gather the clinical information about the patient by asking questions during the history interview and examining the patient during the physical exam. The data collected by a physician should be arranged in a structured, systematic, and scientific fashion so that subsequent clinical decisions based on arguments embodied in the findings are valid.[3] In the new context, the process of doing an H and P is called "data collecting."

Clinical Pearls (Data Decoding Tips)

When the meaning of symptoms and signs is not understood and needs to be explained in order to become applicable information, the process of deciphering the symptoms and signs is called "data decoding."

Preliminary Diagnosis (Data Processing)

Data analysis is the process of gathering, modeling, and transforming data with the goal of highlighting useful information, suggesting conclusions, and supporting decision making.[4] The first step is called "data processing." It may be simple or complex, depending on context. Simple problems may be identified and resolved with few iterations of data collecting and data processing.

Complex problems may require many iterations of data collection from various sources (i.e., results of tests) and interfacing with Decision Support Systems that support diagnosis of complex problems. If the process is complex, requiring input of a physician to arrive at a clinical diagnosis, it is called "data converting."

After formulating a preliminary working diagnosis and a short list of differential diagnoses, as a next step the physician will order the least number of tests to confirm the working diagnosis and to rule out the differential diagnoses.

Extraclinical Investigation by Testing (Data Mining)

According to traditional teachings, the clinical investigation is the bedside H and P. When the patient undergoes testing, it is called extraclinical or paraclinical investigation. This terminology creates an impression that extraclinical investigation is the testing done outside the clinical spectrum, inside the confinement of a laboratory, or literally "outside the patient's body." This is in contrast to the new concept of "data mining."

Definition

In information technology (IT) terminology, the term "data mining" means to extract data from and to look for patterns in a database. The resulting patterns may lead to either asking new questions or finding answers to solve a problem. Applying data mining to medicine means sending a command to look for specific data inside the database, which is the body of a patient. This concept is important because from the view of an Automated DSS or of a physician, all the clinical questions and answers are inside the body of a patient, sitting, lying, or standing in front of the examining physician. The only thing that she or he has to do is to go inside the patient, look for the right data, and extract the right results to solve the medical problems. With this new understanding, the term data mining brings with it new and meaningful perspectives.

This new concept is important because the physicians now know exactly where the answer is. However, the one million dollar question is: How does one get the data from inside the patient in a humane and cost-effective way?

Technique

Data mining involves using analysis techniques that focus on modeling and knowledge discovery for descriptive purposes. The processes of data mining may range from the transparent (rule-based approaches) to the opaque ("neural networks"), through "classification," "clustering regression," and "association rule learning" by using programs or algorithms such as "nearest neighbor," "naive Bayes classifier," or "genetic programming." Data mining leads to "predictive analytics," in which collected information may be analyzed for prognostic outlook.[5]

Differential Diagnosis (Data Filtering)

Data filtering involves ruling out the possibility of other relevant diagnoses. The process occurs by discrimination or parsing between relevant and irrelevant data.

Main Diagnosis (Data Converting)

Data converting involves using medical information to make a definitive diagnosis. This is the main role reserved for a physician. No computers, lay persons, or other health care providers are able to perform this important job. It is the result of a complex process of reasoning and rationalizing by the physician. This action of data converting (making a diagnosis) also imposes on the physician a moral and legal responsibility for his or her clinical decision. A computer program does not bear any legal or moral responsibility. If a physician does not do this data converting job well, or if his or her performance is substandard (making too many wrong diagnoses), then this particular physician does not fulfill his or her duty as assigned by society.

CARDIAC INVESTIGATION AND MANAGEMENT IN THE 21ST CENTURY

When a physician sees a patient, there is a need to define the main question or problem to be solved. The main problem can be a symptom, a sign, or a disease condition, and the goal can be an investigation or disease management.

In this first decade of the 21st century, how can a physician evaluate and manage patients with the time-honored medical tradition combined with the assistance of a computer? The goal is not for a middle-aged cardiologist to behave like today's teenager with an iPhone, iPod, Facebook, or to be connected to the Internet 24/7. These accessories do not bring a cardiologist into the 21st century.

In a hospital or in society, the goal of the new way of working with AI is to improve the quality, safety, and efficiency of medical care by maximizing the use of clinical information technology in key issues, such as complex clinical workflows, usability, controlled terminology, knowledge management, and clinical decision support.

However, in a personal setting, in a face-to-face encounter between a physician and a patient, the new methodology assisted by AI is the new way to scrutinize, dissect, and solve a medical problem (from diagnosis to treatment and prevention) through maximizing the management of knowledge and information technology resources. It is the use of the AI methodologies (and not just the commercial application of AI) that constitute the key success factors for the improvement of efficacy and efficiency in delivering quality cardiac care.

Areas in Focus Based on a Computational Model

At the bedside, while asking questions in the history taking and performing a complete physical examination, how can a physician know that he or she has exhausted all the questions about (subjective) symptoms and all the searches for (objective) signs? Has he or she ordered the least number of tests needed? Has he or she delivered all the best indicated treatments? One of the answers is that the patient needs to be checked from head to toe or that all the systems should be searched on an anatomical basis. Another answer is to use an AI program for data collecting (symptoms and signs) and data mining (laboratory, noninvasive and invasive tests). Which are the different areas to be focused on by an AI program for data collecting and data mining? They are listed in Table 1-3.

In each of these areas, the clinical aspects to be documented include the derangement caused by the index section, failure of the distal segment, compensation of the proximal and distal sections, work-around configuration as a temporary solution, and adaptation to function at lower capacity of the cardiovascular system. Once all data are collected, classified, and integrated, and a diagnosis is pronounced, the physician would suggest a standard treatment plan based on current guidelines, with the assistance of AI. The goal is to determine whether a treatment is beneficial in patients with a given disease, and if so, whether the benefits outweigh the costs and risks. Advanced management consists of a treatment plan tailored to the patient's own characteristics and its gradual modification following the success or failure of each step of the standard treatment.

A Cardiac Computational Model

From an IT perspective, the heart is designed and functions like a sophisticated computer system, incorporated inside a complex supernetwork (which is the body). The anatomical structure of the heart is the hardware. The mechanism running the heart's contractile function is the software. The smooth relation between the heart and other organs,

---

TABLE 1-3: Areas in Focus Based on a Computational Model

- The area of interest or index problem (zone A)
- The area proximal to or upstream to the index problem with hyper-dynamic-producing activities (compensatory state) or overwhelmed compensatory condition (disease state) (zone B)
- The area distal or downstream to the index problem with hyper-dynamic-receiving capacity (compensatory state) or overwhelmed compensatory condition (disease state) (zone C)
- The configuration of the system or network (zone E)
- The work-around configuration (the bypass system) (zone D)
- The system (the cardiovascular system)
- The network (the whole body is a network of systems) (zone F)

such as the lungs and the kidneys, or the interactions between different chambers of the heart, are the results of an elaborate configuration and intricate mechanism.

For example, mitral stenosis is a hardware problem, obstructing blood flow at the level of the mitral valve. Essential hypertension (HTN) is caused by a software problem, because the blood pressure is set abnormally high without any anatomical abnormality. It is similar to a house in summer with the heat blasting because the thermostat is set too high, while the air conditioning would cool the house nicely if it were turned on. If the HTN is secondary to coarctation of the aorta (CoA), then this is a hardware problem. In patients experiencing uncontrolled supraventricular tachycardia and wide QRS complex due to Wolff-Parkinson-White syndrome, the problem is clearly a configuration problem because of the aberrant connections between the atrium and ventricle through abnormal electrical lines.

Interactions and Coupling in a Computational Model

In general, there are two kinds of relations between components of a system: interaction and coupling. Interactions refer to the linear or complex dependencies between components, while coupling refers to the loose or tight flexibility in a system. The systems with simple, linear interactions have components that affect only other components that are functionally downstream. One example is that of a significant lesion in the superficial femoral artery (SFA), which only affects the flow, the nutritional status, and the function of the ipsilateral lower leg downstream.

In contrast, complex system components interact with many other components in different parts of the system. Loosely coupled systems have more flexibility in time constraints, operation sequencing, and assumptions about the environment than do tightly coupled systems. Systems with complex interactions and tight coupling are likely to promote accidents. Complex interactions allow for more complications to develop and make the system hard to understand and predict. Tight coupling also means that the system has less flexibility in recovering when things go wrong. According to these definitions, the cardiovascular system has complex interaction within its components and tight coupling with the pulmonary and renal systems.[6]

To illustrate this new perspective, three examples of system disruption and its corrective mechanism and actions are selected and presented. The first example is a hypothetical Internet application. What happens if there is a failure in its infrastructure? The second example is a patient with coarctation of the aorta. What happens to the patient, and how does the body react? How does a physician of the 21st century investigate the problem? The third example is the case of a patient with acute myocardial infarction (AMI) complicated by heart failure. How are these problems investigated and treated from the perspective of a physician helped by the AI of an Automated DSS ? Many of the AI technologies in current decision support systems don't need the complexity of a high cost computer network. Many can be run on commodity systems that are affordable by comparison.

Corrective Mechanisms in Case of an Interruption of a Hypothetical Large Internet Application Infrastructure

In this example, there is infrastructure failure of an Internet application provider. Typically such applications are constructed with a redundant and loosely coupled architecture. Failure of the server and network components is not a single point of failure. Such components are arranged in *farms* or *clusters*, where the load is more or less evenly distributed. If a single server fails, other servers in the farm or cluster will carry the load by using reserve capacity until they become overloaded. When an overload occurs, the calls in progress do not fail, but they prevent the server from accepting additional calls. Because of the malfunction in the index server, all the activities downstream to it are idle, function at lower capacity, run at slower speed, or shut off (crash or outage).

In the current set-up, the servers in a farm or cluster have little-to-no dependencies on the other servers in the same farm/cluster. That implies *loose coupling,* which allows for expected failures with little-to-no disruption to end-users.

In the event of major disruptions to network infrastructure or entire server farms that do result in outage (or crash), typically there are thorough procedures in place to rapidly "work around" known types of problems and/or to stabilize the system to render it usable until the problem's root cause can be diagnosed and corrected.

Corrective Mechanisms in Case of an Interruption of the Cardiovascular System

Applying the same corrective mechanisms of an IT structure to a computational cardiac model, in the case of CoA, the index lesion is the narrowing area in the isthmus of the thoracic descending aorta (zone A). There is dilation (hyperdynamic compensatory activity) of the segment proximal to the index lesion (zone B). The segment distal to the index lesion is hypoplastic (zone C). Collaterals from the upper body through the internal mammary and the intercostal arteries channel blood to the lower body by the work-around set-up (collaterals) (zone D). Because of CoA, there is high blood pressure and overdevelopment of the upper body while there is low blood pressure and underdevelopment of the lower half of the body. The patient would complain of headache because of high BP and claudication due to insufficient blood below the isthmic narrowing. The lower extremities are cold and the distal pulses

TABLE 1-4: Data Collecting, Mining, and Treatment for Coarctation of the Aorta on a Computational Cardiac Model

Coarctation of the Aorta	Main Area of Interest	Proximal to Index Problem	Distal to Index Problem	Work-around Configuration
Mechanism	Narrowing at isthmus (zone A)	Prestenotic dilation (zone B)	Poststenotic low flow (zone C)	Collaterals (zone D)
Symptoms	None	Headache	Claudication	None
Signs	Pathogno-monic sign: none	HTN in well-developed upper body	Weak pulse, atrophy in lower body	Collaterals, murmur in back
Direct Tests	Aortogram CT of chest	Aortogram CT of chest	Aortogram CT of chest	
Indirect Tests	None	CXR with the reverse 3 image	CXR with the reverse 3 image	CXR with notched rib
Target Treatment	Stent or end-to-end surgery	Control HTN	None	None
Work-around	None	None	None	Bypass graft surgery

CT: computed tomography, CXR: chest x-ray, HTN: hypertension.

are weak. If there are enough collaterals and augmentation from the reflecting wave, then the distal pulses at the ankles can be felt normally. According to the computational cardiac map, the CoA functions with linear interactions and loose coupling. The summaries of data collecting, mining, and treatment for CoA based on a computational cardiac model are listed in Table 1-4.

Assessment and Management of a Patient with Myocardial Infarction and Heart Failure Based on a Computational Cardiac Model

The heart is a major component in the complex cardiovascular system. It has intricate interaction and tight coupling between its own chambers and with other adjacent organs. The functions of the heart governed by different mechanisms include the following:

- The myocardium contracts under the principles of physics.
- The atria and ventricles circulate the blood under the principles of hydraulics.
- The electrical system triggers and stimulates the atrial and ventricular contractions.
- The coronary arteries supply the blood to the myocardium.

All of the four components above function under tight control and coordination of the nervous and hormonal regulatory systems. In the following four sections, the process of soliciting symptoms and signs, testing and treatment based on the seven areas of focus from the computational cardiac model is discussed in detail.

Data Collecting (History Interview)

Applying the same corrective mechanisms on a computational cardiac model to a patient with AMI complicated by heart failure, the main area in focus is the index lesion with acute occlusion of the infarct-related artery (IRA) (zone A). There is prestenotic dilation (hyperdynamic compensatory activity) of the coronary artery segment proximal to the index lesion (zone B). The coronary segment distal to the index lesion could be dilated (positive remodeling) or constricted due to low flow (zone C). There are collaterals from the proximal coronary segment to the distal vasculature (work-around set-up) (zone D). There are no symptoms and signs related to the segment proximal to the index lesion. The patient experiences chest pain because of acute and prolonged occlusion of the index lesion, causing ischemia in the myocardium supplied by the coronary artery segment distal to the index lesion. The pain does not come from the index lesion of the IRA. There are no symptoms from the work-around configuration. The mechanism and origin of chest pain in AMI are illustrated in Table 1-5.

TABLE 1-5: Mechanism and Origin of Chest Pain in AMI

	Index Lesion (zone A)	Proximal Coronary Segment (zone B)	Distal Coronary Segment (zone C)	Myocardium Downstream of the Index Lesion (zone C)
Mechanism	Occlusion at the lesion	Compensatory dilation	Constriction due to slow flow	Ischemia due to lack of blood
Symptom(s) Generated	None	None	None	Chest pain

If the myocardium supplied by the index artery is large, there would be wall motion abnormality with left ventricular dysfunction, lower cardiac output, and mainly lower blood pressure. The response from the upstream section of the left ventricle is to increase the sympathetic drive, causing increased heart rate and blood pressure (BP), which hopefully deliver (1) the amount of blood required for the body metabolism, and (2) better perfuse the distal segment of the IRA. Because of the increased sympathetic output, the patient could feel apprehensive and complain of palpitation (even though the heart rate is not very high yet).

In contrast, at the distal extremities, due to low BP, the patient could feel cold because of vasoconstriction. If the BP is low enough, the effect of low BP will be evidenced in the cerebral system as the patient complains of dizziness, lightheadedness, and syncope. If there is severe LV dysfunction, there are symptoms of shortness of breath due to lung congestion (upstream to the LV). There are no signs from the work-around configuration. The mechanisms and origins of these symptoms are illustrated in Table 1-6.

Data Collecting (Physical Examination)

In the physical examination, there are no objective signs pointing exactly to the acute occlusion of the IRA. The physician can hear an S4, implying that the LV is stiff that there is a need for a stronger boost from a vigorous atrial contraction. The physician tries to listen to an S3 to see

TABLE 1-6: Mechanism and Origin of Symptoms Due to LV Dysfunction

	Index Area (zone A)	Upstream to the Index Area (zone B)	Downstream to the Index Area (System) (zone C)	Downstream to the Area (Network) (zone F)
	Left ventricle	Pulmonary vasculature	Aorta and distal vasculature	Cerebral vasculature
Mechanism of Disease	Left ventricular failure	Fluid overload	Decreased blood pressure	Decreased blood pressure
Symptoms Generated	Sense of palpitation due to increased heart rate	Shortness of breath	Feeling cold in feet	Lightheadedness, dizziness, confusion

whether there is LV dysfunction. However, these S3 and S4 sounds are indirect and inconclusive signs. Further, there are no signs pointing to the fact that an IRA is being recanalized.

If there is severe LV dysfunction, there are signs pointing to the fact that the left heart system is overwhelmed, with low blood pressure (weak pulse), low cardiac output (vasoconstriction in the lower extremities), decreased urine output (in the renal system), and fluid overload (rales in lungs). The signs of right-sided heart failure are elevation of the jugular venous pulse and distention of the external jugular vein. The mechanisms and origin of the signs caused by the LV dysfunction after AMI are summarized in Table 1-7.

Data Mining (Work-up)

In the example of a patient with ST segment elevation (STEMI) complicated by HF, an electrocardiogram (ECG) will document whether or not there is ST elevation in a 12-lead ECG. An ECG does not give exact information about the location, severity, and patency of the IRA. The ECG only reflects the electrical activities of the myocardium as a whole. A coronary angiogram will provide an exact location of the occlusion, its severity, and distal flow (zone A).

An ECG monitor in the intensive care unit will help to track the heart rate or simple or complex premature atrial or ventricular contractions (PACs or PVCs) resulting from an increased compensatory sympathetic output by the upstream regulatory system of the heart.

TABLE 1-7: Mechanism and Origin of Signs Due to LV Dysfunction After AMI

	Index Area (zone A)	Upstream to the Index Area (zone B)	Downstream to the Index Area (System) (zone C)	Downstream to the Index Area (Network) (zone F)
	Left ventricle	Pulmonary vasculature	Aorta and distal vasculature	Renal vasculature
Mechanism of Disease	Left ventricular failure	Fluid overload	Decreased blood pressure	Decreased blood pressure
Signs	S3	Rales in lungs, jugular vein distention	Decreased BP, distal vasoconstriction	Decreased urine output

Brain-type natriuretic peptide (BNP) level would tell us about the fluid status in the right atrium (upstream to the LV) (zone B). In contrast, troponin and creatine phosphate kinase enzyme would tell us about the damage to the myocardium distal to the index lesion (downstream to the obstruction) (zone C). With current technologies, there are no noninvasive tests to detect collaterals of the coronary arteries, only the invasive coronary angiogram (zone D).

In order to assess the LV function, echocardiography would help to discern the LV or RV dysfunction, the wall motion abnormality, and valvular problems. A pulmonary catheter can measure the pressure in the left and right atrium and ventricle (Table 1-8). All the possible tools to investigate the cardiac function for patients with LV dysfunction due to AMI based on a computational cardiac model are listed in Table 1-8.

TABLE 1-8: All Possible Tests for Patients with LV Dysfunction Due to AMI Based on a Computational Cardiac Model

	Area in Focus	Direct Tests	Indirect Tests
Coronary Artery	Coronary artery index lesion (anatomy)	Coronary angiogram	ECG showing ST elevation
	Coronary artery (flow)	Coronary angiogram	Fractional flow reserve
Myocardium	Myocardial damage distal to the index lesion	CK-MB, troponin elevation	Echocardiography: wall motion abnormality
Cardiovascular System	Left ventricular systolic function	Left-sided heart catheterization: LVEDP, echocardiography, LVA	
	Aorta	Left-sided heart catheterization: AO pressure, BP	
	Pulmonary artery	Right-sided heart catheterization: PA mean pressure	Doppler echo: PA systolic pressure
	Right atrium	Right-sided heart catheterization: RA pressure	Doppler echo: RA systolic pressure

LVEDP: left ventricular end-diastolic pressure, LVA: left ventriculogram, AO: aortic, PA: pulmonary artery, RA: right atrium.

Management Based on a Computational Cardiac Model

In the example of AMI, the main treatment is to open the IRA ASAP by fibrinolytic therapy or percutaneous coronary intervention (PCI) and to give antiplatelet or anticoagulant treatment if required. This therapy is aimed directly at the root cause of the problem (zone A). From the proximal end of the index lesion, because the IRA cannot deliver oxygen to the distal myocardium, it is necessary to decrease the oxygen requirement by decreasing demand (zone C). This tactic can be implemented effectively by beta blockade while oxygen supplement by nasal cannula also intuitively helps. The intravenous (IV) nitroglycerin (NTG) decreases preload and thereby decreases oxygen as well. An intra-aortic balloon pump (IABP) works by increasing the blood pressure, which hopefully improves the distal coronary perfusion (zone C).

At the distal segment of the IRA, NTG tries to dilate the distal coronary arteries if the distal coronary vasculature is not at maximal vasodilation (which it usually is). This is why NTG has never been proven to decrease mortality or morbidity (zone C).

Coronary artery bypass graft surgery (CABG) works on the mechanism of work-around to bring the blood to the distal segment without correcting the index lesion.

Looking at the other systems of the body network, if there is lung congestion, the treatment includes relieving fluid congestion by IV diuretic. If there is respiratory failure, oxygen supplement, intubation, and mechanical ventilation are indicated while waiting for the LV function to recover.

During AMI, a patient can develop ventricular tachycardia (VT) or fibrillation (VF). If these conditions are not treated accordingly, the patient can die (cardiovascular system shutdown). Therefore in the case of VT and VF, electrical shock is the treatment of choice. An extrinsic electrical surge crosses the heart and wipes out all the electrical activities for one or two seconds. After that, the heart recovers its intrinsic electrical activities and restarts them from their origin, the sinus node. From it, the electrical activity spreads out again on its regular grid. Using IT terminology, this is called system recovery.

A summary of all possible modalities of treatment for a patient with AMI complicated by HF according to a computational cardiac model is listed in Table 1-9.

PRACTICAL APPLICATIONS

Difference Between the Clinical Approach and the New Method

Using artificial intelligence methodologies to investigate and treat a CV problem is a new and innovative way to work with a familiar subject—the heart. During data collecting, mining, and management, the physicians are *proactively* looking for symptoms and signs based on a

TABLE 1-9: Classification of All Possible Modalities of Treatment for AMI and LV Dysfunction on a Computational Cardiac Model

	Main Area of Interest	Proximal to the IRA	Distal to the IRA	Work-around Configuration
CORONARY ARTERY				
Location	Index lesion at IRA	Prestenotic dilation	Poststenotic dilation	Collaterals
Target Treatment	PCI antiplatelet	Increase perfusion by IABP	Nitroglycerin	Nitroglycerin
Work-around		None	None	CABG
MYOCARDIUM				
Location	Not applicable	Myocardium in adjacent area	Myocardium supplied by the index lesion	None
Target Treatment		Beta blockade to decrease O_2 demand, give O_2 supplement	Beta blockade to decrease O_2 demand, give O_2 supplement	None
Electrical System Recovery	None	Cardioversion if VT or VF	Cardioversion if VT or VF	None
CARDIOVASCULAR SYSTEM				
Location	Left ventricle	Pulmonary venous and arterial system, right ventricle	The aorta and peripheral vasculature	None identified yet
Target Treatment	Vasodilator Diuretic LVAD	Diuretic	Arterial dilator LVAD, IABP	None
System Replacement	Cardiac transplant	None	None	None

CABG: coronary artery bypass surgery, IABP: intra-aortic balloon pump, IRA: infarct-related artery, LVAD: left ventricular assist device, PCI: percutaneous coronary intervention, VF: ventricular fibrillation, VT: ventricular tachycardia.

computational configuration of the cardiovascular system. The physicians have to pinpoint *exactly* the symptoms and signs generated by the index problem or lesion (zone A). Which are the *direct* tests proving the pathology of the index lesion or problem? Which are the direct treatments correcting the abnormality of the index lesion or problem? These questions are applied again on the four other areas of interest including: (1) the area proximal (zone B) and (2) distal to the index lesion or problem (zone C), (3) the work-around configuration (the bypass system) (zone D), and (4) the other pulmonary, renal, or cerebral systems (zone F) interacting with the cardiovascular system (zone E).

When searching for symptoms and signs, selecting tests or delivering treatment, the physician needs to confront the problem head-on, asking for the first-hand data, analyzing the results of the direct tests, and aiming the treatment straight at the target. This approach can be done only after reviewing all the possible clinical scenarios provided by a computational cardiac map.

An example of the diagnostic, testing, and treatment process of a patient with aortic stenosis is summarized in Table 1-10. What makes Table 1-10 special is the fact that the empty cells are showing no identified data. This would stimulate more thinking and observation from physicians to look for new symptoms, signs, or modalities of treatment in the seven areas of interest because "we only see what we are proactively looking for."

This active search is very helpful and fruitful because the physician is following the investigative and treatment trail on a computational cardiac model. This is different than the passive way of asking questions for symptoms, looking for physical signs, and treating patients through a checklist handed down by and memorized from many previous generations of physicians.

Fewer Brain Cells for Storage, More Brain Cells for Thinking

The new methodology is to investigate and treat a cardiac problem through a new computational configuration of the cardiovascular system. This would help physicians to use fewer brain cells for storage and more for thinking. Our brain does not have enough chips to store all the data taught in medical school, which needs to be updated constantly by new discoveries while purging the daily "junk" with which we are bombarded from the print and electronic media. The physicians then formulate the opinions with his own brain cells combined with all the best output of a collective brain called "the artificial intelligence," which is graciously owned collectively by humankind. The advantages of the new thought-generating process while using a computational cardiac model or map are listed in Table 1-11.

TABLE 1-10: Guide for Data Collecting, Mining, and Management of Aortic Stenosis Based on a Computational Cardiac Model

		Area of Interest	Upstream to the Area of Interest	Downstream to the Area of Interest	Work-around Set-up	Other Cardiovascular System
		Aortic valve	Left ventricle	Aorta and peripheries	None identified	Central nervous system
Data Collecting	Symptom	None	SOB because of pulmonary congestion, chest pain	Dizziness because of low BP		Syncope
	Sign	Systolic murmur at 2nd R ICS	Rales in lungs	Pulsus tardus and Parvus	None	None
Data Mining	Direct Tests	LHC echo, Doppler	Echo LHC	BP measurement	None	RHC
	Indirect Tests	None	None	None	None	None
Management	Target Treatment	Percutaneous aortic valve stenting	Diuretic to relieve congestion	Vasodilator is contraindicated	None	Dialysis if renal failure and fluid overload
	Replacement	Surgical aortic replacement	None	None	None	None

BP: blood pressure, ICS: intercoastal space, LHC: left heart catheterization, SOB: Shortness of breath.

TABLE 1-11: Advantages of the Use of a Cardiac Computational Model

- Setting up all the possible clinical scenarios on a computational cardiac model
- Actively seeking symptoms, signs, and testing of the problems located in the three main areas (index, upstream, and downstream) of a computational cardiac model
- Actively looking at the symptom(s), sign of the work-around configuration
- Clearly focusing the treatment on each area of the computational cardiac model
- No missing data and treatment
- No need for checklist or memorization

Critical Thinking and Clinical Judgment

Computer technologies with AI help a great deal in collecting, storing, sorting, processing, and analyzing data. They are extremely helpful in providing physicians with detailed information and facts (verified information). However, data and facts alone do not necessarily lead to solutions. It is the critical analysis of the facts that delivers the correct answers. Medical decisions are made on the basis of *critical thinking*, and *clinical judgments* are based on the relevancy of the collected data. These medical decisions and clinical judgments are the results of the long thought process generated from formal learning, data from guidelines and practice standards, experience, an understanding of the incidence of disease in the population that the patient represents, the relationship of symptoms to specific disease states, and the likelihood of a disease being present in a specific patient.

Even so, at the end of each bedside encounter with a patient, it is the physician *alone* who makes a decision about what is relevant and what is helpful to patients. These decisions come from wisdom and compassion, which can only occur through experience and introspection, unique human traits.

In this book, all the discussed strategies and tactics of data collecting, data mining, data converting, and management are applied in each chapter. At the beginning of each chapter there is a paragraph devoted to strategic programming, detailing the tactics used in the investigating process for that particular CV condition. Next to it, in the data collecting section, there is a paragraph detailing what to look for in the seven areas of interest based on the computational cardiac model. Then at the beginning of each management section, there is a table pinpointing the available treatments in the following four areas: data management, root-cause correction, work-around configuration, and system replacement.

In each chapter, all the possible aspects of a specific CV problem are presented—from symptoms and signs to testing and options in management based on a computational cardiac model. This new view is challenging because it opens new doors and brings us to new horizons.

CONCLUSION

Physicians are faced daily with the challenge of delivering the best care to patients with CV disorders. The expert physician integrates all of the information and each patient's unique status to decide the best investigative plan and therapy. In every case, thorough knowledge of the patient's history, examination, laboratory results, and imaging studies are essential for high-quality care.

In the new way of managing cardiovascular care, with the help of AI methodologies, physicians are able to navigate through a computational cardiac map that encompasses strategic programming for prevention, diagnosis, and treatment of heart disease in a clinical and cost-effective manner. With the time they save, physicians can focus more on performance improvement and having quality time with family and society. The end result is to deliver the best, cost-and time-effective quality cardiac care. These are the noble goals and tools for the delivery of quality cardiac care in the 21st century.

References

1. Bovey, A.: What is a cardiologist? JACC. 2009;53:1730–1731.
2. Zaleski, J.: Balancing Data Quantity with Quality: Techniques for Data Analysis and Reduction. In Zaleski J, ed. Integrating Device Data into the Electrical Medical Record, GWA, Erlangen, Germany: Publicist KommunikationsAgentur GmbH, pp. 131–177.
3. http://en.wikipedia.org/wiki/Data_collection (accessed 6/29/2009).
4. http://en.wikipedia.org/wiki/Data_analysis (accessed 6/29/2009).
5. http://en.wikipedia.org/wiki/Data_mining (accessed 6/29/2009).
6. Perrow, C.: Normal Accidents: Living with High Risk Technologies, New York: Basic Books, 1984.

Futuristic Applications to Today's Management of Cardiovascular Problems

*Thach Nguyen, Timothy Yee,
Hoang Trong Minh Tuan,
Loan Pham, and John Reilly*

Chapter Outline

APPROACHING A CARDIOVASCULAR PROBLEM

Strategic Programming: Doing Business in the 21st Century

When approaching a patient with a possible cardiovascular (CV) problem, should a physician adopt the paternalistic behavior of a traditional patriarchal society? Should the physician approach the CV problem with the zeal of a well-trained specialist, the heart of a country doctor, and the cost-effective approach of a morally responsible business person? The authors prefer the second scenario because the physician is practicing medicine by making the patient healthier within the budgeted share of the gross national product without bankrupting this system.

The goals which guide the physician through the process of investigation and management are to search for the most direct symptoms and exact signs and to aim the treatment directly at the index lesion, or problem in order to bring in a definitive and best solution to a CV problem. This fits the mentality of doing business in the 21st century, where the customer is king (or queen) and everything is available at one's fingertips.

The goal of a well-seasoned customer is to get the best product (not the imitating ones), with the best, lowest price, directly from the source (outlet stores), without having to pay the commission to middlemen. The customer typically does not mind paying for an imitation product if it costs only a fraction of the price of the original one. With the emerging of e-commerce and e-shopping, the interesting question is whether it is better to go to the store and look for the needed item? There are evidences that it is more comfortable for many people (from the elderly women with knee arthritis to the teenagers who are linked 24/7 to Twitter) to go through a catalog presented conveniently on the Internet. By shopping online, users can save their time, see how other customers review the quality of the product, compare the prices, and select the one that is the most affordable.

With the same business strategy of providing the best product at the best price with the least discomfort to the customer, this is how a physician goes through the process of investigating a cardiovascular problem and starting a treatment plan. The physician is asking the same question: What is the single-best symptom and sign I have to search for in order to make a diagnosis in this particular patient? I don't like to collect junk data: they crowd my mind and fill up the patient's medical records for nothing. Suppose the best symptom is identified and a preliminary diagnosis is made; which is the single-best test to confirm my clinical suspicion? With a yes-or-no result, I can tell the patient what problem he or she has, and then I go on with the next case or to the next step. There is nothing rewarding about lingering on an inconclusive case. Once there is a diagnosis, which treatment will fix the problem for good? In which scenario could the treatment fail?

With this working strategy in mind, a physician approaches the problem with three tactics: (1) direct and open access information, (2) transparent strategies, and (3) exact, targeted interventions. Is this the same treatment that a cardiologist would like to receive for himself or herself if she or he were the patient?

Then as the physician starts out along the investigative trail, he or she relies on a CV computational map, which shows the CV system as an irrigation network. However, when observing the CV system in action, the accuracy and efficacy of its function remind us more of a supercomputer or a centralized local area network (LAN). In this chapter, these out-of-the-box thinkings and their practical applications in daily practice are to be discussed, so that the casual or serious readers can be readily convinced.

One Principle: Direct Information and Exact Target Treatment

In the investigation of a CV problem, the goal is to search for the exact sign or the exact symptom caused by the index CV pathology. In management, the goal is to aim directly at and correct the index lesion. This is the main principle that guides the physician through the history and physical examination and subsequent management plan.

When learning about a new disease, the most important question to ask is what the pathognomonic sign of that particular disease is. How can the problem be recognized quickly? The other questions are as

> **TABLE 2-1:** Information Needed for Practicing Physicians in the Diagnosis and Management of a Cardiovascular Condition
>
> 1. What is the pathognomonic sign or symptom?
> 2. What are the typical symptoms and signs?
> 3. What are the atypical symptoms and signs?
> 4. Which is the earliest symptom and sign?
> 5. Which signs and symptoms denote the severity?
> 6. Which signs or symptoms require urgent treatment?
> 7. Which signs and symptoms show that the problem improves or is solved?

follows: What is the main presentation of that specific cardiac condition? What are the typical and atypical symptoms? How do you know whether or not the patient is in dangerous condition (e.g., dissection of the aorta)? What are the signs of an emergency (e.g., chest pain with low blood pressure)? In clinical cardiology, getting the direct and exact information is a main goal in the data collecting process (history taking and physical examination). The information needed is listed in Table 2-1.

DATA DECODING TIPS (CLINICAL PEARLS)
Cost-and Time-Effective Management

On an early Sunday morning, an elderly patient was brought to the hospital because of syncope. At the bedside in the intensive care unit, the patient was examined, and a systolic ejection murmur 3/6 was heard at the second right intercostal space. The patient was thought to have syncope due to aortic stenosis (AS). Right at that moment, the nurse handed the physician the results of the troponin level test. It was significantly elevated. The electrocardiogram (ECG) showed only nonspecific ST-T changes. So did the patient pass out because of AS or because of non-Q myocardial infarction (non-QMI)? There is a need to make a quick decision. If the patient had syncope due to sustained ventricular tachycardia caused by non-QMI, then he or she would need an urgent angiogram for angioplasty and stenting. If the patient passed out because of AS, then the patient would need to recuperate from non-QMI and will have aortic valve replacement (AVR) about a month later (as far as possible in time from the MI). So the physician listened to the heart sound again and tried to focus on the second heart sound. S2 was still sharp, well preserved, not muffled, and not soft (the aortic valve leaflets were still moving, not frozen yet). The AS was considered to be mild-to-moderate and not severe enough to cause syncope. Without having echocardiography, the patient underwent successful angioplasty and stenting of the culprit lesion (the left anterior descending artery). The right-and left-side heart catheterization confirmed the moderate narrowing of the aortic valve area. The patient was followed up for the next five years without further episodes of syncope or the need for AVR.

Data Mining (Single-Best Test)

At the present time, with the wild proliferation of novel technologies, there are many available noninvasive and invasive tests that can confirm a preliminary clinical diagnosis. However, when the patient needs to have a test, the question is which *single* test will give the best result, with a most time-and cost-effective ratio and the least discomfort to the patient. In real life, a test is ordered according to the availability of the tests at the local area, the expertise of the local interpreting specialist, and the affordability of the test by the patient. Now the off-hour interpretation of the tests is solved with the help of local or outsourced telemedicine.

Single-Best Treatment

There are many modalities of treatment for every single CV problem. In general, all the treatments fall into either one of the four strategies: (1) reversing the index abnormality (**zone** A), (2) mimicking or enhancing the compensatory mechanisms (**zones** B and C), (3) bypassing the index abnormality and connecting two healthy areas (**zone** D), and (4) correcting the excesses of the compensatory mechanisms. When the patient needs a treatment, the question to be asked is "What is the direct *single* treatment that will definitively solve the problem?" A patient with coronary artery disease (CAD) can take nitroglycerin, beta blockers, calcium channel blockers, angiotensin-converting enzyme inhibitors (ACEIs), angiotensin receptor blockers (ARBs), a statin, clopidogrel, aspirin, or undergo stenting and open heart surgery. Which one is the *single*, direct, and exact treatment that reverses the index problem? At which part of the problem is each of the modalities of treatment above beneficial? Table 2-2 lists all the possible treatments of CAD. The goal is to identify clearly the treatment that directly targets and corrects the index problem and the secondary, complementary options.

APPROACHING THE CV PROBLEM FROM THE TECHNICAL POINT OF VIEW

Even though it is very interesting to know, to learn about, or to do research about the CV system, the end product after all the efforts and expenses is a patient with healthy cardiac function. In the scale of this book, there are two hypothetical concepts to be discussed.

TABLE 2-2: Classification of All Possible Modalities of Treatment for CAD on a Computational Cardiovascular Model

	Main Area of Interest	Proximal to the Index Lesion	Distal to the Index Lesion	Work-Around Configuration
CORONARY ARTERY				
Location	Index lesion	Proximal segment with prestenotic dilation	Distal segment with poststenotic dilation	Collaterals
Target Treatment	Stenting, antiplatelet drugs, statin	Antiplatelet drugs, statin	Nitroglycerin, antiplatelet drugs, statin	Nitroglycerin, antiplatelet drugs, statin
Work-Around	Statin	Statin	Statin	CABG, statin
MYOCARDIUM				
Location	Not applicable	Myocardium in adjacent area	Myocardium supplied by the index lesion	
Target Treatment	Beta blockade to decrease O_2 demand	Beta blockade to decrease O_2 demand	Beta blockade to decrease O_2 demand	None

CABG: coronary artery bypass graft surgery.

OUT-OF-THE-BOX THINKING: THE HEART AS A PUMPING STATION OF AN IRRIGATION SYSTEM

Observed from a few feet away, with a global bird's eye scan the CV system looks like a closed-circuit irrigation network. There are three major observations on the heart, the lungs and the pulmonary veins.

The Left Ventricle as a Main Pump

The left ventricle (LV) is the main chamber receiving blood from the lungs and pumping blood to the aorta and the distal peripheral arteries. From there, the blood is diffused to the surrounding tissue (Figure 2-1).

The Lungs as a Suction Machine

From the lower legs, the venous blood returns to the lungs through the right side of the heart. The venous return is further aided by the respiratory pump. When the chest cavity expands during inhalation, the

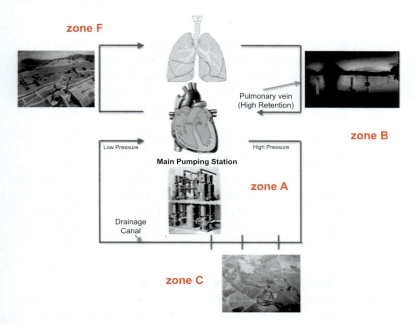

Figure 2-1 The cardiovascular system is designed and functions as an irrigation network. The heart is the main pump. The lungs sucks the blood upwards against the earth's gravity thanks to the intrathoracic negative pressure. The pulmonary veins serve as a retention reservoir for the left ventricle like as do the peripheral veins for the right ventricle and pulmonary arteries.

pressure within the thoracic cage decreases. This negative intrathoracic pressure thereby creates a favorable pressure gradient for the blood to reach the heart (sucking the blood towards the chest), against gravity. During exhalation, the intrathoracic pressure increases, thus decreasing venous return.

The Pulmonary Venous System as a Reservoir

The upstream section of the heart is the pulmonary venous system (PVS), which functions as a retention reservoir. The PVS will expand to receive blood when there is too much blood and will constrict to increase the blood flow when the blood supply decreases. By this accommodation, the left ventricle can increase or decrease its stroke volume as needed. We believe that the PVS expands to contain more blood if the LV cannot use all of the available blood. During diastole, with the mitral valve open and the aortic valve closed, the LV and the PVS become one large container equalizing the blood from the LV to the PVS. During systole, the LV and the aorta become one entity. As the peripheral venous system is a reservoir for the blood to the right side of the heart, the PVS is a reservoir for the LV.

Analogy in Hydraulics: Retention Reservoir

Commonly known as an "*attenuation*" or "*balancing*" reservoir, these are used to prevent flooding to lower lying lands. Flood-control reservoirs collect water at times of unseasonably high rainfall and then release the water slowly over the course of the following weeks or months.

In the CV system, the role of the retention reservoir is also very important because it provides a stable amount of blood flow in times of overload or in times of dehydration. How about a pressure-relief valve? We don't think a closed-circuit piping system can function without fail if it lacks a pressure-relief mechanism. In the case of the heart, we believe that the relief valve is the mitral valve. This is why mitral valve regurgitation is so common; its level of severity changes with time, and only a small percentage of MR becomes significant enough to require surgical valvular replacement.

Analogy in Hydraulics: Pressure Relief Valve

A relief valve is used to control or limit the pressure in a system or vessel that can build up by a process upset, instrument or equipment failure, or a fire. The pressure is relieved by allowing the pressurized fluid to flow from an auxiliary passage out of the system. The relief valve is designed or set to open at a predetermined set pressure to protect pressure vessels and other equipment from being subjected to pressures that exceed their design limits. When the set pressure is exceeded, the relief valve becomes the "path of least resistance" as the valve is forced open and a portion of the fluid is diverted through the auxiliary route. As the fluid is diverted, the pressure inside the vessel will drop. Once it reaches the valve's resetting pressure, the valve will close.[1]

PRACTICAL APPLICATIONS

Searching the Symptoms and Signs of Heart Failure

The CV system is composed of the arterial and venous systems. The arterial system carrying oxygenated blood includes the LV and the distal peripheral system (including the renal arteries and the cerebrovascular system). The right heart system includes the PVS, the pulmonary arterial system, the right ventricle and atrium, the liver and abdominal area, and the peripheral venous system. In each patient with disturbance of the blood flow, which symptoms and signs are originated from each segment mentioned above? An example of identifying the symptoms and signs in patients with heart failure is illustrated in Table 2-3.

TABLE 2-3: Origins of the Symptoms and Signs in Heart Failure

Location	Symptoms	Signs	Mechanisms
Left Ventricle	Heaviness	S3	Stiff LV
Distal Peripheral Arteries	Cold feet	Cold feet and hands	Distal vasoconstriction
Distal Peripheral Veins	Tightness	Edema	Poor absorption
Liver and Abdominal Area	Pain in right upper quadrant	Enlarged liver, pain with percussion of RUQ, edema in the abdominal wall	Congested liver
Right Atrium and Ventricle	Polyuria	Right side S3	Polyuria due to atrial natriuretic peptide
Pulmonary Arteries	Heaviness sensation		Stretching of the pulmonary arteries and RV strain
Pulmonary Veins	Shortness of breath	Rales in lungs, hemoptysis	PVS overload

LV: left ventricle, RUQ: right upper quadrant, RV: right ventricle, PVS: pulmonary venous system.

OUT-OF-THE-BOX THINKING: THE CARDIOVASCULAR SYSTEM AS A SUPERCOMPUTER

From an IT perspective, the heart is designed and functions like a sophisticated computer, incorporated inside a complex supercomputer or network, which is the CV system and other system of the body. The anatomical structure of the heart is the hardware. The mechanism running the heart's contractile function is the software. As the CV system functions as a local area network (LAN) or supercomputer, there is tight coupling between organs/compartments in the CV system, e.g., load balancing and congestion control similarly seen in the interactions between components of a LAN. The smooth relations between the heart and other systems, such as the lungs, the kidneys, or the interactions between different chambers of the heart, assure the best functioning of a human body.

Areas of Interest

When investigating or managing a specific CV problem, there are seven areas of the CV system on a computational model, to be focused on for data collecting, data mining, and management. The area of interest, or index problem, is the main focus (zone A). It is the cause of the cardiac condition. Proximal to the index problem is the upstream area with hyperdynamic-producing activities to overcome the index problem (zone B). Distal to the index lesion is the downstream area with hyperdynamic-receiving capacity (compensatory state) (zone C). When this compensatory mechanism is overwhelmed, then the disease state happens. Another mechanism to overcome the index problem is the bypass (or work-around) system (zone D), which tries to maintain the usual cardiac function at lower capacity without correcting the index (or root cause) problem or while the root cause problem is being fixed. In addition to these four areas, the regular configuration of the cardiovascular system (zone E) needs to be checked. The other systems (pulmonary, renal, cerebral, peripheral venous return) (zone F) are also involved in the production of symptoms and signs of a cardiac condition. The seven areas of interest are listed in Table 2-4 and Figure 2-2.

PRACTICAL APPLICATIONS

Searching for the Symptoms and Signs of CAD

When there is a lesion in a coronary artery, there is dilation of the proximal segment (prestenotic dilation), while there is positive remodeling right at the segment of the index lesion. The distal segment is also dilated (poststenotic dilation). In a patient with CAD, where

TABLE 2-4: Seven Areas to be Investigated When Approaching a Cardiovascular Problem

The area of interest, or index problem (zone A)
The area proximal or upstream to the index problem with hyperdynamic-producing activities (compensatory state) or overwhelmed compensatory condition (disease state) (zone B)
The area distal or downstream to the index problem with hyperdynamic-receiving capacity (compensatory state) or over-whelmed compensatory condition (disease state) (zone C)
The configuration of the system or network (zone E)
The work-around configuration (the bypass system) (zone D)
The system (the cardiovascular system)
The network (the whole body is a network of systems) (zone F)

do the symptoms and signs of angina and its associated symptoms (shortness of breath or dizziness) come from? Which test can give the most information needed? What are the indications of the tests (Table 2-5)?

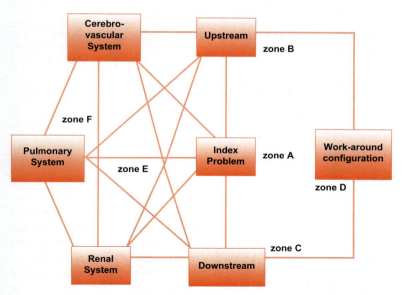

Figure 2-2: This is the schema of the cardiovascular system with interactions between its seven areas of interest.

TABLE 2-5: Single-Best Symptom, Sign, and Test for Patients with CAD Based on a Cardiovascular Computational Map

	Single-Best Symptom	Single-Best Sign	Single-Best Test
Index Lesion	None	None	Coronary angiogram
Prestenotic Segment	None	None	Coronary angiogram
Poststenotic Segment	None	None	Coronary angiogram
Work-Around Configuration	Angina relief when the collaterals open up	None	Coronary angiogram
Prestenotic Myocardium	None	None	None
Poststenotic Myocardium	Angina	None	Stress imaging
Left Ventricular Dysfunction	Easy fatigue	S3	Echocardiography
Pulmonary Venous Congestion	Shortness of breath	Rales in lungs	Chest X-ray
Decreased Cerebral Blood Flow	Dizziness	Low blood pressure	None

One Goal: The Main Priority in Cardiovascular Management

With the care of the cardiac patient, what is the most important goal in solving a CV problem? Is it the coronary artery system or the electrical system? Or is it the myocardium with its efficient contractile function?

A patient without a perfect electrical system can survive easily with the help of a pacemaker. A patient can live without a right coronary artery and a left circumflex artery. A patient can function almost normally with a single patent left anterior descending artery. There are plenty of cases in which patients had occlusion of all native arteries and survived with the remnants and collaterals to the distal segments. If a patient has severe dilated cardiomyopathy, even with a perfect electrical system and perfect coronary arteries, there is no long-term hope. The mortality is still extremely high.

The main function (or focus) of the heart is in its myocardium with its effective contractile function. The electrical system must stimulate the heart to contract on a timely basis. The coronary arteries must supply the oxygenated blood to the myocardium. Without a functioning myocardium, there is no reason for the existence of the coronary arteries or the electrical system. In any situation, the main goal is still the preservation of a good LV contractile performance. Once there is a significant decrease in the systolic function, there is reverberation of blood stagnation at every segment of the cardiovascular system.

PRACTICAL APPLICATIONS
New Classification of Heart Disease

When there is significant obstruction of the blood flow at any single segment of the CV system (seen as a closed-circuit irrigation network), there is disturbance of the blood flow everywhere. If there is obstruction at the aortic valve level, this is aortic stenosis. If the obstruction is at the mitral valve level, then there is mitral stenosis. In the patient with dilated cardiomyopathy and heart failure, the left ventricle is the location of blood stagnation. If the patient has large emboli to the pulmonary arteries, the cardiac output can decrease drastically, causing severe hypotension and death. If there is acute pericardial effusion (obstructing the blood flow of the right ventricle and totally cutting out the cardiac output causing cardiogenic shock), it is called pericardial tamponade. From that concept, a new classification of cardiovascular problems is listed in Tables 2-6 and 2-7.

TABLE 2-6: New Classification of Cardiovascular Problems

Direct Interruption of Blood Circulation	
Clinical Entity	**Level of Obstruction or Stagnation**
Aortic stenosis	Aortic valve
Hypertrophic cardiomyopathy	Aortic outflow tract
Dilated cardiomyopathy	Left ventricle
Mitral stenosis	Mitral valve
Diastolic heart failure	Pulmonary venous system
Primary pulmonary hypertension	Pulmonary arterioles
Pulmonary embolism	Pulmonary arteries
Pulmonic stenosis	Pulmonary valve

(continued)

TABLE 2-6: New Classification of Cardiovascular Problems *(continued)*

Clinical Entity	Level of Obstruction or Stagnation
Cardiac tamponade	Right ventricle
Tricuspid stenosis	Tricuspid valve
Edema in metabolic syndrome	Distal peripheral veins
Hypertensive CV disease	Distal resistance arterioles

Turbulent and Inefficient Blood Flow

Clinical Entity	Level of Obstruction
Aortic regurgitation	Aortic valve
Mitral regurgitation	Mitral valve
Pulmonic regurgitation	Pulmonic valve
Tricuspid regurgitation	Tricuspid valve

Turbulent and Inefficient Blood Flow Caused by System Configuration Abnormalities

Atrial septal defect	Abnormal flow from left atrium to right atrium
Ventricular septal defect	Abnormal flow from left ventricle to right ventricle
Patent ductus arteriosus	Abnormal flow from aorta to pulmonary artery
Tetralogy of Fallot	Atrial septal defect, ventricular septal defect, etc.

Decreased Blood Flow to the Target Organs (Dead-End Section)

Peripheral artery disease	Peripheral arterial disease, coarctation of the aorta, renal artery stenosis
Syncope	Insufficient flow to the cerebral arteries
Cerebral vascular accident	Emboli to the cerebral arterial system
Coronary artery disease	Coronary lesion decreases flow to myocardium

Arrhythmia with LV Dysfunction

Atrial fibrillation
Supraventricular tachycardia
Nonsustained ventricular tachycardia
Ventricular tachycardia, ventricular fibrillation

Obstruction of the Venous Flow Return

Deep vein thrombosis	Thrombotic formation in the deep vein system of the legs
Renal vein thrombosis	Thrombotic formation in the renal vein
Hepatic vein thrombosis	Thrombotic formation in the hepatic vein

Coronary Artery Disease

CAD is the obstruction of the flow in the coronary arteries, which supply blood to the myocardium. This disturbance becomes clinically relevant when there is angina and LV dysfunction. The chest pain is caused by the lesion in the index artery; however, the sensation of pain comes from the downstream myocardium. If there is no angina, there is no need for dilating the index lesion unless the treatment decreases mortality or reverses the LV dysfunction in the myocardium supplied by the index coronary artery. A patient with total occlusion of an artery (CTO) can live without indication for reopening the CTO. CAD becomes more relevant when it compromises the LV function. The symptoms and signs of CAD are listed in Table 2-5 and the single-best test in Table 2-8.

For patients with CAD, the medication that deals directly with the index lesion is antiplatelet medication. Statins shrink the plaques in all vascular segments, including the index lesion. NTG only affects the coronary flow distal to the index lesion. Beta blockers decrease oxygen demand in the myocardium, especially the myocardium supplied by the index lesion. The percutaneous coronary intervention (PCI) reverses the pathologic hold of the index lesion by dilating the lesion and scaffolding the ruptured plaque with stent. CABG provides a bypass conduit to bring blood to the distal segment without correcting any abnormalities of the index lesion. However, the mortality in CAD patients is not due to the index lesion. The lower mortality depends on the size of the ischemic burden (size of the myocardium in jeopardy). All the optional treatments of mild CAD are listed in Table 2-9, while the ones for severe CAD appear in Table 2-10.

⊙ DATA DECODING TIPS (CLINICAL PEARLS)
Difference Between Medical Therapy and Invasive Intervention in CAD

The mechanism of action for all drugs in the treatment of CAD is to decrease oxygen demand (e.g., beta blockers), while the goal of invasive intervention is to increase blood flow to the distal segment. From this understanding, all future medications or invasive procedures are judged and compared.

However, patients who undergo PCI or CABG also receive standard medical therapy, including ASA, beta blockers, and statins. This is why in all clinical trials comparing medical versus invasive therapy, it is in reality a comparison between medical therapy and invasive plus medical therapy. The comparison between PCI and CABG is a comparison between medical therapy plus PCI and medical therapy plus CABG.

TABLE 2-7: Location of Blood Flow Stagnation and Associated CV Abnormalities

Clinical Syndrome	Distal Peripheral Arteries	Aortic Valve	Left Ventricle	Pulmonary Venous System	Pulmonary Arterial System	Right Ventricle	Distal Peripheral Venous System
			LHF	Lung congestion	Pulmonary HTN	RHF	Leg Edema
	Hypertensive CVD		+	+	++	+	
	Dilation	Aortic stenosis	+	+	+	++	++
	Dilation		Dilated CM	++	++	++	++
	Dilation		Normal pressure	Diastolic HF	++	++	++
	Constriction		Low	Low	Pulmonary embolism	++	
	Constriction		Low	Low	Low	Cardiac tamponade	
	Normal		Normal	Normal	Normal	Normal	++ Metabolic syndrome

CM: cardiomyopathy, CVD: cardiovascular disease, HF: heart failure, HTN: hypertension, LHF: left heart failure, RHF: right heart failure.

TABLE 2-8: Single-Best Non-Invasive Test for Diagnosis of CAD

Stable angina	Regular treadmill testing: Best if patient can run up to 12 minutes
Unstable angina	Stress imaging (best with nuclear scan)
Non-Q myocardial infarction	Significantly high troponin level
ST segment myocardial infarction	ECG with ST segment elevation
Coronary spastic syndrome	ECG during pain

ECG: electrocardiogram.

TABLE 2-9: Treatment of CAD with Mild-to-Moderate Lesion

Location	Treatment	Mechanism	Results
Index lesion	Antiplatelet	Prevent accumulation of thrombus	Prevent AMI
	Statin	Prevent rupture of plaque Shrink plaque	
Enhance compensatory mechanism	Nitroglycerin	Dilate distal vasculature	No effect on mortality
	Beta blockade	Decrease oxygen demand	Decrease mortality
Correct excess of compensatory mechanism	None		
Enhance Work-around effect	Nitroglycerin, exercise	Angiogenesis by exercise	Fewer symptoms
Correct abnormality at other system	None		

AMI: acute myocardial infarction.

Heart Failure

In the conventional (and currently correct) thinking, heart failure (HF) is a clinical syndrome resulting from any structural and functional cardiac disorders that impair the capacity of the left ventricle (LV) to fill or to eject the appropriate amount of blood.[2] According to this definition, aortic stenosis, mitral stenosis, hypertrophic cardiomyopathy, and cardiac tamponade all prevent the LV from filling or ejecting the appropriate amount of blood.

According to the new concept with the heart as a main pumping station of a closed-circuit irrigating CV system, HF is a syndrome presented with blood flow stagnation at the level of the left ventricle.

TABLE 2-10: Treatment of CAD with Severe, Significant Lesion

Location	Treatment	Mechanism	Results
Index lesion	PCI Antiplatelet	Unblock the lesion, prevent accumulation of thrombus	Prevent AMI
	Statin	Prevent rupture of plaque Shrink plaque	
Enhance compensatory mechanism	Nitroglycerin	Dilate distal vasculature	No effect on mortality
	Beta blockade	Decrease oxygen demand	Decrease mortality
Correct excess of compensatory mechanism	None		
Enhance work-around effect	CABG Exercise	Bypass the index lesion and bring blood to the distal segment	Fewer symptoms and decreased mortality in 3 VD and LV dysfunction
Correct abnormality at other system	Treat LV dysfunction		

AMI: acute myocardial infarction, CABG: coronary artery bypass surgery, LV: left ventricle, PCI: percutaneous coronary intervention, 3 VD: three-vessel disease.

Before the patient develops frank HF, he or she is clinically stable by various compensatory mechanisms. The first compensatory mechanism is that the distal peripheral arterial system is on a maximal dilating state. In contrast, the patients with acute decompensated HF (ADHF) come to the emergency room with rales in their lungs and cyanotic extremities due to peripheral vasoconstriction.

DATA DECODING TIPS (CLINICAL PEARLS)
Predictor Signs of Heart Failure Correction

Two patients were intubated because of heart failure. One had fluid overload and one had cardiac arrest in the field. Both had low ejection fractions in the 20-30% range. I came to see the patients and checked the capillary flow at the big toe. Both had good flow: The skin of the big toe blanched well with pressure and the capillary flow returned quickly upon release. Both patients were extubated in the next 24 hours without problem. Both recovered from the HF and were discharged.

OUT-OF-THE-BOX THINKING:

A NEW CLINICAL ENTITY: Fluid Overload without Heart Failure

A patient with dilated cardiomyopathy and low ejection fraction can come to the hospital because of SOB and leg edema. The cause can be due high fluid intake for any reason. In the examination, the patient can have some rales and leg edema. However, the capillary refill is normal. There is no vasoconstriction. These patients respond well to a diuretic, and improve and are discharged in 48 hours. Even if the patient has sign of fluid overload, however, there is no inappropriate peripheral vasoconstriction that is the hallmark of HF. This observation can help to distinguish between the sick HF patients who need many days of hospitalization and the stable ones with fluid overload without HF who will go home in 48 hours. This is similar to a patient with normal LV function and having fluid overload. The patient can have leg edema without long-term sequelae of HF.

Distal Peripheral Vasodilation and Vasoconstriction

If an event is caused by lower blood pressure, the reactive compensatory mechanism is vasoconstriction to raise the BP. If there is lower cardiac output, then the first reactive compensatory mechanism is vasodilation in the distal peripheral arteries. In patients with early dilated cardiomyopathy, the examination of the feet should show either prominent vasodilation or at least no vasoconstriction. The diastolic blood pressure is lower. This observation is evidenced clearly in patients with aortic regurgitation. In patients with decompensated HF (e.g., due to chemotherapy, negative inotropic drugs, worsening CAD, fluid overload, or cold environment), vasoconstriction appears and disrupts the precarious balance of compensated LV dysfunction. The same observations of vasodilation in the distal peripheral arteries apply to patients with early aortic stenosis. This observation is reinforced in the explanation of the mechanism of syncope in AS. In patients with AS, there is peripheral vasodilation due to decreased cardiac output, making the patient very vulnerable to dizziness or syncope. Once there is HF in long-standing AS, there is distal vasoconstriction resulting in a lower gradient across the aortic valve even if there is severe AS. The therapeutic options of HF are listed in Table 2-11. Among all the treatments, only beta blockade and ACE inhibition decrease the morbidity and mortality.

TABLE 2-11: Treatment Options for Patients with Heart Failure

Target Location	Treatment	Mechanisms	Results
Left ventricle	Diuretics and arterial dilator, IABP, LVAD	Unload the LV	No change in mortality
	Beta blockers and ACE inhibitors	Beta Blockade and ACE inhibition	Decrease mortality and morbidity
Distal peripheral arteries	Arterial dilators	Enhance the vasodilating compensatory mechanism	No change in mortality
Distal peripheral veins	Diuretics	Fluid removal	No change in mortality
Liver and abdominal area	Diuretics	Fluid removal	No change in mortality
Right atrium and ventricle	Diuretics	Fluid removal	No change in mortality
Pulmonary arteries	Diuretics	Fluid removal	No change in mortality
Pulmonary veins	Diuretics	Fluid removal	No change in mortality

ACE inhibitors: angiotensin-converting enzyme inhibitors, IABP: intra-aortic balloon pump, LV: left ventricle, LVAD: left ventricular assist device.

DATA DECODING TIPS (CLINICAL PEARLS)
Signs of Stability in Heart Failure

How is the peripheral arterial system in patients with severe dilated cardiomyopathy and well-compensated HF? The difference is that in patients with severe dilated cardiomyopathy and well-compensated HF, there is distal peripheral vasodilation, while in patients with decompensated HF, there is vasoconstriction.

For patients with acute decompensated HF (ADHF), upon physical examination, if the patients show good capillary flow at the big toes and fingers without cyanosis (no vasoconstriction), then I believe they are improving. If the patients still have the sign of vasoconstriction at the capillary level, the mechanism causing HF is not reversed yet. This is why in patients with ADHF, ACEI inhibitors should be given before beta blockers. This notion is reinforced by the fact that in clinical trials, beta blockers were given on a background of ACEI inhibitors.

Aortic Stenosis: A Different Form of Heart Failure

Based on the computational CV model proposed in this chapter, the index problem of HF is the obstruction or stagnation of the blood flow at the LV level. This is a hardware problem. The upstream area is the pulmonary vascular system. The downstream area is the aorta and the distal peripheral system. Surprisingly, the stagnation is similar to the ones of severe end-stage aortic stenosis (AS). The difference is that in AS, the blood flow is impeded at the level of the aortic valve, while in HF the whole LV is the location of the blood stagnation. Another difference in the HF patient compared to the patient with AS is that, in AS, the LV functions under high and increasing blood pressure while in HF, the LV operates in high LV end-diastolic pressure with any level of (normal, low, or high) systolic BP. At the early stages, the distal peripheries in patients with AS and HF should be dilated. This is why the common symptoms of AS —dizziness and syncope— are due to over-vasodilation.

In the same line of thinking, in patients with severe end-stage AS and patients with end-stage HF, the treatment is the same with system replacement (aortic valve replacement or cardiac transplant).

🔴 DATA DECODING TIPS (CLINICAL PEARLS)
Aortic Stenosis with and without Dizziness

An elderly, wheelchair-bound patient arrived at the hospital because of orthostatic dizziness. The examination showed severe AS with AVA equal to 0.6 cm^2. The patient had refused surgery previously. The patient was on valsartan, an angiotensin receptor blocker (ARB), and amlodipine, a very popular calcium channel blocker (CCB) for hypertensive elderly patients. Every time the patient sat up or stood up, dizziness developed. Applying the principle that, in AS, there is maximal distal vasodilation, CCB was discontinued. The blood pressure was controlled by increasing the dosage of the ARB. The dizziness disappeared, and the patient went home without any problems.

Metabolic Syndrome

Many severely obese patients have SOB and leg edema. Their ejection fraction is normal. Their pulmonary capillary wedge pressure is normal. Their pulmonary artery pressure is normal. Where is the level of blood flow stagnation? The leg edema is caused by decreased return of the venous blood to the pulmonary vasculature due to poor suctioning function of the lungs. The level of blood flow stagnation is at the level of the peripheral venous system. Other causes of peripheral edema could be due to poor serum reabsorption by the venous or lymphatic systems.

DATA DECODING TIPS (CLINICAL PEARLS)
Severe Morbid Obesity and Leg Edema

Many patients who are severely obese have normal lipid profiles and normal left ventricular systolic function. They do not complain of having leg edema, and they have no lung problems. Usually the patients with COPD or mainly sleep apnea have leg edema. We suspect that in these patients the respiratory pump is not working well and therefore the venous return is not optimal with residual edema in both legs. The treatment is administering diuretics as needed besides moving the lower leg in order to pump the blood upwards.

Diastolic Heart Failure

In patients with diastolic heart failure with good EF, LVH, and high left ventricular end-diastolic pressure (LVEDP), where is the location of blood stagnation? We suspect that it is at the pulmonary venous system.

In systole, the reflecting wave in the distal peripheries builds up the systolic pressure in the aorta. In diastole, the pulmonary venous system bears the reflecting wave from the LV. The pulmonary venous system serves as a retention reservoir to absorb all the excess blood not needed from the LV. In the same way, if the LV needs more blood to be able to increase the stroke volume, then the pulmonary venous system will be able to provide the extra amount of blood. If the pulmonary venous system is overloaded, as in mitral stenosis, then there is pulmonary edema. The fluid overload in the pulmonary arterial system does not cause pulmonary edema; it causes pulmonary hypertension.

We suspect that diastolic heart failure is a form of heart failure with high LVEDP caused by loss of accommodation from the pulmonary venous system and/or vasoconstriction of the pulmonary venous system and/or because the retention capacity of the pulmonary venous system is overwhelmed. When there is too much blood, the LV cannot accommodate much by dilating itself. The main area to accommodate the extra blood is the PVS. This situation is demonstrated clearly in patients with acute aortic regurgitation in which the LVEDP rises very fast in a way similar to that in diastolic dysfunction.

Hypertensive Cardiovascular Disease: A Different Form of Heart Failure

Long-standing uncontrolled essential HTN causes LV hypertrophy. As the LV is upstream to the index problem, so the index lesion causing HTN should be the distal peripheral arteries that are in a state of vasoconstriction. The difference between HCVD and LVF is that in HCVD, the BP is more frequently high.

⊙ DATA DECODING TIPS (CLINICAL PEARLS)
Beta Blockade (BB) in HTN

Because the mechanism of essential HTN is vasoconstriction, the main treatment should be vasodilation (e.g., an ACEI). Recent data showed that the treatment of essential HTN by BBs can be detrimental. However, if the cause of HTN is due to increased adrenergic stimulation, then the treatment of choice will be a BB.[2]

Blood Pressure in Outer Space

In negative-gravity conditions, body fluids, including blood, of the space travelers shift away from the lower body into the upper body, causing blood to pool in the chest and head. Over time, the excess volume is excreted through the kidneys.

When someone stands up too quickly, this causes blood pressure to drop and the person may feel light headed. Usually, the circulatory system makes immediate adjustments in blood pressure to restore flow to the upper body and counteract the effects of gravity. The adjustments include increasing heart rate and vasoconstriction of the peripheral veins. However, if they are not being used, with time, these compensatory mechanisms will become dysfunctional. Many space travelers who spend more than two weeks in space are unable to stand up without getting dizzy due to *orthostatic intolerance.*

In the microgravity of space, body fluids, including blood, shift to the upper regions of the body, eventually leading to a reduction in blood volume. Upon return to earth's gravitational field, the majority of the blood volume shifts back into the lower body.

Arrhythmia

Arrhythmia is irrelevant if it does not cause symptoms and does not interfere with the contractile function of the myocardium. The sense of palpitation is caused by the fast rate of the arrhythmia. The feeling of chest pain comes from a mismatch between oxygen demand and supply in the myocardium; even the coronary arteries are patent. The sense of SOB caused by the arrhythmia is due to stagnation of the blood in the PVS. If there is significant low blood pressure, then the patient can pass out or succumb to cardiac arrest (e.g., ventricular tachycardia, ventricular fibrillation).

DATA DECODING TIPS (CLINICAL PEARLS)

Sustained or Nonsustained Supraventricular and Ventricular Arrhythmia in AV Block

In the context of the CV system as a supercomputer, how does one best explain the problem of arrhythmia? The electrical system is created to time the cardiac contractions. The electrical system does not contract the heart and does not generate any concrete products, such as propelling a volume of oxygenated blood to the distal tissue. The electrical system does not produce anything. Its role is to stimulate the heart to contract on a timely basis. This is why we suspect (and there is weak supporting evidence) compensatory hyperproductive activity of the area above the index lesion. If there is atrioventricular block, there is hyperdynamic function above (frequent premature atrial beats) and below the index lesion (junction rhythm or frequent premature ventricular contractions).

Atrial Fibrillation (AF)

AF is characterized by chaotic electrical activities in the atrium and these chaotic activities also spread to the ventricle. Thus the flow stagnation is at the left atrium or more specifically at the left atrial appendix (LAA). This is why thrombi form at the LAA. If there is stagnation of the flow in the LA, we strongly believe there is flow stagnation at the PVS, which is a retention reservoir. There, thrombi can develop like they do in the deep vein system of the leg.

CASE ILLUSTRATION:

Thrombotic Formation in the Pulmonary Veins

An elderly man with pulmonary vein varix and atrial fibrillation is described. The diagnosis of pulmonary varix, a localized dilatation of the pulmonary vein, was made by transesophageal echocardiography. The patient had chronic atrial fibrillation, and transesophageal echocardiography demonstrated thrombus in the pulmonary varix. In patients with atrial fibrillation, pulmonary varix may be an unusual site for thrombus formation.[3]

CONCLUSIONS

The purpose of this chapter is to explore how the management of biomedical data, information, and knowledge can optimize and advance clinical cardiac care. On a societal level, the specific importance of cardiology informatics is derived from the biological, psychological, social, and cultural needs that distinguish cardiac patients from other populations. These distinctions create complexities in the management of cardiac data and information that make cardiac patients a vulnerable population that requires special care.

At the bedside, on a personal level, as a physician of the 21st century, it is important to proactively search for the symptoms and signs causing the CV problem and to aim the treatment directly at the index problem. If the problem is mild, then the main goal is to prevent worsening of the condition. If the problem is severe enough, then the goal is to reverse the problem for good.

In the search for symptoms and signs of CV disease, the physician-investigator is helped by using a computational model in which the CV system is seen as an irrigating network. The CV system is also believed to function like a local area network (LAN), in which, if there is a failure, there would be compensatory increased activity in the proximal segment of the index lesion and there is a work-around configuration to keep the CV system functioning at near-normal or lower capacity. Many modalities of treatment are modelled along these compensatory mechanisms or aim to correct the non-intended excesses of these mechanisms.

So in the 21st century, a physician should use the methodologies of IT and AI to investigate and manage a cardiovascular problem. This is how a middle-aged physician, born and trained in the 20th century, can practice the medicine of the 21st century.

References

1. http://en.wikipedia.org/wiki/Relief_valve.
2. Lindholm, L. H., Carlberg, B., Samuelsson, O.: Should beta blockers remain first choice in the treatment of primary hypertension? A meta-analysis. Lancet. 2005;366:1545–1553.
3. Bhaktaram, V. J., Asirvatham, S., Sebastian, C., Chandrasekaran, K., et al.: Large pulmonary vein varix diagnosed by transesophageal echocardiography: an unusual site for thrombus in atrial fibrillation. J Am Soc Echocardiogr. 1998;11:213–215.

Cardiac Examination

*Chittur A. Sivaram, Thach Nguyen,
Bao Van Ho, and Phong D Phan*

Chapter Outline

INTRODUCTION

Despite major advances in diagnostic testing, history and cardiac physical examination still occupy a key role in the assessment of patients with suspected heart disease. While it is true that cardiac physical diagnosis has lost some of its traditional importance due to easily available and highly accurate diagnostic tests, the optimal clinical decision-making process still requires a comprehensive history interview and a complete physical examination. The ideal patient interview and physical examination would provide the physician with meaningful information regarding the pathophysiology at play, thereby leading to the selection of the least number of most sensitive and specific diagnostic tests in order to arrive at the most probable diagnosis and plan for the most appropriate treatment. Moreover, the time and effort invested in obtaining a history and performing a physical examination allow the physician to establish the time-honored doctor-patient relationship that still remains the foundation for the delivery of excellent patient care.

In order to exploit the maximum output from a physical diagnosis, the physician needs sound knowledge and strong background in both cardiac anatomy and physiology. While there were few reliable corroborative diagnostic studies available to physicians in the past, in the current age we are able to constantly improve our physical diagnostic skills through comparison with the results of many sophisticated diagnostic tests. Our confidence in physical diagnostic skills would improve through a process of confirmation of our clinical predictions with diagnostic tests on each patient. In fact, this exercise could serve as an example of practice-based learning and improvement.

This chapter is focused on heart disease and the examination of the heart and other abnormalities in the peripheral organs caused by heart disease. The outline is summarized in Table 3-1. A focused examination of the carotid artery is discussed in Chapter 19. The physical examination of the peripheral arterial and venous systems of the lower extremities is discussed in Chapters 18 and 13, respectively.

DATA COLLECTING

History

A patient-provided account of symptoms is a highly important aspect of the initial data collecting process. In addition to providing many clues to the underlying pathophysiologic process, a thorough history summarizes what constitutes the patient's burden. Special features of symptoms in individual conditions will be covered in other chapters of this book. We will, however, review the common symptoms in cardiovascular disease in this chapter.

TABLE 3-1: Cardiac-Focused Physical Examination

History
Vital signs: Blood pressure and heart rate
Comprehensive cardiac examination
Carotid pulse examination
Jugular venous examination
Examination of other organs related to heart disease (e.g., liver, abdomen, spleen, extremities)

Chest Pain

Chest pain is one of the most common symptoms in the cardiac patient.

Typical angina: This condition is characterized by central chest discomfort, described as pressure, tightness, or a squeezing type of discomfort produced by exertion and relieved by rest, radiating to the left or less commonly right arm and often associated with other symptoms, such as shortness of breath, sweating, or dizziness. The likelihood of severe coronary atherosclerosis in the presence of typical angina is very high (more than 90% probability) in elderly American male patients.

Atypical angina: This condition is characterized by the lack of one or more components of the features of chest pain described earlier. For example, the chest pain might be sharp rather than a tightness, but otherwise produced by exertion. The probability of severe coronary atherosclerosis is lower at ~50% in a patient with atypical angina.

Nonischemic chest pain: This diagnosis is characterized by sharp, apical chest pain that is nonexertional. The probability for coronary artery disease is lowest in patients in this group.

Shortness of Breath

Patients who complain of shortness of breath mostly have either cardiac or pulmonary disease. Exertional dyspnea is a very important symptom of left heart failure (HF), where elevated left ventricular filling pressure leads to a higher content of interstitial lung fluid, reduced lung compliance, and increased need for the muscular activity of breathing. Shortness of breath (dyspnea) might be seen in ischemic heart disease, nonischemic cardiomyopathy, valvular heart diseases such as mitral stenosis, or diastolic HF. Many patients with left-sided origin of HF develop characteristic episodes of dyspnea at night that cause them to wake up from sleep and assume an upright sitting position with legs dangling over the edge of the bed. These short-lived episodes subside spontaneously after several minutes and might be accompanied by a dry cough. Such episodes constitute paroxysmal nocturnal dyspnea. Dyspnea that improves upon sitting up is termed orthopnea. Exertional dyspnea, orthopnea, and paroxysmal nocturnal dyspnea share similar pathogenesis and point toward left-sided HF.

While no strict reliable historical point exists distinguishing pulmonary from cardiac dyspnea, the association of wheezing and a productive cough favors pulmonary rather than cardiac origin of dyspnea.

Night-time dyspnea might also be related to obstructive sleep apnea and sleep-disordered breathing. The presence of obesity, snoring, daytime somnolence, and episodic stoppage of breathing at night are clues to obstructive sleep apnea. The association of many cardiac disorders, such as hypertension (HTN), HF, atrial fibrillation, and bradyarrhythmias with sleep apnea has been well documented.

Swelling

Swelling of the extremities and the abdomen results from excessive accumulation of fluid in the body. It is one of the features of right-sided HF, even though other causes for swelling (edema) are frequently present. The common sites where edema might be present are ankles and feet in the ambulatory patient and along the sacral region in the bed-ridden patient due to the effect of gravity on the most dependent part of the body. Ankle edema can be present in tricuspid regurgitation, pulmonary HTN, and chronic constrictive pericarditis.

The noncardiac causes for edema include inferior vena cava obstruction, deep venous thrombosis, chronic liver disease with hypoalbuminemia, and nephrotic syndrome. In lymphedema the edema is nonpitting and the toes also appear edematous along with the ankle, a finding not seen in edema due to venous HTN.

Palpitations

The abnormal awareness of cardiac action results in the symptom of palpitations. Not all patients with palpitations have serious cardiac disease. Palpitations might imply either regular but forceful cardiac contraction or irregular cardiac activity. Conditions such as supraventricular tachycardia produce abrupt onset of regular rapid heart rate and often abrupt termination as well. Atrial fibrillation, in contrast, produces irregular cardiac rhythm, even though some patients might not sense it. Isolated premature beats (ventricular or supraventricular) cause a sensation of thumping or skipping within the chest. Some patients who complain of palpitations have an anxiety disorder or a volume overloaded cardiac lesion.

Loss of Consciousness

Patients with cardiac disease reporting syncope (black-out or loss of consciousness) have episodic critical reduction in cerebral blood flow. Near syncope is a less severe manifestation of a similar problem. Vasovagal syncope, or the common faint, is typically associated with an unpleasant stimulus, such as the sight of blood, and is preceded by a sense of warmth and nausea. The patient recovers completely and spontaneously once assuming a supine position. Vasovagal syncope might also occur during removal of sheaths after cardiac catheterization. Exertional syncope is characteristically seen in left ventricular (LV) outflow tract obstruction (valvular aortic stenosis as well as hypertrophic cardiomyopathy) and due to transient severe decrease in cerebral blood flow from failure of cardiac output to increase with exertion. Syncope not related to effort might be from either tachyarrhythmias (ventricular tachycardia or supraventricular tachycardia) or bradyarrhythmias (complete heart block or sinus arrest). Vertebrobasilar insufficiency produces loss of consciousness, while carotid disease is more likely to produce focal deficits related to the motor or sensory cortex. Loss of consciousness associated with upper extremity exercise is suggestive of subclavian steal syndrome.

Physical Examination

Several simple principles are involved in preparing for the physical examination. These simple points can enhance the accuracy of our diagnosis and when not followed might cause major obstacles to an adequate examination. The patient should be examined in a comfortable bed in a relaxed position with the ideal room temperature. Ambient noises can be a significant cause for errors during auscultation. Both the patient and physician should turn off cell phones to promote focused examination by the physician. The patient should be undressed in order to promote adequate examination, including palpation of lower extremity pulses and for auscultation. Failure to adequately expose regions being examined is a frequent issue in female patients. It might be helpful to the patient to be told in advance of the visit what to wear.

One needs only one instrument, a stethoscope, for adequate cardiac examination. There are a variety of stethoscopes available in the market. The relative additional contribution of the more sophisticated stethoscope remains unproven. The old adage correctly states that what matters more than the stethoscope is what is between its ear pieces.

General Appearance

The patient should be observed for clues for the underlying pathophysiology while the physician is eliciting a history from the patient and as he or she is being prepared for examination. A general physical examination frequently provides information that might be disease-specific or pathophysiology-specific.

Pathophysiology-specific examples of general physical appearance are as follows:

1. A patient who appears to be anxious with increased respiratory rate, sweating, and a tendency to sit upright is common in acute left HF.
2. Markedly swollen lower extremities with prominent jugular venous pulsations and abdominal swelling suggest right-sided HF. Bluish discoloration of skin and mucous membranes associated with clubbing of fingers and toes is consistent with chronic, significant venous-to-arterial blood mixing either due to congenital cyanotic heart disease or pulmonary parenchymal disease.

Disease-specific general physical appearances are as follows:

1. In coronary artery disease, frequently truncal obesity with increased abdominal circumference may be present. Abdominal circumference should be measured at the level of the iliac crests. While normal values have been published for both males

and females, remember that normal values are slightly lower for Asians.

2. In coarctation of the aorta, the lower extremities may be shorter and less well developed compared to the upper extremities. In adults with severe long-standing coarctation, prominent arterial collaterals might be seen on the back of the patient. Webbing of the neck, wide-set nipples, and short stature suggest Turner syndrome, an occasional associated condition of coarctation.

3. In Marfan syndrome, where cardiac lesions of aortic root dilatation, aortic dissection, and chronic aortic regurgitation due to failure of leaflet coaptation secondary to aortic annulus dilatation occur, patients characteristically have long extremities out of proportion to their torso length.

Blood Pressure

Blood pressure (BP) should be measured in the sitting position after about three minutes of rest. The size of the cuff should be two-thirds of the arm circumference. A larger cuff relative to the arm circumference will falsely reduce the recorded blood pressure. If there is a question about peripheral vascular disease, it is advisable to record the blood pressure of all four extremities. The peripheral blood pressure is the result of the central sympathetic drive and peripheral resistance. As such, in some instances, the peripheral BP may be higher or lower than the central BP.

DATA DECODING TIPS (CLINICAL PEARLS)
Discrepancy Between Peripheral and Central Blood Pressure

The amplification is more marked in vasoconstricted states, many of which are clinically important. With impending circulatory shock, a high level of circulating catecholamines exists. Early diagnosis of an impending circulatory shock can be missed if one only pays attention to systolic pressure; the mean arterial and diastolic pressures should be low in this situation. A patient with congestive heart failure (in which peripheral vasoconstriction exists) may exhibit an exaggerated systolic amplification. Arm systolic pressure in subjects running on a treadmill can be markedly higher than the central aortic pressure. With subjects receiving catecholamine infusion or other vasoconstrictors, less amplification of systolic pressure is noted in vasodilated states, including (a) subjects receiving vasodilators, and (b) subjects who have received a contrast dye injection (which has vasodilating effects) during cardiac catheterization.[1]

Pulse Examination

In a pulse examination, the following three characteristics should be evaluated: rate, regularity, and volume. Traditionally, pulse rate is counted at the wrist. The most common causes of an irregular pulse are premature beats (ventricular or atrial) and atrial fibrillation.

The value of documenting a regularly irregular versus an irregularly irregular pulse in the clinical differentiation of atrial fibrillation from ectopics is somewhat an overemphasized point.

Inspection of the Chest

Inspection of the chest in some cardiac patients might reveal evidence of scars from previous surgical procedures. A central sternal scar may be associated with coronary artery bypass surgery, valve replacement or repair surgery, ascending aortic surgery, closure of a congenital cardiac shunt, or pericardectomy or cardiac transplantation. A left thoracotomy scar due to cardiac surgery is indicative of a procedure on the descending thoracic aorta or a Blalock-Taussig procedure in childhood. A bilateral thoracotomy scar is seen when patients undergo surgical ablation for atrial fibrillation. A small left infraclavicular scar is expected after pacemaker or defibrillator implantation.

Other abnormalities of the thoracic cage might produce displacement of the heart and as such deserve notice. These abnormalities include kyphosis, scoliosis, pectus excavatum, and pectus carinatum. Prominent venous collaterals might be present on the anterior chest wall in patients with obstruction of the superior vena cava. Arterial collaterals may rarely be present along the posterior chest wall in coarctation of the aorta.

The part of the chest wall overlying the cardiac area is termed the precordium. Abnormalities of the precordium are rare in today's cardiology practice. A bulging precordium typically signifies a volume overloaded cardiac lesion that has been present from very early in life. Usually this requires a congenital cardiac defect with volume overload physiology. Acquired cardiac defects with volume overload do not produce precordial bulge.

⚬ DATA DECODING TIPS (CLINICAL PEARLS)
Parasternal Movements

Parasternal movements (left, right, or combined) are sometimes best seen by the examiner looking upward from the patient's feet. It is worth underscoring that precordial retraction is more readily seen than felt, whereas outward displacement is generally as readily palpable as seen. When the left ventricle occupies the cardiac apex but retracts in systole, the cause is usually constrictive pericarditis. The retraction is generally most pronounced at the apex but is likely to cover a wider area, sometimes involving most of the precordium.[2]

Palpation of the Chest

Palpation of the precordium is done to check the presence of a thrill, the point of maximal impulse (PMI), and precordial hyperactivity.

The PMI is the location that is lowest and most lateral on the precordium where an impulse can be felt during systole. Three features of the PMI—location, size, and character—should be evaluated.

Location of the PMI should be reported in relation to the intercostal space as well as a superior-inferior landmark line (such as the midclavicular or axillary line). The usual location of the PMI is the fifth left intercostal space slightly medial to the midclavicular line. The location of the PMI must be ascertained with the patient in the supine position; palpation in the left lateral position is helpful in determining the nature of apical impulse, however. The normal PMI makes contact with the palpating hand only briefly, as the left ventricle rotates slightly anteriorly during systole.

DATA DECODING TIPS (CLINICAL PEARLS)
Information to Look for When Palpating the PMI

The PMI is helpful in determining whether the right ventricle (RV) or left ventricle (LV) is dominant. With RV dominance, the impulse is maximal at the lower left sternal border or over the xiphoid process; with LV dominance, the impulse is maximal at the apex. The normal apical impulse is no bigger than the size of a quarter (about 2.5 cm in diameter). If the impulse is more diffuse and slow rising, it is called a *heave*. If it is well localized and sharp rising, it is called a *tap*. Heaves are often associated with volume overload. Taps are generally associated with pressure overload.[1] The presence of a hyperactive precordium characterizes heart disease with volume overload, such as that seen in defects with large left-to-right shunts (patent ductus arteriosus, ventricular septal defect) or heart disease with severe valvular regurgitation (aortic regurgitation, mitral regurgitation [MR]).[2] When an LV impulse is displaced laterally (apart from noncardiac causes), it is generally palpated in the sixth rather than the fifth intercostal space, not because the impulse is necessarily lower but because the ribs slant upward as the anterior axillary line is reached. Accordingly, the sixth interspace at the anterior axillary line is at the same horizontal level as the fifth interspace at the midclavicular line.[2]

Other precordial impulses include right ventricular heave felt in the left lower parasternal region. Because the right ventricle is more medial than the left ventricle, in most patients an abnormally prominent impulse in the left parasternal region will be attributable to right ventricular origin. Rarely a much dilated left atrium in chronic mitral regurgitation might cause a systolic impulse in the left parasternal region. Unlike an impulse due to right ventricular activity, left atrial pulsation is more delayed within systole. In patients with chronic obstructive lung disease causing right ventricular hypertrophy, left parasternal heave may be absent in the presence of significant lung hyperinflation. In such cases, right ventricular impulse may be felt as an epigastric thrust due to the slight downward descent of the heart produced by hyperinflation.

Pulsations felt in the second left intercostal space close to the sternum are due to abnormalities in the pulmonary artery. Prominent pulmonary artery pulsations may be present in left-to-right shunts with increased pulmonary flow or in pulmonary HTN.

All the precordial impulses are significantly masked by obesity and lung hyperinflation. As such, absence of abnormal precordial impulses does not rule out cardiac pathology.

DATA DECODING TIPS (CLINICAL PEARLS)
Role of Cardiac Percussion

Percussion is used to establish the position of the heart, such as visceral situs (either situs solitus with left thoracic heart, solitus with right thoracic heart, or situs inversus). Cardiac percussion is often inaccurate, however, and adds little in the detection of cardiac enlargement.[2]

Cardiac Auscultation

Heart sounds and other audible phenomena should be assessed in a systematic manner with sequential auscultation of the mitral, tricuspid, pulmonic, and aortic areas. The genesis of heart sounds is believed to be the movement and oscillation of the blood column in relation to various events during the cardiac cycle. It is a good idea to have a reliable marker for systole throughout by palpating the carotid pulse for timing of systole. Carotid palpation is also helpful during cardiac auscultation because the timing of the carotid pulse accurately reflects the timing of systole. Auscultatory events that correspond with the carotid pulse are systolic in timing, while diastolic events are slightly more delayed from the carotid pulse. Radial or femoral pulses must not be used for timing of systole in view of the delay caused by the transit time from the heart to the periphery.

JOB DESCRIPTION:
How to Listen to the Heart

Place the stethoscope along the patient's lower left sternal border, thereby providing an overview: First start over the aortic area, remembering that the second heart sound over the aortic area is almost always louder than the first. Listen specifically to the first sound; then the second sound; then systematically listen for sounds in systole, murmurs in systole, sounds in diastole, and murmurs in diastole. Then turn the patient to the left lateral position and palpate with the index and middle fingers of the left hand to locate the point of maximum impulse of the left ventricle. Hold that spot with the fingers, and place the bell of the stethoscope lightly over this localized area; the ventricular (S3) gallop may now be louder and more clearly heard. A faint ventricular (S3) gallop might be overlooked in a patient having an emphysematous chest with an increase in AP diameter due to chronic pulmonary disease. This is true if one listens over the usual areas of the precordium, the lower left sternal border and apex; however, by listening over the xiphoid area or epigastric area, an S3 might be easily detected.[3]

The bell-type chest piece is better suited for detecting low-frequency events, whereas the diaphragm selectively picks up high-frequency events. When the bell is firmly pressed against the chest wall, it acts like the diaphragm by filtering out low-frequency sounds or murmurs and picking up high-frequency events. Using only the diaphragm may result in missing some important low-frequency murmurs or sounds, such as mid-diastolic rumble, pulmonary regurgitation (PR) murmur, and faint Still's innocent heart murmurs.[1]

First Heart Sound

The first heart sound (S1) is related to the closure movement of the mitral and tricuspid valves. It is loudest at the apex compared to the base and coincides with the carotid pulse (Table 3-2 and Table 3-3). Factors that influence the intensity of S1 include (1) the position of the mitral leaflets within the left ventricle at the onset of ventricular systole (wide-open versus partially closed), (2) anatomical integrity of the anterior mitral leaflet, (3) force of ventricular contraction, and (4) the PR interval on a 12-lead electrocardiogram (an inverse relationship).

A variable intensity of S1 occurs in atrial fibrillation (due to irregularly spaced cardiac cycles and differing mitral valve positions at the onset of systole) and complete heart block due to a variable P to QRS complex relationship. In atrial fibrillation the heart rate is irregular and

TABLE 3-2: Causes of Loud S1
Mitral stenosis with pliable leaflets
Hyperdynamic ventricular function
Short PR interval

TABLE 3-3: Causes of Soft S1
Mitral regurgitation due to rheumatic heart disease
Poor ventricular function
Long PR interval

frequently fast, while in complete heart block the heart rate is slow and regular. Thus a slow regular rhythm with variable intensity of S1 would be suggestive of complete heart block.

DATA DECODING TIPS (CLINICAL PEARLS)
First Heart Sound

The mitral component is generally louder than the tricuspid component of the first heart sound. Therefore when the tricuspid component (T1) is louder, two conditions should immediately come to mind: Ebstein's anomaly and atrial septal defect. Wide splitting of the first heart sound can occur with complete left bundle branch block (BBB), complete right BBB, Ebstein's anomaly, and at times with premature ventricular beats.[3]

Second Heart Sound

The second heart sound (S2) is related to the closure of the aortic and pulmonic valves. S2 is louder at the base compared to the apex. While it may be heard well both in the aortic and pulmonic areas, the contribution of aortic closure (A2) to the second heart sound is greater in the aortic area. Pulmonic closure (P2) is similarly better assessed in the pulmonic area.

While the two components of S1 (mitral and tricuspid) are very close to each other and hard to separate under normal conditions, A2 and P2 separate significantly from each other during respiration. Under normal circumstances, there is widening of the interval between A2 and P2 during inspiration. This phenomenon is called physiological splitting of S2 and it is very prominent in children, becoming less prominent in the adult age group.

While it is usual that mild splitting of S2 can be heard during quiet respiration with A2 and P2 heard separately during inspiration, no splitting is normally present during expiration. When splitting of S2 is heard during both inspiration and expiration with widening of the two components—A2 and P2—with inspiration, wide splitting of S2 is present (Table 3-4).

TABLE 3-4: Causes of Wide Splitting of S2

Right bundle branch block
Arial septal defect (causes wide and fixed splitting, with no change in A2-P2 interval with respiration)
Left ventricular pacing
Left ventricular ectopy
Severe mitral regurgitation
Mild to moderate pulmonic stenosis

🔴 DATA DECODING TIPS (CLINICAL PEARLS)
Normal or Pathological Splitting of S2

Splitting of the second heart sound is usually best appreciated over the third left sternal border. With expiration, the splitting becomes closer or may even become single, and coincident with inspiration there is an increase in the degree of splitting. Press firmly with the diaphragm of your stethoscope against the skin of the chest wall at the lower left sternal border and/or apex. When the second heart sound is distinctly split, this raises the possibility of atrial septal defect or bundle branch block. Often the only clue to an ostium primum defect is left axis deviation on the ECG. A simple maneuver is to have the patient sit or stand up: if the second sound then becomes single or very closely split on expiration, this is most likely a normal variant and not the wide splitting of atrial septal defect. However, "never say never".... Occasionally, a small atrial septal defect can have a single or closely split S2 on expiration. Also remember that the absence of a systolic murmur (even faint) heard over the pulmonic area or left sternal border practically eliminates the diagnosis of atrial septal defect.[3]

In atrial septal defect, a characteristic wide and fixed spitting of S2 occurs. Because the left to right atrial shunting provides the right atrium and right ventricle with a larger than normal volume, right ventricular ejection proceeds longer than normal, causing delay in the timing of P2 and wide split S2. Because there is a reciprocal change in the contribution to right atrial filling from the vena cava versus the atrial septal defect during inspiration and expiration, the net volume on the right side of the heart remains unchanged and elevated in atrial septal defect, causing the fixed splitting of S2. Wide fixed S2 splitting is a highly reliable physical finding suggestive of atrial septal defect. All assessments to verify respiratory changes of S2 splitting must be done during normal, quiet respiration.

🔴 DATA DECODING TIPS (CLINICAL PEARLS)
Wide Splitting of S2

Wide splitting of the second heart sound also can be found in patients with anomalous venous return. This defect is often associated with atrial septal defect but, uncommonly, it does occur alone. In such cases, the second heart sound is more likely to have more movement of the split with respiration than that of the typically "fixed splitting" of atrial septal defect. Wider splitting can also occur in patients with large ventricular septal defects; the mechanism is similar to that of mitral regurgitation.[3]

TABLE 3-5: Causes of Reversed or Paradoxical Splitting of S2

Left bundle branch block
Right ventricular pacing
Severe aortic stenosis
Severe left ventricular dysfunction

In patients with severe LV outflow obstruction or left HF, LV ejection is significantly prolonged and completion of ejection markedly delayed, causing A2 to occur after P2. Consequently the respiratory variation of the individual components of S2 (A2 and P2) will now cause a narrowing of the P2-A2 interval during inspiration. This apparent paradoxical nature of the behavior of the two components of S2 is termed reversed or paradoxical splitting (Table 3-5).

Intensity of A2 and P2 is influenced by the pressure in the corresponding great vessel, the size of the great vessel, and the anatomic features of the semilunar valve (pliable or nonpliable; Table 3-6). In aortic and pulmonic stenosis, A2 and/or P2 will become softer as the stenosis becomes more severe.

Third and Fourth Heart Sounds

During the rapid ventricular filling phase of diastole, a diastolic sound might be occasionally heard due to the oscillation of the incoming blood column into the ventricle. This produces a low frequency sound soon after S2 (heard best with the bell of the stethoscope) called S3 or third heart sound. S3 is a normal finding in children and adolescents because the ventricular muscle in younger subjects does not relax rapidly enough to accommodate the diastolic filling. As such, the presence of S3 in a completely asymptomatic young subject does not carry adverse implications. Often this type of S3 is referred to as the physiological third heart sound. Conversely, in older subjects, S3 is always a significant pathological finding and is frequently associated with congestive HF. A small early diastolic outward movement of the apical impulse may be felt with S3 (sometimes referred to as palpable S3).

The fourth heart sound (S4) is produced in late diastole and is associated with forceful contraction of the atria to facilitate filling of a noncompliant ventricle in late diastole. S4 is best heard with the bell of the

TABLE 3-6: Causes of Loud A2

Systemic hypertension
Ascending aortic dilatation and aneurysm

stethoscope with minimal pressure applied to the chest wall. S4 is heard in many older subjects without overt cardiac disease probably due to changes in ventricular compliance and diastolic function that occur with aging. Thus the presence of an S4 in an older subject in and of itself is not abnormal. Prominent S4 is often heard in patients with HTN, aortic stenosis, hypertrophic diomyopathy, and coronary artery disease. Auscultation while the patient is performing isometric handgrip will augment S4. In some patients, S4 will be heard for the first time or might be augmented during episodes of angina and active ischemia as a result of diastolic relaxation abnormalities induced by ischemia. Because S4 is produced by forceful atrial contraction, it will not be heard in the presence of atrial fibrillation. A small outward expansion of the apical impulse may on occasion be felt in patients with a loud S4, especially the patient placed in the left lateral position.

The differentiation between right-sided versus left-sided S3 and S4 is helped by the following:

(1) the location of the abnormal sound (left lower sternal edge favors right-sided S3 or S4, more lateral location favors left-sided origin), and (2) the augmentation of the sound during inspiration are specific for right-sided S3 and S4. Augmentation during expiration, however, is a nonspecific finding for all cardiac findings.

In constrictive pericarditis, an early loud S3 may be heard, referred to as a pericardial knock. This sound shares many features of an S3 described earlier but occurs sooner in diastole than the S3 associated with ventricular failure.

Clicks (Ejection and Nonejection) and Opening Snap

A high-frequency sound heard in systole is referred to as a click. This is best heard with the diaphragm of the stethoscope with firm pressure applied to the chest wall. There are two types of clicks—ejection and nonejection. These differ only in their relative timing after S1 within systole; the ejection click is closer to S1 and the nonejection click occurs a little bit later. The differentiation of an ejection click from a nonejection click requires careful auscultation and ascertaining the approximate distance of the click from S1 while simultaneously palpating the carotid pulse.

Ejection click, also referred to ejection sound, occurs typically with congenital aortic stenosis due to a bicuspid aortic valve, where the valve moves rapidly at the end of isovolumic contraction. Calcified bicuspid aortic valves are not associated with ejection click. Aortic root and ascending aortic dilatation may also be associated with an ejection click. Based on a similar mechanism, ejection sound can be heard in congenital pulmonic stenosis with very mobile valve cusps. The ejection click in pulmonic stenosis is heard only in expiration because during inspiration the S1-to-ejection distance is too brief for one to appreciate the two sounds separately.

Nonejection click, also referred to as midsystolic click, is the hallmark of mitral valve prolapse. A high frequency, sharp sound occurs in systole (much later than the ejection click) in mitral valve prolapse. This sound is produced due to the previously folded segments of the prolapsing mitral leaflet being pushed open in mid-systole. When mitral regurgitation is associated with mitral valve prolapse, the murmur will follow the midsystolic nonejection click. The interval between S1 and the midsystolic click is highly influenced by the filling pressures and ventricular size. Smaller LV volume would shorten the S1 to midsystolic click interval.

The opening snap is heard in mitral stenosis. It is a high frequency, sharp sound heard at the beginning of the rapid filling phase of diastole, coincident with the opening of the mitral valve and its rapid downward descent caused by the elevated left atrial pressure. It is best heard with the diaphragm of the stethoscope with the patient in the left lateral decubitus position. The opening snap disappears when mitral leaflets calcify or undergo fibrosis as the disease advances and the anterior mitral leaflet fails to move rapidly downward in diastole. The interval between S2 and the opening snap is inversely correlated with left atrial pressure and consequently with the severity of mitral stenosis.

The relative position of the various additional sounds within diastole is as follows: opening snap, pericardial knock, S3, and S4.

DATA DECODING TIPS (CLINICAL PEARLS)
Checking for Constrictive Pericarditis

If one hears a sound thought to be the opening snap of mitral stenosis, listen over the PMI of the LV with the patient turned to the left lateral position. If you don't hear a diastolic rumble, you might at first assume that perhaps the bell of the stethoscope is not over the localized spot where a rumble of mitral stenosis would be heard. However, if you listen over various localized spots and double check that the bell of the stethoscope is indeed over the PMI and you still do not hear a rumble but only the extra sound that could be an opening snap of mitral stenosis, do a " double-take." Check the neck veins, and if there is definite distention, constrictive pericarditis is the diagnosis. This cardiac pearl has stood the test of time and can provide an immediate diagnostic clue to constrictive pericarditis. The diagnosis can be suggested even earlier in the physical examination by examining the jugular venous pulse in the neck. The pericardial knock sound of constrictive pericarditis is present in the great majority of patients who have this condition if one carefully searches for it. Pulsus paradoxus can be present with constrictive pericarditis, but it is more likely to occur with cardiac tamponade.[3]

Sound That Cannot be Identified by Cardiac Auscultation

Recognition of a tricuspid opening snap requires secure identification of an accompanying split second heart sound and a mitral snap, or secure evidence that the stenotic mitral valve is immobile so that the snap becomes tricuspid by exclusion. Auscultation, however meticulous, is likely to be inadequate to the task of identifying the split second heart sound and both mitral and tricuspid opening snaps. A phonocardiographic record is needed for this purpose.[2]

Murmurs

A significant focus of the cardiac physical diagnosis is centered on murmurs. Laminar blood flow through cardiac chambers and blood vessels is quiet and inaudible to the stethoscope. When blood flow is transformed from laminar to turbulent, a murmur is produced. As such, all murmurs are indicative of abnormally turbulent flow, either due to a narrowing or an increased volume of flow causing relative narrowing. Occasionally the turbulent flow causing the murmur might also be palpable as a thrill. It is uncommon to palpate thrills in the current cardiology practice. Small ventricular septal defect is a classic lesion that is associated with a thrill. Often a murmur may be heard over a large area over the precordium causing difficulties in determining the site of origin. However, murmurs generally tend to be loudest in the area close to the origin of the turbulent flow. Radiation of the murmur is usually in the direction of the turbulent jet. Thus careful sequential auscultation of the precordium by moving the stethoscope a little each time can help in deciding the origin of a murmur heard over a large precordial area.

Right-sided origin of a murmur is suggested when the murmur intensity increases during inspiration. Because the lungs recede from the anterior surface of the heart during expiration, an expiratory increase can be seen in murmurs originating from the right side as well as the left side. The time for a murmur to reappear after the strain phase of the Valsalva maneuver can also be helpful in determining whether a murmur is right or left sided. Right-sided murmurs disappear during the strain phase due to reduced flow rates but reappear very quickly upon release of the strain, whereas left-sided murmurs return after only six or more cardiac cycles due to the transpulmonary transit time.

A description of a murmur should include its location, timing (systolic, diastolic, or continuous), grade (out of a scale of VI), radiation, and the effect of respiration. Grades of IV, V, and VI murmurs are accompanied by a thrill and tend to be very loud in intensity.

Systolic Murmurs

Systolic murmurs are more common than diastolic murmurs (Table 3-7). Innocent murmurs, also referred to as functional murmurs or physio-

TABLE 3-7: Causes of Systolic Murmurs

Innocent (physiological) murmur
Mitral regurgitation
Mitral valve prolapse with mitral regurgitation
Tricuspid regurgitation
Aortic stenosis
Hypertrophic cardiomyopathy
Pulmonic stenosis
Ventricular septal defect

logical murmurs, are typically due to flows slightly more turbulent than normal. These murmurs are usually midsystolic in timing and are heard over the pulmonic or aortic areas. Physiological murmurs are common in hyperdynamic states, such as in children, pregnancy, anemia, and thyrotoxicosis.

The timing of a systolic murmur is an important feature. Holosystolic murmurs occupy the entire length of systole and occur in conditions such as mitral regurgitation and tricuspid regurgitation with turbulent flow that is present throughout systole between a higher and a lower pressure chamber. In ventricular septal defect, the persistent gradient between left and right ventricles produces a holosystolic murmur. A holosystolic murmur does not necessarily require the same intensity throughout, however.

In patients with coronary artery disease, papillary muscle dysfunction is a frequent cause of mitral regurgitation. The murmur produced by papillary muscle dysfunction can be holosystolic, midsystolic, or early systolic, as determined by the extent of leaflet malcoaptation produced by ventricular dilatation, left atrial pressure, LV end-diastolic pressure, and the degree of papillary muscle dysfunction. When acute myocardial infarction is complicated by papillary muscle rupture, there is usually an early systolic murmur only, because the latter part of systole is associated with a very marked rise in left atrial pressure and the resultant reduction in regurgitant flow from the left ventricle.

In mitral valve prolapse, due to the timing of prolapse in midsystole only after LV ejection has been in progress, mitral regurgitation murmur is heard only in mid-and late systole. The murmur of mitral regurgitation in mitral valve prolapse always follows the midsystolic click. Various bedside maneuvers that reduce LV cavity size cause the murmur of mitral valve prolapse to lengthen and become louder.

The direction of radiation of the systolic murmur is often a clue to the leaflet responsible for mitral regurgitation. When the anterior mitral leaflet is the culprit, the murmur of mitral regurgitation typically will radiate to the back and the axilla. On the other hand, posterior mitral leaflet–generated mitral regurgitation radiates to the front toward the left parasternal region and the aortic area. This phenomenon could cause the murmur to be mistaken for one that is aortic in origin.

Outflow tract obstruction produces a midsystolic, crescendo-decrescendo, ejection type of systolic murmur, coincident with the origin of turbulent flow with the ejection phase of systole. An ejection murmur will start after a gap from S1 that corresponds to the isovolumetric contraction phase. The maximum intensity of the murmur in aortic stenosis is on the right side of the cardiac base (second right intercostal space), while in pulmonic stenosis the murmur is most prominent in the second left intercostal space.

 DATA DECODING TIPS (CLINICAL PEARLS)

Differential Diagnoses of Systolic Murmurs

Always rule out aortic stenosis in a patient with the following findings: A very high-pitched musical systolic murmur that peaks in midsystole and can be heard over the precordium (although it may be detected only at the apex); the heart sounds may be distant or absent. Remember also that almost all pregnant women have innocent grade 2 or 3 early to midsystolic murmurs, which may not be heard before or after pregnancy. A short systolic murmur heard over multiple areas of the back of the chest and often over the right and left anterior chest may afford the first clue about the diagnosis of pulmonary branch arterial stenosis. With very large shunts (5:1 or greater) of atrial septal defect, a systolic murmur similar to the pulmonary arterial branch stenosis (due to increased flow) may be found over the back if searched for. An arteriovenous fistula might be detected by the presence of a continuous murmur.

A systolic murmur of coarctation of almost equal intensity may be heard in the upper back as well as the front. Larger intercostal arteries of coarctation and tetralogy of Fallot may at times be felt and have a systolic murmur. In tetralogy patients, a continuous murmur may also be detected over the intercostal arteries. The transmitted holosystolic murmur of severe mitral regurgitation can be detected at the left posterior lung base. (The murmur has radiated—"band-like"—from the lower left sternal border, apex, and axillary lines to the posterior lung base.)[3]

DATA DECODING TIPS (CLINICAL PEARLS)

Differential Diagnoses Between Mitral Regurgitation and Ventricular Septal Defect

The holosystolic murmur detected along the lower left sternal border and apex brings up the differentiation between mitral regurgitation (MR) and ventricular septal defect. The murmur of ventricular septal defect is usually best heard along the lower left sternal border, although there is radiation of this murmur to the apex. The murmur can be loud and heard in both places; however, if one carefully inches the stethoscope from the lower sternal border to the apex, the murmur is loudest along the lower left sternal area. The papillary muscle rupture causing acute MR is more likely to have the murmur loudest at the apex, with radiation laterally to the axillary lines.[3] If it is a loud systolic murmur and accompanied by a palpable thrill, the ventricular septal defect thrill is along the left sternal border, whereas the mitral regurgitation thrill is at the apex.

Thrills are vibratory sensations that represent palpable manifestations of loud, harsh murmurs. Palpation for thrills is often of diagnostic value.

 JOB DESCRIPTION:

How to Palpate a Thrill

A thrill on the chest is felt better with the palm of the hand than with the tips of the fingers. However, the fingers are used to feel a thrill in the suprasternal notch and over the carotid arteries. Therefore, be sure to use the palm of the hand and the junction of the fingers when searching for a palpable thrill.[3] Thrills in the upper left sternal border originate from the pulmonary valve or pulmonary artery (PA) and therefore are present in pulmonic stenosis, pulmonary artery stenosis, or patent ductus arteriosus (PDA) (rarely). Thrills in the upper right sternal border are usually of aortic origin and are seen in AS. Thrills in the lower left sternal border are characteristic of a ventricular septal defect (VSD). Thrills in the suprasternal notch suggest AS but may be found in PS, PDA, or coarctation of the aorta (COA).[3]

Diastolic Murmurs

The presence of a diastolic murmur is a highly significant finding on physical examination because it is always indicative of a serious cardiac pathology (Table 3-8). Mid-diastolic murmur occurs due to turbulence during the rapid filling phase of diastole through the mitral or tricuspid valve. A common mechanism for such turbulence is mitral stenosis due to rheumatic valve disease or mitral valve obstruction due to other processes, such as a left atrial myxoma. Positional variation in the intensity of the diastolic murmur is found in left atrial myxoma, unlike rheumatic mitral stenosis, and occurs due to the variable obstruction of the mitral valve induced by body positions. Tricuspid stenosis is a rare disease again causing a mid-diastolic murmur. Murmurs due to mitral and tricuspid stenosis have a low frequency quality, termed a diastolic rumble, and are best audible with the bell. In severe mitral stenosis

TABLE 3-8: Causes of Diastolic Murmurs

Mid-diastolic
    Mitral stenosis
    Tricuspid stenosis
    Mitral valve obstruction due to left atrial myxoma
    Increased mitral flow due to ventricular septal defect or severe mitral regurgitation
    Austin-Flint murmur in severe aortic regurgitation
    Carey-Coombs murmur in acute rheumatic valvulitis
Early diastolic
    Aortic regurgitation
    Pulmonic regurgitation

the diastolic rumble builds in intensity in late diastole with a presystolic accentuation. Mid-diastolic murmur may also be caused by increased flow through a nonstenotic mitral valve in severe mitral regurgitation. In atrial septal defect the left-to-right atrial shunt causes increased flow through the tricuspid valve and may result in a mid-diastolic murmur in the left lower sternal edge. In severe aortic regurgitation, a mid-diastolic mitral murmur might be produced by the regurgitant flow through the aortic valve, causing partial closure of the mitral valve during diastole (referred to as the Austin-Flint murmur). A diastolic murmur heard during the acute phase of rheumatic carditis due to inflammation of mitral leaflets (called the Carey-Coombs murmur) is now very rare due to the declining rate of acute rheumatic fever and carditis worldwide.

Aortic and pulmonic regurgitation produce an early diastolic decrescendo murmur coincident with S2. In both aortic and pulmonic regurgitation, the rate of abnormal flow is highest at the beginning of diastole, with progressive decline as diastole proceeds. The length of early diastolic murmur of aortic regurgitation is inversely related to the severity of the regurgitant lesion. With the patient in the sitting position leaning forward with his or her breath held in end expiration, aortic regurgitation murmur is frequently more audible.

A wide pulse pressure (the difference between systolic and diastolic blood pressure) is seen in chronic severe aortic regurgitation. Isometric hand grip will cause the blowing early diastolic murmur of aortic regurgitation to become more prominent.

⚪ DATA DECODING TIPS (CLINICAL PEARLS)
Differences Between Aortic Insufficiency and Pulmonic Regurgitation

Can one distinguish the diastolic murmur of aortic regurgitation from that of hypertensive pulmonary regurgitation? Yes. The aortic regurgitation murmur is accompanied by the palpation of a "quick rise or flip" (collapsing) type of peripheral arterial pulse, whereas the pulmonary regurgitation murmur is not.[3]

Musical Murmurs

Musical quality of a murmur implies rapid oscillation of a freely mobile structure. It is seen in murmurs resulting from valve perforations in infective endocarditis and cardiac trauma. Musical overtones of the systolic murmur are characteristic of calcific aortic stenosis in the elderly. Calcification causes the aortic valve cusps to become rigid and immobile, while the free edges of the leaflets remain highly mobile in calcific aortic stenosis. During rapid ejection, the vibration of the mobile cusp edges imparts a low frequency, musical quality to the murmur of calcific aortic stenosis.

Continuous Murmurs

Compared to systolic and diastolic murmurs, continuous murmurs are relatively less frequent. A murmur starting in systole and extending into diastole by spilling over S2 is termed a continuous murmur. Thus it is not required for a murmur to occupy the entire systole and diastole to be labeled continuous. Moreover, a continuous murmur might be louder or softer at different times within the cardiac cycle rather than of sustained loudness. The presence of a continuous murmur implies turbulent flow that occurs between a higher and a lower pressure chamber beyond the semilunar valves (Table 3-9).

TABLE 3-9: Causes of Continuous Murmurs

Patent ductus arteriosus
Aortopulmonary window
Arteriovenous fistula
Rupture of sinus of Valsalva aneurysm into right atrium or right
    ventricle

🔵 DATA DECODING TIPS (CLINICAL PEARLS)
Continuous Murmur of PDA

The continuous murmur of a large patent ductus is generally loud and of low frequencies, with so-called "eddy" sounds. A palpable continuous thrill is generally present. Murmurs from small caliber patent ducti are often faint and of higher frequencies. Firm pressure with the diaphragm of one's stethoscope on the chest wall is helpful and often necessary to isolate this murmur. A very faint continuous murmur from a small patent ductus may become louder and more easily heard by using the isometric handgrip maneuver.[3]

A jugular venous hum might be heard in children. This produces a continuous murmur heard at the root of the neck caused by hyper-dynamic venous flow, frequently present in otherwise normal healthy children. This may be mistaken for a serious organic cardiac diagnosis. Jugular venous hum is influenced by neck position and may be completely eliminated by turning the neck sideways. It also disappears on applying compression to the root of the neck above the stethoscope. A phasic inspiratory increase in the intensity of the jugular venous hum also helps differentiate it from other causes of continuous murmur.

Dynamic Auscultation

Applying various bedside maneuvers to obtain additional physiological information about murmur genesis can be a very important step toward establishing a correct diagnosis. The rationale for use of bedside maneuvers is that, by altering LV size, murmur genesis can be characteristically altered. This concept is highly practical and relevant for the bedside diagnosis of mitral valve prolapse and hypertrophic cardiomyopathy.

In mitral valve prolapse a smaller LV cavity size promotes earlier displacement and billowing of the prolapsing leaflet into the left atrium and creates the milieu for greater mitral regurgitation. As such, maneuvers that reduce LV size cause earlier occurrence of the non-ejection click, a shorter S1-to-click interval, and longer duration with greater intensity of the mitral regurgitation murmur. Thus auscultation while the patient is standing causes S1-to-click distance to decrease and the mid- and late-systolic murmur of mitral regurgitation to become louder in mitral valve prolapse. In other etiologies of mitral regurgitation, such changes in the systolic murmur do not occur.

In patients suspected of having pericardial effusion, it is important to hear a rub. If a rub is not heard in the supine position, the patient should be put in the left lateral position or in the sitting position while leaning forward. Milder degrees of effusion may not muffle the heart sounds and murmurs. Very severe degrees of pericardial effusion can be clinically suspected without having to turn the patient in this position.

JOB DESCRIPTION:

How to Hear a Rub

To detect a pericardial friction rub: Use the flat diaphragm of the stethoscope: Listen along the third and fourth left sternal borders. Exert firm pressure with the patient sitting upright, breath held in deep expiration. Note the following three component friction rub abbreviations: as = Atrial systolic component, vs = Ventricular systolic component, vd = Ventricular diastolic component. This procedure can be particularly helpful in diagnosing moderate-to-severe effusion.[2]

 JOB DESCRIPTION:

How to Check Pulsus Paradoxicus and Pulsus Alternans

To elicit the paradoxical pulse, the patient should be positioned comfortably with the trunk raised to a level that minimizes increased respiratory excursions. Specific instructions should be given to breathe as regularly and quietly as comfort permits. The examiner's thumb should be applied to the brachial arterial pulse with enough compression to elicit the maximal systolic impact. Compression is gradually released while the examiner observes the patient's respiratory movements by glancing at the chest or abdomen. As pressure on the brachial artery decreases in a gradual stepwise fashion, a level is reached at which the pulse diminishes or even vanishes during inspiration.[2] If the presence of pulsus paradoxus is checked with a blood pressure cuff, the method is as follows: (a) The cuff pressure is raised about 20 mm Hg above the systolic pressure. (b) The pressure is lowered slowly until Korotkoff sound 1 is heard for some but not all cardiac cycles, and the BP reading is noted. (c) The pressure is lowered further until systolic sounds are heard for all cardiac cycles, and the BP is noted. (d) If the difference between readings A and B is greater than 10 mm Hg, pulsus paradoxus is present.[1] If pulsus alternans is present, the Korotkoff sounds initially appear at a rate that is half the pulse rate. On further deflating the cuff, the rate of Korotkoff sounds will suddenly double and equal the pulse rate.[2] Because mechanical alternans tends to be exaggerated as the pulse wave moves peripherally, the radial and femoral pulses tend to be more revealing than the carotids and brachials. With the thumb applied to a femoral artery or the thumb or finger applied to a radial artery, compression is gradually increased until the impact of the pulse is maximal.[2]

In hypertrophic cardiomyopathy, a smaller LV cavity causes a greater degree of systolic anterior motion of the mitral valve, more outflow tract

TABLE 3-10: Maneuvers That Reduce Left Ventricular Size

Standing
Strain phase of Valsalva maneuver

TABLE 3-11: Maneuvers That Increase Left Ventricular Size

Passive leg raising
Isometric hand grip
Squatting

obstruction, and a louder systolic murmur. In contrast, a larger LV cavity is accompanied by less outflow tract obstruction and a less prominent systolic murmur. Standing causes a relatively smaller LV size due to reduced venous return and ventricular filling. Squatting causes LV size to increase due to the effect of arterial compression on afterload (Table 3-10 and Table 3-11).

DATA CONVERTING TIPS (CLINICAL PEARLS)
Diagnosing Hypertrophic Cardiomyopathy

Now let's shake hands again with another patient, and then put our palpating fingers over the radial pulse. We note a quick rise of the pulse; this is called a "flip." It is a sensation obtained when one flips the middle finger of one hand against the middle finger of the other. This brief contact against the stationary finger produces a sensation that we have termed a flip. Even a little flip produces a quick-rise sensation. The quick-rise pulse (also termed Corrigan or waterhammer pulse) is consistent with aortic regurgitation, a diagnostic possibility to be ruled in or out. Now search for the aortic diastolic murmur, listening with the patient sitting upright, leaning forward, and in deep expiration. Listening with the flat diaphragm of the stethoscope pressed firmly against the chest wall at the third left sternal border. We expect to hear the early blowing diastolic murmur of aortic regurgitation; however, we don't hear it. Instead there is a systolic murmur. Even at this point, we should think of hypertrophic cardiomyopathy. The next step is to use the squatting maneuver. On the patient's squatting, the murmur decreases in intensity (on rare occasions it may even disappear). The murmur becomes louder again on standing, and the diagnosis of hypertrophic cardiomyopathy is made.[3]

The Valsalva maneuver can also be helpful in diagnosing hypertrophic cardiomyopathy. While listening along the left sternal border or apex, have the patient take a deep breath, blow the breath out, and then strain as if having a bowel movement. The murmur may increase in intensity, indicating a positive response.

However, some patients, such as the elderly, may have difficulty in performing this maneuver. A simpler way is to have the patient place his or her or index finger in the mouth, seal it with the lips, exhale, and at the point of a deep expiration, "blow hard" on the finger. This usually works.[3]

Examination of the Neck

The goals of a vascular examination of the neck include evaluation of the carotid pulse upstroke, of a pulsatile mass in the neck, and the search for a carotid bruit. The examination of the neck vein includes evaluation of the venous pressure and waveform analysis in patients with severe left and right HF and pericardial disease. However, not every patient can have the neck examined for a variety of reasons.

DATA DECODING TIPS (CLINICAL PEARLS)
When the Neck Exam Is Not Feasible

In some adults, the carotid artery is undesirable for analysis of waveform because of atherosclerotic obstruction, kinking, or the presence of a marked thrill or shudder. In some patients, a short neck precludes the use of carotid arterial palpation for routine assessment of waveform. Similarly, in adults with short, thick, or obese necks, the venous pulse may not be transmitted through the overlying tissue to the skin.[2]

Examination of the Carotid Artery

Locating the proper pulse for assessment of pulse upstroke is important. The carotid pulse is the most appropriate pulse for this purpose, while radial pulse is a poor choice. The carotid pulse can be found on the medial border of the sternomastoid muscle. The bifurcation of common carotid into external and internal carotid pulses occurs at the level of the thyroid cartilage. As such, carotid pulsations felt medial to the sternomastoid muscle below the thyroid cartilage originate from the common carotid artery, while above that level the external carotid pulsations are felt. Normal carotid pulse upstroke is accompanied by a small degree of external displacement. While this is a relatively subjective assessment, by practicing the palpatory technique on many patients, one can learn how to gauge the upstroke.

DATA DECODING TIPS (CLINICAL PEARLS)
Differentiating the Pulse of the Neck

Normally the carotid pulsation is not visible. However, it may be prominent at the base of the right side of the neck in thin patients with long-standing HTN. Even in the setting of internal carotid artery occlusion, there is generally a palpable common carotid pulse, as the external carotid artery often remains patent. A diminished or absent common carotid pulsation suggests significant proximal occlusive disease at the origin of the carotid artery in the chest. The presence of a temporal artery pulse anterior to the ear indicates a patent common and external carotid artery. Palpation itself cannot differentiate between carotid aneurysm and carotid body tumor, both of which may present as a pulsatile mass in the neck. Enlarged lymph nodes often have similar findings, and differentiation in the setting of a pulsatile neck mass requires duplex ultrasonography, computed tomography (CT), or magnetic resonance imaging (MRI). The vertebral artery is not accessible to palpation; it lies deep at the posterior base of the neck and is surrounded by cervical bone for most of its course. Pulsatile masses at the base of the neck or in the supraclavicular fossa generally originate from the subclavian artery.[4]

Conditions that produce poor carotid upstroke include low cardiac output and aortic valve stenosis (Table 3-12). In aortic regurgitation, pulse upstroke is brisk since the stroke volume is increased and the systemic vascular resistance is low. Brisk pulse upstroke may also be present in other conditions characterized by a hyperdynamic circulation (patent ductus arteriosus, arteriovenous fistula, and beriberi heart disease) (Table 3-13).

Carotid palpation should be attempted gently without excessive pressure in order to avoid development of vagally mediated bradycardia as well as to prevent vigorous palpation from dislodging plaque. The

TABLE 3-12: Causes of Reduced Carotid Pulse Upstroke

Low cardiac output states
Valvular aortic stenosis (slow rising small volume pulse—pulsus parvus et tardus)

TABLE 3-13: Causes of Brisk Carotid Pulse Upstroke

Aortic regurgitation
Patent ductus arteriosus
Aortopulmonary window
Arteriovenous fistula
Hyperdynamic circulation
   Beriberi heart disease
   Thyrotoxicosis
   Pregnancy

carotid arteries should not only be palpated one at a time, but the examining thumb should also be applied in the lower half of the neck to avoid carotid sinus stimulation, especially in the elderly patient.[3] However, the overall risk for either complication is quite low. In some patients with advanced age and/or atherosclerosis, the carotid artery might be tortuous and might appear more prominent on palpation on one side versus the opposite side.

Carotid artery bruits indicate the presence of underlying vascular disease and stenosis. A systolic bruit over the carotid artery is highly predictive of future risk for transient ischemic attacks, including stroke, despite the fact that the bruit might originate in the external carotid artery. Systolic and diastolic bruits occurring together indicate more critical stenosis of an artery compared to systolic bruit alone. Transmitted murmurs, particularly from the aortic and pulmonic areas, might be heard over the carotids and might cause confusion with carotid bruits. A helpful differentiating feature is that transmitted murmurs are much louder close to the source of their origin (aortic area or pulmonic area) rather than over the carotid artery.

DATA DECODING TIPS (CLINICAL PEARLS)
Assessing the Carotid Bruit

The presence of a cervical bruit does not necessarily mean that a carotid stenosis is present. In fact, only half of patients with carotid bruits will have stenoses of 30% or more, and only a quarter will have stenoses of more than 75%. Additionally, the severity of underlying carotid stenosis does not correlate with the loudness of the bruit.[4]

Examination of the Neck Veins

Examination of the neck veins provides a large body of diagnostic and physiological clues. The value of the jugular venous examination is based on the fact that the right side of the heart is connected to the jugular vein without an intervening valve and, as such, provides an easy opportunity to measure and assess right heart dynamics.

Venous Waveform Analysis

For the assessment of venous pulse, the internal jugular vein is the preferred vessel, and the external jugular vein, despite being easily visible may, if at all, only be used for venous pulse waveform analysis. Locating the venous pulse can be difficult. The internal jugular vein lies behind the belly of the sternomastoid muscle, while the external jugular vein crosses the sternomastoid muscle. For evaluation of the jugular venous pressure, the patient should be positioned with the head adequately elevated to demonstrate the top of the pulsating jugular venous column. Any tight abdominal binders such as belts should be fully released in order to avoid overestimation of venous pressure. Observation of venous pressure and pulse should be performed during normal quiet respiration. The differentiating features of venous pulse from arterial pulse are the following:

Arterial pulse is seen and felt equally well, while venous pulse is better seen than felt due to its low pressure characteristics.

The more lateral to the sternomastoid the pulse location is, the more likely that it is venous.

Venous pulse has multiple deflections or waves per cardiac cycle, while arterial pulse has a single outward movement.

Venous pressure responds phasically to respiration, while arterial pulse does not.

Abdominal compression causes venous pressure to rise, whereas it does not affect arterial pressure.

Venous pressure is influenced by the position of the patient, with a pressure drop in the sitting position; arterial pulse and pressure do not change with the position of the patient.

Nonpulsating venous engorgement in the neck should be a clue to superior venacaval compression. This is often accompanied by suffusion of the face and conjunctiva, pitting edema of the eyes and upper extremities, and, rarely, venous collaterals draining the upper extremity flow to the inferior vena caval territory.

Venous pressure is measured as the vertical height of the top of the pulsating venous column from the sternal angle (the angle of Louis). The sternal angle is a bony ridge located at the junction of the manubrium with the body of the sternum, a point that is approximately 5 cm in front of and above the center of the right atrium. Venous pressure should be expressed in centimeters of water (remember that for conversion into mm of mercury, this number is divided by 1.7). The venous pressure reading obtained from the sternal angle will remain constant in a given patient irrespective of the incline of the patient; raising the head of the patient is done only to identify the top of the venous pulse. Normal venous pressure should be between 0 to 5 mm Hg (Table 3-14).

TABLE 3-14: Causes of Elevated Venous Pressure

Right ventricular failure due to left-sided heart failure
   RV myocardial infarction
    Chronic pulmonary hypertension due to lung pathology
Tricuspid valve obstruction
Pericardial effusion and tamponade
Constrictive pericarditis

JOB DESCRIPTION:

How to Look for the Crest of the Jugular Vein

Begin with the patient's head elevated 30 to 45 degrees above the horizontal position and then lower or elevate it from there. The higher the central venous pressure, the greater the required elevation above horizontal. If oscillations of the internal jugular vein are not seen at an angle of 0 to 15 degrees, gentle abdominal compression with the flat of the hand serves to increase venous return, transiently revealing the oscillations of the jugular pulse. In addition to selecting the appropriate elevation of the trunk, the examiner must properly position the patient's chin to relax the right sternocleidomastoid muscle. The patient's head should be adjusted from a neutral position slightly upward or downward or to either side by gently moving the chin, but the head should not be tilted too far upward or too sharply to the left; these maneuvers tense the right sternocleidomastoid muscle and compress or obliterate the underlying internal jugular vein.[2]

Venous pulse waveform should be assessed next. In order to perform this adequately, one needs an understanding of cardiac physiology and a landmark for timing systole. Carotid pulse is an excellent marker for systole, since the time taken for cardiac systole to transmit to carotid is minimal as opposed to the femoral pulse. As such the radial and femoral pulses should never be used for timing of systole. The typical venous pulse is characterized by two positive deflections or waves —'A' and 'V'—and two negative deflections— 'X' and 'Y'. The A wave occurs in association with atrial systole and atrial contraction (Table 3-15). The X descent is related to a drop in atrial pressures coincident with atrial diastole and relaxation. The V wave occurs during systole as the venous return to the atrium causes a rise in the right atrial pressure since the tricuspid valve is closed at this time (Table 3-16). The Y descent is due to the drop in the right atrial pressure during early diastole as the right ventricle fills from the right atrium. Generally the A wave is seen in the

TABLE 3-15: Causes of Prominent 'A' Waves

Tricuspid valve obstruction
   Tricuspid stenosis
   Tricuspid atresia
Reduced right ventricular compliance
   Pulmonic stenosis
   Pulmonary hypertension
   Right ventricular myocardial infarction

TABLE 3-16: Causes of Prominent 'V' Waves
Tricuspid regurgitation

neck as a prominent pulse that travels from below upwards. The V wave, however, usually produces an expansile lateral deflection.

Large A waves in the neck veins are present with each cardiac cycle in conditions such as tricuspid atresia, and these are called giant A waves. These should be distinguished from cannon A waves, a finding present in complete heart block; these large A waves occur not with each cardiac cycle but off and on when the atrial and ventricular contractions coincide by chance, resulting in the force of atrial contraction's failing to transmit to the right ventricle due to the closed tricuspid valve.

Normally the venous pressure falls during inspiration and rises slightly with expiration. Paradoxical inspiratory rise in the venous pressure is termed Kussmaul's sign; this might be present in severe right ventricular dysfunction and in conditions with abnormal right ventricular compliance, such as right ventricular myocardial infarction.

When the rise in venous pressure is borderline and the diagnosis of right HF is doubtful, hepatojugular reflux should be tested. Sustained pressure over the abdomen causes an increase in venous pressure in positive hepatojugular reflux due to the failure of the right ventricle to accommodate the additional venous return. Under normal circumstances a transient elevation of venous pressure may be seen with abdominal pressure; the distinction from a positive hepatojugular reflux is made by the persistence of venous pressure elevation for more than ~30 seconds. In a patient with clearly elevated venous pressure, the value of hepatojugular reflux is dubious; when venous pressure elevation is only marginal, hepatojugular reflux confirms the presence of right ventricular failure. Hepatojugular reflux also establishes the patency of the superior vena cava because, when obstruction of the SVC is present, abdominal compression cannot transmit to upper extremity veins. In patients who do not have a clear view of the internal jugular crest, can we estimate the right atrial pressure with the external jugular vein?

DATA DECODING TIPS (CLINICAL PEARLS)
Measuring Right Atrial Pressure with the External Jugular Vein

The external jugular vein is, as a rule, not pulsatile but instead often presents as a visible column that distends to a crest, which could be a reliable measure of the mean right atrial pressure. The internal jugular vein accurately reflects both right atrial waveform and phasic pressure.

Accordingly, it is the right rather than the left internal jugular vein that is more important in the physical examination, because the right provides a more accurate reflection of right atrial activity. A more prominent left rather than right internal jugular pulse occurs in situs inversus.[3]

Examination of the Abdomen

Examination of the abdomen is done to check the fluid congestion in the liver (hepatomegaly), spleen (splenomegaly), abdominal wall area, genitalia (scrotal and vulvar edema), peritoneal cavity (ascites), and hemorrhoidal vein (hemorrhoids).

Certain anatomic features related to the aorta and iliac arteries should be considered when one palpates the abdomen. The aorta bifurcates into the common iliac arteries at about the level of the umbilicus and, in order to assess the infrarenal aortic segment, one must palpate deeply above this surface landmark.

◉ DATA DECODING TIPS (CLINICAL PEARLS)
How to Palpate the Aorta

With the patient bending the knees, relaxing the abdominal musculature, and exhaling slowly and fully, you should be able to facilitate the exam. It should also be remembered that, unless the patient is obese, an aortic pulse should normally be palpable above the umbilicus, especially if the abdominal wall is relaxed. The normal aorta is approximately the width of the patient's thumb, or 2 cm in diameter. An aortic aneurysm should be suspected when the aortic pulse feels expansile and larger than 4 cm. Elderly patients may have a tortuous, anteriorly displaced aorta that can be mistaken for an aneurysm.[4]

Because the sensitivity of abdominal palpation is limited, an aortic ultrasound should be ordered as an easy and noninvasive test in patients in whom there are any questions about aortic diameter. In addition to size, other characteristics of an aneurysm may be identified by palpation. If the enlarged aorta extends high to the xiphoid or costal margins, a suprarenal or thoracoabdominal aortic aneurysm should be suspected. Aneurysm tenderness on palpation is a sign indicating pending rupture, aneurysm leak, or the presence of an inflammatory aneurysm. Because of the anatomic location of the iliac arteries deep within the pelvis, aneurysms in this location are often not palpable.[4]

DATA DECODING TIPS (CLINICAL PEARLS)
Auscultation of the Abdomen

Auscultation commonly reveals bruits when significant occlusive disease of the aorta or its branches is present. Aortoiliac occlusive disease causes bruits in the middle and lower abdomen and the femoral region. Bruits secondary to isolated renal artery stenosis are faint and localized in the upper abdominal quadrants lateral to the midline. Mesenteric artery occlusive disease may be associated with epigastric bruits.[4]

Asymptomatic abdominal bruits are an occasional incidental finding on abdominal examination of young adults, especially thin women. If the patient is not hypertensive and does not have intestinal angina or leg claudication, these bruits may be considered benign. The bruits may originate from impingement of the diaphragmatic crura on the celiac axis.[4]

Examination of the Arterial System of the Extremities
The blood pressure is measured in both arms. A difference in arm pressures of more than 10 mm Hg indicates a hemodynamically significant innominate, subclavian, or axillary artery stenosis on the side with the diminished pressure. When coarctation of the aorta obstructs the orifice of the left subclavian artery, the left brachial pulse is diminished or absent, while the right brachial pulse is increased. In supravalvular aortic stenosis, the right brachial pulse is increased, while the left brachial pulse is normal.[2]

Examination of the upper extremity arteries should include comparison of blood pressure in both arms, auscultation of the supraclavicular fossa for bruits, and examination for ischemia due to obstructive arterial disease.

DATA DECODING TIPS (CLINICAL PEARLS)
Differentiating Ischemia in the Upper Extremities

Pink fingertips with a capillary refill time of less than 3 seconds are a sign of good perfusion. In contrast, the acutely ischemic upper extremity is pallid and may have neurologic compromise in the form of motor or sensory deficits. The main change in appearance of the extremity with chronic arterial ischemia is muscle atrophy, especially in the forearm and proximal hand. Embolization or small-vessel disease may be recognized by painful mottled areas or ulcerations of the fingertips. Raynaud's phenomenon presents as a triphasic color change (white, blue, red) in the hands and fingers following an inciting event such as cold exposure or emotional stress. The fingers first appear pallid or white, then cyanotic or blue, and last hyperemic or red as circulation is restored.[4]

However, does every patient with subclavian artery stenosis have no peripheral pulse?

DATA DECODING TIPS (CLINICAL PEARLS)
Severe Proximal Stenosis with Normal Radial Pulse

Because collateral flow to the arm is extensive, a proximal subclavian stenosis may be present in an asymptomatic individual with palpable pulses at the wrist. If the patient has symptoms suggesting arm claudication, the arm should be exercised for 2 to 5 minutes and the brachial pressures rechecked. With this provocative maneuver, the brachial pressure will decrease if a significant arterial stenosis exists. When pulses are not palpable, continuous wave Doppler ultrasound can be used to assess arterial signals and measure arm and forearm pressures.[3]

DATA DECODING TIPS (CLINICAL PEARLS)
Decipher the Abnormal Pulses in CoA

Simultaneous palpation of the radial and femoral pulses should be done to assess the femoral pulse delay. The explanation for the delay is the arrival of the pulse wave at the femoral artery through collateral vessels originating from the aorta proximal to the obstruction. In many patients with coarctation, the femoral pulse volume is reduced or may even be absent. However, delay of the femoral pulse relative to the radial pulse is more important than the abnormalities of femoral pulse volume per se in coarctation. While absent or weak femoral pulse might be caused by aortoiliac atherosclerotic disease, delay of femoral pulse is not seen in the latter condition.[4] Both the dorsalis pedis and posterior tibial pulses might be absent unilaterally in some patients without serious adverse consequences.[4] If a good pedal pulse is felt, coarctation of the aorta (COA) is effectively ruled out, especially if the blood pressure in the arm is normal. Weak leg pulses and strong arm pulses suggest COA. If the right brachial pulse is stronger than the left brachial pulse, the cause may be COA occurring near the origin of the left subclavian artery or supravalvular aortic stenosis (AS). A right brachial pulse weaker than the left suggests an aberrant right subclavian artery arising distal to the coarctation. In an occasional adult with iliac obstruction and in an occasional younger patient with COA, collateral circulation is so abundant that dorsalis pedis and posterior tibial pulses are palpable even though the proximal lower extremity (femoral) pulses are diminished.[1] Bounding pulses are found in aortic run-off lesions, such as PDA, aortic regurgitation (AR), large systemic arteriovenous fistula, or persistent truncus arteriosus (rarely).[1]

TAKE-HOME MESSAGE

The approach to bedside cardiac physical diagnosis should be systematic, with the awareness that many clues to the pathophysiology are available through physical findings without any additional cost or risk to the patient. Often the clinician will need to slightly modify the physical examination in each patient to detect the necessary clues for a specific diagnosis. Findings that do not adequately correlate with the diagnostic tests should be carefully considered by the clinician for any other potential explanation and the need for additional testing. This approach is much more logical rather than ignoring the presence of an unexplained finding altogether. Lastly, clinicians who seek constant corroboration of their physical findings from all available additional tests become more skilled diagnosticians through a process of practice-based learning improvement.

References

1. Park, M. K.: Pediatric Cardiology for Practitioners, Philadelphia, PA: Mosby Elsevier, 2008.
2. Perloff, J.K.: Physical Examination of the Heart and Circulation, Shelton, CT: People's Medical Publishing House, 2009.
3. Harvey, W. P.: Cardiac Pearls, Fairfield, NJ: Leannec Publishing, 1993.
4. Rasmussen, T. E., Clouse, W. D., Tonnessen, B. H., eds.: Handbook of Patient Care in Vascular Diseases, 5th ed., Philadelphia, PA: Lippincott Williams & Wilkins, 2008.

Further Reading

Braunwald's Heart Disease: A Textbook of Cardiovascular Medicine. Philadelphia, PA: W.B. Saunders Company, 2008.

Clinical Guidelines on the Identification, Evaluation and Treatment of Overweight and Obesity in Adults: Evidence Report, NHLBI. www.nhlbi.nih.gov/guidelines.

The Seventh Report of the Joint National Committee on Prevention, Detection, Evaluation, and Treatment of High Blood Pressure. www.nhlbi.nih.gov/guidelines/hypertension.

Vascular Medicine: A Companion to Braunwald's Heart Disease. Philadelphia, PA: Saunders Elsevier, 2006.

Section II

Cardiovascular Risk Factors

Prevention of Cardiovascular Disease

Thach Nguyen, John Huynh, Adolphus Anekwe, Huy V. Tran, Tung Mai, and Mario Maranhao

Chapter Outline

DEFINITION

Cardiovascular disease (CVD) is a group of major cardiac and vascular diseases with end organ failure, including myocardial infarction (MI), stroke, dilated cardiomyopathy, hypertrophic cardiomyopathy, critical limb ischemia, and renal dysfunction. CVD is predisposed by two groups of risk factors that are listed in Table 4-1.

TABLE 4-1: Risk Factors for Cardiovascular Disease

Risk Factors for Cardiovascular Atheroslerosis

Uncontrolled hypertension (HTN)
Hypercholesterolemia
Overweight
Diabetes mellitus (DM)
Chronic kidney disease (CKD)
Arthritis

Risk Factors for Cardiomyopathy

Valvular insufficiency or stenosis
Atrial fibrillation, uncontrolled supraventricular arrhythmia
Uncontrolled HTN
Alcohol abuse
Coronary artery disease
Diabetes mellitus

Patient Population at Risk

There are billions of people in the world who are currently healthy and do not have any form of cardiovascular abnormality. These people need to be protected from developing CVD.

Strategic Programming

The best strategy for preventing CVD is to identify the patients with risk factors as early as possible through data collecting with a comprehensive history and physical examination. The following two major risk factors need to be detected and prevented early: DM type 2 and CKD. The reason is that there are no definitive cures or complete reversal of DM or CKD. Once a patient has diabetes, the prognosis is as serious and equivalent to having an acute MI. The next step is to perform data mining. Tests may be ordered (fasting lipid profile, fasting glucose level, blood urea nitrogen (BUN), creatinine level, and electrocardiogram) in order to confirm (data converting) the diagnoses of hypercholesterolemia, DM, CKD, and metabolic syndrome. Prevention of CVD also requires a comprehensive effort because the integrative nature of atherosclerosis (as a global disease) and cardiomyopathy (with its vast numbers of affected patients) mandates transcendence of traditional specialty boundaries. The management strategies for prevention of CV disease are summarized in Table 4-2.

DATA COLLECTING

History

When a patient is coming in for a cardiology visit, the physician should look for the presence of risk factors and early manifestations of CVD. The components of a comprehensive interview are listed in Table 4-3.

Queries About Diet

The physician should ask about dietary habits, including how salty the patient's foods are and how much salt is added to foods when cooking.

TABLE 4-2: Management Strategies for Prevention of Cardiovascular Disease
Screen and detect subjects at risk by the history and physical examination.
Confirm the preliminary diagnosis by appropriate testing.
Set up a comprehensive corrective and preventive plan.
Initiate diet, exercise, and healthy lifestyle changes, teaching compliance.
Apply evidence-based medicine and cost-effective treatment.

TABLE 4-3: Components of an Interview of a Healthy Person
General Health Condition

Level of physical activity
  Level of activity without shortness of breath
  Symptoms with strenuous activities
  History of easy fatigue or shortness of breath with activities
Awareness of CVD risk factors
Awareness of need for CVD prevention

Risk Factors for Atherosclerosis
History of smoking History of dietary habits (high-cholesterol diet) Family history of sudden cardiac death at an early age Family history of CVD at an early age Symptoms of arthritis Symptoms of unrecognized DM (too good appetite, weight gain, weight   loss, polyuria, polydipsia) Symptoms of erectile dysfunction at age <50 History of recurrent or chronic infection History of vaccination
Risk Factors for Cardiomyopathy
History of alcohol abuse Family history of sudden cardiac death Symptoms of valvular disease Symptoms of unrecognized DM (too good appetite, weight gain, weight   loss, polyuria, polydipsia) Symptoms of anemia
CVD: cardiovascular disease, DM: diabetes mellitus.

Does the patient have a salt shaker on the table? Does the patient have a low-cholesterol diet? Does the patient use canned foods? How does the patient buy foods? Does the patient drink alcohol? In cases of heavy alcoholism, it is better to ask these patient whether they drank excessively in the past because they tend to deny drinking alcohol or minimize the amount of daily alcohol intake.

SMART THINKING:

Novel Risk Factor: Is Rheumatoid Arthritis a Risk Factor for CVD?

Goal: To investigate the first-ever incidence of acute MI and stroke in a community-based rheumatoid arthritis (RA) cohort compared with the general population. ***Methods:*** The RA cohort consisted of all patients in a local RA register in Malmö, Sweden (n = 1022). The patients were recruited from private and hospital-based rheumatology practices and made up the absolute majority of patients with RA in the city. The general population of Malmö, aged 16 and above, served as controls. From the Swedish National Hospital Discharge Register and the national Swedish Causes of Death Register, information about all first-ever MIs and strokes in Malmö residents between July 1997 and December 1999 was retrieved. The age- and sex-adjusted standardized morbidity ratio (SMR) of the two cohorts was calculated. *Results:* Fifty-four patients with RA had first-ever MIs or strokes during the study period, compared with 3862 subjects in the general population. The age- and sex-adjusted SMR was 161 (95% confidence interval [CI] 121 to 210). The first-ever incidence of CV disease was increased among female and male patients when studied separately. The increase of CV events in the RA cohort was mainly due to an excess of MIs (n = 36; SMR = 176 (95% CI 123 to 244). *Practical Applications:* Patients with RA in Malmö had an increased first-ever incidence of MI or stroke compared with the general population. This confirms that CV comorbidity is of major importance in RA.[1]

Physical Examination

In a patient coming for a CV visit, besides the usual measurements of blood pressure (BP), weight, waist circumference, and optic fundi exam, the focuses of a physical examination are listed in Table 4-4.

TABLE 4-4: Focuses of a Cardiovascular Examination

Signs of Cardiovascular Disease
Old myocardial infarction
Old stroke
Peripheral arterial disease
Cardiomyopathy and heart failure
Signs of Risk Factors
Uncontrolled hypertension
Dyslipidemia
Cigarette smoking
Diabetes mellitus
Alcohol abuse
Signs of novel risk factors
Rheumatoid arthritis

The physician should look for heart murmur, carotid artery murmur, status of the peripheral pulse (femoral, pedis dorsalis, and posterior tibial), pulsation in the mid-abdominal area to rule out abdominal aortic aneurysm, murmur of renal artery stenosis, and swelling of the joints from arthritis.

However, it is vital to recognize the physical signs of unrecognized early manifestations of risk factors, such as HTN, dyslipidemia, cigarette smoking, DM, and alcohol abuse.

DATA DECODING TIPS (CLINICAL PEARLS)
How to Detect the Early Manifestations of DM, HTN, Dyslipidemia, Cigarette Smoking, or Alcohol Abuse

For patients with early DM, there may be a concern about excellent (or excessive) appetite and/or high food intake without gaining weight. Some would complain of losing weight, with more urination and thirst. Patients with HTN can be detected early at regular check-ups with BP taken during these visits. There are neither signs nor symptoms of early dyslipidemia. For a patient who smokes, look at the yellowish stain on the fingers. The skin on the face has a ground, glassy look. Early signs of alcohol abuse are that the patient is not punctual at work and requires many days off (absenteeism) from work.

Examination of an Obese Person

Obesity can be defined as an excess of body fat. A surrogate marker for body fat content is body mass index (BMI), which is determined by weight (kilograms) divided by height squared (square meters). In clinical terms, a BMI of 25–29 kg/m^2 is called overweight; higher BMIs ($\geq$30 kg/m^2) are termed obese. The best way to estimate obesity in clinical practice is to measure the waist circumference.

JOB DESCRIPTION:
How to Measure the Waist Circumference

Locate the top of the right iliac crest. Place a measuring tape on a horizontal plane around the abdomen at the level of the iliac crest. Before reading the tape measure, be sure that the tape is parallel to the floor and snug but does not compress the skin. Measurement is made at the end of a normal expiration.

Among subjects who are equally overweight, those with more abdominal cavity fat (visceral adipose tissue) compared to those with excessive subcutaneous adipose tissue are at greater risk for CV disease. The waist circumference is a crude but simple measure of abdominal fat. Is the body-mass index as good as the waist circumference?

SMART THINKING:

Waist Circumference Versus BMI

In a study of metabolic syndrome (MetS) patients with successful reduction of visceral fat, was waist circumference or BMI a surrogate marker of success? ***Methodology:*** Included were patients with waist circumferences ≥90 cm, triglycerides >150 mg/dL, and high-density lipoprotein (HDL) cholesterol levels <40 mg/dL; after screening with an oral glucose-tolerance test, patients with DM were excluded. In total, 144 patients were randomized to the lifestyle-intervention program and 26 patients to the usual clinical care. ***Results:*** The results showed that the lifestyle-modification program resulted in significant improvements in many components of the MetS. Compared with baseline, plasma triglyceride levels were down significantly and HDL-cholesterol levels were increased. The waist circumferences decreased approximately 9 cm with lifestyle modification, even though body weight remained unchanged in some patients. Visceral fat was cut by more than half at one year. ***Practical Applications:*** In the treatment of patients who are overweight, the decrease of waist circumference is a more reliable measure than the weight itself.[2]

DATA MINING (WORK-UP)

There is a need to confirm the preliminary diagnosis of dyslipidemia, DM, or early CKD. Then the early presence of many major clinical end-organ problems also needs to be detected. They are (1) dilated cardiomyopathy from alcohol abuse (ETOH) and coronary artery disease (CAD), (2) atrial fibrillation (very common), (3) hypertrophic cardiomyopathy (nonobstructive) due to long-standing uncontrolled HTN or aortic stenosis (AS), (4) diastolic LV dysfunction, and (5) valvular insufficiency and stenosis. There are other subclinical or laboratory abnormalities that are precursors of future major CVD. They include high fibrinogen, microalbuminuria, or glomerular filtration rate <60 mL/min, impaired glucose tolerance, and impaired fasting glucose levels.[3] The size and function of the left (LV) and right ventricle (RV), left atrium (LA) and right atrium (RA), and the pressure of the pulmonary artery need to be checked. These abnormalities clearly need to be identified so that prevention measures can be started. They are listed in Table 4-5.

DATA CONVERTING (FORMULATING THE MAIN DIAGNOSIS)

Once the patient has a complete history, physical examination, and a basic set of tests, a diagnosis can be made. It is important to rule in or to rule out the presence of some important CVDs, or risk factors, which are shown in Table 4-6.

TABLE 4-5: Subclinical and Laboratory Abnormalities to be Identified as Targets for Prevention of CVD

Precursor Targets	Clinical Conditions
HbA1c >6.1	Diabetes type 2
GFR <90 mL%	CKD
LVH	Diastolic HF, Right HF
Dilated left ventricle	Dilated cardiomyopathy
Left atrium enlargement	MR
RV dilation or hypertrophy	RV or LV failure, pulmonary HTN

HbA1c: hemoglobin A1c, GFR: glomerular filtration rate, LVH: left ventricular hypertrophy, AF: atrial fibrillation, MR: mitral regurgitation, RV: right ventricle, LV: left ventricle.

TABLE 4-6: Cardiovascular Diagnoses and Risk Factor Targets for Prevention

Risk Factors for CAD
Uncontrolled HTN, smoking, uncontrolled DM, CKD, arthritis, AF
Risk Factors of Dilated or Hypertrophic Cardiomyopathy
Aortic stenosis, mitral regurgitation, AF, ETOH abuse, aortic regurgitation, uncontrolled DM, uncontrolled HTN, hypothyroidism, hyperthyroidism
End-Organ Failure
CAD, CVA, PAD, erectile dysfunction, TIA, pulmonary HTN, retinopathy
Significant Comorbidities
Anemia, collagen vascular disease
Abnormal Lifestyle
No exercise
Biomarkers
HbA1c >6.1, GFR <90 mL%, high C-reactive protein level, homocysteinemia, albuminuria

AF: atrial fibrillation, CAD: coronary artery disease, CVA: cerebro-vascular accident, CVD: cardiovascular disease, CKD: chronic kidney disease, DM: diabetes mellitus, ETOH: alcohol, GFR: glomerular filtration rate, HbA1c: hemoglobin A1c, HTN: hypertension, PAD: peripheral arterial disease, TIA: transient ischemic attack.

Diagnostic Criteria for Obesity

A BMI of 25 to 29 kg/m^2 is called overweight; higher BMIs ($\geq$30 kg/m^2) are called obesity. The best way to estimate obesity in clinical practice is to measure the waist circumference. For American patients, abdominal obesity is defined as a waist circumference of +102 cm for men and +88 cm for women according to the National Cholesterol Education Program (NCEP) Expert Panel on Detection, Evaluation, and Treatment of High Blood Cholesterol in Adults (Adult Treatment Panel III).[4] In other countries, the International Diabetes Federation (IDF) has defined the waist circumference values according to gender and ethnic group (not country of residence) (Table 4-7).[5]

Diagnostic Criteria for Metabolic Syndrome

Obesity is a major component of the metabolic syndrome (MetS), which is defined as a constellation of interrelated risk factors of metabolic origin that appear to directly promote the development of atherosclerotic CVD as well as increase the risk for developing type 2 diabetes. The ATP III criteria required no single factor for diagnosis but instead

TABLE 4-7: Ethnic Specific Values for Waist Circumference

Country/Ethnic Group		Waist Circumference
Europids	Male	$\geq$ 94 cm
	Female	$\geq$ 80 cm
In the US the ATP III values (102 cm male; 88 cm female) are likely to continue to be used for clinical purposes.		
South Asians and Chinese	Male	$\geq$ 90 cm
Based on a Chinese, Malay, and Asian-Indian population	Female	$\geq$ 80 cm
Japanese	Male	$\geq$ 85 cm
	Female	$\geq$ 90 cm
Ethnic South and Central Americans	Use South Asian recommendations until more special data are available	
Sub-Sahara Africans	Use European data until more special data are available	
Eastern Mediterranean and Middle East (Arab) populations	Use European data until more special data are available	

TABLE 4-8: Criteria for Clinical Diagnosis of Metabolic Syndrome

(Any three of five constitute diagnosis of metabolic syndrome.)

Elevated Waist Circumference

102 cm (40 inches) in men
88 cm (35 inches) in women

Elevated Triglycerides

150 mg/dL (1.7 mmol/L)
or on drug treatment for elevated triglycerides

Reduced HDL-cholesterol

<40 mg/dL (1.03 mmol/L) in men
<50 mg/dL (1.3 mmol/L) in women
or on drug treatment for reduced HDL-cholesterol

Elevated Blood Pressure

130 mm Hg systolic blood pressure
or 85 mm Hg diastolic blood pressure
or on antihypertensive drug treatment in a patient with a history of
  hypertension

Elevated Fasting Glucose Levels

100 mg/dL,
or on drug treatment for elevated glucose

made the presence of three of five factors the basis for establishing the diagnosis. The American Heart Association and National Heart, Lung and Blood Institute recently reaffirmed the utility of ATP III criteria, with minor modifications (Table 4-8).[6]

Once the patient is diagnosed with obesity, metabolic syndrome, hypertension, or having a strong family history of premature CV disease, there is a need to clarify whether or not the patient belongs to the high-risk group who need the special focus of aggressive preventive measures.

Risk Stratification

An assessment of CV risk is the key point in the evaluation of seemingly healthy subjects and people with risk for developing CVD. The assessment has the following three objectives: (1) to classify patients at low, medium, or high-risk for a CV event in the next 10 years, (2) to assess the presence or absence of target-organ damage, and (3) to assess lifestyle and identify other CV risk factors or associated disorders in order to find comprehensive prevention and treatment plans for CVD risk factors.

PROGRAMMED MANAGEMENT

Strategic Programming

The main goal in the prevention of CV disease is the prevention of acute MI, stroke, loss of limb from ischemia, and end-stage renal disease requiring hemodialysis. The main strategy is to treat and prevent the risk factors, including HTN, hypercholesterolemia, metabolic syndrome, diabetes, and CKD. Once the patient develops any of these risk factors, there is a strong indication to aggressively treat them.

The treatment of HTN is discussed in Chapter 7, hypercholesterolemia in Chapter 5, and diet in Chapter 6. However, how much money, time, or people skills must be expended to prevent a single event of AMI or stroke? Below is an analysis of the cost and need for societal resources in the prevention of CVD (Table 4-9).

 SMART THINKING:

Is it Worth the Money to Prevent Myocardial Infarction and Stroke?

Methodology: To assess whether drug treatment in common practice can prevent disease, four preventive CV randomized clinical trials (RCTs), were analyzed and expressed as efficacy by one-year Number Needed to Treat (NNT) in RCT, common practice effectiveness by the Disease Impact Number (DIN) in all subjects at risk, and by the Population Impact Number (PIN) in the entire population (based on a Swedish population survey). Adjustments were made for nonadherence. Calculations were made of alternative one-year drug costs and the number of years an average general practitioner (GP) would need to work in order to prevent one event using the actual treatment.[7] The results are listed in Table 4-10. *Practical Applications:* The results in the study showed that it is cost-effective to do secondary prevention of MI or to do primary prevention of AMI in high-risk patients (elderly patients and patients with CAD, peripheral vascular disease, CKD). It is more costly for primary prevention in low-risk patients.

Lifestyle Changes

All healthy subjects or patients at all stages of CAD, heart failure (HF), DM, HTN, CKD, and MetS benefit from a normal lifestyle and behavior changes, which are the cornerstone of any treatment plan for primary or secondary prevention of CVD. A lifestyle change program includes a well-balanced diet with low salt, reduced saturated fat and cholesterol, increased aerobic physical activity, not smoking, and weight

TABLE 4-9: Management Master Plan

Data Management	Lifestyle change Exercise Low-salt, low-cholesterol diet
System Configuration Correction	None
Root Cause Treatment	No alcohol consumption Stop cigarette smoking Lowering cholesterol drugs Control hypertension
Work-around Management	None
System Replacement	None

reduction in obese and overweight individuals. The concrete instructions are highlighted in Table 4-11.

Exercise

Substantial evidence exists that physical activity exerts a beneficial effect on multiple CV risk factors. A plausible explanation is that physical activity tends to lower BP and weight, enhance vasodilatation, improve glucose tolerance, and promote CV health. Through lifestyle modification, exercise can minimize the need for more intensive medical and pharmacological interventions or enhance treatment endpoints. While being physically active was found to be associated with a decrease in risk of coronary heart disease (CHD), a question was raised about whether the intensity or the amount of exercise accounted for the greatest reduction in risk.

SMART THINKING:

Short Power Exercise or Longer Time Exercising?

Methodology: This is an observational registry of a cohort of 44,452 U.S. men who were enrolled in the Health Professionals' Follow-up Study. *Results:* The results showed that total exercise, running, weight training and rowing were all associated with a decreased risk of future CHD. However, running for more than an hour per week was associated with a 42% decreased risk compared with not running; lifting weights for 30 minutes or more per week was associated with a 23% decrease. Walking briskly for half an hour a day was also associated with an 18% decreased risk of CHD. *Practical Applications:* The intensity of the physical activity was more re-

TABLE 4-10: Cost-Effective Analysis of Primary and Secondary Prevention for Myocardial Infarction and Stroke

	Number Needed To Treat	Disease Impact Number	Patient Impact Number	GP Work Time (year)	Cost ($Euro)
Secondary Prevention of MI by simvastatin	37	93	2657	2.7	1020-13,595
Primary Prevention of stroke by antihypertensive meds in high-risk patients (elderly with BP>169 mm Hg)	167	239	11,950	6	6905-51,567
Primary Prevention of MI by pravastatin	208	2080	24,470	12.2	5736-117,676
Primary Prevention of stroke by antihypertensive drug treatment in low-risk subjects (diastolic blood pressure 90-99 mm Hg)	1667	3334	116,982	58.5	60,895-511,718

BP: blood pressure, GP: general practitioner, MI: myocardial infarction.

lated to a decreased CHD risk than the amount of time spent exercising. Working out until breaking a sweat is the goal to apply in daily life.[8]

The usual recommendation is that an increase in physical activity is an important part of any weight management program. Most weight loss occurs because of decreased caloric intake. Sustained physical activity is most helpful in the prevention of weight regain. In addition, exercise has the benefit of reducing risks of CV disease and diabetes, beyond that produced by weight reduction alone. The exercise can be done all at one time or intermittently throughout the course of the day.

Concrete Instruction: How to Exercise

For the beginner, activity level can begin at a very light level and would include an increase in standing activities, special chores like room painting, pushing a wheelchair, yard work, ironing, cooking, and playing a musical instrument.

The next level would be light activity, such as slow walking of 24 minutes per mile (walking is particularly attractive because of its safety and accessibility), garage work, carpentry, house cleaning, child care, golf, sailing, and recreational table tennis.

The next level would be moderate activity, such as walking a 15-minute mile, weeding and hoeing a garden, carrying a load, cycling, skiing, tennis, and dancing.

High activity level would include walking a 10-minute mile or walking with a load uphill, heavy manual digging, basketball, climbing, or soccer/kickball.

TABLE 4-11: Concrete Instructions About Therapeutic Lifestyle Changes

Low-salt diet	Low-salt diet, 1.5 gram/day Read labels about salt when buying foods. No salt shaker on table. Use salt substitute for food seasoning.
Low-cholesterol diet	Select foods high in polyunsaturated fat Avoid foods with high levels of monosaturated fat.
Moderate fluid intake	3000 cc/day
Avoid high glycemic or high protein diet	
Daily weight	Weigh yourself every morning on the same scale.
Exercise	Exercise at home or in a health club.

Start exercising slowly and gradually increase the intensity. Trying too hard at first can lead to injury and discouragement.[9]

Moderation in Alcohol Consumption

Observational studies consistently show a J-shaped relation between alcohol consumption and total mortality. The lower mortality appears to be related to CHD death because CHD accounts for a significant proportion of total deaths. Case-control, cohort studies indicate lower risk for CHD at low-to-moderate alcohol intake.[10] A moderate amount of alcohol can be defined as no more than one drink per day for women or lighter-weight persons and no more than two drinks per day for men. A drink is defined as 12 ounces of beer, 5 ounces of wine, and 1.5 ounces of 80-proof liquor.[4]

Stop Cigarette Smoking

Epidemiological evidence has unequivocally confirmed that active smoking is a risk factor for CVD and the leading cause of preventable death. The risk of death from CVD is elevated at least two-fold among smokers when compared with nonsmokers. There is evidence that exposure to smoke, or passive smoking, also increases the risk of CV disease, including stroke.[11] Smoking just one or two cigarettes a day or just 30 minutes of secondhand smoke exposure is enough to jumpstart the biological processes leading to atherosclerosis.[12]

Concrete Instruction: How to Stop Smoking

First-line therapies include nicotine replacement and/or bupropion. Second-line treatments include clonidine and nortriptyline. Additional treatment strategies, with less proven efficacy, include monoamine oxidase inhibitors, selective serotonin reuptake inhibitors, opioid receptor antagonists, bromocriptine, antianxiety drugs, nicotinic receptor antagonists (mecamylamine), and glucose tablets. Social support and skills training have been proven to be the most effective approaches for quitting.[13]

Compliance

Despite accumulating evidence of the benefits of BP and LDL lowering over the past two decades, initiation of treatment and long-term compliance with therapy remain far from optimal. Lack of compliance is causing individuals to miss the risk-reducing benefit of treatment and is creating enormous costs in the health system to treat CV events that could have been prevented. Therefore, effective strategies for compliance are needed for the success in prevention of CVD (Table 4-12).

ADVANCED MANAGEMENT

Detection

In order to effectively prevent CVD, there is a need to detect atherosclerosis as early as possible. Various methods have been proposed to

TABLE 4-12: How to Improve Compliance
Main Strategy
Keep the medication regimen as simple as possible.
Give the patient clear instructions.
Involve patient in own care through self-monitoring.
Follow-up
Discuss compliance for at least a minute at each visit.
Concentrate on those who don't reach treatment goals.
Always call patients who miss visit appointments.
Strategies
Use two or more strategies for those who miss treatment goals.
Use systems to reinforce compliance and maintain contact with patient.
Develop a standardized treatment plan to structure care.
Use feedback from past performance to foster change in future care.
Encourage the support of family and friends.

detect and quantify subclinical atherosclerosis in asymptomatic patients. They include the ultrasound measurement of carotid intima-media thickness (IMT), coronary calcification assessed by electron-beam CT, and measurement of carotid plaque by ultrasound and reactive hyperemia (RH) in the peripheral arteries.

Intima-Media Thickness

The combined thickness of the intima and media of the carotid artery has proved to be associated with increased prevalence of CV disease. Noninvasive measurements of the intima and media of the common and internal carotid arteries could predict the future CV event. In the ARIC study, IMT was measured with high-resolution ultrasonography.[15] CV events (new MI or stroke) served as outcome variables in subjects without prior clinical CV disease (4476 subjects) over a median follow-up period of 6.2 years. The results showed that the incidence of CV events correlated with measurements of carotid-artery intima–media thickness. The relative risk of MI or stroke increased with intima–media thickness (P < 0.001). The association between CV events and intima–media thickness remained significant after adjustment for traditional risk factors.[14-15]

Flow-Mediated Dilation of the Brachial Artery

All physiological assessments incorporate a stimulus that activates nitric oxide–dependent vasodilation mediated by the endothelium. Flow-mediated dilation (FMD) of the brachial artery with ultrasonographic assessment has become the most widely published standard in the assessment of endothelial dysfunction. Briefly, arterial occlusion with a blood pressure cuff for five minutes and subsequent release lead to reactive hyperemia and local endothelial activation. When this is performed on the patient's arm, increased shear stress leads to endothelium-dependent dilation of the brachial artery, which can be measured and quantified by ultrasound.[16]

Peripheral Arterial Tonometry Measuring Reactive Hyperemia

A more practical method of assessing endothelial function is peripheral arterial tonometry measuring reactive hyperemia (RH-PAT). This Food and Drug Administration (FDA)-approved office-based technique uses a finger probe to assess digital volume changes accompanying pulse waves after inducing reactive hyperemia with a blood pressure cuff on the upper arm (Endo-PAT 2000, Itamar Medical Ltd. Framingham MA). RH-PAT has been extensively correlated with early and clinically relevant CAD. For instance, RH-PAT results were significantly impaired in patients with exercise-induced myocardial ischemia. RH-PAT results have also been found to correlate well with coronary endothelial function. RH-PAT is a 15-minute noninvasive assessment that can be performed in an office setting, Furthermore RH-PAT, when compared to FMD, requires less specialized training, and the results are not operator-dependent.[17]

Coronary Artery Calcification

In a general population of individuals without known CAD, coronary artery calcification (CAC) by CT scan can be used to predict future MI. A recent MESA study found that CAC was an independent predictor of incident heart disease across different racial subgroups in the United States.[18] The results of a new study (the Heinz Nixdorf Risk Factors Evaluation of Coronary Calcium and Lifestyle [Recall] study) were presented at the scientific meeting of the American College of Cardiology in April 2009.

 SMART THINKING:

The RECALL Study

Methodology: This study randomly selected 4487 participants without known CAD. NCEP categories were computed from CV risk factors. The CAC-Agatston score was calculated using electron beam CT. The primary endpoint was fatal and nonfatal MI. The age range was 45 to 75 years, and 52% were women. Follow-up information was obtained from 99.1% of participants after a median of five years. *Results:* Cardiac death and nonfatal MI were observed in 90 participants (2.2%). The relative risk of CAC >75th versus ≤25th percentile was 3.35 (95% CI: 1.35-8.35, P = 0.006) for women and

11.09 (95% CI: 3.42-35.92, P <0.0001) for men. The odds ratio (OR) for the highest versus the lowest NCEP category was 3.18 (95% CI: 1.81-5.58, P <0.0001) and the OR for the highest versus lowest CAC quartile was 4.59 (95% CI: 2.24-9.38, P <0.0001).[19]

Practical Applications: The current study confirms the results from the MESA study in a low-risk European population. However, whether CAC should be used as a screening tool still remains an area of debate due to concerns about disease prevalence and radiation exposure. CAC scoring can help predict who is likely to have an MI or cardiac death among those who are at intermediate risk of coronary events according to traditional risk-factor assessment. The findings appeared to be more pertinent for men, who had almost a 10-fold greater risk of cardiac death or MI if they were in the highest CAC quartile compared with the lowest. Women were at twice the risk. Among those who were deemed intermediate risk, addition of the CAC score into the assessment showed that 14% should be reclassified as high risk and just over 60% could be shifted to low risk. Even though these data seem to reallocate exact level of risk, CAC is not inexpensive, and there is some radiation exposure.[19]

Treatment

Pharmacological Prevention of CVD

Despite the epidemiological importance of CAD, CV events are rare from the individual viewpoint. There is considerable uncertainty as to when to start medical treatment. A given risk factor modification results in a relative risk reduction independent of the global risk. Therefore the global risk determines the absolute benefit of a preventive measure. The global risk can be estimated using different scoring systems.

 SMART THINKING:

Is it Worth the Money to Use Medication in Order to Prevent Heart Disease?

Methodology: Using the global risk and the expected relative risk reduction, the number needed to treat (NNT) to avoid one event or cardiac death can be calculated. The NNT is a measure for the usefulness of a preventive intervention. *Results:* An NNT of <200 appears acceptable for primary prevention. This can be achieved with pharmacological preventive strategies if the global risk of 10 years is ≥ 20%. As age is one of the most important risk predictors, the need for treatment at comparable risk factor constellations is age-dependent. Risk stratification with estimation of the NNT is therefore important for the decision to treat or not to treat.[20]

SMART THINKING:

Prevention of Atherosclerosis in the Prediabetic Patient

People with impaired glucose tolerance (IGT) and/or impaired fasting glucose (IFG) are at increased long-term risk for CV disease. Effects of angiotensin-converting enzyme inhibitor (ACEI) and of thiazolidinedione (TZD) on vascular disease in this population are unknown. The aim of this study was to evaluate the effects of the ACEI ramipril and the TZD rosiglitazone on carotid intima-media thickness (CIMT) in people with IGT and/or IFG. *Methodology:* This is a double-blind randomized trial. Some 1425 people with IGT and/or IFG but without CV disease or DM were randomized to ramipril 15 mg/day or its placebo and to rosiglitazone 8 mg/day or its placebo with a 2 x 2 factorial design. *Results:* There were no differences in the primary and secondary outcomes between the ramipril and placebo groups. Compared with placebo, rosiglitazone reduced the primary CIMT outcome, but the difference was not statistically significant (difference = 0.0027 ± 0.0015 mm/year; P = 0.08) and significantly reduced the secondary CIMT outcome (difference = 0.0043 ± 0.0017 mm/year; P = 0.01). *Practical Applications:* In people with IGT and/or IFG without CV disease and diabetes, treatment with ramipril had a neutral effect on CIMT, whereas rosiglitazone modestly reduced CIMT progression.[21]

Efficacy of Surgery for Obesity

Until now, there have been no effective new drugs specifically for obesity available. Bariatric surgery may lead to improvement in patients with Class II/III obesity: significant weight loss (> 44 kg), decreased SBP and DBP, total cholesterol decreased by 45 mg/dL, and LDL decreased by 40 mg/dL.[22] However, do the cardiac abnormalities reverse after weight loss?

SMART THINKING:

Reversal of Cardiac Abnormality After Bariatric Surgery

Methodology: Data from 38 adolescents (13 to 19 years) were evaluated before and after bariatric surgery. Left ventricular mass (LVM), left ventricular (LV) geometry, and systolic and diastolic function were assessed by echocardiography *Results:* Weight and body mass index decreased postoperatively (mean weight loss 59 ± 15 kg, preoperative body mass index 60 ± 9 kg/m² vs. follow-up 40 ± 8 kg/m², P < 0.0001). Change in LVM index (54 ± 13 g/m²·⁷ to 42 ± 10 g/m²·⁷, P < 0.0001) correlated with weight loss (r = 0.41, P = 0.01). Prevalence of concentric left ventricular hypertrophy (LVH) improved from 28% preoperatively to only 3% at follow-up (P = 0.007), and normal LV geometry improved from 36% to 79% at follow-up (P = 0.009). *Practical Applications:* Elevated LVM index, concentric LVH, altered diastolic function, and cardiac workload significantly improve following surgically induced weight loss in morbidly obese adolescents. Large weight loss due to bariatric surgery improves predictors of future CV morbidity in these young people.[23]

Prevention of CAD by Treatment of Diabetes Mellitus

There was little to no hard evidence that glucose control altered the risk of CV events. Some studies, including the United Kingdom Prospective Diabetes Study (UKPDS),[24] suggested improvements in microvascular endpoints, but there were no effects on hard clinical endpoints, such as mortality or MI. The Action in Diabetes and Vascular Disease (ADVANCE) trial[25] showed a reduction in the progression of albuminuria with intensive glucose control but no effect on CV event rates. The Action to Control Cardiovascular Risk in Diabetes (ACCORD) trial,[26] on the other hand, was stopped early because of an increased risk of death in patients who underwent intensive blood glucose lowering. In order to clarify the question of treatment of DM for prevention of CAD, the results of the Veterans Affairs Diabetes Trial (VADT) are presented below.

SMART THINKING:

Treatment of Diabetes for Prevention of Coronary Artery Disease

Methodology: 1791 military veterans with diabetes who had a suboptimal response to medical therapy were randomized to intensive glucose control or standard glucose control. At the time of randomization, median HbA_{1c} levels were 9.4%. In addition, nearly 75% of patients had hypertension, 40% had a previous CV event, and patients had been diagnosed with DM for a mean of 11.5 years. In both study groups, obese patients were started on two drugs, metformin and rosiglitazone. Nonobese patients were started with glimepiride plus rosiglitazone. Patients in the intensive arm started on maximal doses. Insulin was added to most participants to achieve HbA_{1c} levels less than 6.0% in the intensive-treatment arm and less than 9.0% in the standard-therapy arm. *Results:* After a median follow-up of 6.5 years, median HbA_{1c} levels were reduced to 8.4% in the standard-lowering arm and to 6.9% in the intensive-glucose-control arm. During this time, 264 patients in the standard-therapy group and 235 patients in the intensive-therapy group experienced a major CV event, the composite primary endpoint consisting of MI, stroke, death from CV causes, congestive heart failure, vascular surgery, inoperable coronary disease, and amputation for ischemic gangrene.

Practical Applications: The ACC/AHA/ADA report emphasizes the importance of controlling nonglycemic risk factors, such as blood pressure and lipids (using statins), as well as using aspirin and lifestyle modifications as the primary strategies for reducing the burden of CV disease in people with diabetes.[28]

Lowering HbA$_{1c}$ levels to <7% to reduce microvascular and neuropathic complications in type 1 and 2 DM remains a class I recommendation. Less than 7% is also a reasonable target for reducing the risk of macrovascular complications, a class IIb recommendation, at least until more evidence becomes available. The guideline also emphasized the importance of treating blood pressure and lipid abnormalities to reduce the risk of CV and microvascular complications from diabetes. For those with a short duration of disease, long life expectancy, and no significant CV disease, a more aggressive HbA$_{1c}$ goal might be appropriate. For older patients and those with advanced microvascular and macrovascular disease, less stringent targets are recommended.[28]

 SMART THINKING:

Treatment of Arthritis to Prevent CAD

The prevalence of CV disease in patients with rheumatoid arthritis (RA) and its association were analyzed with traditional CV risk factors, clinical features of RA, and the use of disease-modifying antirheumatic drugs (DMARDs) in a multinational cross-sectional cohort of nonselected consecutive outpatients with RA (The Questionnaires in Standard Monitoring of Patients with Rheumatoid Arthritis Program, or QUEST-RA). *Methodology:* This is a retrospective cross-sectional review involving a clinical assessment by a rheumatologist and a self-report questionnaire by patients. *Results:* The prevalence for lifetime CV events in the entire sample was 3.2% for MI, 1.9% for stroke, and 9.3% for any CV event. There was an association between any CV event and age and male gender and between extra-articular disease and MI. Prolonged exposure to methotrexate (HR 0.85; 95% CI 0.81 to 0.89), leflunomide (HR 0.59; 95% CI 0.43 to 0.79), sulfasalazine (HR 0.92; 95% CI 0.87 to 0.98), glucocorticoids (HR 0.95; 95% CI 0.92 to 0.98), and biological agents (HR 0.42; 95% CI 0.21 to 0.81; P < 0.05) was associated with a reduction of the risk of CV morbidity; analyses were adjusted for traditional risk factors and countries. *Practical Applications:* Prolonged use of treatments such as methotrexate, sulfasalazine, leflunomide, glucocorticoids, and tumor necrosis factor-alpha blockers appears to be associated with a reduced risk of CV disease. In addition to traditional risk factors, extra-articular disease was associated with the occurrence of MI in patients with RA.[24]

TROUBLE-SHOOTING AND DEBUGGING

Prevention of CVD is the responsibility of each health care provider and layperson. When the results are not achieved as expected, the management requires the expertise of a consultant cardiologist. The common questions from the referring physicians to the consultant cardiologist in the prevention of CVD are discussed below.

What is the Role of Vitamin Supplements in the Prevention of CVD?

Vitamin supplements are a major source of nutritional intake for many patients. Is there benefit of vitamin C or E for prevention of CVD? This question was answered by the results of the Physicians' Health Study II. *Methodology:* The Physicians' Health Study II was a randomized, double-blind, placebo-controlled 2 x 2 x 2 x 2 factorial trial of vitamin E (400 IU of synthetic alpha-tocopherol) or placebo every other day, vitamin C (500 mg synthetic ascorbic acid) or placebo every other day, or a multivitamin or placebo daily for the prevention of cancer and CVD. The study enrolled 14,641 U.S. male physicians aged 50 years and older at the study outset. Men with a history of MI, stroke, or cancer were eligible to enroll, and 754 men (5.4%) of the cohort had prevalent CVD at randomization. *Results:* During a mean follow-up of 8 years and a total of 120,000 person-years of follow-up, 1245 confirmed CV events occurred. Almost identical numbers of events occurred in both supplementation and placebo groups. For the vitamin E versus placebo comparison, there were 10.9 events per 1000 person-years in both groups. Among those treated with vitamin C, there were 10.8 events per 1000 person-years and 10.9 events for those receiving placebo, again almost identical outcomes. *Harms:* Treatment with vitamin E was associated with an increased risk for hemorrhagic stroke, although the association was only marginally significant. This is something that has been seen in one other trial but no other vitamin E trials.[30] *Practical Application:* Neither vitamin E nor vitamin C had any effect on total mortality.

How Effective Is Primary Prevention for Chronic Kidney Disease?

Chronic kidney disease (CKD) is a worldwide public health problem. In the United States, there is an increasing incidence and prevalence of renal failure with poor outcome and high costs and an even higher prevalence of earlier stages of CKD (approximately 80 times greater than ESRD prevalence). Moreover, CKD is associated with elevated CV morbidity and mortality. Therefore, strategies that are aimed at identifying, preventing, and treating CKD and its related risk factors are needed. The patients at risk for CKD include those with diabetes or HTN or close relatives with ESRD. The risks in these categories are markedly amplified in African-American, Native-American, and Hispanic groups. The tools for screening are cost-effective and include spot urine samples for protein-creatinine ratio (obviating the need for 24-hour urine collections) and a urine-free calculation of GFR requiring a serum creatinine measurement and anthropometric measures of the patient.[3] The main plan for prevention of CKD is to control HTN, prevent diabetes, maintain a low-protein diet, exercise, and achieve a lower cholesterol level. Does beta blockade reduce the incidence of microalbuminuria in patients with a high risk for CKD? The results were answered in the Glycemic Effects in Diabetes Mellitus Carvedilol-Metoprolol Comparison in Hypertensives (GEMINI) trial presented below. *Methodology:* This is an RCT with a prespecified secondary endpoint of the trial, which was to examine the effects of different beta blockers on changes in albuminuria in the presence of renin-angiotensin system blockade. Participants with HTN and type 2 DM were randomized to either metoprolol tartrate (n = 737) or carvedilol (n = 498) groups in blind fashion. *Results:* A greater reduction in microalbuminuria was observed for those randomized to carvedilol ($-16.2\Delta\%$; 95% confidence interval, -25.3, -5.9; P = 0.003). Of those with normoalbuminuria at baseline, fewer progressed to microalbuminuria on carvedilol versus those on metoprolol (6.6% versus 11.1%, respectively; P = 0.03). *Mechanism of Difference:* Microalbuminuria development was not related to differences in BP or achievement of BP goal (68% carvedilol versus 67% metoprolol).[32] *Practical Applications:* The apparent advantage of carvedilol over other agents includes a protective effect on the kidney against the development of microalbuminuria, which is a major risk factor for CV events and death in this population. Not only cardiologists but also nephrologists and diabetologists now have a new goal—to prevent patients who have DM from progressing to nephropathy, the final aim being to limit CV events and death.[33]

Is Vitamin D Deficiency Causing CVD?

Vitamin D deficiency is a highly prevalent condition, present in approximately 30 to 50% of the general population. A growing body of data suggest that low 25-hydroxyvitamin D levels may adversely affect CV health. Vitamin D deficiency activates the renin-angiotensin-aldosterone system and can predispose patients to hypertension and left ventricular hypertrophy. Additionally, vitamin D deficiency causes an increase in parathyroid hormone, which increases insulin resistance and is associated with diabetes, hypertension, inflammation, and increased CV risk. Epidemiological studies have associated low 25-hydroxyvitamin D levels with coronary risk factors and adverse CV outcomes. Vitamin D supplementation is simple, safe, and inexpensive. Large randomized controlled trials are needed to firmly establish the relevance of vitamin D status to CV health. In the meanwhile, monitoring serum 25-hydroxyvitamin D levels and correction of vitamin D deficiency are indicated for optimization of musculoskeletal and general health.[34]

Does Vaccination Against Pneumonia Prevent CVD?

The answer or not the right answer was quoted frequently by a study from Canada. The validity of the results should be evaluated by the methodology of the study. *Methodology:* This is a hospital-based case-control (propensity score analysis) study that included patients considered to be at risk for MI. Health databases were obtained for hospital diagnoses and vaccination status. Patients who had been admitted for treatment of MI were compared with patients admitted to a surgical department in the same hospital for reasons other than MI between 1997 and 2003. *Results:* A total of 43,209 patients were at risk; of these, 999 cases and 3996 controls were matched according to age, sex, and year of hospital admission. Cases were less likely than controls to have been vaccinated (adjusted odds ratio [OR] 0.53, 95% confidence interval [CI] 0.40–0.70). This putative protective role of the vaccine was not observed for patients who had received the vaccine up to one year before MI (adjusted OR 0.85, 95% CI 0.54–1.33). In contrast, if vaccination had occurred 2 years or more before the hospital admission, the association was stronger (adjusted OR 0.33, 95% CI 0.20–0.46). *Practical Applications:* Pneumococcal vaccination was associated with a decrease of more than 50% in the rate of MI two years after exposure.[35] *Caveat:* However, the methodology used in this study is very weak. We believe that the analysis using propensity score is fatally flawed and give it little credence. There is a need for a better study before we can convince ourselves and our patients that vaccination against pneumonia prevents heart disease.[36]

TAKE-HOME MESSAGE

Data Collecting Collect all the data about the patient's history (including smoking, high-salt, high-cholesterol diet, alcohol abuse, lack of exercise, HTN, DM, and high cholesterol level), family history (of early sudden death due to heart disease and history of early CAD), social history (work and behaviors) and from a complete physical examination (signs of prior stroke, CAD, PAD, carotid murmur, weak peripheral pulses), all of which add weight to the clinical decision-making process.

Data Mining Recommend safe, appropriate, and efficacious investigation, including fasting lipid profile, fasting blood glucose, BUN and creatinine levels, weight, BMI, and waist circumference.

Management Recommend safe, appropriate, and efficacious therapy to maintain the stable health status of the patient over time (low-salt, low-cholesterol diet, stopping smoking, losing weight, no drinking alcohol, exercising).

Patient-Centered Care Get patients involved in their own lifestyle modification to increase compliance with diet, exercise, medication, office visits, and testing, in order to provide continuity of care.

References

1. Turesson, C., Jarenros, A., Jacobsson, L.: Increased incidence of cardiovascular disease in patients with rheumatoid arthritis: results from a community based study. Ann Rheum Dis. 2004;63:952–955.
2. Després, J. P., on behalf of the SYNERGIE investigators. Lifestyle management of abdominal obesity and related cardiometabolic risk: the SYNERGIE trial. EAS 2008: 77th European Atherosclerosis Society Congress; Istanbul, Turkey; April 27, 2008.
3. Neaton, J. D., Wentworth, D.: Serum cholesterol, blood pressure, cigarette smoking, and death from coronary heart disease: Overall findings and differences by age for 316,099 white men. Multiple Risk Factor Intervention Trial Research Group. Arch Intern Med. 1992;152: 56–64.
4. Third Report of the National Cholesterol Education Program (NCEP) Expert Panel on Detection, Evaluation, and Treatment of High Blood Cholesterol in Adults (Adult Treatment Panel III) final report. Circulation. 2002;106:3143–3421.
5. International Diabetes Federation: The IDF consensus worldwide definition of the metabolic syndrome, 2006. Available at www.idf.org/webdata/docs/IDF_Meta_def_final.pdf.
6. Grundy, S. M.: Metabolic Syndrome Scientific Statement by the American Heart Association and the National Heart, Lung, and Blood Institute. Arterioscler Thromb Vasc Biol. 2005;25:2243–2244.
7. Melander, A., Lindberg, G., Nilsson, J. L.: Can drug treatment prevent disease in common practice? Z Arztl Fortbild Qualitatssich. 2007; 101(5):326–332.
8. Tanasescu, M., Leitzmann, M. F., Rimm, E. B., Willett, W. C.: Exercise type and intensity in relation to coronary heart disease in men. JAMA. 2002;288:1994–2000.
9. National Heart, Lung, and Blood Institute. Guide to Physical Activity. Available at http://www.nhlbi.nih.gov/health/public/heart/obesity/lose_wt/phy_act.htm.
10. Criqui, M. H.: Alcohol and coronary heart disease: consistent relationship and public health implications. Clin Chim Acta. 1996;246: 51–57.
11. Raupach, T., Schäfer, K., Konstantinides, S., Andreas, S.: Secondhand smoke as an acute threat for the cardiovascular system: a change in paradigm. EHJ 2006;27:386–392.
12. Barua, R. S., Ambrose, J. A., Eales-Reynolds, L. J., DeVoe, M. C.: Heavy and light cigarette smokers have similar dysfunction of

endothelial vasoregulatory activity: an in vivo and in vitro correlation. J Am Coll Cardiol. 2002;39:1758–1763.

13. Sacco, R. L., Adams, R., Albers, G., et al.: Guidelines for Prevention of Stroke in Patients With Ischemic Stroke or Transient Ischemic Attack A Statement for Healthcare Professionals From the American Heart Association/American Stroke Association Council on Stroke: Co–Sponsored by the Council on Cardiovascular Radiology and Intervention: The American Academy of Neurology affirms the value of this guideline. Stroke. 2006;37:577–617.

14. O'Leary, D. H., Polak, J. F., Wolfson, S. K., Jr., et al.: Use of sonography to evaluate carotid atherosclerosis in the elderly: the Cardiovascular Health Study. Stroke. 1991;22:1155–1163.

15. Chambless, L. E., Heiss, G., Folsom G, et al.: Association of coronary heart disease incidence with carotid arterial wall thickness and major risk factors: the Atherosclerosis Risk in Communities (ARIC) Study, Am J Epidemiol. 1997;146:483–494.

16. Corretti, M. C., Anderson, T. J., Benjamin, E. J., et al.: Guidelines for the ultrasound assessment of endothelial-dependent flow-mediated vasodilation of the brachial artery: a report of the International Brachial Artery Reactivity Task Force. J Am Coll Cardiol. 2002;39: 257–265.

17. Chouraqui, P., Schnall, R. P., Dvir, I., et al.: Assessment of peripheral artery tonometry in the detection of treadmill exercise-induced myocardial ischemia. J Am Coll Cardiol. 2002;40:2195–2200.

18. Detrano, R., Guerci, A. D., Carr, J. J., et al.: Coronary calcium as a predictor of coronary events in four racial or ethnic groups. N Engl J Med. 2008;358:1336–1345.

19. Erbel, R.A., et al.: The Nixdorf Risk Factors Evaluation of Coronary Calcium and Lifestyle (Recall) study, presented at the late-breaking clinical-trials session of the American College of Cardiology (ACC) 58th Annual Scientific Session. March 2009, Orlando, FL.

20. Gohlke, H., von Schacky, C.: Total risk for cardiovascular disease. At what point is medical prophylactic medication useful? Z Kardiol. 2005;94 Suppl 3:III/6–10.

21. Lonn, E. M., Gerstein, H. C., Sheridan, P., on behalf of the DREAM (Diabetes REduction Assessment with ramipril and rosiglitazone Medication) and STARR (STudy of Atherosclerosis with Ramipril and Rosiglitazone) Investigators. Effect of ramipril and of rosiglitazone on carotid intima-media thickness in people with impaired glucose tolerance or impaired fasting glucose: J Am Coll Cardiol. 2009;53: 2036–2038.

22. Batsis, J. A.: Effects of bariatric surgery on cardiovascular risk factors and predicted effect on CV events and mortality of class II/III obesity. Abstract #842–848. Presented at the American College of Cardiology Scientific Session Atlanta, Georgia, March 11–14, 2006.

23. Ippisch, H. M., Inge, T., Daniels, S. R., et al.: Reversibility of cardiac abnormalities in morbidly obese adolescents. J Am Coll Cardiol. 2008; 51:1342–1348.

24. Holman, R. R., Paul, S. K., Bethel, M. A., et al.: Ten-year follow-up of intensive glucose control in type 2 diabetes. N Engl J Med. 2008; 359:1577–1589.
25. The ADVANCE Collaborative Group. Intensive blood glucose control and vascular outcomes in patients with type 2 diabetes. N Engl J Med. 2008;358:2560–2572.
26. The Action to Control Cardiovascular Risk in Diabetes Study Group. Effects of intensive glucose lowering in type 2 diabetes. N Engl J Med. 2008;358:2545–2559.
27. Duckworth, W., Abraira, C., Mortiz, T., et al.: Glucose control and vascular complications in veterans with type 2 diabetes. N Engl J Med. 2009;360:129-139
28. Skyler, J. S., Bergenstal, R., Bonow, R. O., et al.: Intensive glycemic control and the prevention of cardiovascular events: Implications of the ACCORD, ADVANCE, and VA Diabetes Trials. A position statement of the American Diabetes Association and a scientific statement of the American College of Cardiology Foundation and the American Heart Association. Circulation. 2008;DOI:10.1161/CIRCULATIONAHA. 108.191305. Available at http://circ.ahajournals.org.
29. Naranjo, A., Sokka, T., Descalzo, M. A., et al.: Cardiovascular disease in patients with rheumatoid arthritis: results from the QUEST-RA study. Arthritis Res Ther. 2008;10:R30.
30. Sesso, H. D., Buring, J. E., Christen, W. G., et al.: Vitamins E and C in the prevention of cardiovascular disease in men: The Physicians' Health Study II Randomized Controlled Trial. JAMA. 2008;300:2123–2133.
31. Eddy, A. A.: Interstitial nephritis induced by protein-overload proteinuria. Am J Pathol.1998;135:719–733.
32. Bakris, G. L., Fonseca, V., Katholi, R. E., et al.: for the GEMINI Investigators Differential Effects of Beta–Blockers on Albuminuria in Patients With Type 2 Diabetes. Hypertension. 2005;46:1309–1315.
33. Remuzzi, G., Macia, M., Ruggenenti, P.: Prevention and treatment of diabetic renal disease in type 2 diabetes: The BENEDICT Study. J Am Soc Nephrol. 2006;17:S90–S97.
34. Lee, J. H., O'Keefe, J. H., Bell, D., et al.: An Important, Common, and Easily Treatable Cardiovascular Risk Factor? J Am Coll Cardiol. 2008;52:1949–1956.
35. Lamontagne, F., Garant, M. P., Carvalho, J. C., et al.: Pneumococcal vaccination and risk of myocardial infarction. Can Med Assoc J. 2008; 179:773–777.
36. DeMaria, A. N.: Lies, Damned Lies, and Statistics. J Am Coll Cardiol. 2008;52:1430–1431.

Hypercholesterolemia

Huy V. Tran, Hung Canh Phan,
Dayi Hu, Timothy Yee,
Thach Nguyen, and Andy Kates

Chapter Outline

DEFINITION

Hypercholesterolemia is the presence of a high level of cholesterol in the blood. It may be related to diet, genetic factors, and/or the presence of other diseases.

Population in Focus

In order to detect hypercholesterolemia at the early stage, all adults aged 20 years or older should undergo a lipoprotein profile measurement once every five years. For individuals with coronary artery disease (CAD) or other atherosclerotic disease, lipoprotein analysis is the initial assessment.

Strategic Programming

The strategy is about identifying the patients with hypercholesterolemia through data collecting with a comprehensive history and physical examination. The overall risk of CAD should be assessed and categorized. The causes of high blood cholesterol should be investigated. Using the method of data mining, tests could be ordered (e.g., fasting lipid profile, fasting glucose, liver enzyme, thyroid function test) in order to confirm (data converting) the main diagnosis of hypercholesterolemia and its possible etiologies.

DATA COLLECTING

History

For any adults aged 20 years or older, a history of a high-cholesterol diet, obesity in the family, or any particular negative dietary habits should be investigated. There is a need to find out about a history of cardiovascular (CV) disorders such as CAD, peripheral artery disease (PAD), carotid artery disease, and stroke, for example. The history of other medical conditions causing high cholesterol should also be investigated, including diabetes mellitus; hypothyroidism; nephrotic syndrome; obstructive liver disease; or the use of drugs such as progestins, anabolic steroids, corticoids, beta blockers, or diuretics.

Physical Examination

There are no abnormal clinical manifestations of early and short-term hypercholesterolemia. Once hypercholesterolemia is severe and long-standing (longer than three decades), some physical findings such as corneal arcus, corneal opacification, xanthelasma, or xanthomas may be seen. The clinical peripheral manifestations of atherosclerosis, such as decreased peripheral pulses and vascular bruits, should be carefully assessed. Other problems to look at are coronary artery disease, abdominal aortic aneurysm, carotid artery disease, sequelae of transient ischemic attacks, or stroke of carotid origin. The clinical findings of diabetes mellitus, hypothyroidism, nephrotic syndrome, obstructive liver disease, or hypercholesterolemia due to the use of drugs such as progestins, anabolic steroids, corticoids, beta blockers, or diuretics should be investigated.

DATA MINING (WORK-UP)

Once the patient is suspected of having hypercholesterolemia, he or she should undergo selective laboratory tests, including a fasting lipid profile, apolipoprotein B, urinalysis, serum albumin, fasting glucose, liver and renal function, thyroid-stimulating hormone (TSH), creatinine, high-sensitivity C-reactive protein, uric acid, and creatine phosphokinase (CPK). If the testing opportunity is nonfasting, only the values for total cholesterol and HDL cholesterol will be usable to calculate non-HDL cholesterol.

DATA CONVERTING (FORMULATING A MAIN DIAGNOSIS)

LDL Cholesterol

The relationship between LDL cholesterol levels and CAD risk is continuous over a broad range of LDL levels. Therefore, the Adult Treatment Panel (ATP) III adopts the classification of LDL, total, and HDL cholesterol levels as shown in Table 5-1.[1]

Non-HDL Cholesterol

Although LDL cholesterol is the primary target of therapy, other lipid risk factors in addition to elevated LDL also affect CAD risk. Among these are low HDL cholesterol, elevated triglycerides (especially very low-density lipoprotein [VLDL] remnants), and possibly small LDL particles. This "lipid triad" has been called *atherogenic dyslipidemia*. Therefore, the ATP III introduced a secondary target of therapy, namely, non-HDL cholesterol, in patients with elevated triglycerides (>200 mg/dL). VLDL+LDL cholesterol, termed non-HDL cholesterol, equals

TABLE 5-1: ATP III Classification of LDL, Total, and HDL Cholesterol (mg/dL)

LDL Cholesterol

Optimal: <100
Near optimal/above optimal: 100-129
Borderline high: 130-159
High: 160-189
Very high: ≥190

Total Cholesterol

Desirable: <200
Borderline high: 200-239
High: ≥240

HDL Cholesterol

Low: <40
High: ≥60

total cholesterol minus HDL cholesterol, which represents *atherogenic cholesterol*. Relations among the different lipoprotein fractions are as follows:

$$\text{Total cholesterol} = \text{LDL} + \text{VLDL} + \text{HDL}$$
$$\text{Total cholesterol} - \text{HDL} = \text{LDL} + \text{VLDL} = \text{non-HDL}$$

The non-HDL cholesterol goal is 30 mg/dL higher than the LDL cholesterol goal. Non-HDL cholesterol was added as a secondary target of therapy to take into account the atherogenic potential associated with remnant lipoproteins in patients with hypertriglyceridemia.[1-2] In recent years, there has been new evidence showing that non-HDL cholesterol is better in predicting future cardiovascular disease (CVD) events than LDL cholesterol.[2]

Risk Stratification

Risk determinants in addition to LDL cholesterol include the presence or absence of CAD, other clinical forms of atherosclerotic disease, and the major risk factors other than LDL. LDL is not counted among the risk factors in Table 5-2 because the purpose of counting those risk factors is to modify the treatment of LDL.[1]

CAD risk equivalents include clinical manifestations of noncoronary forms of atherosclerotic disease (peripheral arterial disease, abdominal aortic aneurysm, and carotid artery disease, transient ischemic attacks or stroke of carotid origin, or <50% obstruction of a carotid artery), diabetes, and two or more risk factors with a 10-year risk for hard CAD ≥ 20% by using the Framingham scores.

TABLE 5-2: Major Risk Factors (Excluding LDL Cholesterol)

Cigarette smoking
Hypertension (BP ≥140/90 mm Hg or on antihypertensive medication)
Low HDL cholesterol (<40 mg/dL)
Family history of premature CAD (CAD in male first degree relative
   <55 years; CAD in female first degree relative <65 years)
Age (men ≥45 years; women ≥55 years)

The very high risk category includes patients with established CAD in addition to (1) multiple major risk factors (especially diabetes), (2) severe and poorly controlled risk factors (especially continued cigarette smoking), (3) multiple risk factors of the metabolic syndrome (especially high triglycerides of 200 mg/dL plus non-HDL cholesterol of 130 mg/dL with low-HDL cholesterol [40 mg/dL]), and (4) acute coronary syndrome (ACS).[2]

C-Reactive Protein (CRP)

CRP is an inflammatory marker that predicts the intensity of the atherosclerotic process but not its extent and may be useful for further stratifying coronary heart disease (CHD) risk.[3] It is produced by the liver in response to inflammation but also amplifies the inflammatory response, thus becoming a potential target for therapy. CRP is increased in conditions associated with or with risk factors that are associated with CHD; however, it may be increased by infections and other inflammatory disorders. It is also clear, for instance, that the increase in CRP in childhood obesity does not indicate the presence of atherosclerosis or of increased short-term risk of CHD events but probably predicts endothelial dysfunction.

The American Heart Association has recommended that CRP values be stratified as follows: low risk, <1 mg/liter; average risk, 1–3 mg/liter; and high risk, >3 mg/liter.[4]

PROGRAMMED MANAGEMENT

Goals

The treatment goal of hypercholesterolemia is to achieve the maximum reduction in the long-term total risk of cardiovascular (CV) events from atherosclerotic diseases. Based on evaluation of the recently available evidence, the consensus panel of the American Diabetes Association (ADA) and the American College of Cardiology (ACC) Foundation concluded that routine calculation and use of non-HDL cholesterol constitute a better index than LDL cholesterol for identifying high-risk patients. That does not mean, however, that LDL cholesterol should not

TABLE 5-3: Treatment Goal Recommendations of the Consensus Panel of the ADA/ACC

Patients	Goal		
	LDL-C (mg/dL)	Non-HDL C (mg/dL)	Apo B (mg/dL)
Highest Risk	<70	<100	<80
High Risk	<100	<130	<90

Highest Risk: Known CVD or diabetes plus one or more additional major CVD risk factors. High Risk: No diabetes or known clinical CVD but two or more additional major CVD risk factors or type 2 diabetes but no other major CVD risk factors.

be measured and used to guide therapy. The treatment goal recommendations are listed in Table 5-3.[4]

Strategic Programming

Therapeutic lifestyle changes (TLC) consisting of diet and exercise are critical components in the management of patients with hypercholesterolemia. Consideration of drug therapy often occurs simultaneously with the decision to initiate TLC. Thus weight reduction and exercise may begin at the same time as drug treatment. After six weeks, the response to therapy should be assessed. If the LDL cholesterol goal is still not achieved, further intensification of therapy should be considered, with re-evaluation in another six weeks. Once the LDL-C goal has been attained, attention turns to other lipid risk factors when present. If triglycerides are high (≥200 mg/dL), the secondary target of treatment becomes non-HDL cholesterol. If the LDL-C goal has been attained but not the non-HDL cholesterol goal, the following two alternative approaches are appropriate: (1) the dose of the LDL-lowering drug can be increased to reduce both LDL and VLDL, or (2) consideration can be given to adding a triglyceride-lowering drug (fibrate or nicotinic acid) to LDL-lowering therapy, which will mainly lower VLDL. Once the patient has achieved the treatment goal(s), follow-up intervals may be reduced to every four to six months. The primary focus of these visits is encouragement of long-term compliance with therapy and checking for side effects.[1-2, 5]

Lifestyle Modification

Lifestyle changes are the first mode of treatment, including dietary changes, smoking cessation, weight reduction (if overweight), and exercise.

With respect to dietary principles, the standard recommendations for LDL cholesterol lowering have focused on lowering saturated and *trans* fat to <7% of calories and dietary cholesterol to <200 mg/day, lowering excess body weight by at least 5–10%, and increasing soluble

TABLE 5-4: Management Master Plan

Data Management	Lower cholesterol level Lower blood pressure level Lifestyle changes Exercise Diet Moderation in alcohol consumption Stop cigarette smoking
System Configuration Correction	None
Root Cause Treatment	Cholesterol-lowering drugs
Work-Around Management	None
System Replacement	None

fiber consumption. Weight reduction and weight maintenance are best achieved by a combination of caloric reduction and increased physical activity. Lifestyle changes are the most cost-effective means to reduce risk for CAD. (Table 5-4) Lifestyle modification program is discussed in detail in Chapter 4. Diet is discussed in Chapter 6.

Pharmacologic Treatment- Primary Prevention

The benefit and safety of cholesterol-lowering therapy in the primary prevention of CAD in patients with hypercholesterolemia is well established. Individuals with multiple risk factors have a greater potential for benefit. The latest information comes from the results of the Justification for the Use of Statins in Primary Prevention: An Intervention Trial Evaluating Rosuvastatin (JUPITER) Trial presented below. The question is whether a statin is beneficial in the treatment of healthy people who have normal LDL cholesterol levels but high CRP?

 EVIDENCE-BASED MEDICINE:

The JUPITER Trial

Methodology: This was a randomized, double-blind, placebo-controlled, multicenter trial in which. 17,800 apparently healthy men and women with LDL cholesterol levels of < 130 mg/dL (3.4 mmol per liter) and high-sensitivity C-reactive protein (hs CRP) levels of 2.0 mg per liter or higher were randomized to rosuvastatin, 20 mg daily, or placebo. *Benefits:* Rosuvastatin reduced LDL cholesterol levels by 50% and hs CRP levels by 37%. The rates of the primary endpoint were 0.77 and 1.36 per 100 person-years in the rosuvastatin and placebo groups, respectively (hazard ratio for rosuvastatin, 0.56; 95%

confidence interval [CI], 0.46 to 0.69; P<0.00001), with corresponding rates of 0.17 and 0.37 for MI (hazard ratio, 0.46; 95% CI, 0.30
to 0.70; P = 0.0002), 0.18 and 0.34 for stroke (hazard ratio, 0.52;
95% CI, 0.34 to 0.79; P = 0.002), 1.00 and 1.25 for death from any
cause (hazard ratio, 0.80; 95% CI, 0.67 to 0.97; P = 0.02).[6-7] *Harms:*
The rosuvastatin group did not have a significant increase in myopathy or cancer but did have a higher incidence of physician-reported diabetes.[7] *Cost-Effectiveness Analysis:* In the United States, if JUPITER
is adopted in clinical practice, one in five (20%) middle-age adults
newly eligible for statin therapy correspond to rosuvastatin costs of
$1200 per year; the yearly cost is $8.9 billion. If a generic statin is
used, the yearly cost is $443 million.[8-10] *Practical Applications:* Al-
though the results of JUPITER are impressive for LDL, it did not
prove or disprove whether CRP elevation can be used as a marker for
risk reduction with statin. All it proved was that in individuals with
normal LDL who had elevated CRP, there is a reduction in risk. What
it did not prove was if the CRP had been normal whether they would
still have had the same benefit or no benefit.

Other studies, including the Pravastatin or Atorvastatin Evaluation
and Infection Therapy (PROVE-IT) and the Reversal of Atherosclerosis with Lipitor (REVERSAL) trials showed that lower CRP levels were
associated with fewer cardiovascular events, independent of LDL cholesterol levels. However, infection, cancer, arthritis, any inflammation,
any flu, cold, and sleep apnea can raise CRPs. So one has to be certain
that the CRP seems attributable to coronary vascular risk before taking
an aggressive approach to treatment with atorvastatin. Another note of
caution about the JUPITER trial, while its results are very interesting, in
real world practice, physicians still have to focus on treating high cholesterol.[11]

Secondary Prevention

The use of statins was studied in secondary prevention trials to determine if these agents would reduce subsequent cardiac events. The
studies that have documented benefit from LDL cholesterol reduction
in secondary prevention include the Scandinavian Simvastatin Survival Study (4S),[11a] the Medical Research Council Heart Protection
Study,[11b] Pravastatin or Atorvastatin Evaluation, Infection Therapy–
Thrombolysis in Myocardial Infarction 22 (PROVE-IT-TIMI-22),[12]
Treating to New Targets (TNT),[13] and Incremental Decrease in End
Points through Aggressive Lipid Lowering (IDEAL).[14] The number
needed to treat (NNT) of these trials were 56.8 (2 years), 55.5 (4.9
years), and 79.8 (4.8 years), respectively.[11] However, at what level
should LDL be lowered, and for what benefits? The answers are in the
meta-analysis that follows.

SMART THINKING:

Intensive versus Standard Therapy

Methodology: This is a meta-analysis for cardiovascular outcomes comparing high-dose statin therapy to standard dosing from the data of four RCTs, including TNT, IDEAL, PROVE-IT-TMI-22, and A–Z (Aggrastat-to-Zocor) with a population of 27,548 patients. *Results:* There was a significant 16% odds reduction in coronary death or MI (P < 0.00001) as well as a significant 16% odds reduction of coronary death or any CV event (P < 0.00001).[15] These trials achieved final mean LDL cholesterol levels of 62–81 mg/dL (1.6–2.1 mmol/L), which are well below the current 100 mg/dL (2.6 mmol/L) guideline target for patients at elevated CV risk.[1] No difference was observed in total or noncardiovascular mortality, but there was a trend toward decreased cardiovascular mortality (odds reduction 12%; P < 0.054).[15] *Practical Applications:* Intensive therapy for LDL lowering does provide additional clinical CV benefit to 'standard' intervention with these statins. However, these benefits are modest, and the potential for further benefits may be limited. In addition, for some patients, increased cost or emergence of side effects may limit the practicability of intensive statin therapy.

Selection of Drug

There are many drugs available for the treatment of hypercholesterolemia. The majority of patients achieve treatment goals with statins. Based on available evidence, there were no data on clinical events to suggest the superiority of any one statin over the others in reducing cardiovascular events. Therapy should usually be initiated with the most affordable, lowest cost drug.[16] The major classes of drugs for consideration are listed in Table 5-5. A brief summary of effects, side effects, and contraindications of the drugs used for hypercholesterolemia is provided in Table 5.5.

TABLE 5-5: Major Class of Drugs for Hypercholesterolemia

- HMG CoA reductase inhibitors (statins)—lovastatin, pravastatin, simvastatin, fluvastatin, atorvastatin, rosuvastatin
- Bile acid sequestrants—cholestyramine, colestipol, colesevelam
- Nicotinic acid—crystalline, timed-release preparations
- Fibric acid derivatives (fibrates)—gemfibrozil, fenofibrate, clofibrate
- Cholesterol absorption inhibitors – ezetimibe

ADVANCED MANAGEMENT
Efficacy Comparison of Statin
In a meta-analysis, the Cholesterol Treatment Trialists (CTT) showed that a 40-mg/dL reduction in LDL cholesterol resulted in a 21% reduction in the risk of vascular events and a 12% reduction in mortality. This is RELATIVE risk reduction — not absolute — that depends upon the study population (higher risk, higher absolute reduction).

Formula of Absolute Statin Reduction Translating into Clinical Benefit

**40 mg LDL decrease = 20% decrease in risk of vascular events
= 10% decrease in risk of total mortality**

Based on those findings, the "real benefits" of lowering LDL cholesterol by approximately 50 mg/dL over two years in JUPITER would be expected to yield a 20 to 30% reduction in the risk of ischemic events and a 10% reduction in total mortality.[11]

Efficacy of Statin
LDL cholesterol reduction by percentage change according to statin and daily dose from 164 randomized placebo controlled trials is seen in Table 5-6.[20]

Side Effects
There was no evidence that statins increased the incidence of cancer overall or at any particular site. In meta-analysis of 23 statin trials with over 309,000 person-years, no significant relationship between percent LDL-C lowering and elevated liver enzymes ($R^2 < 0.001$, $P = 0.91$),

TABLE 5-6: Percentage of LDL Reduction According to Daily Dose of Statin[20]

Percentage of LDL Reduction					
	5 mg	10 mg	20 mg	40 mg	80 mg
Lovastatin		21%	29%	37%	45%
Pravastatin	15%	20%	24%	29%	33%
Fluvastatin	10%	15%	21%	27%	33%
Simvastatin	23%	27%	32%	37%	42%
Atorvastatin	31%	37%	43%	49%	55%
Rosuvastatin	38%	43%	48%	53%	58%

rhabdomyolysis ($R^2 = 0.05$, $P = 0.16$), or rates of cancer ($R^2 = 0.09$, $P = 0.92$) were observed.

Significantly higher rates of elevated liver enzymes were noted in the high-dose statin recipients compared with the intermediate or low-dose statin treatment groups ($P < 0.001$ for all pair-wise comparisons).[17–18] A drug safety alert has been issued on the increased risk of hemorrhagic stroke associated with high doses of atorvastatin in people with recent hemorrhagic stroke.

The following new warning was issued by the Federal Drug Administration (FDA) on 8/8/08: There is an increased risk of rhabdomyolysis when simvastatin is prescribed with amiodarone, and doses of simvastatin higher than 20 mg per day should be avoided in patients taking amiodarone.[19] A brief summary of effects, side effects and contraindications for the drugs used for hypercholesterolemia is provided in Table 5-7.

Follow-Up Enzyme Testing

In some patients, CPK testing allows one to document the baseline value, which is occasionally high and can be misleading if only measured when the common complaint of myalgias or arthralgias raise the issue of muscle toxicity.[18] If there are no symptoms later, there is no value in monitoring the CPK. Alanine aminotransferase (ALT) and aspartate aminotransferase (AST) should be assessed within 8 to 12 weeks after starting a statin, changing dose, or adding another drug that might interfere with statin clearance. If the ALT or AST increase is above three times the upper limit of normal, the patient should be questioned about symptoms and the values should be repeated within a few days.

Combination Therapy

Statins are currently the most prescribed lipid-altering drugs because of their efficacy in favorably altering blood lipid levels, safety, tolerability, and proven benefits in reducing atherosclerotic CAD events. However, some patients require combination lipid-altering treatment to achieve their LDL cholesterol and non-HDL cholesterol goals. Should a patient have higher dose statin monotherapy or a combination of two different classes of drugs? The lipid-altering agents most commonly used in combination with statins include niacin, bile acid sequestrants, fibrates, fish oils, and ezetimibe. The needs for combination therapy are listed in Table 5-8.

Statin and Omega 3

Omega-3 polyunsaturated fatty acids inhibit triglycerides synthesis and augment triglyceride clearance. They lower triglycerides by about 45% and increase HDL by about 13%. The major issue with omega-3 agents is a lack of outcomes-based data. Additionally, they can increase LDL and cause dyspepsia and nausea and may increase bleeding time.

TABLE 5-7: Effects, Side Effects, Contraindications for the Drugs Affecting Lipoprotein Metabolism

Drug Class	Lipid/Lipoprotein Effects	Side Effects	Contraindications	Clinical Trial Results
HMG-CoA reductase inhibitors (statins)	LDL ↓18%-55% HDL ↑5%-15% TG ↓7%-30%	Myopathy; increased liver enzymes	Absolute: active or chronic liver disease Relative: concomitant use of certain drugs	Reduced major coronary events, CAD deaths, need for coronary procedures, stroke, and total mortality
Bile acid sequestrants	LDL ↓15%-30% HDL ↑3%-5% TG No change or increase	Gastrointestinal distress; constipation; decreased absorption of other drugs	Absolute: dysbetalipoproteinemia; TG .400 mg/dL; Relative: TG .200 mg/dL	Reduced major coronary events and CAD deaths
Nicotinic acid	LDL ↓5%-25% HDL ↑15%-35% TG ↓20%-50%	Flushing; hyperglycemia; hyperuricemia (or gout); upper gastrointestinal distress; hepatotoxicity	Absolute: chronic liver disease; severe gout Relative: diabetes; hyperuricemia; peptic ulcer disease	Reduced major coronary events, and possible total mortality
Fibric acids	LDL ↓5%-20% (may be increased in patients with high TG) HDL ↑10%-20% TG ↓20%-50%	Dyspepsia; gallstones; myopathy; unexplained non-CAD deaths in WHO study	Absolute: severe renal disease; severe hepatic disease	Reduced major coronary events
Ezetimibe	LDL ↓18% HDL ↑1% TG ↓10%	Headache and/or diarrhea, joint pains, and tiredness	Hypersensitivity to any component of this medication	Not yet determined

CAD: coronary artery disease, HDL: high density lipoprotein, LDL: low density lipoprotein, TG: triglycerides, WHO: World Health Organization.

TABLE 5-8: Indications for Combination Therapy

- Failure of statin monotherapy to achieve treatment goals
- Intolerance and adverse drug interactions with higher-dose statin monotherapy
- Complementary benefits toward further reduction in CAD risk

The Japan Eicosapentaenoic acid (EPA) Lipid Intervention Study (JELIS) showed the effects of long-term use of EPA of 1800 mg per day in addition to a statin in Japanese patients with hypercholesterolemia. In the secondary prevention patients, EPA was associated with a significant 19% reduction in major coronary events compared with the control group. Unstable angina was also significantly reduced in the EPA group, by 28%. Nonsignificant reductions were seen in fatal MI, nonfatal MI, and CABG/PCI, and in combined endpoints. A higher incidence of adverse events, especially gastrointestinal disorders, skin disorders, and abnormal liver function tests, was recorded in the EPA group than in the control group (25.3% vs. 21.7%, P < 0.0001). Most of these adverse events were mild.[21]

 SMART THINKING:

Conflicting Data on Fish Oil After AMI

The Italian GISSI-Prevenzione trial found a 50% reduction in sudden cardiac death in those who took omega-3 in the first months after an acute MI. In the OMEGA trial, 3827 patients from 104 German centers were randomized to one year of treatment with omega-3-acid ethylesters 90 (460 mg eicosapentaenoic acid [EPA] and 380 mg docosahexaenoic acid [DHA]) 1 g daily, or to placebo (1 g of olive oil) within 3 to 14 days of their heart attack. In addition, they received the best possible medical care. *Results:* At one year, there was no difference in the rate of the primary endpoint—sudden cardiac death—which occurred in 1.5% of patients in both groups. Nor were there any differences in any secondary endpoints, which included total mortality (4.2%), reinfarction (4.4%), stroke (1.4%), and revascularization. *Mechanism of Difference:* There were very clear differences in treatment following AMI between OMEGA and Gissi-Prevenzione, which likely explain the results. Some 80% of the OMEGA patients received acute revascularization, 90% got clopidogrel, and half had GP IIb/IIIa inhibitors, while those in GISSI-Prevenzione had none of these. In addition, more than 90% of those in the OMEGA trial were prescribed aspirin, beta blockers, and statins, and more than 80% received ACE inhibitors. *Practical Applications:* In patients who have suffered an acute MI and are receiving optimal medical care, omega-3 fatty acids—the kind found in oily fish—offer no additional benefits. The AHA/ACC recommendations for secondary prevention are: 1 gm for all with CAD and 3 to 4 gm for those with CAD and high TGs. The main practical point is that the patient is to receive 1 gm of total EPA and DHA.[22]

Statin and Ezetimibe

Ezetimibe blocks the synthesis of a key protein in the intestinal villi, thus preventing the absorption of cholesterol.

In the Ezetimibe Study with 628 patients diagnosed with primary hypercholesterolemia, ezetimibe 10 mg plus 10 mg of atorvastatin were more effective than atorvastatin 10 mg, 20 mg, or 40 mg in lowering LDL-C levels. In fact, the LDL cholesterol lowering efficacy of 10 mg of ezetimibe plus 10 mg of atorvastatin was similar to 80 mg of atorvastatin (the "formula" of "10 + 10 = 80")[23]

SMART THINKING:

Efficacy Comparison Between Ezetimibe plus Atorvastatin (20 mg) versus Uptitration of Atorvastatin (to 40 mg)

The aim of this study was to evaluate the efficacy and safety of ezetimibe 10 mg added to atorvastatin 20 mg compared with doubling atorvastatin to 40 mg in patients with hypercholesterolemia at moderately high risk for coronary heart disease who did not reach low-density lipoprotein (LDL) cholesterol levels <100 mg/dL with atorvastatin 20 mg. *Methodology:* In this six-week, multicenter, double-blind, randomized, parallel-group study, 196 patients treated with atorvastatin 20 mg received atorvastatin 20 mg plus ezetimibe 10 mg or atorvastatin 40 mg for six weeks. *Results:* adding ezetimibe 10 mg to atorvastatin 20 mg produced significantly greater reductions in LDL cholesterol than increasing atorvastatin to 40 mg (-31% vs. -11%, P <0.001). Significantly greater reductions were also seen in non–high-density lipoprotein cholesterol, total cholesterol, and apolipoprotein B (P <0.001). Significantly more patients reached LDL cholesterol levels <100 mg/dL with atorvastatin 20 mg plus ezetimibe compared with atorvastatin 40 mg (84% vs. 49%, P <0.001). The two treatment groups had comparable results for high-density lipoprotein cholesterol, triglycerides, apolipoprotein A-I, and high-sensitivity C-reactive protein. The incidences of clinical and laboratory adverse experiences were generally similar between groups.[24] *Practical Applications:* The addition of ezetimibe 10 mg to atorvastatin 20 mg was generally well tolerated and resulted in significantly greater lipid-lowering efficacy compared with doubling atorvastatin to 40 mg in patients with hypercholesterolemia at moderately high risk for coronary heart disease.

Evidence of Mortality Benefits on Surrogate Endpoints or Harms

No studies of ezetimibe alone or the combination of ezetimibe and simvastatin or atorvastain have examined cardiovascular morbidity or mortality or all-cause mortality.

The Effect of Combination Ezetimibe and High-Dose Simvastatin vs. Simvastatin Alone on the Atherosclerotic Process in Patients with Heterozygous Familial Hypercholesterolemia (ENHANCE) trial, conducted in 720 patients with heterozygous familial hypercholesterolemia, showed no significant difference in the primary endpoint—mean change in the intima media thickness (IMT) measured at three sites in the carotid arteries—between patients treated with ezetimibe/simvastatin 10/80 mg versus patients treated with simvastatin 80 mg alone over a two-year period. The reduction in LDL-cholesterol levels, however, was statistically significant, reduced by 56% and 39% in the ezetimibe/simvastatin and simvastatin treatment arms, respectively.[25] So the LDL-cholesterol lowering efficacy of 10 mg of ezetimibe plus 10 mg of atorvastatin was similar to 80 mg of atorvastatin (thus the "formula" of "10+10=80").

The Intensive Lipid Lowering with Simvastatin and Ezetimibe in Aortic Stenosis (SEAS) trial also showed a failure in primary outcome. Simvastatin and ezetimibe did not reduce the composite outcome of combined aortic valve events and ischemic events in patients with aortic stenosis. Cancer occurred more frequently in the simvastatin–ezetimibe group (105 vs. 70, P = 0.01).[26]

However, in the analyses of cancer data from three ezetimibe trials, including SEAS, and the two large ongoing trials of this regimen—the Study of Heart and Renal Protection (SHARP) with 9264 patients (mean follow-up, 2.7 years) and the Improved Reduction of Outcomes: Vytorin Efficacy International Trial (IMPROVE-IT)—no credible evidence was provided of any adverse effect of ezetimibe on rates of cancer.[27] The FDA issued a statement reaffirming that the results from ENHANCE do not change the FDA's position. Based on current available data, patients should not stop taking ezetimibe or other cholesterol-lowering medications.[28]

Statin and Nicotinic Acid

Nicotinic acid, or "niacin," has moderate LDL-lowering capabilities but a relatively high capacity to raise HDL, with a nonlinear dose-related increase in HDL cholesterol of ~20% following the use of modest doses of nicotinic acid (~1 g per day). Several clinical trials supported the efficacy of nicotinic acid for reduction of CAD risk, both when used alone and in combination with statins. The combination of a statin with nicotinic acid produces a marked reduction of LDL cholesterol and a striking rise in HDL cholesterol. Although the majority of patients can tolerate nicotinic acid therapy, a sizable minority are intolerant because of a variety of side effects such as hot flashes and burning. Currently, prolonged-release formulation of nicotinic acid shows identical efficacy, superior tolerability, and comparable antiatherogenic benefits compared with the immediate-release formulation. The safety and tolerability profiles of prolonged-release nicotinic acid did not differ in patients who were and were not taking a statin.[29–30]

Nicotinic acid in combination with a bile-acid binding resin or a statin was associated with regression of atherosclerosis and reduced CVD events in several studies.[31-32] Until now, there have been no long-term outcome data for the combination of niacin with statin. Two on-going trials, the Atherothrombosis Intervention in Metabolic Syndrome with Low HDL/High Triglycerides and Impact on Global Health (AIM-HIGH) and the Heart Protection Study 2–Treatment of HDL to Reduce the Incidence of Vascular Events (HPS2-THRIVE), will address the outcomes and safety of statin plus niacin combination therapy, and the results of these trials are expected by 2012.

Statin and Fibrate

Although the evidence base to support fibrate therapy is not as strong as that for statins, fibrates may have an adjunctive role in the treatment of patients with high triglycerides/low HDL, especially in combination with statins. Concern about development of myopathy with this combination has been lessened somewhat by the recent finding that one fibrate, fenofibrate, does not interfere with catabolism of statins and thus likely does not substantially increase the risk for clinical myopathy in patients treated with moderate doses of statins.[33]

A statin-fibrate combination can reduce both LDL cholesterol and VLDL cholesterol (non-HDL cholesterol) in patients with elevated triglycerides. The atorvastatin-fenofibrate combination has been shown to have a highly beneficial effect on lipid parameters in patients with type 2 diabetes and hypercholesterolemia. The atorvastatin-fenofibrate combination reduced total cholesterol by 37%, LDL cholesterol by 46%, and triglycerides by 50% and increased HDL-C by 22%. These changes were significantly better than those of both monotherapies.[34]

The additive effects of simvastatin and fenofibrate on lipid parameters have been documented in the Simvastatin Plus Fenofibrate for Combined Hyperlipidemia (SAFARI) trial.[35] Simvastatin monotherapy (20 mg/day) was compared with combination therapy (simvastatin 20 mg/day plus fenofibrate 160 mg/day) in patients with CAD. The mean LDL levels were significantly decreased with combination therapy compared with monotherapy (31.2 and 25.8%, respectively; P <0.001). In addition, mean HDL cholesterol levels significantly increased with combination therapy compared with monotherapy (18.6 and 9.7%, respectively; P <0.001).

Historically, however, fibrate-statin combination therapy has been a source of safety concerns. Although there is an increase in reports of rhabdomyolysis with statin–fibrate combined therapy, this risk appears to be about 15 times higher for gemfibrozil than for fenofibrate when used with statins.[36] Data from the several recent trials suggest that combining fenofibrate with statins does not significantly increase the risk of myopathy.[34-35] Since the primary aim of cholesterol management is LDL reduction, statin therapy usually will be introduced before fibrates. In some patients with high triglycerides, both LDL and non-HDL goals can be attained with higher doses of statins or by an alternative approach with statin and fibrate.[1] However, there was no robust evidence for incremental benefits or risks of combination therapy.

TROUBLE-SHOOTING AND DEBUGGING

Treatment of hypercholesterolemia is standard for any physician in the care of patients with hypercholesterolemia. When the problems are not controlled as expected, management requires the expertise of a consultant cardiologist. Common questions from the referral physicians to the consultant cardiologist in the management of hypercholesterolemia are discussed below.

How to Treat Elevated Triglycerides

Elevated triglyceride levels, especially in individuals with additional lipoprotein abnormalities, predict higher cardiovascular disease risk. However, there is a lack of data regarding the benefits of strategies directly targeting elevated triglyceride levels. Factors contributing to elevated triglycerides include obesity and being overweight, physical inactivity, cigarette smoking, excess alcohol intake, high-carbohydrate diets (60% of energy intake), several diseases (type 2 diabetes, chronic renal failure, nephrotic syndrome), certain drugs (corticosteroids, estrogens, retinoids, higher doses of adrenergic-blocking agents), and genetic disorders (familial combined hyperlipidemia, familial hypertriglyceridemia, and familial dysbetalipoproteinemia). The classification and treatment strategies for high triglycerides are listed in Table 5-9.

For many patients with mild increase in triglycerides, a lifestyle program alone will normalize the triglyceride levels. The limitation of the intake of complex carbohydrates can be very beneficial in lowering triglyceride levels.[37] When lifestyle modification cannot achieve the desired triglyceride goal, pharmacological therapy will need to be considered. Triglyceride values higher than 500 mg/dL usually require drug therapy. The fibric acid derivatives are most commonly used for isolated hypertriglyceridemia, although these agents typically lower triglyceride levels only about 30%.[1] Omega-3 fatty acids in the form of dietary fish or fish oil supplements can help to lower triglyceride levels. Prospective data and clinical trial evidence in

TABLE 5-9: ATP III Classification of Triglyceride Levels and Treatment Strategies

Normal	150 mg/dL (170 mmol/L)	None
Borderline-high	150 to 199 mg/dL (170 to 2.25 mmol/L)	Achieve LDL-C goal, lifestyle changes.
High	200 to 499 mg/dL (2.26 to 5.64 mmol/L)	Achieve LDL-C goal and non-HDL-C goal, lifestyle changes.
Very high	≥500 mg/dL (5.65 mmol/L)	Triglyceride lowering to prevent acute pancreatitis (first priority).

secondary CAD prevention suggest that higher intakes of n-3 fatty acids reduce the risk for coronary events or coronary mortality.[38] Doses of 4 grams of omega-3 fish oils a day may be needed to achieve about a 30% reduction in triglyceride levels.

How to Treat Low HDL Cholesterol

Low HDL cholesterol levels (<40 mg/dL) may be due to a genetic disorder or to secondary causes. HDL-cholesterol levels are inversely correlated with CAD risk. Strategies to raise HDL cholesterol have also been studied. Nonpharmacologic therapy such as exercise, weight loss, and smoking cessation should be stressed. Exercise increases HDL about 3 to 9%, but the increase is related to the frequency and intensity of the exercise. Smoking cessation will increase HDL by about 4 mg/dL. Weight loss is another effective way to increase HDL, but the degree of increase is related to the number of pounds lost and kept off. Niacin therapy has the greatest potential to raise HDL cholesterol levels. Niacin is available as a short-acting supplement or as a prolonged release preparation to attempt to avoid cutaneous side effects such as flushing. High doses of niacin can raise HDL cholesterol more than any other currently available therapy. There have been few outcome studies, however, that document cardiovascular risk reduction with niacin. The Coronary Drug Project conducted between 1966 and 1975 evaluated the long-term efficacy of 3 grams of niacin daily in a group of men who had had a previous MI.[39] No further studies with niacin have been performed that clearly show risk reduction.

Niacin is difficult to take and nearly 50% of individuals cannot tolerate the drug because of side effects. Niacin is used in lower doses in combination with statins in the hope that a combined effect of lowering LDL cholesterol with the statin and raising HDL cholesterol with niacin will translate into further risk reduction. Combining lovastatin with extended-release niacin can lower LDL cholesterol from 30% to 42% and raise HDL cholesterol up to 30% with currently available doses. Studies will need to be done to determine if these favorable lipid changes bring about further event reduction. Nicotinic acid should be used with caution in persons with active liver disease, recent peptic ulcer, hyperuricemia and gout, and type 2 diabetes. The maximum dose of extended release niacin should not exceed 2000 mg/d to avoid hepatotoxicity, and doses of 1000–1500 mg/d are most reasonable, particularly because its role is to supplement or amplify therapy with an LDL cholesterol-lowering agent.[1] As a general rule, lower doses are required for increasing HDL-C than for reducing LDL cholesterol and triglyceride levels.

The fibrates are a class of medications that lower triglyceride levels and mildly raise HDL cholesterol. They may lower LDL cholesterol, although if there is a substantial decrease in triglyceride levels, it may increase slightly in some patients. This increase in LDL cholesterol may be due to an increase in the size and thus the cholesterol content of the LDL particles and not an increase in the absolute number of LDL particles. These less dense LDL particles may be less atherogenic than small dense LDL particles.[5]

How to Treat Hypercholesterolemia in Patients with Liver Disease

Biliary obstruction can lead to severe hypercholesterolemia that is resistant to conventional cholesterol-lowering drugs. The only effective therapy is treatment of the underlying liver or biliary tract disease.[1] In patients with borderline elevation of liver enzymes, if the patient needs to be on medication, the patient should be on a statin with more frequent checks of liver enzymes. If there is persistent and substantial elevation of liver enzymes, then the statin should be discontinued.[40] Different tactics for how to use statins in patients with baseline elevation of liver enzymes are listed in Table 5-10.

How to Treat Hypercholesterolemia in HIV Patients Taking Protease Inhibitors

Dyslipidemia associated with the treatment of HIV infection, particularly with the use of protease inhibitors (PIs), can raise cholesterol and triglyceride (TG) levels to the thresholds indicated for intervention. Diet and exercise should be tried first. If results are not satisfactory, other options include switching antiretroviral agents and starting lipid-lowering drugs. Selection of drug therapy for lipid lowering depends on the type of predominant dyslipidemia and the potential for drug interactions. The use of statins is recommended for the treatment of patients with elevated LDL cholesterol levels. Gemfibrozil or fenofibrate is recommended for patients with elevated TG concentrations. Because atorvastatin and some antiretroviral drugs

TABLE 5-10: Tactics for Treatment of Hypercholesterolemia in Patients with Liver Disease

Measure baseline electrolyte, liver function, renal function, and thyroid-stimulating hormone.

- Look for nondrug causes of elevation of aminotransferase (ALT or AST) such as alcohol use, non-immune hepatitis, infectious hepatitis, or non-alcoholic fatty liver disease.
- Statin can be started if the ALT and AST levels are not > 3 times the upper limit of normal.
- After starting a statin, monitor ALT and AST every 6 and 12 weeks and after dose increase.
- If the levels of AST and ALT are elevated >3 times of normal during monitoring, repeat measurement in one week.
- If level is still high, decrease the dose or stop the medication if the patient has chronic liver disease or chronic alcohol abuse.
- If decreasing the dose, repeat measurement in 2 to 4 weeks.
- If level returns to baseline, continue lower dose and monitor.
- If statin is discontinued, consider reissuing the same statin at a lower dose or another statin.[40]

are metabolized by the same cytochrome C-450 isoenzyme, CYP3A4, inhibition of the isoenzyme may result in an excessively high level of statin (raising the risk of rhabdomyolysis). Simvastatin and lovastatin should be avoided, while atorvastatin should be used at lower dose. Pravastatin can be used; however, its efficacy is questioned. Rosuvastatin is a better choice for patients receiving antiretroviral drugs because it may have slightly more CYP3A4 activity.[41–42] Ezetimibe alone reduces LDL cholesterol in HIV-infected patients receiving combination antiretroviral therapy.[43] Its high tolerability and the lack of interactions with the cytochrome CYP3A4 indicate that ezetimibe will not increase the risk of toxicity or pharmacokinetic interactions with antiretrovirals.

How to Treat Children and Young Adults in a Family of Patients with Hypercholesterolemia

The process of atherosclerotic CVD begins early in life and is progressive throughout the life span. Clinical evidence suggests that serum cholesterol measured at 22 years of age is predictive of the risk of CAD over the next 30 to 40 years.[44] The National Cholesterol Education Program (NCEP) recommends screening children older than 2 years of age with parental hypercholesterolemia or a first-degree family history of premature cardiovascular disease.[45] For patients 8 years and older with an LDL concentration of ≥ 190 mg/dL (or ≥160 mg/dL with a family history of early heart disease; or <2 additional risk factors present; or ≥130 mg/dL if diabetes mellitus is present), pharmacologic intervention should be considered. The initial goal is to lower LDL concentration to <160 mg/dL. However, targets as low as 130 mg/dL or even 110 mg/dL may be warranted when there is a strong family history of CVD, especially with other risk factors including obesity, diabetes mellitus, metabolic syndrome, and other higher-risk situations.[46] The American Heart Association has recommended that triglyceride concentrations of >150 mg/dL and HDL concentrations of <35 mg/dL be considered abnormal for children and adolescents.[47] Treatment of hypercholesterolemia during childhood and adolescence is based on dietary treatment and lifestyle modification. Drug therapy should be limited to children with levels above the 99th percentile who fail to reduce their levels after 6–12 months. Successful treatment is considered to be any reduction of LDL-C cholesterol accompanied by changes to an appropriate lifestyle and healthy eating habits. Lovastatin is the only statin currently approved for children, but simvastatin, pravastatin, and atorvastatin have also been used. LDL-C decreased by 17% on 10 mg/d and by 27% on 40 mg/d of lovastatin in boys 10–14 years of age[48] without an adverse effect on growth and development. LDL-C was reduced by 41% and Apo-B by 34% with 40 mg/d of simvastatin[49] in 173 boys and girls with heterozygous hypercholesterolemia.

How to Treat Hypercholesterolemia in Patients with Renal Disease

Patients with chronic kidney disease (CKD) and end-stage renal disease (ESRD) are at increased CAD risk. Various dyslipidemias are common and no doubt contribute to this risk. Hypertriglyceridemia and low HDL cholesterol levels are the most frequently described lipid abnormalities with chronic renal failure and hemodialysis. Therefore, if hypercholesterolemia persists despite specific treatment for renal disease, consideration can be given to use of cholesterol-lowering drugs. Although several lipid-lowering agents appear to modify elevated lipid levels, statins are particularly effective. It has always been assumed that patients with chronic renal failure would benefit from hypolipidemic therapy, but most patients had suboptimum changes in lipoproteins, and it was not clear whether CAD events would be reduced. A post hoc analysis of 1711 patients in the Cholesterol and Recurrent Events (CARE) trial with chronic renal insufficiency (creatinine clearance, <75 mL/min), half of whom received 40 mg pravastatin/d and the other half placebo, revealed a 28% reduction in major CAD events and a 35% reduction in the need for revascularization.[50] Benefits were independent of the severity of renal insufficiency, and the therapy was well tolerated.[50] One reason that these studies in dialysis and transplant patients have shown only mixed results and not clear benefits may be that these patients have had such long-standing CKD and diabetes that their CVD has become so advanced that it is less responsive to such interventions. As glomerular filtration rate (GFR) falls, the dosages of many of the drugs that are used for the treatment of hypercholesterolemia need to be modified. In general, however, atorvastatin and fluvastatin dosages do not have to be modified.[51–52] In general, combinations of statins and fibrates should be avoided, and fenofibrate should be avoided in all patients with decreased GFR levels.[52]

SMART THINKING:

The AURORA Trial (A Study to Evaluate the Use of Rosuvastatin in Subjects On Regular Haemodialysis: an Assessment of Survival and Cardiovascular Events)

Methodology: A total of 2776 patients on hemodialysis for at least three months prior to the study received rosuvastatin (Crestor) 10 mg daily (n = 1391) or placebo (n = 1385).The patients' ages ranged from 50 to 80 years. Patients tolerated rosuvastatin very well, and there was no difference in adverse events between placebo- and rosuvastatin-treated patients. *Results:* Despite a 43% reduction in LDL-cholesterol and an 11% reduction in CRP in the patients in the statin group, there was no beneficial treatment effect on the composite cardiovascular endpoint or on any of the secondary endpoints with rosuvastatin. *Mechanism of Difference:* Patients who were on dialysis treatment for up to four years could have produced greater calcification of the coronary arteries, a known side effect of hemodialysis. *Practical Applications:* Even though the results of AURORA were negative, dialysis patients should still get a statin if they have other risk factors associated with the coronary arteries or other parts of their vascular tree. These patients don't die from a heart attack or stroke, they die of kidney failure from their end-stage renal disease. If the patients can avoid dying of coronary disease, they may live to receive a kidney transplant.[53]

How to Treat Hypercholesterolemia in Asian People

The pattern of lipid abnormalities and their relative impact on CVD risk might vary among ethnic groups.[54–71] Asians experience the largest proportion of the worldwide burden of CVD. Further, Asians include several distinct ethnic subpopulations, who may differ in their lipid profiles.[55] These differences may be the result of both genetic and environmental factors (e.g., high-carbohydrate diets, reduced physical activity.)[60] In a case-control study, 65 centers in Asia recruited 5731 cases of a first AMI and 6459 control subjects. Among both cases and controls, mean LDL-C levels were about 10 mg/dL lower in Asians compared with non-Asians. A greater proportion of Asian cases and controls had LDL-C ≤100 mg/dL (25.5% and 32.3% in Asians vs. 19.4% and 25.3% in non-Asians, respectively). HDL-C levels were slightly lower among Asians compared with non-Asians. There was a preponderance of people with low HDL-C among South Asians (South Asia vs. rest of Asia: cases 82.3% vs. 57.4%; controls 81% vs. 51.6%; P < 0.0001 for both comparisons). However, despite these differences in absolute levels, the risk of AMI associated with increases in LDL-C and decreases in HDL-C was similar for Asians and non-Asians. Among South Asians, changes in apolipoprotein (Apo) A1 predicted risk better than HDL-C. ApoB/ApoA1 showed the strongest association with the risk of AMI. Therefore, it is necessary to rethink treatment thresholds and targets in this population.[62] In the treatment, a low dose of statin may reduce the risk of CAD, just as higher doses have been shown to be effective in Europe and the US.[63]

TAKE-HOME MESSAGE

Data Collecting Collect all the data about the patient's history (of smoking, high salt, high cholesterol diet, alcohol abuse, lack of exercise, HTN, DM, high cholesterol level), family history (of early sudden death due to heart disease, of early CAD), social history (work and behaviors), and from a complete physical examination (signs of prior stroke, CAD, PAD, carotid murmur, weak peripheral pulses)—all of which add weight to the clinical decision-making process.

Data Mining Recommend safe, appropriate, and efficacious investigation (including fasting lipid profile, fasting blood glucose, BUN and creatinine levels, weight, BMI, and waist circumference). Optimal lipids levels are as follows: LDL cholesterol, below 70 mg/dL; HDL cholesterol, above 40 mg/dL; and triglycerides, below 150 mg/dL.

Management Recommend safe, appropriate, and efficacious therapy to maintain the stable health status of the patient over time (low salt, low cholesterol diet, stopping smoking, losing weight, not drinking alcohol, exercise). TLC consisting of diet and exercise is a critical component of the management of patients with hypercholesterolemia. It should precede or occur with pharmacological therapy, depending on the clinical urgency.

Management means reducing LDL cholesterol, non-HDL cholesterol to ATP III goals as well as panel consensus of ADA/AHA goals. Reduction of LDL cholesterol by 50–70% is possible with statin monotherapy or the use of statins in combination with other hypolipidemic agents.

Patient-Centered Care Get the patients involved in their own lifestyle modification to increase compliance with diet, exercise, medication, office visits, and testing in order to provide continuity of care.

References

1. Third Report of the National Cholesterol Education Program (NCEP) Expert Panel on Detection, Evaluation, and Treatment of High Blood Cholesterol in Adults (Adult Treatment Panel III) final report. Circulation. 2002;106:3143–3421.

2. Grundy, S. M., Cleeman, J. I., Merz, C. N. B., et al.: Implications of recent clinical trials for the National Cholesterol Education Program Adult Treatment Panel III guidelines. Circulation. 2004;110:227–239.

3. Ridker, P. M.: Clinical application of C-reactive protein for cardiovascular disease detection and prevention. Circulation 2003;107:363–369.

4. Brunzell, J. D., Davidson, M., Furberg, C. D., et al.: Lipoprotein Management in Patients With Cardiometabolic Risk: Consensus Conference Report From the American Diabetes Association and the American College of Cardiology Foundation. J Am Coll Cardiol. 2008;51:1512–1524.

5. Huy Van Tran, et al.: Intergrated primary prevention of cardivascular disease. Management of complex cardiovascular problems. 2007; 129–189.

6. Ridker, P.M., Fonseca, F. A., Genest, J., et al.: Baseline characteristics of participants in the JUPITER trial, a randomized placebo-controlled primary prevention trial of statin therapy among individuals with low low-density lipoprotein cholesterol and elevated high-sensitivity C-reactive protein Am J Cardiol. 2007;100:1659–1664.

7. Ridker, P. M., Danielson, E., Fonseca, F. A. H., et al. for the JUPITER Study Group: Rosuvastatin to prevent vascular events in men and women with elevated C-reactive protein. N Engl J Med. 2008;359:2195–2207.

8. Hlatky, M.A.: Expanding the Orbit of Primary Prevention Moving Beyond JUPITER. Engl J Med. 2008;359:2280–2281.

9. Spatz, E. S., Canavan, M. E., Desai, M. M.: From here to JUPITER. Identifying New Patients for Statin Therapy Using Data from the 1999–2004 National Health and Nutrition Examination Survey Circ Cardiovasc Qual Outcomes. 2009;2:41–48.

10. Ridker, P. M., Danielson, E., Fonseca, F. A., et al.: Reduction in C-reactive protein and LDL cholesterol and cardiovascular event rates after initiation of rosuvastatin: A prospective study of the JUPITER trial. Lancet. 2009;DOI: 10.1016/S0140-6736(09)/60447-5. Available at: http://www.thelancet.com/.

11. Yusuf, S., Lonn, E., Bosch, J.: Lipid lowering for primary prevention. Lancet. 2009;373;1152–1155.

11a. Scandinavian Simvastatin Survival Study Group. Randomised trial of cholesterol lowering in 4444 patients with coronary heart disease: the Scandinavian Simvastatin Survival Study (4S). Lancet. 1994;344:1383–1389.

11b. Heart Protection Study Collaborative Group. MRC/BHF Heart Protection Study of cholesterol lowering with simvastatin in 20,536 high–risk individuals: a randomized placebo-controlled trial. Lancet. 2002;360(9326):7–22.

12. Cannon, C. P., Braunwald, E., McCabe, et al.: Pravastatin or Atorvastatin Evaluation and Infection Therapy-Thrombolysis in Myocardial Infarction 22 Investigators. Intensive versus moderate lipid lowering with statins after acute coronary syndromes. N Engl J Med. 2004;350: 1495–1504.

13. Shepherd, J., Barter, P., Carmena, R., et al.: Treating to New Targets Investigators: Effect of lowering LDL cholesterol substantially below currently recommended levels in patients with coronary heart disease and diabetes. Diabetes Care. 2006;29:1220–1226.

14. Pedersen, T. R., Faergeman, O., Kastelein, J. J. P., et al.: High-dose atorvastatin vs. usual dose simvastatin for secondary prevention after myocardial infarction: the IDEAL Study: a randomized controlled trial. JAMA. 2005;294:2437–2445.

15. Christopher, P., Cannon, Benjamin A., et al.: meta-analysis of cardiovascular outcomes trials comparing intensive versus moderate statin therapy. J Am Coll Cardiol. 2006;48:438–445.

16. NICE. Statins for the prevention of cardiovascular events assessment report: coronary heart disease-statins. http://www.nice.org.uk/pdf/statins_ assessment_report.pdf. 20082005. Accessed October 14, 2008.

17. Alsheikh-Ali, A, Maddukuri, P. V., Han, H., et al.: Effect of the magnitude of lipid lowering on risk of elevated liver enzymes, rhabdomyolysis, and cancer: insights from large randomized statin trials. J Am Coll Cardiol. 2007;50:409–418.

18. Kapur, N. K., Musunuru, K.: Clinical efficacy and safety of statins in managing cardiovascular risk. Vasc Health Risk Manag. April 2008; 4(2):341–353.

19. FDA ALERT: Recommendations and Information for Healthcare Professionals to Consider When Prescribing Simvastatin to Patients Taking Amiodarone. [08/08/2008]: http://www.fda.gov/medwatch/report/hcp.htm.

20. Law, M. R., Wald, N. J., Rudnicka, A. R.: Quantifying effect of statins on low density lipoprotein cholesterol, ischemic heart disease, and stroke: systemic review and mete-analysis. BMJ. 2003;326;1423–1430.

21. Yokoyama, M., Origasa, H., Matsuzaki, M., et al.: Effects of eicosapentaenoic acid on major coronary events in hypercholesterolaemic patients (JELIS): A randomised open-label, blinded end point analysis. Lancet. 2007;369:1090–1098.

22. Senges, J.: The OMEGA study at a late-breaking clinical trials session at the American College of Cardiology. 2009; Scientific Sessions in Orlando. FL.

23. Ballantyne, C. M., Houri, J., Notarbartolo, A., et al.: for the Ezetimibe Study Group. Effect of ezetimibe coadministered with atorvastatin in 628 patients with primary hypercholesterolemia: a prospective, randomized, double–blind trial. Circulation. 2003;107;2409–2415.

24. Conard, S., et al.: Efficacy and safety of ezetimibe added on to atorvastatin 20 mg versus uptitration of atorvastatin to 40 mg in hypercholesterolemic patients at moderately high risk for coronary heart disease. Am J Cardiol. 1489–1494.

25. Kastelein, J. J., Akdim, F., Stroes, E. S., et al.: Simvastatin with or without ezetimibe in familial hypercholesterolemia. N Engl J Med. 2008; 358:1431–1443.
26. Rossebo, A. B., Pedersen, T. R., Boman, K., et al.: Intensive lipid lowering with simvastatin and ezetimibe in aortic stenosis. N Engl J Med. 2008;359: 1343–1356.
27. Nissen, S. E., Collins, R., Peto, R.: Analyses of cancer data from three ezetimibe trials. NEJM. 2008;360:86–87.
28. Food and Drug Administration: Update of safety review—follow-up to the January 25, 2008 early communication about an ongoing data review for ezetimibe/simvastatin (marketed as Vytorin), ezetimibe (marketed as Zetia), and simvastatin (marketed as Zocor). January 8, 2009. Available at: http://www.fda.gov/cder/drug/early_comm/ezetimibe_ simvastatin200901.htm.
29. Taylor, A. J., Sullenberger, L. E., Lee, H. J., et al.: 1:Arterial Biology for the Investigation of the Treatment Effects of Reducing Cholesterol (ARBITER) 2: A double-blind, placebo-controlled study of extended-release niacin on atherosclerosis progression in secondary prevention patients treated with statins. Circulation. 2004;110: 3512–3517.
30. Vogt, A., Kassner, U., Hostalek, U., et al.: on behalf of the NAUTILUS Study Group. Safety and tolerability of prolonged-release nicotinic acid combined with a statin in NAUTILUS. Br J Cardiol. 2006;13(4): 273–277.
31. Brown, B. G., Zhao, X. Q., Chait, A., et al.: Simvastatin and niacin, antioxidant vitamins, or the combination for the prevention of coronary disease. N Engl J Med. 2001;345:1583–1592.
32. Bays, H. E., Dujovne, C. A., McGovern, M. E., et al.: ADvicor vs. Other Cholesterol-Modulating Agents Trial Evaluation. Comparison of once-daily, niacin extended-release/lovastatin with standard doses of atorvastatin and simvastatin (the ADvicor vs. Other Cholesterol-Modulating Agents Trial Evaluation [ADVOCATE]). Am J Cardiol. 2003;91: 667–672.
33. Prueksaritanont, T., Tang, C., Qiu, Y., et al.: Effects of fibrates on metabolism of statins in human hepatocytes. Drug Metab Dispos. 2002; 30:1280–1287.
34. Athyros, V. G., Papageorgiou, A. A., Athyrou, V. V., et al.: Atorvastatin and micronized fenofibrate alone and in combination in type 2 diabetes with combined hyperlipidemia. Diabetes Care. 2002;25(7): 1198–1202.
35. Grundy, S. M., Vega, G. L., Yuan, Z., et al.: Effectiveness and tolerability of simvastatin plus fenofibrate for combined hyperlipidemia (the SAFARI trial), Am J Cardiol. 2005;95(4):462–468.
36. Davidson, M.H., Reducing residual risk for patients on statin therapy: the potential role of combination therapy. Am J Cardiol. 2005;96(9A): 3K–13K, discussion 34K–35K.
37. Neil, H. A. W., Cooper, J., Betteridge, D. J., et al.: Reductions in all-cause, cancer and coronary mortality in statin-treated patients with heterozygous familial hypercholesterolaemia: a prospective registry study. Eur Heart J. 2008;29:2625–2633.

38. Wang, C., Harris, W. S., Chung, M., et al.: N-3 Fatty acids from fish or fish-oil supplements, but not alpha-linolenic acid, benefit cardiovascular disease outcomes in primary- and secondary-prevention studies: a systematic review. Am J Clin Nutr. July 2006; 84(1):5–17.

39. Canner, P. L., Berge, K. G., Wenger, N. K., et al.: Fifteen year mortality in Coronary Drug Project patients: Long–term benefit with niacin. J Am Coll Cardiol. 1986;8:1245–1255.

40. Vasudevan, A., Hamirani, Y., Jones, P.: Safety of statin: Effects on the muscle and liver. CCJM. 2005;72:990–1000.

41. Martinez, E., Tuset, M., Milinkovic, A., et al.: Management of dyslipidemia in HIV–infected patients receiving antiretroviral therapy. Antivir Ther. Oct 2004;9(5):649–663. Review.

42. Calza, L., Colangeli, V., Manfredi, R., et al.: Rosuvastatin for the treatment of hyperlipidemia in HIV-infected patients receiving protease inhibitors: a pilot study. AIDS. July 2005;19(10): 1103–1105.

43. Wohl, D. A., Waters, D., Simpson, R. J. Jr., et al.: Ezetimibe alone reduces low-density lipoprotein cholesterol in HIV-infected patients receiving combination antiretroviral therapy. Clin Infect Dis. Oct 15 2008;47(8):1105–1108.

44. Klag, M. J., Ford, D. E., Mead, L. A., et al.: Serum cholesterol in young men and subsequent cardiovascular disease. N Engl J Med. 1993;328: 313–318.

45. National Cholesterol Education Program Coordinating Committee. Report of the Expert Panel on Blood Cholesterol in Children and Adolescents. Bethesda, Md: National Heart, Lung and Blood Institute; 1991. NIH Publication no. 91-2732.

46. Daniels, S. R., Greer, F. R., and the Committee on Nutrition. Lipid Screening and Cardiovascular Health in Childhood. Pediatrics. 2008; 122;198–208.

47. Kavey, R. E., Daniels, S. R., Lauer, R. M., et al.: American Heart Association guidelines for primary prevention of atherosclerotic cardiovascular disease beginning in childhood. Circulation. 2003;107(11): 1562–1566; copublished in J Pediatr. 2003;142(4):368–372.

48. McCrindle, B. W., Helden, E., Cullen-Dean, G., et al.: A randomized crossover trial of combination pharmacogenic therapy in children with familial hyperlipidemia. Pediatr Res. 2002;51:715–721.

49. Stein, E. A.: Statins in children. Why and when? Nutr Metab Cardiovasc Dis. 11(Suppl 5);2001:24–29.

50. Tonelli, M., Moyer, L., Sacks, F. M., et al.: for the Cholesterol and Recurrent Events (CARE) Trial Investigators 2003. Pravastatin for secondary prevention of cardiovascular events in persons with mild renal insufficiency. Ann Intern Med. 138;98–110.

51. Molitch, M. E.: Management of dyslipidemias in patients with diabetes and chronic kidney disease. Clin J Am Soc Nephrol. 1:2006;1090–1099.

52. Ritz, E., Wanner, C.: Lipid abnormalities and cardiovascular risk in renal disease. J Am Soc Nephrol. June 1, 2008;19(6):1065–1070.

53. Fellstroem, B. C., Jardine, A. G., Schmieder, R. E., et al.: Rosuvastatin and cardiovascular events in patients undergoing emodialysis. N Engl J Med. 2009;360;1395–1407.

54. Huy, V., Tran, M. T., Truong, Thach Nguyen.: Prevalence of metabolic syndrome in adults in Khanh Hoa, Viet Nam. J Geriatr Cardiol. 2004; 1(2):9–100.

55. McKeigue, P. M., Miller, G. J., Marmot, M. G.: Coronary heart disease in South Asians: a review. J Clin Epidemiol. 1989;42:579–609.

56. Heng, D. M., Lee, J., Chew, S. K., et al.: Incidence of ischemic heart disease and stroke in Chinese, Malays, and Indians in Singapore: Singapore Cardiovascular Cohort Study. Ann Acad Med Singapore. 2000; 29:231–236.

57. Pan, W. H., Chiang, B. N.: Plasma lipid profiles and epidemiology of atherosclerotic diseases in Taiwan—a unique experience. Atherosclerosis. 1995;118:285–295.

58. Thomas, I., Gupta, S., Sempos, C., et al.: Serum lipids in Indian physicians living in the US compared to US born physicians. Atherosclerosis. 1986;61:99–106.

59. Ko, G. T., Cockram, C. S., Woo, J., et al.: Obesity, insulin resistance and isolated low high-density-lipoprotein cholesterol in Chinese subjects. Diabet Med. 2001;18:663–666.

60. Chambers, J. C., Kooner, J. S.: Diabetes, insulin resistance and vascular disease among Indian Asians and Europeans. Semin Vasc Med. 2002;2:199–214.

61. Radhika, G., Ganesan, A., Sathya, R. M., et al.: Dietary carbohydrates, glycemic load and serum high-density lipoprotein cholesterol concentrations among South Indian adults. Eur J Clin Nutr. Nov 7, 2007 [Epub ahead of print].

62. Karthikeyan, G., Koon, K., et al.: Lipid Profile, Plasma Apolipoproteins, and Risk of a First Myocardial Infarction Among Asians: An Analysis From the INTERHEART Study. J Am Coll Cardiol. 2009;53:244–253.

63. Nakamura, H., Arakawa, K., Itakura, H., et al.: Primary prevention of cardiovascular disease with pravastatin in Japan (MEGA Study): a prospective randomised controlled trial. Lancet. 2006;368:1155–1156.

CHAPTER

6

Diet

Thach Nguyen, Timothy Yee, Tung Mai, Tuongman Phan, and Peter McCullough

Chapter Outline

GENERAL DIETARY GUIDELINES FOR HEALTHY PEOPLE

Assuming an environment where there are adequate caloric sources from a variety of foods, what are the modern-day priorities for an optimal diet? From the point of view of preventive cardiology, "optimal" could be defined as without causing excess adiposity, metabolic syndrome, DM, or heart disease. Figure 6-1 presents a healthy eating pyramid,

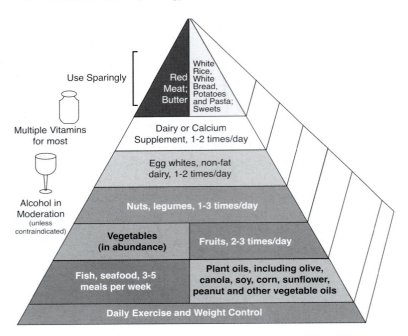

Figure 6-1 Optimal food pyramid for the prevention of obesity, metabolic syndrome, type 2 diabetes, and heart disease.

which summarizes the concepts in this chapter and goes beyond current dietary recommendations from most societies (Figure 6-1).

Protein

First, there is an absolute need for essential amino acids in high-quality sources of protein. The daily intake of protein can vary between 40 to 110 grams per day according to body size, food preferences, and diet composition. The caloric density of protein is 4 kcal/gram. Since many sources of animal and plant protein provide these essential amino acids (isoleucine, leucine, lysine, methionine, phenylalanine, threonine, tryptophan, valine, arginine, histidine), it is important to consider the "package" in which the protein is delivered. The optimal package is fish, because the protein is present with unsaturated omega-3 fatty acids, which are highly favorable for cardiovascular protection.

Next on the priority list are beans, legumes, and nuts, because these foods contain protein along with unsaturated fat and fiber. Following these are nonfat dairy products (fat-free milk, yogurt, etc.) and egg whites, which are excellent sources of protein without adverse macronutrients. Poultry, pork, and red meats all provide sources of protein, but at the cost of introducing saturated fat into the diet. Thus, the package in which the protein is presented is less desirable and becomes fat-promoting.

Fat

The next macronutrient to consider is fat. At 9 kcal/gram, sources of fat can be the most obesity-promoting food of all. Yet, like amino acids, there are essential fatty acids needed for metabolism. There are two families of essential fatty acids—omega-3 or n-3 and omega-6 (n-6). Fats from each of these families are essential, as the body can convert one omega-3 to another omega-3, for example, but cannot create an omega-3 de novo. As cited above, fish and fish oil are the richest and most appropriate sources of omega-3 fatty acids. Multiple epidemiologic studies have found a protective effect within diets high in fish consumption.[1] In addition, randomized trials have conclusively found that fish oil supplementation with ~1 gram of omega-3 fatty acids (eicosapentaenoic acid or EPA, docosahexaenoic acid or DHA) reduced cardiac death in patients with established CAD.[2] The omega-6 fatty acids include gamma-linolenic acid, dihomo-gamma-linolenic acid, and arachidonic acid. Some food sources of omega-3 and omega-6 fatty acids include fish and shellfish, flaxseed (linseed), hemp oil, soy oil, canola (rapeseed) oil, chia seeds, pumpkin seeds, sunflower seeds, leafy vegetables, and walnuts. Beyond these food sources, fats are found to be polyunsaturated and saturated. As a general rule, the greater the degree of saturation, the more likely the source of fat is to promote adiposity, dyslipidemia, and atherogenesis. Trans fat is the common name for a type of unsaturated fat with trans-isomer fatty acid(s). Trans fats may be monounsaturated or polyunsaturated. Most trans fats consumed today are industrially created by partially hydrogenating plant oils—a process developed in the early 1900s and first commercialized as Crisco™ shortening in 1911. The goal of partial hydrogenation is to add hydrogen atoms to unsaturated fats, making them more saturated. These more saturated fats have a higher melting point, which makes them attractive for preserving at room temperature and baking and extends their shelf-life. Given the danger of trans fats and their lack of any nutritional value, there is a considerable public health initiative to remove these types of fat from consumption.

Carbohydrate

Carbohydrates are commonly referred to as sugar and starch, which is the assembly of multiple sugar molecules into a chain. These chains are readily broken down in saliva and the gastrointestinal tract for nearly complete absorption of the base component, sugar. Common forms of starch include rice, potatoes, and foods made from flour (e.g., baked goods, bread, cookies, pasta, bagels).

Another important form of carbohydrate is fiber, which is the third major dietary priority. Fiber is considered a form of carbohydrate (4 kcal/gram); however, forms of soluble and insoluble fiber are not readily absorbed in the gastrointestinal tract and thus offer a much lower caloric load, if any, on the body. The optimal sources of fiber are low-starch fresh fruits and vegetables. There have been a multitude of studies conferring that these sources of food are protective against the development of obesity, metabolic syndrome, and DM.[3] Thus, if forms of carbohydrates that are predominately fiber make up 50–60% of the calories in an 1800 kcal per day diet, 225 to 270 grams of fresh fruits and vegetables per day (5 or 6 servings) are advised.

Assuming adequate resources in most geographic areas, a simple adult multivitamin is advised to handle micronutrient requirements as well as the need for trace metals in the human body.

Foods to Be Avoided or Markedly Restricted

The American Heart Association recommends limiting total fat intake to less than 25–35% of total calories each day (50-70 grams for an 1800 kcal/day diet), saturated fat intake to less than 7% of total daily calories (14 grams), and trans fat intake to less than 1% of total daily calories. Forms of saturated fat in poultry, pork, and red meat should be eaten once or twice per week at most. Foods from animals include beef, beef fat, veal, lamb, pork, lard, poultry fat, butter, cream, milk, cheeses, and other dairy products made from whole milk. All of these foods also contain dietary cholesterol, which should be limited to <300 mg/day. Foods from plants that contain saturated fat include coconut, coconut oil, palm oil, palm kernel oil (often called tropical oils), and cocoa butter. The problem with carbohydrates will be discussed later in the section about diet and diabetes.

DATA MANAGEMENT TIPS (CLINICAL PEARLS)
The Myth of Whole Grains

Whole grains, if not ground and filtered, may impede the breakdown of the starch component in oats, barley, wheat, etc. Whole grains contain no essential amino or fatty acids, are not a satisfactory source of fiber or micronutrients, and are an excess source of calories. Therefore, countering popular recommendations, one approach is to avoid or limit whole grains as they are closer to simple carbohydrates than fruits or vegetables. Whole wheat pasta, baked goods, and other foods simply are not much better than products made from white flour. Rather, they contribute to worsening obesity in those who believe these are healthy choices. Instead of whole grains, more fresh fruits and vegetables are readily advised.

SPECIFIC DIET FOR PREVENTION OF HEART DISEASE

From a CVD point of view, which diet could prevent the occurrence of and progression to CAD, hypertensive CVD, diabetes, CKD, obesity, and diastolic dysfunction (Table 6–1)?

Low-Salt Diet

A diet with 1500 mg of salt is considered a low-salt diet. It is intended for patients who really need to cut down their salt intake, such as patients with HF, CKD, aortic stenosis (AS) or HTN. Lowering sodium to the levels of 1.2 g/day, as achieved in the lowest sodium intake group of the Dietary Approaches to Stop Hypertension (DASH)-Sodium Trial, would be nearly impossible without changes in the food industry, as 75% of sodium intake comes from additions made in food processing.[4-5]

 DATA DECODING TIPS (CLINICAL PEARLS)
Compliance with Low-Salt Diet

One way to know that a patient is adhering to his or her low-sodium diet is when he or she says: "The food is too salty when I eat in restaurants or away from home." I have heard this unsolicited from many patients. (W. Proctor Harvey.)

Low-Carbohydrate Diet[5]

A low-carbohydrate diet, of which the Atkins diet is most representative, recommends two weeks of extreme carbohydrate restriction, followed by gradually increasing carbohydrates to 35 g/day. The Atkins' diet has 68% of total calories from fat, 27% from protein, and 5% from carbohydrates.[6] Low-carbohydrate diets recommend limiting complex and simple sugars, causing the body to oxidize fat to meet energy requirements. During the initial carbohydrate restriction, the body resorts

TABLE 6-1: Diet for Prevention of Cardiovascular Disease

Type of Diet	Clinical Entities to be Prevented
Low-salt diet	HTN, HF
Fluid restriction	HTN, HF
Low-cholesterol diet	CAD, stroke, PAD, metabolic syndrome
Low-protein diet	CKD
Low-glycemic index diet	DM 2
Low-calorie diet	Diastolic dysfunction due to aging, metabolic syndrome, obesity

CAD: coronary artery disease, CKD: chronic kidney disease, DM2: diabetes type 2, HTN: hypertension, HF: heart failure, PAD: peripheral artery disease.

to ketosis for energy needs. Ketones are excreted in the urine with fluid. Rapid initial weight loss may occur from this diuretic effect,[7,8] which can be encouraging. A drastic reduction in carbohydrates also leads to an overall decrease in caloric intake.[9] Weight loss can be sustained by this reduction in caloric intake. Although palatable for the short term, low-carbohydrate diets raise several nutritional and cardiovascular concerns, including a high-protein diet (with adverse effect on liver and kidneys); atherogenesis (because it is high in saturated fat and cholesterol); and lack of fruits, vegetables, and whole grains. Low-carbohydrate diets may increase HDL cholesterol, decrease triglyceride levels, and improve glycemic control, but there appears to be no significant difference in weight loss compared with a low-fat diet at one year.[5, 8]

Diet for Prevention of Diabetes

After a meal, beyond approximately 20 grams of glucose intake, the glucose receptors in the skeletal muscles and liver become oversaturated. The high glycemic load in the bloodstream triggers the release of insulin. It is insulin and insulin-like growth factors from the liver that promote adipocyte growth and proliferation. Importantly, these factors stimulate the uptake of excess nutrients, glucose, and free fatty acids into adipocytes, directly promoting abdominal adiposity (the necessary element in the genesis of the metabolic syndrome and type 2 DM). Simple carbohydrates, such as white rice, have been directly linked to the obesity pandemic, especially in Asia.[9] In addition, it is clear that the glycemic load in the diet is the strongest dietary link to obesity, DM, and heart disease (Figure 6-2).[10]

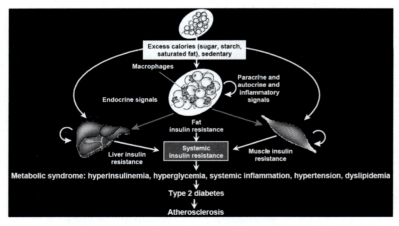

Figure 6-2 Pathogenesis of metabolic syndrome, type 2 diabetes, and atherosclerosis as primarily diseases of diet and inactivity.

SMART THINKING:

The Insulin Resistance Atherosclerosis Study

Question: Are food intake patterns associated with incidence of type 2 diabetes? *Methodology:* This is a post-hoc analysis of 880 middle-aged adults initially free of diabetes from the Insulin Resistance Atherosclerosis Study cohort. At the five-year follow-up, 144 individuals had developed diabetes. The usual dietary intake was ascertained with a 114-item food frequency questionnaire. Using reduced rank regression, a food pattern maximizing the explained variation in PAI-1 and fibrinogen could be identified. Subsequently, the food pattern-diabetes association was evaluated using logistic regression. *Results:* High intake of the food groups of red meat, low-fiber bread and cereal, dried beans, fried potatoes, tomato and vegetables, eggs, cheese, and cottage cheese, and low intake of wine characterized the pattern, which was positively associated with both biomarkers. With increasing pattern score, the odds of diabetes increased significantly (P trend < 0.01). After multivariate adjustment, the odds ratio comparing extreme quartiles was 4.3 (95% CI 1.7-10.8). Adjustment for insulin sensitivity and secretion and other metabolic factors had little impact. *Practical Applications:* The findings in this study provide support for potential behavioral prevention strategies, as a food intake pattern that was strongly related to PAI-1 and fibrinogen and independently predicted type 2 diabetes was identified.[11]

Concrete Instruction: How to Select Foods with Low Sugar Content[5]

For any packaged food, one can simply take the total carbohydrates and subtract the fiber to estimate the sugar and starch (net carbohydrate content). A reasonable heuristic to follow is at any given meal to keep the net carbohydrate content to less than 20 grams to avoid hyperinsulinemia. Another way to check the carbohydrate content is the concept of the glycemic index (GI),[8] which is proposed to guide carbohydrate consumption by ranking the foods based on their rate of conversion to glucose within the human body. The GI uses a scale of 0 to 100, with higher values given to foods that cause the most rapid rise in blood sugar. Pure glucose serves as a reference point and is given a GI of 100. If the blood glucose rises too fast after ingestion (high GI), the pancreas needs to secrete more insulin to bring the blood glucose down by converting the excess glucose to stored fat. Then, the greater the rate of increase in blood glucose, the higher the level of excess insulin will be, which can cause hypoglycemia. The theory behind the GI is to simply minimize insulin-related problems by identifying and avoiding foods that cause too much swing in blood glucose (and insulin level).[5]

However, it is not the high-GI foods that would lead to the increased blood glucose level. The glycemic response depends on both the type *and* the amount of carbohydrate consumed. This concept is known as glycemic load and calculated as follows:

$$GL = GI/100 \times Net\ Carbs$$

(Net Carbs are equal to the Total Carbohydrates minus Dietary Fiber)

Therefore, a patient can control the glycemic response by consuming only low-GI foods and/or a smaller amount of foods.[12] Table 6-2 shows values of the glycemic index (GI) and glycemic load (GL) for a few common foods. GIs of 55 or below are considered low, and 70 or above are considered high. GLs of 10 or below are considered low, and 20 or above are considered high. For complete information, please visit the following website: http://www.nutritiondata. com/glycemic-index.html.[5] A high-GI diet was believed to increase the risk of obesity, diabetes, and CVD.[12]

TABLE 6-2: Glycemic Index and Glycemic Load for Common Foods

Food	GI	Serving Size	Net Carbs	GL
Peanuts	14	4 oz (113 g)	15	2
Bean sprouts	25	1 cup (104 g)	4	1
Grapefruit	25	1/2 large (166 g)	11	3
Pizza	30	2 slices (260 g)	42	13
Low-fat yogurt	33	1 cup (245 g)	47	16
Apples	38	1 medium (138 g)	16	6
Spaghetti	42	1 cup (140 g)	38	16
Carrots	47	1 large (72 g)	5	2
Oranges	48	1 medium (131 g)	12	6
Bananas	52	1 large (136 g)	27	14
Potato chips	54	4 oz (114 g)	55	30
Snickers Bar	55	1 bar (113 g)	64	35
Brown rice	55	1 cup (195 g)	42	23
Honey	55	1 tbsp (21 g)	17	9
Oatmeal	58	1 cup (234 g)	21	12
Ice cream	61	1 cup (72 g)	16	10
Macaroni and cheese	64	1 serving (166 g)	47	30
Raisins	64	1 small box (43 g)	32	20
White rice	64	1 cup (186 g)	52	33
Sugar (sucrose)	68	1 tbsp (12 g)	12	8
White bread	70	1 slice (30 g)	14	10
Watermelon	72	1 cup (154 g)	11	8
Popcorn	72	2 cups (16 g)	10	7
Baked potato	85	1 medium (173 g)	33	28
Glucose	100	(50 g)	50	50

Very Low-Fat Diet

Very low-fat (VLF) diets allow less than 15% of total calories from fat (with an equal distribution of saturated, monounsaturated, and polyunsaturated fats), 15% from protein, and 70% from carbohydrates.[8] The VLF diet includes variations of vegetarian diets that may contain eggs and dairy foods. The VLF diet and intense lifestyle changes produce significant results in terms of reducing risk factors and cardiac event rates. To check the fat content of each food, please visit the following website: http://www.nutritiondata.com/nutrient-search.html.[13]

Concrete Instruction: How to Select Polyunsaturated Fat

Saturated fat is a fat or fatty acid that becomes hard at room temperature. Common saturated fats include butter, lard, palm oil, coconut oil, cottonseed oil, cream, cheese, and red meat. The alternatives to saturated fats are monosaturated fats, such as olive oil. Polyunsaturated fats such as canola oil and corn oil can still cause high total and LDL cholesterol (LDL-C). The goal of a low-fat diet is to substitute unsaturated fats for saturated fats. To learn how to buy foods with low saturated and high polyunsaturated fat content, please visit the following website: http://www.prevention.com/pdf/PV_ShoppingList.pdf.[5]

The Mediterranean Diet[5]

The Mediterranean diet establishes a pattern of eating characterized by the use of olive oil for cooking and little use of dairy fats. Other characteristics of this diet include increased intake of oily fish, fruit, vegetables, nuts (and occasionally low-fat dairy products and red wine), and a lower intake of processed foods, meat, meat products, and hard fats compared with a typical European or U. S. diet.

Although a Mediterranean-style diet has demonstrated greater weight reduction compared to control diets in randomized, controlled trials,[13] the most impressive benefits of the diet are related to lower cardiovascular morbidity and mortality. No isolated aspect of the Mediterranean diet explains these benefits, but much has focused on the omega-3 polyunsaturated fatty acids (N-3 FA). Patients on a Mediterranean diet have been shown to lose more weight, have lower C-reactive protein levels, less insulin resistance, lower total cholesterol and triglycerides, higher HDL levels, and a decreased prevalence of MetS.[5]

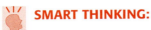

SMART THINKING:

Does the Mediterranean Diet Prevent Heart Disease?

Methodology: The Melbourne Collaborative Cohort Study was a prospective cohort study (mean follow-up: 10.4 years) of 40,653 volunteers aged 40 to 69 years. *Results:* The Mediterranean diet was inversely associated with CVD and ischemic heart disease (IHD) mortality in models adjusting for diabetes, waist-to-hip ratio, BMI, and HTN. For IHD, the hazard ratio (HR) for the highest compared with the lowest quartile of consumption was 0.59 (95% CI: 0.39, 0.89; P for trend 0.03). Associations persisted in analyses excluding people with prior CVD (HR: 0.51; 95% CI: 0.30, 0.88; P for trend 0.03). *Practical Applications:* Among people at high risk for cardiac events, the large absolute reductions in serious vascular events are associated with the Mediterranean diet.[15]

Diet for Losing Weight[5]

Excess adiposity (BMI ≥25 kg/m² with abdominal protuberance) promotes a host of physiologic and metabolic changes that make the human body more susceptible to greater and more rapid weight gain. Apparently obese individuals may have enhanced gastric responsiveness to the hunger hormone ghrelin that is secreted from the stomach and small intestine.[16] In addition, they have markedly reduced production of neuropeptide PYY (3-36) after eating, and thus less satiety with food as compared with normal body weight individuals.[17] Another major physiologic change that occurs in the obese individual is leptin resistance.[18] Leptin is a human hormone produced by the adipocyte that signals the hypothalamus to reduce food intake. When there is a critical increase in body fat, again typically beyond a BMI ≥ 25 kg/m² with abdominal protuberance, leptin resistance develops at the level of the central nervous system, attenuating the satiety signal to reduce food intake. In addition, there is a reduction in the secretion of adiponectin, an adipokine that normally works to regulate adipocyte mass and preserve insulin sensitivity.

Many psychological factors contribute to excess food consumption, including stress, anxiety, and depression. Binge-eating disorder, however, is considered a discrete condition defined as eating to excess, resulting in discomfort and remorse, on two or more occasions per week.[19] There are other psychosocial situations that have been related to eating styles that may lead to excess caloric intake and obesity, including "emotional eating" (eating in response to feelings), "fast food" (eating the most available, processed, high-calorie food), "stress eating" (eating as a response to life stressors), "task snacking" (eating while doing other activities), and "eating alone."[20]

Thus, it is important for patients to understand that there is not one single cause of obesity, and most can see one or more of these six components of the perfect storm as contributing to their obesity problem. It follows then that the most desirable course is to avoid excess adiposity altogether. With the avoidance of excess body fat, the preponderance of evidence would suggest elimination of metabolic syndrome, type 2 DM, and a markedly reduced chance of developing heart disease (Table 6–3).

TABLE 6-3: "Perfect Storm" Theory Explaining the Origins of the Modern-Day Obesity Pandemic and Secondary Epidemics of Metabolic Syndrome and Diabetes

Factor	Explanation
Genetic factors	Permissive genes allow growth of adipose tissue in periods of greater access to food
Expanding adipose tissue alters gut hormone physiology	↑Gut sensitivity to hunger hormone ghrelin ↓Gut secretion of satiety hormone PYY (3-36)
Loss of adipokine control of fat mass	Leptin resistance ↓Adiponectin secretion by adipocytes
Individual psychological factors	Stress eating Emotional eating Binge eating disorder Depression and anxiety as a result of obesity worsens these behaviors
Cultural "food insecurity"	Children urged to eat all food on their plates, even if not hungry Eating behavior pattern continued into adulthood
Societal changes	↑Work hours and productivity Both spouses working ↑Single mothers working ↓Home meal preparation Development of trans-fats and improved preservation techniques ↑Fast food inside and outside the home ↓Obligatory physical activity with labor/activities of daily living

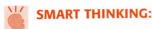

SMART THINKING:

What Diet to Lose Weight?

The possible advantage for weight loss of a diet that emphasizes protein, fat, or carbohydrates has not been established, and there are few studies that extend beyond one year. *Methodology:* One of four diets was randomly assigned to 811 overweight adults; the targeted percentages of energy derived from fat, protein, and carbohydrates in the four diets were 20, 15, and 65%; 20, 25, and 55%; 40, 15, and 45%; and 40, 25, and 35%, respectively. The diets consisted of similar foods and met guidelines for cardiovascular health. The participants were offered group and individual instructional sessions for two years. The primary outcome was the change in body weight after two years in two-by-two factorial comparisons of low fat versus high fat and average protein versus high protein and in the comparison of highest and lowest carbohydrate content. *Results:* At six months, participants assigned to each diet had lost an average of 6 kg, which represented 7% of their initial weight; they began to regain weight after 12 months. By two years, weight loss remained similar in those who were assigned to a diet with 15% protein and those assigned to a diet with 25% protein (3.0 and 3.6 kg, respectively); in those assigned to a diet with 20% fat and those assigned to a diet with 40% fat (3.3 kg for both groups); and in those assigned to a diet with 65% carbohydrates and those assigned to a diet with 35% carbohydrates (2.9 and 3.4 kg, respectively) (P > 0.20 for all comparisons). *Mechanisms of Difference:* Among the 80% of participants who completed the trial, the average weight loss was 4 kg; 14 to 15% of the participants had a reduction of at least 10% of their initial body weight. Satiety, hunger, satisfaction with the diet, and attendance at group sessions were similar for all diets; attendance was strongly associated with weight loss (0.2 kg per session attended). The diets improved lipid-related risk factors and fasting insulin levels. *Practical Applications:* Reduced-calorie diets result in clinically meaningful weight loss regardless of which macronutrients they emphasize.[21]

Low-Caloric Food Selections

Caloric intake from protein, carbohydrate, and fat, along with energy expenditure during rest and activity, provide the basis for estimation of caloric balance.[22] Some foods have very high and nearly complete rates of caloric absorption, including refined sugar, starch (most baked goods), and saturated fat. However, other foods have much lower rates of caloric absorption because of high levels of soluble and insoluble fiber.[23] For example, beans, nuts, and some fruits and vegetables, despite being calorically dense, have not been linked to obesity because of their lower rates of gastrointestinal absorption and the body's inability to fully utilize their caloric content.[24] Furthermore, there is a person-to-person variation in caloric energy utilization of 7 to 9% (only 2% accounted for by measurement techniques).[25] Having considered these factors, studies of caloric balance indicate that ~3500 kcal excess (intake > expenditure) results in a one pound gain of adipose tissue. Most obese patients are in a state of caloric imbalance due to both excess energy intake and reduced caloric expenditure. Thus, modest caloric restriction alone would have little impact on reducing body weight and fat stores. In order to select the foods correctly, there is a need to look at the fullness factor.

Concrete Instruction: How to Eat without Gaining Weight[5]

The fullness factor (FF) is calculated from the food's nutrient content, using values from those nutrients that have been shown experimentally to have the greatest impact on satiety. The values of the FF range from 0 to 5, with the FF for white bread being 1.8. That means that for servings of equal calories, those foods with FF's above 1.8 are more likely to fill you up faster than white bread, and foods with FF's below 1.8 are less likely to fill you up faster than white bread.

Foods that contain large amounts of fat, sugar, and/or starch have low FFs, which people have a higher tendency to overeat. Foods that contain large amounts of water, dietary fiber, and/or protein have the highest FF. These high-FF foods, which include most vegetables, fruits, and lean meats, do a better job of satisfying hunger. Most liquid foods will have above average FF due to their high water content. By simply selecting foods with high FFs, people can improve the chances of consuming fewer calories while simultaneously minimizing their hunger (Table 6-4). For complete information, please visit the following website: http://www. nutritiondata. com/fullness-factor.html.[5]

However, a low fat diet *alone* cannot prevent CVD in a high risk patient, because CVD is result of many other risk factors besides high cholesterol level. This concern is confirmed in the following study.

 SMART THINKING:

Is Dieting Enough?

Methodology: 48,835 postmenopausal women aged 50 to 79 years who participated in the Women's Health Initiative Dietary Modification Trial were randomly assigned to an intervention (19,541) or comparison group (29,294) in a free-living setting. The intervention included intensive behavior modification in group and individual

TABLE 6-4: Fullness Factors for Common Foods

Food	FF	
Bean sprouts	4.6	
Watermelon	4.5	
Grapefruit	4.0	
Carrots	3.8	More filling per Calorie
Oranges	3.5	
Fish, broiled	3.4	Less filling per Calorie
Chicken breast, roasted	3.3	
Apples	3.3	
Sirloin steak, broiled	3.2	
Oatmeal	3.0	
Popcorn	2.9	
Baked potato	2.5	
Low-fat yogurt	2.5	
Banana	2.5	
Macaroni and cheese	2.5	
Brown rice	2.3	
Spaghetti	2.2	
White rice	2.1	
Pizza	2.1	
Peanuts	2.0	
Ice cream	1.8	
White bread	1.8	
Raisins	1.6	
Snickers Bar	1.5	
Honey	1.4	
Sugar (sucrose)	1.3	
Glucose	1.3	
Potato chips	1.2	
Butter	0.5	

sessions designed to reduce total fat intake to 20% of calories and increase intakes of vegetables/fruits to five servings/d and grains to at least six servings/d. The comparison group received diet-related education materials. ***Results:*** By year six, mean fat intake decreased by 8.2% of energy intake in the intervention versus the comparison group, with small decreases in saturated (2.9%), monounsaturated (3.3%), and polyunsaturated (1.5%) fat. LDL cholesterol levels, diastolic blood pressure, and factor VIIc levels were significantly reduced by 3.55 mg/dL, 0.31 mm Hg, and 4.29%, respectively; levels of HDL cholesterol, triglycerides, glucose, and insulin did not significantly differ in the intervention versus comparison groups. There was no difference in the numbers who developed CHD, stroke, and

CVD. Annualized incidence rates were 0.63%, 0.28%, and 0.86% in the intervention group and 0.65%, 0.27%, and 0.88% in the comparison group. The diet had no significant effects on incidence of CHD, stroke, or CVD.[26] *Practical Applications:* A dietary intervention that reduced total fat intake and increased intakes of vegetables, fruits, and grains ALONE did not significantly reduce the risk of CHD, stroke, or CVD in postmenopausal women and achieved only modest effects on CVD risk factors, suggesting that more focused diet, lifestyle interventions, and drugs may be needed to improve risk factors and reduce further CVD in high risk patients.[25]

Diet for Prevention of CKD

In order to prevent CKD in a patient with a normal creatinine level, the diet required is the "renal diet," synonymous with the low-protein diet. It is critical to note that by Stage 3 CKD and beyond, there is no benefit of a low-protein diet. Such protein restriction will not delay the progression toward end-stage renal disease (ESRD) at Stage 3 CKD. The target protein intake is approximately 0.8–1.0 g/ kg/day and sodium intake is 1500–2000 mg/day.[27]

TAKE-HOME MESSAGE

The recommendations in this chapter go far beyond current guidelines, as they should! Under commonly recommended dietary practices, the world has witnessed a runaway obesity pandemic. Understanding the dietary priorities of high-quality sources of protein with fresh fruits and vegetables is critical. By achieving these priorities, one is guaranteed plenty of essential amino and fatty acids.

By eliminating or markedly restricting the three "S's," or sugar, starch, and saturated fat, one not only easily achieves caloric restriction to 1800–2200 kcal/day, but also avoids hyperinsulinemia and the promotion of abdominal adiposity and all of the downstream sequelae.

After accomplishing these macronutrient goals, then limiting cholesterol to < 300 mg/day (not eating egg yolks and liver) and avoiding fried foods adds extra insurance against adiposity and disease.

Adding an adult multivitamin per day and plenty of hydration handles the rest of the essentials for long-term dietary health. Allowing up to one drink of alcohol per day is also advised given the generally supportive information on elevation of high-density lipoprotein cholesterol and associations with reduced rates of heart disease.[28]

Combining the optimal diet with an intense aerobic and strength program over the course of adulthood is the pathway for a lean, strong, and healthy body free of excess adiposity, the metabolic syndrome, type 2 DM, and cardiovascular disease.

References

1. Kris-Etherton, P. M., Harris, W. S., Appel, L.J.: American Heart Association. Nutrition Committee. Fish consumption, fish oil, omega-3 fatty acids, and cardiovascular disease. Circulation. 2002;106:2747–2757.

2. Wang, C., Harris, W. S., Chung, M., Lichtenstein, A. H.: n-3 Fatty acids from fish or fish-oil supplements, but not alpha-linolenic acid, benefit cardiovascular disease outcomes in primary- and secondary-prevention studies: a systematic review. Am J Clin Nutr. 2006;84:5-17.

3. O'Keefe, J. H., Gheewala, N. M., O'Keefe, J. O.: Dietary strategies for improving post-prandial glucose, lipids, inflammation, and cardiovascular health. J Am Coll Cardiol. 2008;51:249–255.

4. Lichtenstein, A. H., et al.: Diet and lifestyle recommendations revision 2006: A scientific statement from the American Heart Association Nutrition Committee. Circulation. 2006 4;114(1):e27.

5. Huy, T., et al.: Integrated primary prevention of cardiovascular disease. In: Management of Complex Cardiovascular Disease, New York, NY: Blackwell Futura, 2009, pp. 129–190.

6. St. Jeor, S. T., Howard, B. V., Prewitt, T. E., et al.: Dietary protein and weight reduction: a statement for healthcare professionals from the Nutrition Committee of the Council on Nutrition, Physical Activity, and Metabolism of the American Heart Association. Circulation. 2001;104: 1869–1874.

7. Bonow, R. O., Eckel, R. H.: Diet, obesity, and cardiovascular risk. N Engl J Med. 2003;348:2057–2058.

8. Parin, P., Michael, C. M., Dominique, A., et al.: Diets and Cardiovascular Disease. J Am Coll Cardiol. 2005;45:1379–1387.

9. Villegas, R., Liu, S., Gao, Y. T., Yang, G., et al.: Prospective study of dietary carbohydrates, glycemic index, glycemic load, and incidence of type 2 diabetes mellitus in middle-aged Chinese women. Arch Intern Med. 2007;167:2310–2316.

10. Ludwig, D. S.: The glycemic index: physiological mechanisms relating to obesity, diabetes, and cardiovascular disease. JAMA. 2002;287: 2414–2423.

11. Liese, A. D., Weis, K. E., Schulz, M., Tooze, J. A.: Food intake patterns associated with incident type 2 diabetes: the Insulin Resistance Atherosclerosis Study. Diabetes Care. 2009;32:263–268

12. Foster-Powell, K., Holt, S. H.A., Brand-Miller, J. C.: International table of glycemic index and glycemic load values. 2002; Am J Clin Nutr. 2002;76:5–56.

13. Howard, B.V., Horn, L.V., Hsia, J., et al.: Low-fat dietary pattern and risk of cardiovascular disease: The women's health initiative randomized controlled dietary modification trial. JAMA. 2006;295:655–666.

14. Kris-Etherton, P. M., Harris, W. S., Appel, L. J., et al.: Fish consumption, fish oil, omega-3 fatty acids, and cardiovascular disease. Circulation. 2002;106:2747–2757.

15. Hu, F.B.: The mediterranean diet and mortality – olive oil and beyond. N Engl J Med. 2003;348;2595-2596.

16. Cremonini, F., Camilleri, M., Vazquez Roque, M., et al.: Obesity does not increase effects of synthetic ghrelin on human gastric motor functions. Gastroenterology. 2006;131:1431–1439.
17. Le Roux, C. W., Batterham, R. L., Aylwin, S. J., et al.: Attenuated peptide YY release in obese subjects is associated with reduced satiety. Endocrinology. 2006;147:3–8.
18. Zhang, Y., Scarpace, P. J.: The role of leptin in leptin resistance and obesity. Physiol Behav. 2006;88:249–256.
19. Yanovski, S. Z.: Binge eating disorder and obesity in 2003: could treating an eating disorder have a positive effect on the obesity epidemic? Int J Eat Disord. 2003;34;Suppl:S117–120.
20. Scherwitz, L., Kesten, D.: Seven eating styles linked to overeating, overweight, and obesity. Explore (NY). 2005;1:342–359.
21. Sacks, F. M., Bray, G. A., Carey, V. J., et al.: Comparison of weight-loss diets with different compositions of fat, protein, and carbohydrates. N Engl J Med. 2009;360:859–873.
22. Vanhecke, T. E., Franklin, B. A., Lillystone, M. A., et al.: Caloric expenditure in the morbidly obese using dual energy x-ray absorptiometry. J Clin Densitom. 2006;9:438–444.
23. Baer, D. J., Rumpler, W. V., Miles, C. W., et al.: Dietary fiber decreases the metabolizable energy content and nutrient digestibility of mixed diets fed to humans. J Nutr. 1997;127:579–586.
24. Miles, C. W.: The metabolizable energy of diets differing in dietary fat and fiber measured in humans. J Nutr. 1992;122:306–311.
25. Elia, M., Stratton, R., Stubbs, J.: Techniques for the study of energy balance in man. Proc Nutr Soc. 2003;62:529–537.
26. Howard, B. V., Horn, L. V., Hsia, J., et al.: Low-Fat Dietary Pattern and Risk of Cardiovascular Disease: The Women's Health Initiative Randomized Controlled Dietary Modification Trial. JAMA. 2006;295:655–666.
27. Teta, D., Phan, O., Halabi, G., et al.: Chronic renal failure: what diet? Rev Med Suisse. 2006;55:566–569.
28. Goldberg, I. J., Mosca, L., Piano, M. R., et al.: Nutrition Committee, Council on Epidemiology and Prevention, and Council on Cardiovascular Nursing of the American Heart Association. AHA Science Advisory: Wine and your heart: a science advisory for healthcare professionals from the Nutrition Committee, Council on Epidemiology and Prevention, and Council on Cardiovascular Nursing of the American Heart Association. Circulation. 2001;103:472–475.

Section III

Disturbances to the Blood Circulation

Hypertensive Cardiovascular Disease

CHAPTER

7

Huy V. Tran, Timothy Yee, Jose Agusti, Tuongman Phan, and Dayi Hu

Chapter Outline

DEFINITION

Hypertension (HTN) is defined as an elevated blood pressure (BP) level, which produces a variety of structural changes in the arteries that supply blood to the brain, heart, kidneys, and elsewhere.

Population in Focus

The risks of stroke, ischemic heart disease, renal failure, and other diseases are high in patients with high BP and recently, the risks have been found to be high even among people with average and below-average BP.[1] For the majority of the adult population, systolic blood pressure (SBP) is a stronger predictor of cardiovascular (CV) risk than diastolic blood pressure (DBP).[2] However, in the Framingham Heart Study, for participants less than 50 years of age, DBP better predicts the development of coronary artery disease (CAD). Between the ages of 50 and 59, there is a transition period, with DBP and SBP assuming comparable risks. After the age of 60, the risk of CAD remains positively correlated with SBP but is inversely related to DBP.[3]

Strategic Programming

Based on a computational cardiac model, the index problem of HTN is the status of morbidly elevated blood pressure in the CV system. This is a software problem. There are no upstream areas because the status of elevated high blood pressure permeates every segment of the CV system.

In the investigation of patients with HTN, the strategy is to identify patients with HTN through data collection of a blood pressure measurement, a comprehensive history, and a physical examination. The next step is to perform data mining by checking the urine analysis, electrolytes, BUN, and creatinine level in order to confirm (data converting) the main diagnosis of HTN and to rule out (data filtering) the different possible secondary causes of HTN.

DATA COLLECTING
Investigation Master Plan

When a physician comes to see a patient suspected of having HTN, there are seven main areas of interest for data collecting (history and physical examination), based on a computational cardiac model. These areas are summarized in Table 7-1.

The main area of interest is high blood pressure. In general, a patient with HTN is asymptomatic. There are no subjective symptoms or physical findings directly related to HTN. This is a software problem causing hardware derangement (structural changes) in the CV system only after long years of exposure to uncontrolled HTN. In patients with HTN, the blood pressure was programmed (set) at a high level. It is similar to the situation of the temperature in a house with the thermostat set too high in summer, despite the fact that the air conditioning system works perfectly if turned on. This is only a futuristic speculation.

There are no upstream areas for essential HTN. Unless the HTN is caused by stenosis of the renal artery or pheochromocytoma, the upstream areas are the kidneys or the adrenal glands. However, there are no signs or symptoms from the kidneys or adrenal glands per se. The downstream area is the aorta and the distal peripheral arteries.

As for the system configuration, HTN is caused by a software problem. There is nothing wrong with the configuration of the CV system. The work-around configuration is not applicable here.

If there is long-standing uncontrolled HTN, the cardiovascular system is an end-organ which bears the direct effect of high blood pressure by having left ventricular hypertrophy. Acute myocardial infarction and heart failure are indirectly affected by uncontrolled HTN. The symptoms and signs are of the end-organ damage or failure and not due to HTN per se.

With regard to the network (the whole body), long-standing uncontrolled HTN can cause stroke, transient ischemic attack (TIA), peripheral arterial disease, and kidney failure in the cerebral, peripheral, and renal vasculature.

History

For a patient coming to you because of high blood pressure or with high BP first discovered during an office visit, the data needed for a comprehensive history to be captured are listed in Table 7-1.

Physical Examination

The physical examination includes an appropriate measurement of BP, with verification in the contralateral arm. An accurate device is fundamental to all BP measurement techniques. Details of devices and the practice guidelines for accurate noninvasive BP measurement can be obtained at www.dableducation.org. SBP should be noted as the appearance of Korotkoff (K1) and DBP with the disappearance of sounds (K4); when sounds persist down to zero, muffling of sounds (phase 4) should be recorded for DBP and need to be written clearly K1/0/K4.[4]

DATA COLLECTING TIPS (CLINICAL PEARLS)
Estimate the Blood Pressure without A Sphygmomanometer

The systolic pressure can be estimated by the amount of brachial arterial compression—mild, moderate or marked—required to obliterate the ipsilateral radial pulse palpated by the examiner's other hand. When relatively mild brachial arterial compression obliterates the radial artery in adults, the systolic pressure is around 120 mm Hg or less. When considerable compression is required to achieve this, the systolic pressure usually exceeds 160 mm Hg.[4]

DATA COLLECTING TIPS (CLINICAL PEARLS)
Inaudible Korotkoff Sounds

If cuff deflation is too slow, venous congestion serves to elevate diastolic pressure and to decrease the intensity of Korotkoff sounds; systolic pressure is underestimated, while diastolic pressure is overestimated. The cuff should be deflated rapidly after the diastolic blood pressure is determined, and at least one minute should pass before blood pressure determinations are repeated on the same limb. If the Korotkoff sounds are difficult to hear in the brachial artery, audibility can be improved by having the patient open and close hes or her fist vigorously a half dozen times.[4]

TABLE 7-1: Investigation Master Plan

	Mechanism	Symptoms	Signs	Findings
Index Problem: Essential Hypertension	Software problem	None	None	High BP by sphygmomanometer
HTN caused by renal artery stenosis	Hardware problem	None	None	Renal artery stenosis
Upstream		None	None	None
Downstream		Look at cardiovascular system	Look at cardiovascular system	Look at cardiovascular system
System Configuration	Normal	None	None	None
Work Around	Normal	None	None	None
Cardiovascular System	The CV system bears all the adverse effects of uncontrolled HTN	Symptoms of LV dysfunction, HF	Signs of LVH, LVD, HF	LVH, HF
Network (Other Systems)	The pulmonary vascular system, the kidneys, and the brain bear all the adverse effect of uncontrolled HTN	Symptoms of pulmonary congestion, RHF, stroke, TIA, renal failure	Signs of pulmonary congestion, RHF, stroke, TIA, renal failure	Pulmonary congestion, RHF, stroke, TIA, renal failure

BP: blood pressure, CV: cardiovascular, HF: heart failure, HTN: hypertension, LV: left ventricle, LVD: left ventricular dysfunction, LVH: left ventricular hypertrophy, RHF: right heart failure, TIA: transient ischemic attack.

⚕ DATA COLLECTING TIPS (CLINICAL PEARLS)
How to Measure the Blood Pressure if the Cuff Is Small?

If the only available cuff does not adequately encircle the arm, it can be used on the forearm, while the stethoscope is applied to the radial artery for detection of Korotkoff sounds. The technique is appropriate for a forearm of relatively uniform circumference (cylindrical) but not when a conical forearm prevents uniform cuff application. Properly determined forearm blood pressure is a reasonable estimate of brachial arterial blood pressure.[4]

JOB DESCRIPTION:

How to Measure the Blood Pressure in the Leg

Upper extremity blood pressure is routinely taken in the supine position, but lower extremity blood pressure using the popliteal artery is recorded with the patient prone. The popliteal pulse is sometimes difficult to feel even in normal subjects. The thigh cuff is then inflated slowly to a level just above the brachial arterial systolic pressure. It is important to emphasize that slow inflation is important in order to avoid discomfort and pain induced by rapid compression of the thigh. Systolic and diastolic pressures are estimated by auscultation of Korotkoff sounds, as described for the brachial artery. If this technique proves unsatisfactory, the patient can be returned to the supine position and a cuff of appropriate size (often an arm cuff) applied to the lower half of the calf. Korotkoff sounds can then be sought by applying the bell of the stethoscope to the dorsalis pedis or posterior tibial arteries after they have been identified by palpation.[4]

The only direct effect of uncontrolled HTN is by the examination of the optic fundi, which shows hypertensive retinal changes. The examinations looking for comorbidities and findings of other components of cardiovascular disease to be sought are listed in Table 7-2.

DATA PROCESSING (FORMULATING A PRELIMINARY DIAGNOSIS)

The diagnosis of HTN is made when the SBP is >120 mm Hg and the diastolic BP is >80 mm Hg.

DATA MINING (WORK-UP)

When a physician comes to see a patient with HTN, there is no test for HTN per se. The physician needs to check the status of the end-organ

TABLE 7-2: Focuses of the Physical Examination
Looking for Comorbidities of HTN
Calculation of the body mass index (BMI) and measure of the waist circumference
Palpation of the thyroid gland
Findings for Other Components of Cardiovascular Disease
Auscultation for carotid, abdominal, and femoral bruits
A thorough examination of the heart and lungs
Examination of the abdomen for enlarged kidneys, masses, distended urinary bladder, and abnormal aortic pulsation
Palpation of the lower extremities for edema and pulses
Neurological assessment

failure caused by long-standing uncontrolled HTN or investigate the secondary causes of HTN.

The selective tests to investigate the causes of HTN and the effects of HTN on target organs are listed in Table 7-3. Serum creatinine values should also be used to estimate the creatinine clearance with the Cockroft Gault formula or glomerular filtration rate (GFR) by the Modification of Diet in Renal Disease (MDRD) formula. The formula to calculate GFR is available at www.hdcn. com/calcf/gfr.htm. Optional tests include measurement of urinary albumin excretion or albumin/creatinine ratio (ACR). When secondary HTN is suspected, the work-up is included as listed in Table 7-3.

Ambulatory BP Monitoring

The growing availability of ambulatory BP monitoring (ABPM) or self-monitored home BP measurement (SBPM) in combination with conventional clinic BP measurement (CBPM) has allowed the identification of four different patterns when describing the BP status. These include true normotension, sustained HTN, white-coat HTN, and masked HTN. Indications for ABPM and SBPM are listed in Table 7-4.

DATA CONVERTING (FORMULATING THE DEFINITIVE DIAGNOSIS)

The Joint National Committee (JNC) on Prevention, Detection, Evaluation and Treatment of High BP provides guidelines for HTN classification and management. The seventh report from this committee reclassified BP for adults aged 18 years or older, as shown in Table 7-5.[4]

TABLE 7-3: Laboratory Tests for HTN

Test to investigate the causes of HTN

Urinalysis
Is renal failure the cause of HTN?

Plasma glucose
Is diabetic nephropathy the cause of HTN?

Serum creatinine
Does renal failure cause HTN?

Test to investigate the extent of target organ damage

Serum potassium
Is there hypokalemia from diuretics?
Is there hyperkalemia from CKD?

Hematocrit
Does the patient have anemia from CKD?

Chest radiography
Is the heart enlarged?
Does the patient have CHF from uncontrolled HTN?

Electrocardiogram (ECG)
Does the patient have LVH or prior MI?

CHF: congestive heart failure, CKD: chronic kidney disease, HTN: hypertension, LVH: left ventricular hypertrophy, MI: myocardial infarction.

TABLE 7-4: Indications for ABPM and SBPM

Clinical Situations in Which ABPM May be Helpful[6]

Suspected white-coat HTN in patients with HTN and no target organ damage
Apparent drug resistance (office resistance)
Hypotensive symptoms with antihypertensive medication
Episodic HTN
Autonomic dysfunction

SBPM Should Be Encouraged in Order to:[7]

Provide information on the BP lowering effect of treatment at trough
Improve patient's adherence to treatment regimen
Rule out doubts about technical reliability/environmental conditions of ambulatory BP data

SBPM Should Be Discouraged Whenever:[7]

It causes anxiety in the patient
It induces self-modification of the treatment regimen

TABLE 7-5: Classification of Blood Pressure for Adults[4]

BP Classification	Systolic BP (mm Hg)	Diastolic BP (mm Hg)
Normal	< 120	and < 80
Prehypertension	120–139	or 80-89
Stage 1 HTN	140–159	or 90-99
Stage 2 HTN	≥ 160	or ≥ 100

TYPES OF HYPERTENSION

HTN includes sustained HTN, white-coat HTN, masked HTN, pre-HTN, isolated systolic HTN, and systolic and diastolic HTN.

Sustained Hypertension or Clinic Hypertension

BP levels for initial detection of sustained HTN should be based on the average of two or more readings, separated by two minutes taken at each of two or more visits after an initial screening by a physician or a nurse, unless it is a hypertensive crisis.

White-Coat Hypertension or Isolated Clinic Hypertension (ICH)

This is a condition in which an individual is hypertensive (systolic/diastolic BP>140/90 mm Hg) when measured in the doctor's office (CBPM), but pressures measured outside the medical environment by ABPM or SBPM technique are normal. The prevalence of ICH is about 15% of the general population.[7]

Masked Hypertension or Isolated Ambulatory Hypertension (IAH)

This phenomenon refers to patients in whom CBPM is normal but ABPM or SBPM is increased. Although no definitive data are available, IAH has been estimated to occur in approximately 10 to 30% of individuals. Outcome studies have suggested that IAH increases the CV risk, which appears to be close to that of in- and out-of-office HTN.[6] One recent meta-analysis indicates that the incidence of CV events is not significantly different between ICH and true normotension, whereas the outcome is worse in patients with masked or sustained HTN.[7]

Prehypertension

The new category of prehypertension was proposed because of the observation that patients with high BP have two times the risk of developing definite HTN in their lifetime. Prehypertension is defined as shown in Table 7-5.

Isolated Systolic Hypertension

Elderly patients may develop a form of HTN referred as isolated systolic HTN that is defined as a SBP = 140 mm Hg or greater in the absence of an elevated diastolic BP (DBP less than 90 mm Hg). Isolated systolic HTN is a pathologic process due to loss of compliance of the arterial system and is associated with an increased CV risk. The prevalence of isolated systolic HTN increases with age, and 65% of patients over the age of 60 years will have this form of HTN.[4]

Confirmation of Causes of HTN

The most common cause of HTN is still not fully understood and is classified as primary or essential HTN. This category accounts for about 90% of all hypertensive patients. Secondary causes of HTN should be considered in HTN that is severe, begins at a young age, or is resistant to standard therapy. Common causes of secondary HTN are listed in Table 7-6.[4] Chronic kidney disease (CKD) can be subdivided into patients with fibromuscular dysplasia (usually seen in young women) and patients with atherosclerotic disease. Endocrine diseases (especially adrenal and thyroid disorders) are associated with HTN. Diabetes is frequently associated with HTN, as nearly 70% of diabetic patients will develop HTN during the course of the disease. With the obesity epidemic, obstructive sleep apnea has become more common and can be associated with a resistant form of HTN, at least until hypoxia is corrected.

Comprehensive Definition of HTN

HTN is not just a number to be lowered. A high blood pressure reading is part of a clinical entity called hypertensive cardiovascular disease. The

---

TABLE 7-6: Identifiable Causes of Secondary Hypertension[4]

Chronic kidney disease
Coarctation of the aorta
Cushing's syndrome and other glucocorticoid excess states including
    chronic steroid therapy
Drug-induced or drug-related HTN
Obstructive uropathy
Pheochromocytoma
Primary aldosteronism and other mineralocorticoid excess states
Renovascular HTN
Sleep apnea
Thyroid or parathyroid disease

relationship between BP and the risk of future CV events is continuous, consistent, and independent of other risk factors. The higher the BP, the greater is the chance of MI, heart failure (HF), stroke, and kidney diseases. Therefore, an assessment of global CV risk is the key point in the evaluation of apparently healthy subjects or people with potential for having HTN or CVD in the strategies of integrated primary prevention of HTN and CV events. Management of all risk factors is essential and should be followed for controlling these coexisting problems that contribute to the overall CV risk.

The CV risk factors include the traditional major risk factors (HTN, dyslipidemia, cigarette smoking, DM, age, and family history of premature CVD).[4] The other confirmed risk factors include obesity (especially central obesity) (BMI $\geq$30 kg/m²), fibrinogen, micro-albuminuria or estimated glomerular filtration rate <60 mL/min, impaired glucose tolerance (IGT), impaired fasting glucose (IFG), alcohol abuse, lack of physical activity, and ethnicity.[4] The cluster of three out of five risk factors among abdominal obesity, elevated fasting blood glucose, BP > 130/85 mm Hg, low HDL-cholesterol, and high TG (as defined previously) indicates the presence of metabolic syndrome.[8]

Risk Stratification

The 2003 World Health Organization/International Society Hypertension (WHO/ISH) statement classified the total CV risk in three categories.[5] The terms "low," "moderate," and "high" risk are used to indicate an approximate risk of CV morbidity and mortality as estimated by the Framingham[8] or the SCORE (Systematic COronary Risk Evaluation) models[9] or the 2007 WHO charts.[10] The three major risk categories with progressively increasing absolute likelihood of developing a major CV event (fatal and nonfatal stroke and MI within the next 10 years) include: (1) low risk – less than 15%; (2) medium risk – 15–20%; and (3) high risk – greater than 20%. These are listed in Table 7-7.

Markers of Early Hypertensive CVD and of Severity of Hypertensive CVD

Early markers of hypertensive CVD may become evident in patients at BP levels between 120/80 and 139/89 mm Hg (Table 7-8). The presence of these early markers would classify patients as stage 1 HTN of the Hypertension Writing Group of the American Society of Hypertension (WGASH).[11] The subclinical damage and clinical conditions are listed in Table 7-9.

TABLE 7-7: WHO/ISH Stratification of Risk to Quantify Prognosis[5]

Other Risk Factors Disease History	Blood Pressure (mm Hg)		
	Grade 1 SBP 140–159 or DBP 90–99	Grade 2 SBP 160–179 or DBP 100–109	Grade 3 SBP ≥180 and or DBP ≥110
No other risk factors	Low	Medium	High
One or two risk factors	Medium	Medium	High
≥3 risk factors or TOD or ACC	High	High	High

ACC: associated clinical condition, DBP: diastolic blood pressure, SBP: systolic blood pressure, TOD: target organ damage.

PROGRAMMED MANAGEMENT

Strategic Programming

The primary goal of treatment of the hypertensive patient is to achieve the maximum reduction in the long-term total risk of CV and renal morbidity and mortality. In most patients, the target of controlled BP

TABLE 7-8: Early Markers of Hypertensive CVD[13]

System	Physiologic Alterations
Blood-Pressure	Loss of nocturnal BP dipping
	Exaggerated BP response to exercise
	Salt sensitivity
	Widened pulse pressure
Cardiac	Left ventricular hypertrophy (mild)
	Increased atrial filling pressure
	Decreased diastolic relaxation
Vascular	Increased central arterial stiffness or pulse wave velocity
	Small artery stiffness
	Increased systemic vascular resistance
	Increased wave reflection and systolic pressure augmentation
	Increased carotid intima-media thickness
	Coronary calcification
	Endothelial dysfunction
Renal	Microalbuminuria (urinary albumin excretion 30–300 mg/d)
	Elevated serum creatinine
	Reduced estimated GFR (60–90 mL/min)
Retinal	Hypertensive retinal changes

TABLE 7-9: Hypertensive Target Organ Damage and Overt CVD[13]

System	Evidence of Target Organ Damage and CVD
Cardiac	Left ventricular hypertrophy (moderate to severe)
	Systolic or diastolic cardiac dysfunction
	Symptomatic heart failure
	Myocardial infarction
	Angina pectoris
	Ischemic heart disease or revascularization
Vascular	Peripheral arterial disease
	Carotid arterial disease
	Aortic aneurysm
	Wide pulse pressure (> 65 mm Hg)
Renal	Albuminuria (> 300 mg/d)
	Chronic kidney disease (GFR < 60 mL/min) or ESRD
Cerebrovascular	Stroke
	Transient ischemic attack

CVD: cardiovascular disease, GFR: glomerular filtration rate, ESRD: end-stage renal disease.

is under 140/90 mm Hg along with concurrently controlling all other coexisting modifiable CV risk factors, as indicated by the current guidelines. In the special groups of patients, this target is under 130/80 mm Hg.[4] In most current guidelines, these groups are diabetic patients or those with chronic kidney disease. Some other groups of patients who fall under this target are those with CAD, metabolic syndrome, microalbuminuria, and heart failure[11] (Table 7-10).

Lifestyle Modification

A lifestyle modification program is recommended for all individuals with prehypertension and HTN, including a well-balanced diet with

TABLE 7-10: Management Master Plan

Data Management	Keep BP below 140/90 or 120/80 mm Hg
	Low-salt diet
	Pharmacologic therapy
	Preventive measures
Root-Cause Correction	Denervation of the renal artery
	Stenting of the renal artery stenosis
System Configuration Correction	None
Work-Around Management	Not applicable
System Replacement	Kidney transplant

low sodium, reduced saturated fat and cholesterol, increased aerobic physical activity, no smoking, and weight reduction in obese and over-weight individuals.

Diet

Patients with HTN benefit from a healthy diet by adoption of the Dietary Approaches to Stop Hypertension (DASH) eating plan, which is a diet high in fruits, vegetables, low-fat dairy products, whole grains, nuts, fish, and poultry as well as reduced total and saturated fats. Reduced intake of red meat, sweets, and sugar-containing beverages is encouraged, which results in a diet high in potassium, calcium, magnesium, and fiber. This dietary approach has been shown to lower BP by 10 mm Hg.[12]

Low-Sodium Diet

A diet with 1.5 g/day sodium is recommended for patients who really need to cut down their sodium intake (including patients with HTN). However, in view of the readily available high-sodium food supply and the currently high levels of sodium consumption, a reduction in sodium intake to 1.5 g/day (65 mmol/day) is not easily achievable. In the in-terim, an achievable recommendation is 2.4 g/day sodium (100 mmol/day) or 6.4 g/day sodium chloride (salt).[13]

Stop Smoking

All hypertensive patients should be asked about their smoking habits and advised and assisted with the effort to stop smoking. Follow-up, referral to special programs, or pharmacotherapy (including nicotine replace-ment and pharmacological treatment) should be arranged. Exposure to environmental tobacco smoke at home and work should be avoided.[13]

Weight Loss

Weight loss of as little as 10 lb (4.5 kg) reduces BP and/or prevents HTN in a large proportion of overweight persons, although the ideal is to maintain a consistently normal body weight. Most weight loss occurs because of decreased caloric intake. The initial goal of weight loss ther-apy should be to reduce body weight by approximately 10% from base-line. With success, further weight loss can be attempted if indicated by further assessment.[13]

Exercise

The National Heart, Lung and Blood Institute (NHLBI) recommend an increase in physical activity as an important part of any weight man-agement program. Sustained physical activity is most helpful in the prevention of weight regain. For all patients, 30 to 60 minutes of mod-erate-intensity aerobic activity, such as brisk walking, on most, prefer-ably all, days of the week, supplemented by an increase in daily lifestyle activities (e.g., walking breaks at work, gardening, household work)

TABLE 7-11: Lifestyle Modifications for Patients with Hypertension*[4]

Modification	Recommendation	Approximate SBP Reduction (Range)[†]
Weight reduction	Maintain normal body weight (body mass index 18.5–24.9 kg/m^2).	5–20 mm Hg/10 kg
Adopt DASH eating plan	Consume a diet rich in fruits vegetables and low-fat dairy products with a reduced content of saturated and total fat.	8–14 mm Hg
Dietary sodium reduction	Reduce dietary sodium intake to no more than 100 mmol per day (2.4 g sodium or 6 g sodium chloride).	2–8 mm Hg
Physical activity	Engage in regular aerobic physical activity, such as brisk walking (at least 30 minutes per day, most days of the week).	4–9 mm Hg
Moderation of alcohol consumption	Limit consumption to no more than 2 drinks (24 oz beer, 10 oz wine, or 3 oz of 80-proof whiskey) per day in most men and no more than one drink per day in women and lighter-weight persons	2–4 mm Hg

DASH, Dietary Approaches to Stop Hypertension; SBP, systolic blood pressure.
*For overall CV risk reduction, stop smoking.
[†]The effects of implementing these modifications are dose- and time-dependent and could be greater for some individuals.

is recommended. The lifestyle therapeutic measures and level of BP reduction are summarized in Table 7-11.[4]

Pharmacologic Treatment
Strategic Programming

Therapy should be started gradually, and target BP achieved progressively. Choice of drug monotherapy or combination therapy aims to control BP through evidence-based studies with lower CV events and death while minimizing side effects or toxicity. These drugs may improve control of HTN by being affordable and available at low cost, thus improving compliance. A single daily dose provides 24-hour efficacy.

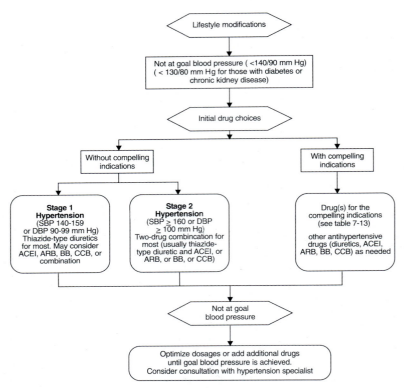

Figure 7-1 Algorithm for treatment of HTN. ACEI, angiotension converting enzyme inhibitor, ARB, angiotensin receptor blocker; BB, beta blocker; CCB, calcium channel blocker; DBP, diastolic blood pressure; SBP, systolic blood pressure.

The algorithm for treatment of HTN is summarized in Figure 7-1.[4] Based on medical evidence, the national and international guidelines have advised use of the following four major classes of antihypertensive agents: thiazide diuretics, calcium antagonists (CCBs), angiotensin-converting enzyme inhibitors (ACEIs), and angiotensin receptor blockers (ARBs) in the initiation and maintenance of antihypertensive treatment, as a single drug or in combination.[4] A brief summary of drugs used for the essential HTN is provided in Table 7-12.

Treatment can start with a single drug, which should initially be administered at a low dose. If blood pressure is not controlled, either a full dose of the initial agent can be given or patients can be switched to an agent of a different class. However, use of more than one agent is necessary to achieve target BP in the majority of patients.[4]

TABLE 7-12: Outline of Drugs Used to Treat Hypertension

Class	Common Generic Names[1]	Mode of Action	Duration of Action	Usage Notes
Thiazide-type diuretic	Hydroclorothiazide	Vasodilatation and moderate diuresis	Commonly once daily morning use	Low-dose thiazide-type diuretics produce (near) maximum BP lowering. Generally well tolerated.
Potassium-sparing diuretics	Spirinolactone	Weakly diuretic, given in addition to or in combination with a thiazide to retain potassium	Once or twice a day	Few side effects. Used to prevent or treat low level potassium in the blood. Not to be used with potassium supplements. Use with an ACEI can cause high potassium levels
Beta blockers (not as first choice alone)	Atenolol, bisoprolol, metoprolol, propanolol, sotalol, carvedilol	Blocking beta receptors in the heart slows down and decreases the force of contraction of the heart	Vary by drug from once to bid	Contraindicated with asthma, heart-block or a rate-limiting calcium-channel blocker. Caution applies to patients with diabetes or peripheral vascular diseases.
Calcium-channel blockers	Dihydropyridines amlodipine, felodipine, lacidipine, nifedipine, 'rate-limiting' diltiazem, verapamil	Reduced flow of calcium to vascular smooth muscle, reducing contraction efficiency and relaxing vasculature Additionally affect the conduction system, slowing the heart rate	Vary by drug from once to bid	Reported side effects include initial headaches, palpitations, facial flushing, and ankle swelling. Caution against use in heart failure or with beta blockers.

(continued)

TABLE 7-12: Outline of Drugs Used to Treat Hypertension *(continued)*

Class	Common Generic Names[1]	Mode of Action	Duration of Action	Usage Notes
Angiotensin converting enzyme (ACE) inhibitors	Catopril, enalapril, lisinopril, perindopril, ramipril, trandolapril	Prevent conversion of the protein angiotensin I to angiotensin II, which raises BP	Vary by drug from once to bid	Dose titration and monitoring are necessary. Contraindicated in pregnancy and some kidney diseases. Caution when initiating in a patients on a diuretic or in renal failure.
Angiotensin receptor blockers (ARBs) or angiotensin II receptors antagonists	Candesartan, irbesartan, losartan, valsartan, telmisartan	Block the action of angiotensin II (which raises BP) by directly blocking the receptor site	Once daily	Contraindications and side-effect profile similar to that of ACE-inhibitors, but ARBs are not associated with the persistent dry cough.
Alpha receptor blockers	Doxazosin, prazosin, terazosin	Block receptor sites in blood vessel wall, relaxing vessels	Vary by drug from once to bid	These tend to be used as adjunctive treatment. Beneficial side effect on lipid profile. Most common side effects are initial dizziness, headache, flushing, nasal congestion, fluid retention, and a rapid heart beat.
Direct renin inhibition	Aliskiren	Blocks the action of renin/pro-renin	Once daily	Similar to that of ARBs at doses up to 300 mg daily. At the 600-mg dose, an increased incidence of diarrhea occurs.

Compelling Indications

Compelling indications for specific therapy involve high-risk conditions that can be a direct sequel of HTN (HF, CAD, CKD, recurrent stroke) or that are commonly associated with HTN (diabetes, high CAD risk). The choices of drugs for these compelling indications are indicated by favorable outcome data from the clinical trials. Therapeutic decisions in such individuals should be directed at both the compelling indication and BP lowering. If a drug is not tolerated or is contraindicated, then one of the other classes proven to reduce CV events should be used instead.[4] The compelling indications and possible contraindications to use of antihypertensive drugs are listed in Table 7-13 and Table 7-14.[4,5]

Follow-Up

Most patients should return for follow-up and adjustment of medications at approximately monthly intervals until the BP goal is reached.

TABLE 7-13: Compelling Indications for Specific Antihypertensive Drugs[5]

Compelling Indication	Preferred Drug	Primary Endpoint
Elderly with isolated systolic hypertension	Diuretic	Stroke
	DHCCB	Stroke
Renal Disease		
Diabetic nephropathy type 1	ACE inhibitor	Progression of renal failure
Diabetic nephropathy type 2	ARB	Progression of renal failure
Nondiabetic nephropathy	ACE inhibitor	Progression of renal failure
Cardiac Disease		
Post-MI	ACE inhibitor	Mortality
Left ventricular dysfunction	Beta blocker	Mortality
	ACE inhibitor	Heart failure
	ACE inhibitor	Mortality
CHF (diuretics almost always included)	Beta blocker	Mortality
	Spironolactone	Mortality
Left ventricular hypertrophy	ARB	Cardiovascular morbidity and mortality
Cerebrovascular disease	ACE inhibitor + diuretic	Recurrent stroke
	Diuretic	Recurrent stroke

ACE: angiotensin-converting enzyme, ARB: angiotensin receptor blocker, CHF: congestive heart failure, DHCCB: dihydropyridine calcium channel blocker, MI: myocardial infarction.

TABLE 7-14: Compelling and Possible Contraindications of Antihypertensive Drugs[4]

	Compelling Contraindications	Possible Contraindications
Thiazide diuretics	Gout	Metabolic syndrome Glucose intolerance Pregnancy
Beta blockers	Asthma atrio-ventricular block (grade 2 or 3)	Peripheral artery disease Metabolic syndrome Glucose intolerance Athletes and physically active patients Chronic obstructive pulmonary disease
Calcium antagonists (dihydropyridines)		Tachyarrhythmia Heart failure
Calcium antagonists (verapamil, diltiazem)	Atrio-ventricular block (grade 2 or 3) Heart failure	
ACE inhibitors	Pregnancy Angioneurotic edema Hyperkalemia Bilateral renal artery stenosis	
Angiotensin receptor antagonists	Pregnancy Hyperkalemia Bilateral renal artery stenosis	
Diuretics (antialdosterone)	Renal failure Hyperkalemia	

More frequent visits will be necessary for patients with Stage 2 HTN or with complicating comorbid conditions. Serum potassium and creatinine should be monitored at least once or twice each year. After BP is at goal and stable, follow-up visits can usually be at three- to six-month intervals (Table 7-15).[4]

ADVANCED MANAGEMENT

Therapeutic Approaches in Special Conditions

The patient with HTN and certain special conditions requires individual attention and follow-up by the clinician.

TABLE 7-15: Recommendations for Follow-Up[4]

Initial BP (mm Hg)	Follow-up Recommended
Normal	Recheck in 2 years
Prehypertension	Recheck in 1 year
Stage 1 hypertension	Confirm within 2 months
Stage 2 hypertension	Evaluate or refer to source of care within 1 month. For those with higher pressures (e.g., >180/110 mm Hg), evaluate and treat immediately or within 1 week, depending on clinical situation and complications.

Prehypertension

Prehypertension is considered a precursor to Stage 1 HTN and a predictor of excessive CV risk. The question is whether pharmacologic treatment of prehypertension prevents or postpones Stage 1 HTN. The answer is shown by the Trial of Preventing Hypertension (TROPHY)[14] that follows.

 EVIDENCE-BASED MEDICINE:

The TROPHY Trial

Methodology: This is a double-blind, randomized clinical trial. Some 800 participants with repeated measurements of systolic pressure of 130–139 mm Hg and diastolic pressure of 89 mm Hg were randomly assigned to receive two years of candesartan (409) or placebo (400), followed by two years of placebo for all. *Results:* During the first two years, HTN developed in 154 participants in the placebo group and 53 of those in the candesartan group (relative risk reduction, 66.3%; P< 0.001). After four years, HTN had developed in 240 participants in the placebo group and 208 of those in the candesartan group (relative risk reduction, 15.6%; P <0.007). Over a period of four years, Stage 1 HTN developed in nearly two-thirds of patients with untreated prehypertension (the placebo group).[14] *Practical Applications:* Treatment of prehypertension with candesartan appeared to be well tolerated and reduced the risk of HTN during the study period. Thus, treatment of prehypertension appears to be feasible and effective in preventing the occurrence of Stage 1 HTN.

Coronary Artery Disease and Hypertension

Hypertensive patients are at increased risk for MI or other major coronary events and may be at higher risk of death following an acute MI. Lowering both SBP and DBP reduces ischemia and prevents CVD events in patients with CAD, in part by reducing myocardial oxygen demand.[4]

However, the existence of the so-called J curve—a paradoxical increase in morbidity and mortality with an excessive decrease in blood pressure—has been argued about for years. In the International Verapamil-Trandolapril (INVEST) Study, 22,576 patients with hypertension and coronary artery disease found that excessively lowering diastolic blood pressure was harmful. An analysis of the Treating to New Targets (TNT) study compared with the reference blood pressures, systolic >130 to 140 mm Hg and diastolic >70 to 80 mm Hg, found that patients with systolic blood pressure ≤110 mm Hg had a threefold increased risk of cardiovascular events, whereas those with diastolic blood pressure ≤60 mm Hg had a 3.3-fold increased risk of events. Therefore, treatment of HTN in CVD needs to avoid harm for a lower threshold level—around 120 mm Hg systolic and 70 mm Hg diastolic.

For patients with stable angina and silent ischemia, unless contraindicated, pharmacologic therapy should be initiated with a BB. If angina and BP are not controlled by BB therapy alone, or if BBs are contraindicated (as in the presence of severe reactive airway disease, severe peripheral arterial disease [PAD], high-degree atrioventricular block, or sick sinus syndrome), either ACEIs or long-acting dihydropyridine or nondihydropyridine-type calcium channel blockers (CCBs) may be used.[15] If angina or BP is still not controlled on this two-drug regimen, nitrates can be added. Short-acting dihydropyridine CCBs should not be used because of their potential to increase mortality, particularly in the setting of acute MI.[4]

Heart Failure and Hypertension

For patients with HTN and HF, ACEIs and BBs are the drugs of choice.[16] In patients intolerant to ACEIs, ARBs may be used. For further BP control, aldosterone antagonists may be of value for both conditions. Aldosterone antagonists may provide additional benefit in patients with severe LV dysfunction, usually late-stage C (NYHA class III–IV). In the Randomized Aldactone Evaluation Study (RALES), low-dose spironaldactone (25 mg daily), when added to standard therapy, decreased mortality by 34%.[17] In the Eplerenone Post-Acute Myocardial Infarction Heart Failure Efficacy and Survival Study (EPHESUS), eplerenone reduced mortality by 15% in patients following a recent MI with left ventricular ejection fraction (LVEF) ≤ 40%, 90% of whom had HF symptoms.[18] However, hyperkalemia is a risk with aldosterone antagonists, even at low doses (especially since most patients are also taking ACEIs or ARBs), but the risk incidence can be reduced by limiting therapy to patients with serum creatinine < 2.5 mg/dL and by carefully monitoring serum potassium.[4] BP targets in HF have not been firmly established, but lowering SBP (110–130 mm Hg) is almost uniformly beneficial.[16]

Diabetes and Hypertension

The coexistence of HTN in diabetes is particularly deleterious because of the strong linkage of the two conditions with all CVD and stroke, progression of renal disease, and diabetic retinopathy. Regarding the selection of medications, clinical trials with diuretics, ACEIs, BBs, ARBs, and CCBs have shown a demonstrated benefit in the treatment of HTN in both type 1 and type 2 diabetics.[19] Thiazide-type diuretics are beneficial in diabetics, either alone or as part of a combined regimen.[20]

Of potential concern is the tendency for thiazide-type diuretics to worsen hyperglycemia, but this effect tended to be small and did not produce more CV events compared to the other drug classes.[20] The American Diabetes Association (ADA) has recommended ACEIs for diabetic patients older than 55 at high risk for CVD, and BBs for those with known CAD.[19] With respect to microvascular complications, the American Diabetes Association has recommended both ACEIs and ARBs for use in type 2 diabetic patients with CKD because these agents delay the deterioration in GFR and the worsening of albuminuria.[19]

Chronic Kidney Disease and Hypertension

CKD is defined as either (1) reduced excretory function with an estimated GFR <60 mL/min/1.73 m^2 (approximately corresponding to a creatinine level of >1.5 mg/dL in men or >1.3 mg/dL in women); or (2) the presence of albuminuria (>300 mg/day or 200 mg/g of creatinine). Urinary albumin excretion has diagnostic and prognostic value equivalent to that of reduced estimated GFR. To avoid inaccuracies associated with 24-hour urine collections, spot urine samples may be used and the albumin/creatinine ratio (ACR) determined. Microalbuminuria is present when the spot urine ACR is between 30 and 200 mg albumin/g creatinine. ACR values >200 signify the presence of CKD.[4]

Treatment of HTN in CKD should include specification of target BP levels (<130/80 mm Hg), nonpharmacologic therapy, and specific antihypertensive agents for the prevention of progression of CKD and development of CVD.[13] Many drugs can be used safely in chronic renal failure, but ACEIs and ARBs were most frequently selected thanks to their renoprotection effects.[21] The Irbesartan Microalbuminuria Type 2 DM in Hypertensive Patients (IRMA 2) study showed that the progression from macroalbuminuria to ESRD can be prevented by inhibition of the renin-angiotensin system with an ARB.[22] Other antihypertensive drugs can be combined with ACEIs or ARBs, such as diuretics, dihydropyridine CCBs, and BBs.

When treating HTN in patients with nondiabetic kidney disease, use of combined therapy with ACEIs and ARBs may offer more renoprotection than with either class of medication alone. Thiazide diuretics may be used if estimated GFR < 30 mL/min/1.73 m^2, but loop diuretics are usually needed for patients with lower kidney function.[4] Potassium-sparing diuretics should be avoided in patients with CKD. A stable increase of serum creatinine—as much as 35% above baseline after ACEI or ARB initiation—may be tolerated as long as hyperkalemia does not occur. ACEI or ARB should be discontinued, or other potentially reversible causes of kidney failure investigated if progressive and rapid rise of serum creatinine continues.

Hypertension and Cerebrovascular Disease

The risk of clinical complications of cerebrovascular disease, including ischemic stroke, hemorrhagic stroke, and dementia increases as a function of BP levels. Given the population distribution of BP, most ischemic strokes occur in individuals with pre-HTN or Stage 1 HTN. The incidence of ischemic or hemorrhagic stroke is reduced substantially by treatment of HTN. No specific agent has been proven to be clearly superior to all others for stroke protection.

In the Losartan Intervention for Endpoint Reduction in Hypertension Study (LIFE), there were fewer strokes in the losartan-treated group than in the group treated with atenolol.[23] In the Antihypertensive and Lipid-Lowering Treatment to Prevent Heart Attack Trial (ALLHAT-LLT), the stroke incidence was 15% greater with ACEI than with thiazide-type diuretics or dihydropyridine CCBs, but the BP reduction in the lisinopril group was also less than with chlorthalidone or amlodipine.[20]

The Anglo-Scandinavian Cardiac Outcomes Trial (ASCOT) trial compared conventional BP lowering based on treatment with a BB (atenolol) with or without a thiazide (bendroflumethiazide-K) with a more contemporary regimen based on a CCB (amlodipine) with or without an ACEI (perindopril). The results show significantly lower rates of coronary and stroke events in individuals allocated to an amlodipine-based combination drug regimen than in those allocated to an atenolol-based combination drug regimen (HR 0.86 and 0.77, respectively).[24] With respect to the prevention of recurrent stroke, the Perindopril Protection Against Recurrent Stroke Study (PROGRESS) trial demonstrated that addition of the diuretic, indapamide, to the ACEI, perindopril, caused a 43% reduction in stroke occurrence. No significant reduction was present in those on perindopril alone whose BP was only 5/3 mm Hg lower than in the control group.[25]

Beta Blockers as Initial Medication for Uncomplicated HTN

In the last few years, questions have been raised about the use of BBs as first-line therapy for HTN. A number of large studies and meta-analyses have suggested that patients with uncomplicated HTN may be at greater risk of stroke with no benefit for the endpoints of all-cause mortality and CV morbidity and mortality.[26–28]

BENEFITS, HARMS, AND COST-EFFECTIVENESS ANALYSIS

Methodology: This is a meta-analysis evaluating 13 randomized controlled trials (n = 105,951) of BBs compared to other antihypertensive drugs. *Results:* The relative risk of stroke was 16% higher for BBs (95% confidence interval [CI] 4-30%) than for other drugs and there was no difference in terms of MI.[29] In a 2006 analysis, compared to placebo, BBs reduced the risk of stroke (relative risk 0.80; 95% CI 0.66-0.96) with a marginal fall in total CV events (0.88, 0.79-0.97) but had no effect on all-cause mortality (0.99, 0.88-1.11), coronary heart disease (0.93, 0.81-1.07), or CV mortality (0.93, 0.80-1.09).[30] *Harms:* The side effects from beta blockers include 1. precipitation of diabetes; 2. little effect on regression of left ventricular hypertrophy; 3. likely failure to improve endothelial function; 4. weight gain; and 5. decrease in exercise endurance. The higher mortality rate is associated with the too-slow heart rate they induce.[31] *Practical Applications:* Except for the compelling indication, BBs are not the first choice for uncomplicated HTN.

Are All Beta Blockers Alike?

This is an important question with the recent controversy surrounding their role as a first-line treatment of HTN. This class of drugs is heterogeneous. The sympathetic nervous system (SNS)—the presumed main target of BB activity—is one of the central pathways in the pathophysiology of HTN, both through its own effects on the heart and vasculature and through its interactions with the RAAS. The BBs are defined by and exert their influence through blocking catecholamine binding to the β_1-, β_2-, and α_1-adrenergic receptors. Traditional BBs (atenolol, metoprolol, propranolol) affect only the β-adrenergic receptors, whereas carvedilol and labetalol mediate vasodilation through blockade of the α_1-adrenergic receptor. Other drugs like nebivolol may exert vasodilation via stimulation of nitric oxide. Vasodilation may be important not only for blood pressure reduction but also for tolerability. The importance of SNS activation in the pathogenesis of HTN and the utility of BBs in certain compelling indications for cardiovascular disease indicate that these drugs still have an important role for many patients in the management of HTN.

Patients Undergoing Surgery

Uncontrolled HTN is associated with wider fluctuations of BP during induction of anesthesia and intubations and may increase the risk for perioperative ischemic events. BP levels of >180/110 mm Hg should be controlled prior to surgery. For elective surgery, effective BP control can be achieved over several days to weeks of outpatient treatment. In urgent situations, rapidly acting parenteral agents, such as sodium nitroprusside, nicardipine, and labetalol, can be utilized to attain effective control very rapidly. Surgical candidates with controlled HTN should maintain their medications until the time of surgery, and therapy should be reinstated as soon as possible postoperatively.[4]

Hypertension in African Americans

Hypertension is more prevalent and severe in populations of African descent living outside of Africa than in any other populations. African Americans with HTN predominantly have a low serum/plasma renin level and consequently a low serum/plasma angiotensin II concentration; conversely, this is associated with robust tissue renin and angiotensin II levels, and therefore large doses of ACEI and ARBs are required to block these vasoactive substances.[32]

Response to ACEIs and BBs is blunted in African Americans when used as monotherapy. A combination regimen, including a diuretic, narrows the response in this racial divide. African Americans exhibit the most profound response of lower BP to diuretics, followed by CCBs.[33] Use of ACEIs or ARBs in adequate doses with other classes of antihypertension medications translates into improved renal and cardiac indices and prevents or stems the progression of new onset diabetes. CCBs are not deleterious to CV outcomes.[20]

Hypertensive Crises

These include hypertensive emergencies and urgencies. Hypertensive emergencies are characterized by severe elevations in BP (>180/120 mm Hg) complicated by evidence of impending or progressive target organ dysfunction. They require immediate BP reduction (not necessarily to normal level) to prevent or limit target organ damage.[4] Patients may require hospitalization and parenteral drug therapy (Table 7-16). The initial goal of therapy in hypertensive emergencies is to reduce mean arterial BP by no more than 25% (within minutes to one hour); then if the patient is stable, to 160/100–110 mm Hg within the next two to six hours.

Hypertensive Urgencies

Hypertensive urgencies are those situations associated with severe elevations in BP without progressive target organ dysfunction. Examples include upper levels of Stage 2 HTN associated with severe headache, shortness of breath, epistaxis, or severe anxiety. The majority of these patients present as noncompliant or inadequately treated hypertensive individuals, often with little or no evidence of target organ damage.[5] The initial goal of therapy should be to achieve a diastolic BP of 100–110 mm Hg in the several hours following admission. Normal BP can be attained gradually over several days as tolerated by the individual patient. Excessive or rapid decrease in BP should be avoided to minimize the risk of cerebral hypoperfusion or coronary insufficiency.[13]

TABLE 7-16: Parenteral Drugs for Treatment of Hypertensive Emergency[4]

Drug	Dose*	Onset of Action	Duration of Action	Adverse Effects[†]	Special Indications
Vasodilators					
Sodium nitro-prusside	0.25–10 µg/kg/min as IV infusion	Immediate	1–2 min	Nausea, vomiting, muscle[‡] twitching, sweating, thio-cyanate and cyanide in-toxication	Most hypertensive emergencies; caution with high intracranial pressure or azotemia
Nicardipine hydrochloride	5–15 mg/hr IV	5–10 min	15–30 min; may exceed 4 hr	Tachycardia, headache, flushing, local phlebitis	Most hypertensive emergencies except acute heart failure; caution with coronary ischemia
Fenoldopam mesylate	0.1–0.3 µg/kg per min IV infusion	<5 min	30 min	Tachycardia, headache, nausea, flushing	Most hypertensive; emergencies; caution with glaucoma
Nitroglycerin	5–100 µg/min as IV infusion	2–5 min	5–10 min	Headache, vomiting,[‡] methemoglobinemia, tolerance with prolonged use	Coronary ischemia
Enalaprilat	1.25–5 mg every 6 hr IV	15–30 min	6–12 hr	Precipitous fall in pressure in high-renin states; variable response	Acute left ventricular failure; avoid in acute myocardial infarction

(continued)

TABLE 7-16: Parenteral Drugs for Treatment of Hypertensive Emergency[‡] (continued)

Drug	Dose*	Onset of Action	Duration of Action	Adverse Effects[†]	Special Indications
Hydralazine hydrochloride	10–20 mg IV 10–40 mg IM	10–20 min IV 20–30 min IM	1–4 hr IV 4–6 hr IM	Tachycardia, flushing, headache, vomiting, aggravation of angina	Eclampsia
Adrenergic Inhibitors					
Labetalol hydrochloride	20–80 mg IV bolus every 10 min 0.5–2.0 mg/min IV infusion	5–10 min	3–6 hr	Vomiting, scalp tingling, bronchoconstriction, dizziness, nausea, heart block, orthostatic hypotension	Most hypertensive emergencies except acute heart failure
Esmolol hydrochloride	250–500 µg/kg/min IV bolus, then 50–100 µg/kg/min by infusion; may repeat bolus after 5 min or increase infusion to 300 µg/min	1–2 min	10–30 min	Hypotension, nausea, asthma, first degree heart block, heart failure	Aortic dissection, perioperative
Phentolamine	5–15 mg IV bolus	1–2 min	10–30 min	Tachycardia, flushing, headache	Catecholamine excess

hr, hour; IM, intramuscular; IV, intravenous; min, minute(s).
*These doses may vary from those in the Physicians' Desk Reference (51st ed.).
[†]Hypotension may occur with all agents.
[‡]Require special delivery system.

Resistant Hypertension

The term "resistant hypertension" is used for the persistence of a BP that is usually above 140/90 mm Hg despite a combination of three or more antihypertensive drugs at full doses, including a diuretic.[29, 33] After excluding potential identifiable causes of resistant HTN (see Table 7-17), physicians should carefully explore reasons why the patient is not at target BP. Successful treatment requires identification and reversal of lifestyle factors contributing to treatment resistance; diagnosis and appropriate treatment of secondary causes of HTN; and use of effective multidrug regimens. Usually, the patients show edema in the extremities and abdominal wall. Ascites and fluid overload (or insufficient diuretic dosage) are the causes of resistant HTN. Otherwise, recommendations for the pharmacologic treatment of resistant HTN remain largely empirical due to the lack of systematic assessments of three or four drug combinations. The diagnostic and treatment recommendations for resistant HTN are summarized in Figure 7-2.[29]

TABLE 7-17: Causes of Resistant Hypertension[4]
Improper BP Measurement
Volume overload and pseudo-tolerance Excess sodium intake Volume retention from kidney disease Inadequate diuretic therapy
Drug-Induced or Other Causes
Noncompliance Inadequate doses Inappropriate combinations NSAIDs; cyclooxygenase-2 inhibitors Cocaine, amphetamines, other illicit drugs Sympathomimetics (decongestants, anorectics) Oral contraceptives Adrenal steroids Cyclosporine and tacrolimus Erythropoietin licorice (including some chewing tobacco) Selected over-the-counter dietary supplements and medicines (ephedra, ma huang, bitter orange)
Associated Conditions
Obesity Excess alcohol intake
BP: blood pressure, NSAIDs: non-steroidal anti-inflammatory drugs.

Confirm Treatment Resistance
Office blood pressure >140/90 or 130/80 mm Hg in patients
with diabetes or chronic kidney disease
and
Patient prescribed three or more antihyperstensive medications at
optimal doses, including a diuretic if possible
or
Office blood pressure at goal but patient requires four or more
antihypertensive medications

Exclude Pseudoresistance
Does patient adhere to prescribed regimen?
Obtain home, work, or ambulatory blood pressure readings to
exclude white coat effect

Identify and Reverse Contributing Lifestyle Factors
Obesity
Physical inactivity
Excessive alcohol ingestion
High salt, low fiber diet

Discontinue or Minimize Interfering Substances
Nonsteroidal anti-inflammatory agents
Sympathomimetics (diet pills, decongestants)
Stimulants
Oral contraceptives
Licorice
Ephedra

Figure 7-2 Resistant hypertension: diagnostic and treatment
recommendations. *(Continued)*

Screen for Secondary Causes of Hypertension
Obstructive sleep apnea (snoring, witnessed apnea,
excessive daytime sleepiness)
Primary aldosteronism (elevated aldosterone/renin ratio)
Chronic kidney disease (creatinine clearance <30 mL/min)
Renal artery stenosis (young female, known
atherosclerotic disease, worsening renal function)
Pheochromocytoma (episodic hypertension, palpitations,
diaphoresis, headache)
Cushing's syndrome (moon facies, central obesity,
abdominal striae, interscapular fat deposition)
Aortic coarctation (differential in brachial or femoral
pulses, systolic bruit)

Pharmacologic Treatment
Maximize diuretic therapy, including possible addition of
mineralocorticoid receptor antagonist
Combine agents with different mechanisms of action
Use of loop diuretics in patients with chronic kidney
disease and/or patients receiving potent
vasodilators (e.g., minoxidil)

Refer to Specialist
Refer to appropriate specialist for known or suspected
secondary cause(s) of hypertension
Refer to hypertension specialist if blood pressure remains
uncontrolled after 6 months of treatment

Figure 7-2 (Continued)

Catheter-Based Renal Sympathetic Denervation for Resistant Hypertension

Renal sympathetic hyperactivity is associated with hypertension and its progression, chronic kidney disease, and heart failure. A proof-of-principle trial of therapeutic renal sympathetic denervation was started in patients with resistant HTN (systolic blood pressure ≥160 mm Hg on three or more antihypertensive medications, including a diuretic) to assess safety and blood-pressure reduction effectiveness.

Methodology: Fifty patients were enrolled (five patients were excluded for anatomical reasons, mainly on the basis of dual renal artery systems) and received percutaneous radiofrequency catheter-based treatment, with subsequent follow-up at one year. The effectiveness of renal sympathetic denervation was assessed with renal noradrenaline spillover in a subgroup of patients. Primary endpoints were office blood pressure and safety data before and at 1, 3, 6, 9, and 12 months after the procedure. *Results:* In treated patients, baseline mean office blood pressure was 177/101 mm Hg (SD 20/15), (mean four to seven antihypertensive medications); estimated glomerular filtration rate was 81 mL/min/1·73 m² (SD 23); and mean reduction in renal noradrenaline spillover was 47% (95% CI 28–65%). Office blood pressures after the procedure were reduced by −14/−10, −21/−10, −22/−11, −24/−11, and −27/−17 mm Hg at 1, 3, 6, 9, and 12 months, respectively. In the five nontreated patients, the mean BP rose rather than decreased. *Harms:* One intraprocedural renal artery dissection occurred before radiofrequency energy delivery, without further sequelae. There were no other renovascular complications. *Practical Applications:* Catheter-based renal denervation causes substantial and sustained blood pressure reduction without serious adverse events in patients with resistant hypertension. Prospective randomized clinical trials are needed to investigate the usefulness of this procedure in the management of resistant HTN.[30]

Treatment of HTN During Acute Stroke

Blood pressure is often elevated in the immediate poststroke period and is thought to be a compensatory physiologic response to improve cerebral perfusion to ischemic brain tissue. Both elevated and low blood pressures are associated with poor outcome after stroke. For every 10 mm Hg increase >180 mm Hg, the risk of neurologic deterioration increased by 40% and the risk of poor outcome increased by 23%.[31] Therefore, treatment should start when SBP >180 mm Hg. A systolic blood pressure >185 mm Hg or a DBP >110 mm Hg is a contraindication to intravenous administration of tissue plasminogen activator (tPA) within the first three hours of an ischemic stroke. Based on general consensus, the American Heart Association and American Stroke Association (AHA/ASA) listed the recommended medications and doses included in Table 7-18.[31] When treatment is indicated, lowering the

TABLE 7-18: Approach to Arterial Hypertension in Acute Ischemic Stroke[31]

Indication that patient is eligible for treatment with intravenous rtPA or other acute reperfusion intervention

BP Level

Systolic >185 mm Hg or diastolic >110 mm Hg
Labetalol 10 to 20 mg IV over 1 to 2 minutes, may repeat x1;
or
Nitropaste 1 to 2 inches;
or
Nicardipine infusion, 5 mg/h, titrate up by 2.5 mg/h at 5- to 15-minute intervals, maximum dose 15 mg/h; when desired BP attained, reduce to 3 mg/h
If BP does not decline and remains >185/110 mm Hg, do not administer rtPA
Management of BP during and after treatment with rtPA or other acute reperfusion intervention
Monitor BP every 15 minutes during treatment and then for another 2 hours, then every 30 minutes for 6 hours, and then every hour for 16 hours

BP Level

Systolic 180 to 230 mm Hg or diastolic 105 to 120 mm Hg
Labetalol 10 mg IV over 1 to 2 minutes, may repeat every 10 to 20 minutes, maximum dose of 300 mg;
or
Labetalol 10 mg IV followed by an infusion at 2 to 8 mg/min

Systolic >230 mm Hg or diastolic 121 to 140 mm Hg
Labetalol 10 mg IV over 1 to 2 minutes, may repeat every 10 to 20 minutes, maximum dose of 300 mg;
or
Labetalol 10 mg IV followed by an infusion at 2 to 8 mg/min;
or
Nicardipine infusion, 5 mg/h, titrate up to desired effect by increasing 2.5 mg/h every 5 minutes to maximum of 15 mg/h
If BP not controlled, consider sodium nitroprusside

blood pressure should be done cautiously. Some strokes may be secondary to hemodynamic factors, and a declining blood pressure may lead to neurologic worsening. A reasonable goal would be to lower blood pressure by 15% to 25% within the first day.[31] For intracerebral hemorrhage (ICH), 2007 AHA/ASA guidelines included recommendations for treating elevated BP.[38] See Table 7-19 and Table 7-20.

TABLE 7-19: Recommended Guidelines for Treating Elevated BP in Spontaneous ICH[38]

If SBP is >200 mm Hg or MAP is >150 mm Hg, consider aggressive reduction of BP with continuous intravenous infusion, with frequent BP monitoring every five minutes.

If SBP is >180 mm Hg or MAP is >130 mm Hg and there is evidence of or suspicion of elevated ICP, consider monitoring ICP and reducing BP using intermittent or continuous intravenous medications to keep cerebral perfusion pressure <60 to 80 mm Hg.

If SBP is >180 mm Hg or MAP is >130 mm Hg and there is no evidence of or suspicion of elevated ICP, consider a modest reduction of BP (e.g., MAP of 110 mm Hg or target BP of 160/90 mm Hg) using intermittent or continuous intravenous medications to control BP, and clinically reexamine the patient every 15 minutes.

SBP: systolic BP, MAP: mean arterial pressure, ICH: intra-cranial hemorrhage, ICP: intra-cranial pressure.

TABLE 7-20: Intravenous Medications That May Be Considered for Control of Elevated Blood Pressure in Patients with ICH[38]

Drug	Intravenous Bolus Dose	Continuous Infusion Rate
Labetalol	5 to 20 mg every 15 min	2 mg/min (maximum 300 mg/d)
Nicardipine	NA	5 to 15 mg/h
Esmolol	250 μ/kg IVP loading dose	25 to 300 μ/kgx^{-1} x min^{-1}
Enalapril	1.25 to 5 mg IVP every 6 h*	NA
Hydralazine	5 to 20 mg IVP every 30 min	1.5 to 5 $\mu g/kgx^{-1}$ x min^{-1}
Nipride	NA	0.1 to 10 $\mu g/kgx^{-1}$ x min^{-1}
Nitroglycerin	NA	20 to 400 μg/min

IVP: intravenous push, NA: not applicable, ICH: intra-cranial hemorrhage.
*Because of the risk of precipitous BP lowering, the enalapril first test dose should be 0.625 mg.

TROUBLE-SHOOTING AND DEBUGGING

Does Correction of HTN Reverse Left Ventricular Hypertrophy?

Left ventricular hypertrophy (LVH) can occur in endurance athletes with normal or supranormal systolic function, large end-diastolic volumes, and elongation of myofibrils (eccentric hypertrophy). LVH due to long-standing uncontrolled HTN is usually characterized by "concentric" hypertrophy with circumferential hypertrophy of myofibrils, normal or increased contractility, increased relative wall thickness, normal or low end-diastolic volumes, and at times, impaired relaxation ("diastolic dysfunction"). In untreated or poorly treated individuals, LVH becomes a major risk factor for dilated cardiomyopathy and HF.

The JNC 7 report says that weight loss, salt restriction, and BP lowering with most antihypertensive agents all produce LVH regression and that selection of individual drugs appears to be less important.[4] The report acknowledges that the results of a number of studies have revealed trends favoring treatment with ACEIs and ARBs, and to a lesser extent, diuretics and CCBs. In the LIFE study,[23] LVH, defined by echocardiography, was reduced significantly more by a losartan-based than an atenolol-based regimen, despite equivalent lowering of BP. Inhibition of the renin-angiotensin-aldosterone system (RAAS) is now regarded as potentially more effective in regressing LVH than other antihypertensive treatment strategies.

Is it Beneficial to Combine Drugs for HTN?

The JNC 7 report recommends that physicians should consider initiating therapy with two drugs, either as separate prescriptions or in fixed-dose combinations, when BP is > 20 mm Hg above SBP goal or > 10 mm Hg above DBP goal.[4] Initiation of therapy with more than one drug increases the likelihood of achieving blood pressure goals in a more timely fashion and the use of multidrug combinations often produces greater blood pressure reduction at lower doses of the component agents, resulting in fewer side effects. One of these drugs should be a diuretic. Consideration of combination therapy is recommended in high-risk individuals, such as those with BP markedly (> 20 mm Hg SBP or > 10 mm Hg DBP) above the HTN threshold and those with milder degrees of BP elevation associated with multiple risk factors, subclinical organ damage, diabetes, and renal or associated cardiovascular disease.

The ASCOT,[24] and the LIFE Study[23] showed that combination amlodipine and perindopril, losartan and thiazide were respectively better than atenolol and thiazide in outcomes. Recently, the ACCOMPLISH (Avoiding Cardiovascular Events through COMbination Therapy in Patients LIving with Systolic Hypertension) trial showed that the combination of ACEI/CCB was superior to ACEI/thiazide-type diuretics.[34] However, the ONgoing Telmisartan Alone and in combination with Ramipril Global Endpoint Trial (ONTARGET) showed that the combination treatment of telmisartan and ramipril was not superior to ramipril alone.[35]

How Much Does an Antihypertensive Agent Cause Orthostatic Hypotension (OH)?

Normally, standing is accompanied by a small increase in DBP and a small decrease in SBP when compared to supine values. Orthostatic hypotension is present when there is a supine-to-standing BP decrease >20 mm Hg systolic or >10 mm Hg diastolic. There is more OH in diabetic individuals. There is a strong correlation between the severity of OH and premature death as well as increased incidents of falls and fractures.[36] The causes of OH include severe volume depletion, baroreflex dysfunction, autonomic insufficiency, and certain venodilator antihypertensive drugs, especially alpha blockers and alpha-beta blockers. Diuretics and nitrates may further aggravate OH. In treating older hypertensive patients, clinicians should be alert to potential OH symptoms, such as postural unsteadiness, dizziness, or even fainting. Lying and standing BPs should be obtained periodically in all hypertensive individuals over age 50. OH is a common barrier to intensive BP control. Appropriate instruction on sitting up slowly from a lying position or standing up slowly from a sitting position while holding on to something firm should be discussed with patients.[4]

Do Statins Decrease BP?

Statins reduce the risk of cardiovascular events in people with hypertension. This benefit could arise from a beneficial effect of statins on central aortic pressures and hemodynamics. The Conduit Artery Function Evaluation–Lipid-Lowering Arm (CAFE-LLA) study, an ASCOT substudy, investigated this hypothesis in a prospective placebo-controlled study of treated patients with hypertension. *Methods:* CAFE-LLA recruited 891 patients randomized to atorvastatin 10 mg/d or placebo from five centers in the United Kingdom and Ireland. Radial artery applanation tonometry and pulse-wave analysis were used to derive central aortic pressures and hemodynamic indices at repeated visits over 3.5 years of follow-up. *Results:* Atorvastatin lowered low-density lipoprotein cholesterol by 32.4 mg/dL (95% CI, 28.6 to 36.3) and total cholesterol by 35.1 mg/dL (95% Confidence Interval, 30.9 to 39.4) relative to placebo. Time-averaged brachial blood pressure was similar in CAFE-LLA patients randomized to atorvastatin or placebo (change in brachial systolic blood pressure, –0.1 mm Hg [95% CI, –1.8 to 1.6], P = 0.9; change in brachial pulse pressure, –0.02 mm Hg [95% CI, –1.6 to 1.6], P = 0.9). Atorvastatin did not influence central aortic pressures (change in aortic systolic blood pressure, –0.5 mm Hg [95% CI, –2.3 to 1.2], P = 0.5; change in aortic pulse pressure, –0.4 mm Hg [95% CI, –1.9 to 1.0], P = 0.6) and had no influence on augmentation index (change in augmentation index, –0.4%; 95% CI, –1.7 to 0.8; P = 0.5) or heart rate (change in heart rate, 0.25 bpm; 95% CI, −1.3 to 1.8; P = 0.7) compared with placebo. The effect of statin or placebo therapy was not modified by the blood pressure-lowering treatment strategy in the factorial design. ***Practical Applications:*** Statin therapy sufficient to significantly reduce cardiovascular events in treated hypertensive patients in ASCOT did not influence central aortic blood pressure or hemodynamics in a large representative cohort of ASCOT patients in CAFE-LLA.[37]

TAKE-HOME MESSAGE

Data Collecting Collect all the data about the patient's history (smoking, high-salt, high-cholesterol diet, alcohol abuse, lack of exercise, DM, high cholesterol level), family history (of early, sudden death due to heart disease, history of stroke, and early CAD), social history (work and behaviors) and perform a complete physical examination (signs of prior stroke, CAD, PAD, carotid murmur, weak peripheral pulses), all of which add weight to the clinical decision–making process.

Data Mining Recommend safe, appropriate, and efficacious investigation (including fasting lipid profile, fasting blood glucose, BUN and creatinine levels, weight, BMI, waist circumference), and echocardiography to detect LVH.

Management Recommend safe, appropriate, and efficacious therapy to maintain the stable health status of the patient over time (low-salt, low cholesterol diet; stopping smoking; losing weight; no drinking alcohol; exercise; and medications).

Patient-Centered Care Get the patients involved in their own lifestyle modification to increase compliance with diet, exercise, medication, and office visits and testing in order to provide continuity of care.

References

1. World Health Organization, The World Health Report 2002: Reducing Risks, Promoting Healthy Life. Geneva: World Health Organization. Available at: http://www.who.int/whr/2002/en/index.html.
2. Asia Pacific Cohort Studies Collaboration. Systolic blood pressure, diabetes and the risk of cardiovascular diseases in the Asia–Pacific region. J Hypertens. 2007;25:1205–1213.
3. Franklin, S. S., Jacobs, M. J., Wong, N. D., et al.: Predominance of isolated systolic hypertension among middle-aged and elderly U. S. hypertensives. Hypertension. 2001;37:869–874.
4. Chobanian, A. V., et al. Complete Report: The Seventh Report of the Joint National Committee on Prevention, Detection, Evaluation, and Treatment of High Blood Pressure. NIH Publication No. 04–5230. August 2004.

5. World Health Organization, International Society of Hypertension Writing.Group. 2003 World Health Organization (WHO)/International Society of Hypertension (ISH) statement on management of hypertension. J Hypertens. 2003; 21; 1983–1992.
6. Vinyoles, E., Felip, A., Pujol, E., Sierra, A. et al.: on behalf of the Spanish Society of Hypertension ABPM Registry. Clinical characteristics of isolated clinic hypertension. J Hypertens. 2008:26(3):438–445.
7. Fagard, R. H., Cornelissen, V.A.: Incidence of cardiovascular events in white-coat, masked and sustained hypertension versus true normotension: a meta-analysis. J Hypertens. 2007;25:2193–2198.
8. Expert Panel on Detection, Evaluation, and Treatment of High Blood Cholesterol in Adults. Third report of the National Cholesterol Education Program (NCEP) Expert Panel on Detection, Evaluation, and Treatment of High Blood Cholesterol in Adults (Adult Treatment Panel III): Final Report. Circulation. 2002;106:3143–421.
9. Conroy, R. M. et al.: SCORE project group. Estimation of ten-year risk of fatal cardiovascular disease in Europe: the SCORE project. Eur Heart J. 2003;24(11):987–1003.
10. World Health Organization Prevention of Cardiovascular Disease. Guidelines for assessment and management of cardiovascular risk. Geneva. 2007
11. Giles, T. D., Berk, B. C., Black, H. R., et al. Expanding the definition and classification of hypertension. J Clin Hypertens. 2005;7: 505–512.
12. Champagne, C. M.: Dietary interventions on blood pressure: the Dietary Approaches to Stop Hypertension (DASH) Trials. Nutr Rev. 2006;64(2 Pt 2):S53–56.
13. Huy, V. T., Olabode, O., Nguyen, H. T., et al.: Integrated primary prevention of cardiovascular disease. Management of complex cardiovascular problems. Blackwell Futura. New York, NY: 2007; 129-189.
14. Julius, S., Nesbitt, S. D., Egan, B. M., et al.: for the Trial of Preventing Hypertension (TROPHY) Study Investigators Feasibility of Treating Prehypertension with an Angiotensin-Receptor Blocker. N Engl J Med. 2006;534:1685–1697.
15. The European Trial on Reduction of Cardiac Events with Perindopril in Stable Coronary Artery Disease Investigators. Efficacy of perindopril in reduction of cardiovascular events among patients with stable coronary artery disease: Randomised, doubleblind, placebo-controlled, multicentre trial (the EUROPA study). Lancet. 2003;362: 782–788.
16. Hunt, S. A., Baker, D. W., Chin, M. H., et al.: ACC/ AHA 2005 Guideline Update for the Diagnosis and Management of Chronic Heart Failure in the Adult: A Report of the American College of Cardiology/ American Heart Association Task Force on Practice Guidelines. American College of Cardiology. Available at: http://www. acc.org/clinical/guidelines/failure//index.pdf.
17. Pitt, B., Zannad, F., Remme, W. J., et al.: The effect of spironolactone on morbidity and mortality in patients with severe heart failure. Randomized Aldactone Evaluation Study Investigators. N Engl J Med. 1999;341:709–717.

18. Pitt, B., Zannad, F., Remme, W.J., et al.: The effect of spironolactone on morbidity and mortality in patients with severe heart failure. Randomized Aldactone Evaluation Study Investigators. N Engl J Med. 1999;341:709-17.

19. Adler, A. I., Stratton, I. M., Neil, H. A., et al.: Association of systolic blood pressure with macrovascular and microvascular complications of type 2 diabetes (UKPDS 36): prospective observational study. BMJ. 2000;321:412–419.

20. The ALLHAT Officers and Coordinators for the ALLHAT Collaborative Research Group. Major outcomes in high–risk hypertensive patients randomized to angiotensin-converting enzyme inhibitor or calcium channel blocker vs diuretic: The Antihypertensive and Lipid-Lowering Treatment to Prevent Heart Attack Trial (ALLHAT–LLT). JAMA. 2002;288:2981–2997.

21. Sharma, A. M., Hollander, A., Koster, J.: Efficacy and Safety in Patients with Renal Impairment; treated with Telmisartan (ESPRIT) Study Group. Telmisartan in patients with mild/moderate hypertension and chronic kidney disease. Clin Nephrol. 2005;63(4).

22. Sasso, F. C., Carbonara, O., Persico, M., et al.: Irbesartan reduces the albumin excretion rate in microalbuminuric type 2 diabetic patients independently of hypertension: A randomized double–blind placebo–controlled crossover study. Diabetes Care. 2002. Nov;25(11): 1909–1913.

23. Dahlof, B., Devereux, R. B., Kjeldsen, S. E., et al.: Cardiovascular morbidity and mortality in the Losartan Intervention For Endpoint Reduction in Hypertension Study (LIFE): A randomized trial against atenolol. Lancet. 2002;359:995–1003.

24. Dahlof, B., Sever, P. S., Poulter, N. R., et al.: ASCOT Investigators. Prevention of cardiovascular events with an antihypertensive regimen of amlodipine adding perindopril as required vs. atenolol adding bendroflumethiazide as required, in the Anglo–Scandinavian Cardiac Outcomes Trial–Blood Pressure Lowering Arm (ASCOT–BPLA): A multicentre randomised controlled trial. Lancet. 2005;366(9489): 895–906.

25. PROGRESS Collaborative Group. Randomised trial of a perindopril-based blood–pressure–lowering regimen among 6,105 individuals with previous stroke or transient ischaemic attack. Lancet. 2001;358: 1033–1041.

26. Lindholm, L. H., Carlberg, B., Samuelsson, O.: Should beta blockers remain first choice in the treatment of primary hypertension? A meta-analysis. Lancet, 2005;366:1545–1553.

27. Bradley, H. A., Wiysonge, C. S., Volmink, J. A., et al.: How strong is the evidence for use of beta blockers as first-line therapy for hypertension? Systematic review and meta-analysis. J. Hypertens. 2006;24:2131–2141.

28. Kaplan, N.: Beta blockers in hypertension. J Am Coll Cardiol. 2008;52:1490–1491.

29. David, A. C., Daniel, J., Stephen, T., et al.: Resistant Hypertension: Diagnosis, Evaluation, and Treatment. A Scientific Statement From the American Heart Association Professional Education Committee of the

Council for High Blood Pressure Research. Circulation. 2008 Jun 24;117(25):e510-26.

30. Krum, H., Schlaich, M., Whitbourn, R., et al.: Lancet. 2009; 373:1275–1281.

31. Adams, H. P., Jr., Adams, R. J., Brott, T., et al.: Guidelines for the early management of patients with ischemic stroke: Stroke. 2007;38:1655–1711.

32. Douglas, J. G.: Clinical guidelines for the treatment of hypertension in African Americans. Am J Cardiovasc Drugs. 2005;5(1):1–6.

33. Kaplan, N.M.: Resistant hypertension. J Hypertens. 2005;23:1441–1444.

34. Jamerson, K., Weber, M. A., Bakris, G. L., et al.: Benazepril plus amlodipine or hydrochlorothiazide for hypertension in high-risk patients. N Engl J Med. 2008;359:2417–2428.

35. Yusuf, S., Teo, K. K., Pogue, J., et al.: for the ONTARGET investigators. Telmisartan, ramipril, or both in patients at high risk for vascular events. N Engl J Med. 2008:358:1547–1559.

36. Masaki, K. H., Schatz, I. J., Burchfiel, C. M., et al.: Orthostatic hypotension predicts mortality in elderly men: The Honolulu Heart Program. Circulation. 1998;98:2290–2295.

37. Williams, B., Lacy, P. S., Cruickshank, J. K., for the CAFE and ASCOT Investigators Impact of Statin Therapy on Central Aortic Pressures and Hemodynamics: Principal Results of the Conduit Artery Function Evaluation–Lipid-Lowering Arm (CAFE-LLA) Study. Circulation. 2009; 119:53–61.

38. Joseph, B., Sander, C., Edward, F., et al.: Guidelines for the Management of Spontaneous Intracerebral Hemorrhage in Adults 2007 Update. Stroke. 2007;38:2001-2023.

Patients with High Risk of/or with Left Ventricular Dysfunction

Thach Nguyen, James Nguyen,
Tam D. Bui, Hung D Huynh,
Olabode Oladeinde, and Dayi Hu

Chapter Outline

DEFINITION

Heart failure (HF) is a clinical syndrome resulting from any structural and functional cardiac disorder that impairs the capacity of the left ventricle (LV) to fill or to circulate the appropriate amount of blood to the general vascular system.[1]

Patient Population in Focus

According to the ACC/AHA classification, in Stage A, patients are totally asymptomatic without structural cardiac abnormality; however, they have a high risk factor for HF. In Stage B, patients have left ventriclular (LV) remodeling without symptoms or signs of HF. The asymptomatic patients of Stages A and B and the mildly symptomatic patients of early Stage C are the focus of this chapter.[1] The population usually consists of patients with early stages of alcoholic cardiomyopathy, patients after acute myocardial infarction (AMI) treated on time with percutaneous coronary intervention (PCI), or very young patients (20–30 years old) having mild cardiomyopathy with well-preserved pulmonary, hepatic, renal, or cerebral function.

Strategic Programming

Based on a computational cardiac model, the index problem of HF is the obstruction or stagnation of the blood flow at the LV level (zone A). This is a hardware problem. The immediate upstream area is the pulmonary venous system (zone B). The downstream area consists of the aorta and the distal peripheral arteries (zone C).

The strategy is to identify the patients through data collecting with a comprehensive history and physical examination. The patients of Stages A and B should be evaluated for signs and symptoms of early, uncontrolled, or severity of the risk factors. In Stage C patients with mild LV dysfunction, besides looking for the risk factors, the signs and symptoms of (1) fluid retention, or (2) exercise intolerance should be searched diligently. Afterward, the etiologies, extent of LV dysfunction, risk of severe arrhythmias, risk of sudden death, and chances for relapse in these patients should be evaluated. The next step is to perform data processing in order to formulate a preliminary diagnosis and a short list of differential diagnoses (COPD, pulmonary embolism). Then, using the method of data mining, tests could be ordered (echocardiography, stress testing, coronary angiography) in order to confirm (data converting) the main diagnosis of HF and to rule out (data filtering) the differential diagnoses.

DATA COLLECTING

Investigation Master Plan

When a physician comes to see a patient suspected of having CHF, there are seven main areas of interest for data collecting (history and physical examination).

The main area of interest is the left ventricle. In general, the patient with Stage A and Stage B HF is asymptomatic. There are no subjective symptoms. The physical findings are directly related to LV dysfunction (zone A).

The upstream area for HF is the pulmonary venous system with signs or symptoms of lung congestion (Stage C) (zone B).

The downstream area is the distal peripheral arteries with vasodilation in asymptomatic patients and vasoconstriction in severe or decompensated HF (Stage C) (zone C).

The system configuration. There is nothing wrong with the configuration of the system (zone E).

The work-around configuration: There is no work-around configuration identified yet (zone D).

The cardiovascular system: The index location of the problem is at the LV, which is a major part of the CV system.

The network (the whole body): Long-standing HF can cause poor renal perfusion in the renal vasculature or dizziness due to low blood pressure to the central nervous system (zone F).

History: Typical Symptoms

The patients of Stages A and Stage B are asymptomatic. At the beginning, for the patients of Stage C with mild LV dysfunction, the predominant sign and symptom is fluid retention. This is because the patient is usually unaware of the need for or does not adhere to a low-salt diet and fluid restrictions. Once the fluid overload is controlled, then symptoms of exercise intolerance become prominent. This is the most common scenario in which the patient with mild LV dysfunction presents at the first office visit.

Dyspnea
Dyspnea is the main symptom of heart failure of Stage C due to interstitial pulmonary edema leading to increased airway resistance. Dyspnea is defined as a condition in which the patient is aware of making an effort to breathe.[2]

Intolerance to Strenuous Activities
In Stage C, once the patient has fluid overload controlled, he or she may quickly become SOB or fatigued with activities that he or she used to enjoy.

Atypical Symptoms
Cough
HF patients may have a cough at night, upon lying down. The mechanism is the same as orthopnea. Another explanation is that the shifting of pleural fluid stimulates the cough reflex. Angiotensin-converting enzyme inhibitors (ACEIs) can cause a cough in about 5% of patients; they have a dry and persistent cough but not necessarily only when lying down. Once the ACEI is discontinued, the cough should disappear within 48 hours. The mechanism of the cough is the build-up of kinins in the lung as a result of kininase (ACE) inhibition. Therefore, the angiotensin receptor blocker (ARB) is not expected to cause coughing.

Nocturia
HF patients have nocturia due to shifting of the extravascular fluid into the intravascular compartment in the supine position. Many (>2) trips to the bathroom at night are subtle symptoms of fluid removal upon prolonged exposure to the supine position.

Gastrointestinal Symptoms
The patients with fluid overload may have a sense of fullness or pain in the right upper quadrant due to stretching of the liver capsule, fullness or pain in the left upper quadrant due to splenic enlargement, or a bloating sensation due to mesenteric edema (which can decrease absorption of cardiac drugs triggering acute HF). Many patients may have nausea, anorexia, or early fullness (satiety) after a small meal. Others may have a heavy feeling in the abdominal area due to fluid infiltration. Liver congestion could cause lack of energy (no pep) or a poor sense of well-being (not feeling well).

Family History

Many details in the family history may suggest a genetic predisposition, such as sudden cardiac death (SCD), coronary artery disease (CAD), dilated or hypertrophic cardiomyopathy, and skeletal myopathies.

Physical Examination
Typical Signs
Vital Signs

In general, a patient with mild HF should show no obvious clinical abnormalities. The pulse pressure may diminish due to a lower cardiac output; the diastolic pressure may be higher because of peripheral vasoconstriction.

Jugular Vein Distention

At this early Stage C with mild LV dysfunction, the patient usually has no jugular venous distention.

Pulmonary Auscultation

The air entry is usually adequate. In patients with early Stage C, crackles which result from transudation of fluid into the alveoli may be heard at the bases of the lungs. Expiratory wheezing, in the case of severe decompensated HF, may also be detected.

Cardiovascular Examination

In patients in Stage A, the cardiac exam should be normal. S4 may be heard, but not in patients over 40 years of age. In Stage B and Stage C, S3 may be heard.

Examination of the Abdomen

The first sign of liver congestion is minimal pain on percussion in the right lower rib cage. It is also tender to deep palpation.

Examination of the Extremities

Bilateral, symmetrical edema in the lower extremities can be seen, especially in patients who do not adhere to a low-salt diet and fluid restrictions.

 JOB DESCRIPTION:

How to Detect Fluid Retention in Patients without Rales or Leg Edema

In a well-managed, early stage HF patient, it is rare to see the conventional signs of HF: rales and leg edema. The patient needs to retain at least 5 liters of fluid before the development of ankle edema. So, at any phase of HF, the status of fluid in different parts of the body, such as the lungs, liver, spleen, abdominal wall, or jugular vein, should be checked in order to assess the severity of fluid retention or the success of fluid removal following treatment.

Critical Thinking: Distal Vasodilation or Vasoconstriction in HF

If an event is caused by lower blood pressure, then the reactive compensatory mechanism is vasoconstriction to raise the BP. If there is lower cardiac output, then the reactive compensatory mechanism is vasodilation in the distal peripheral arteries. In patients with early dilated cardiomyopathy, the examination of the feet should show either prominent vasodilation or at least no vasoconstriction. When a patient becomes decompensated, then vasoconstriction prevails. The same observations of vasodilation or vasoconstriction in the distal peripheral arteries apply to patients with aortic stenosis.

DATA MINING (WORK-UP)

Laboratory Testing

Laboratory tests include Na, K, BUN, and creatinine. It is important to follow the levels of Na and K, which can be depleted by diuretics. Brain-type natriuretic peptide (BNP) can be mildly elevated or even normal in well-compensated HF.

Chest X-Ray

The chest x-ray (CXR) is normal in Stage A. There could be cardiomegaly in Stage B and Stage C.

Echocardiography

The echocardiogram will show the chambers' size, type of remodeling (eccentric or concentric hypertrophy), the extent of the dilation, and segmental wall motion abnormalities of the LV. Ejection fraction gives important information about current exercise tolerance status and prognosis. Valvular problems, pericardial effusion, or pulmonary hypertension can also be easily assessed by echocardiogram.

Holter Monitoring

Holter monitoring may reveal the presence of paroxysmal atrial fibrillation, nonsustained ventricular tachycardia, or supraventricular tachycardia. These arrhythmias can decompensate the LV and precipitate symptomatic HF.

Stress Imaging

Any middle-aged person (especially American or European patients) should undergo nuclear stress testing to rule out CAD as a cause of dilated or ischemic cardiomyopathy.

DATA CONVERTING (FORMULATING THE DIAGNOSIS)

HF is diagnosed by using the Framingham criteria, which require the presence of at least two major criteria or one major criterion and two minor criteria. Minor criteria are acceptable if they cannot be attributed to another medical condition (e.g., pulmonary hypertension, chronic lung disease, cirrhosis, ascites, or nephrotic syndrome). The Framingham criteria are listed in Table 8-1.[3]

Confirmation of Etiologies

The history, physical examination, and work-up could help to confirm the causes of cardiomyopathy. A list of possible causes is shown in Table 8-2.

TABLE 8-1: Major and Minor Framingham Criteria for Heart Failure

Major Criteria

Paroxysmal nocturnal dyspnea or orthopnea
Neck vein distention
Rales in lung auscultation
Cardiomegaly
Acute pulmonary edema, S3 gallop
Increased venous pressure (>16 cm H_2O)
Hepatojugular reflux

Minor Criteria

Ankle edema, night cough
Dyspnea on exertion
Hepatomegaly
Pleural effusion
Vital capacity decreased one third from maximal capacity
Tachycardia (>120/min)

Minor or Major Criterion

Weight loss >4.5 kg in 5 days in response to treatment

TABLE 8-2: Causes of Heart Failure

Uncontrolled hypertension	Diabetes mellitus
Coronary artery disease	Valvular heart disease
Myopathy	Old age
Rheumatic fever	Mediastinal radiation
Exposure to cardiotoxin agents	Alcohol
Collagen vascular disease	Thyroid disorder
Pheochromocytoma	

PROGRAMMED MANAGEMENT

Strategic Programming

The management plan for HF includes risk-factor modification, administration of outcome-proven medications, and prevention of clinical deterioration. All preventive and therapeutic modalities are applied to all patients to various degrees because each stage requires a different level of intensive or preventive care. These are outlined in Table 8-3.

Lifestyle modifications and prevention of risk factors are the two main treatment modalities for Stage A and Stage B patients. All medications or situations that can precipitate or aggravate HF should be clearly identified so they can be effectively avoided or removed. Usually, beta blockers (BBs), angiotensin-converting enzyme inhibitors (ACEIs), or angiotensin receptor blockers (ARBs) are optional medications for Stage A patients, whereas they are essential for Stage B and Stage C patients.

PROGRAMMED MANAGEMENT OF STAGE A PATIENT

Patients at High Risk for Heart Failure without Structural Abnormality

At this stage, patients are without any cardiovascular structural abnormalities. The main management is to screen asymptomatic patients at high risk for ventricular remodeling and to treat any underlying clinical diseases (e.g., hypertension, diabetes, hypercholesterolemia, alcohol abuse, tobacco addiction, obesity) while applying all generic preventive measures (lifestyle changes, low-salt, low-cholesterol diet, exercise, and HF awareness teachings). The pathologic targets are to prevent the occurrence of atrial or ventricular hypertrophy or dilation. The ultimate goal is to prevent remodeling of any cardiac chamber, which is the most important and clinically relevant end result of any cardiac injury. Any entity that can lead to the end result of remodeling and its preventive or corrective measures is listed in Table 8-4.

TABLE 8-3: Management Master Plan

Location	Mechanism	Presentation	Early Stage	Late Stage	Treatment
Left ventricle	Elevated LVEDP	Poor exercise tolerance	No symptoms	Fatigue because of low cardiac output	Diuretic, ACEI, BB
Pulmonary veins	Filling capacity at maximum	SOB			Diuretics
Pulmonary arteries	Increased pulmonary pressure	Chest pain because of strain in RV			Diuretics can cause high BUN levels because the LV function depends on preload
Distal peripheral arteries			Vasodilation	Vasoconstriction	ACEI
Distal lymphatic system		Leg edema			Diuretics
Distal venous system	Vasoconstriction	Abdominal wall edema, leg edema			Diuretics

ACEI: angiotensin-converting enzyme inhibitor, BB: beta blocker, BUN: blood urea nitrogen, LV: left ventricle, LVEDP: left ventricular diastolic pressure, RV: right ventricle, SOB: shortness of breath.

TABLE 8-4: Entities Leading to Ventricular Remodeling and Preventive Measures

Clinical Entity	Pathology	Preventive Measure
Diabetes	Dilated cardiomyopathy	Diet and drug
Uncontrolled HTN	LV hypertrophy, dilation	Diet and drug
CKD	LV hypertrophy, dilation	Diet and drug
Coronary artery disease	Ischemic cardiomyopathy	Drug and revascularization
Valvular stenosis		
Mitral stenosis	Pulmonary HTN, Right HF	Valvuloplasty
Aortic stenosis	LV hypertrophy	Valve replacement or valvuloplasty
Valvular insufficiency		
Aortic insufficiency	LV dilation	Surgery
Mitral regurgitation	Left atrial and LV dilation	Surgery
Toxin (ETOH, drugs)	Dilated cardiomyopathy	Treat cause
Aging	Diastolic dysfunction	Diet??
Viral infection	Dilated cardiomyopathy	Drug ????
Obesity	Diastolic dysfunction	Weight loss
Postpartum cardiomyopathy	Dilated cardiomyopathy	????
Uncontrolled arrhythmias	Dilated cardiomyopathy	Treat cause

CKD: chronic kidney disease, ETOH: alcohol, HF: heart failure, HTN: hypertension, LV: left ventricle.

ACEIs for Asymptomatic Patients at High Risk for CVD

For a Stage A patient who has only a high risk for SVD without any cardiac pathology, is there a benefit to taking an ACEI to prevent cardiovascular disease? The results of the Heart Outcomes Prevention Evaluation (HOPE) trial that follows may provide an answer.[4]

 BENEFITS, HARMS, AND COST-EFFECTIVENESS ANALYSES:

ACEIs in Asymptomatic Patients with Preserved LV Function

Methodology: This is an RCT that enrolled 9297 people at high risk of cardiovascular events owing to preexisting vascular disease or diabetes plus at least one other cardiovascular risk factor. *Results:* Ramipril 10 mg daily reduced the composite primary outcome of cardiovascular death, MI, or stroke compared with placebo over

TABLE 8-5: ACEI in Asymptomatic Patients at High Risk for CVD

Endpoint	Risk Reduction (RR)	Confidence Interval (CI)	Number Needed to Treat (NNT)
Composite Outcome	0.78	95% 0.70-0.86	27
Cardiovascular Death	0.74	95% 0.64-0.87	45
Myocardial Infarction	0.80	95% 0.70-0.90	42
Stroke	0.68	95% 0.56-0.84	67
All Causes	0.84	95% 0.75-0.95	56

an average of 4.7 years. The results of other endpoints are listed in Table 8-5.[4] *Harms:* The major adverse effects reported when comparing an ACEI with placebo were cough (ARI 5–10%), dizziness, hypotension (ARI 5–10%), renal failure (ARI <3%), hyperkalemia (ARI <3%), angina, syncope, and diarrhea (ARI 2%).[5] *Practical Applications:* ACEIs should be used in patients when the benefits outweigh the risks. There is a need to individualize the treatment of these asymptomatic Stage A patients, especially the diabetic patients who have no proven modality to prevent the occurrence of cardiomyopathy (Table 8-5).

PROGRAMMED MANAGEMENT OF STAGES B AND C PATIENTS

Stage B patients are asymptomatic patients with structural abnormalities, while Stage C patients are mildly symptomatic with LV dysfunction. These patients have stable CAD, valvular disease, or a dilated LV without causing any HF symptoms. One such patient is the patient with acute myocardial infarction aborted by an expedited angiopalsty or stenting, or CAD lesion treated by stent. The patients with mildly reduced ejection fraction can still enjoy a highly active lifestyle. Because these patients are asymptomatic, the management strategies are (1) prevention of clinical worsening, (2) reduction of morbidity and mortality, and (3) reversal of ventricular remodeling (Table 8-6).

TABLE 8-6: Management Strategies for Asymptomatic HF Stage B Patients

Detect and treat the causes of HF.
Maintain asymptomatic status by diet, exercise, and medications.
Prevent and treat precipitating and exacerbating factors.
Prevent progression of HF at the cellular level.
Reverse ventricular remodeling by diet, exercise, and medications.

Lifestyle Changes and Education

The first step in the treatment plan for asymptomatic HF patients is lifestyle changes in the form of a low-salt, low-cholesterol diet, fluid restriction (<2000 cc/day = 64 ounces of fluid = 8 CUPS of fluid), no smoking, and increased exercise. For asymptomatic patients, prevention and education are the main focus.

 DATA COLECTING TIPS (CLINICAL PEARLS)
How to Know that the Patient Is Adhering to a Low Sodium Diet

A key to knowing that a patient is adhering to a low-sodium diet is when he or she says: "The food is too salty when I eat in restaurants or away from home."[2]

Data Management (Pharmacologic Therapy)

Angiotensin-converting enzyme inhibition (ACEI) and beta blockade (BB) are the main treatments of HF. They should be given to all patients with asymptomatic LV dilation or hypertrophy, especially in patients with prior MI, even those with normal EF. ACEIs and BBs are used to reduce mortality and to prevent, delay, or reverse LV remodeling. With appropriate treatment for congestion and low cardiac output, the HF patient can be asymptomatic for a long time.

Angiotensin-Converting Enzyme Inhibitors

Since ACEIs are very effective in patients with symptomatic LV dysfunction, are they effective in patients with asymptomatic LV dysfunction? The answer lies in the results of the SOLVD Prevention trial below.

 EVIDENCE-BASED MEDICINE:

The SOLVD Prevention Trial

Question: Does the ACEI enalapril reduce the total mortality and mortality from cardiovascular causes, the development of HF, and hospitalization for HF among patients with asymptomatic left ventricular dysfunction? *Methodology:* This is an RCT in which patients were randomly assigned to receive either placebo (n = 2117) or enalapril (n = 2111) at doses of 2.5 to 20 mg per day in a double-blind fashion. *Results:* There were 334 deaths in the placebo group as compared with 313 in the enalapril group (reduction in risk, 8% by the log-rank test, P = 0.30). In addition, fewer enalapril patients died or were hospitalized for HF (434 in the enalapril group vs. 518 in the placebo group; risk reduction, 20%; 95% CI, 9 to 30%

P<0.001).[6] *Cost-Effectiveness Analysis:* ACE inhibitors significantly reduced mortality (number need to treat [NNT] = 17 people treated for about two years to prevent one death) and admission to the hospital for HF (NNT = 28).[7] *Harms:* Dizziness or fainting (46% with enalapril vs. 33% with placebo) and cough (34% with enalapril vs. 27% with placebo) were reported more often in the enalapril group (significance not reported for any outcome). The incidence of angioedema was the same in both groups (1%).[7] *Evidence-Based Applications:* The ACEI enalapril significantly reduced the incidence of HF and the rate of related hospitalizations as compared with placebo among patients with asymptomatic left ventricular dysfunction.[6]

Beta Blockers

The evidence that proved the benefits of BBs on HF Stage C patients was in the Carvedilol U. S. Heart Failure trial, which randomized a large group of patients with mild, moderate, and severe HF. The data that focused on patients with mild HF are shown below.

 EVIDENCE-BASED MEDICINE:

The U.S. Carvedilol Heart Failure Trial

Methodology: The trial enrolled 1094 patients with mild, moderate, or severe HF with an EF ≤ 0.35. The mild patients are today's Stage C HF patients. They were randomly assigned to receive either placebo (n = 398) or carvedilol (n = 696) on a background therapy with digoxin, diuretics, and ACEIs. *Results:* After 12 months of observation (for the group with mild HF), the overall mortality rate was 7.8% in the placebo group and 3.2% in the carvedilol group; the reduction in risk attributable to carvedilol was 65% (95% confidence interval, 39 to 80%; P<0.001). In addition, as compared with placebo, carvedilol therapy was accompanied by a 27% reduction in the risk of hospitali.zation for cardiovascular causes (19.6% vs. 14.1%, P = 0.036), as well as a 38% reduction in the combined risk of hospitalization or death (24.6% vs. 15.8%, P<0.001).[8]

With evidence from the trial above, BB therapy is recommended even if there is concomitant diabetes, chronic obstructive lung disease (COPD), or peripheral vascular disease. BB therapy should be used with caution in patients with resting limb ischemia or diabetes with recurrent hypoglycemia. Considerable caution should be exercised if BBs are initiated in patients with marked bradycardia (<55 beats/min) or marked hypotension (systolic blood pressure <80 mm Hg).[8] BB is not recommended in patients with bronchospasm being treated regularly with bronchodilating inhalers.

Exercise

Physical activity with moderate-intensity aerobic activity, such as brisk walking of 30 to 60 minutes, seven days per week (minimum five days per week) is recommended. It should also be supplemented by an increase in daily activities, such as walking breaks at work, gardening, or household work).[12]

In the Heart Failure and A Controlled Trial Investigating Outcomes of exercise traiNing (HF-ACTION) study, 960 patients with moderate-to-severe chronic heart failure were randomly assigned to either guideline-based therapy alone or guideline-based therapy plus supervised and home-based exercise. Patients were asked to ride a bicycle or walk on the treadmill for 30-40 minutes, three days a week under supervision, for a goal of 36 sessions. Exercise intensity was set at 60 to 70% of heart rate reserve, a moderate-intensity program. This is enough to modestly lower the risk of hospitalization or death for patients with heart failure.[9]

Prevention of Precipitating Factors

Prevention and Treatment of Precipitating Factors

The compensated condition in Stages A and B can change quickly when any precipitating factors tip over the precarious clinical balance (Table 8-7). Prevention of any precipitating or aggravating factors is the second most important strategy in this group of asymptomatic patients.

TABLE 8-7: Precipitating Factors for Heart Failure

Fluid and sodium impropriety
Infection
Brady- or tachyarrhythmia
Myocardial ischemia or MI
Physical (doing too much at home) or emotional (worry about anything or any member of the family) stress
Pulmonary embolism
High-output states, such as anemia, thyrotoxicosis, Paget's disease, pregnancy, beriberi, and arteriovenous fistula
Cardiac infection and inflammation (myocarditis, infective endocarditis)
Comorbidities (renal, liver, thyroid, respiratory insufficiency)
Cardiac toxin (chemotherapy, cocaine, alcohol)

TROUBLE-SHOOTING AND DEBUGGING

Treatment is standard for any physician caring for a patient with mild HF. When the problems are not controlled as expected, the management requires the expertise and experience of a consultant cardiologist.

The common questions from the referral physicians to the consultant cardiologist in the management of mild HF follow.

What is the Direct Imaging of Sympathetic Downgrading in HF?

Myocardial scintigraphy is a nuclear imaging modality that evaluates the integrity of the sympathetic nerves supplying the heart. It has been known for a long time that the sympathetic nerves are damaged in heart failure. The radioactive tracer ^{123}I meta-iodobenzylguanidine (^{123}I mIBG), which is a physiologic analog of norepinephrine, is taken up into the sympathetic nerves. Lower uptake of ^{123}I mIBG is direct molecular evidence of HF and is associated with poorer outcomes. *Methodology:* In this trial, 964 patients with Class 2 and Class 3 HF were given ^{123}I mIBG by IV injection and underwent nuclear imaging. Quantification of cardiac uptake of the tracer was expressed as the ratio of counts between the heart and the upper mediastinum—the H/M ratio. Normal, healthy individuals would have an H/M ratio of around 2, and the sickest patient with heart failure would have an H/M ratio of 1. In this study, a cutoff value of 1.6 was used, with higher values denoting high uptake. *Results:* The composite endpoint, the first occurrence of NYHA HF class progression, potentially life-threatening arrhythmic event, or cardiac death occurred significantly more frequently (37%) in patients who had low uptake of the tracer than in the higher uptake patients (15%) (P <0.0001). The test was particularly effective in identifying those with the worst prognosis, with the group who were in the lowest 10% for uptake having a death rate of 19.1% (10 times) and those in the highest 20% uptake with a death rate of 1.8%.

The patients with the lowest uptakes (H/M ratio <1.2) tended to die more from HF progression, whereas arrhythmic events tended to occur in patients with H/M ratios in the 1.2 to 1.6 range.[10]

Can Cardiac Structural Abnormalities Be Reversed by BBs?

It is important to correct the underlying disease that causes ventricular remodeling, such as CAD, arrhythmias, and alcohol (ETOH) abuse. The beneficial evidence of BB or any treatment is the reversal of remodeling (LVH or dilation) by the drug. What is the concrete evidence of BBs in remodeling reversal? The answer may be found in the Reversal of Ventricular Remodeling With Toprol-XL (REVERT) trial that follows.[11]

Does extended-release metoprolol succinate reverse cardiac remodeling in asymptomatic HF patients (New York Heart Association [NYHA] class I) with LV systolic dysfunction? *Methodology:* The REVERT trial is a multicenter, double-blind, placebo-controlled study in which 164 patients were randomized to metoprolol 25 mg titrated over 2 months to a target dose of 50 mg or 200 mg or to placebo. *Results:* At 12 months, the results showed that the mean

TABLE 8-8: Conditions in Which Ventricular Remodeling Could be Reversed

Viral cardiomyopathy
Postpartum cardiomyopathy
Atrial fibrillation–induced cardiomyopathy
Aortic stenosis with LV hypertrophy
Mitral regurgitation with dilated left ventricle
Alcohol–induced dilated cardiomyopathy
Dilated left ventricle from metabolic syndrome
Left ventricular hypertrophy after long-standing uncontrolled hypertension
Stress-induced cardiomyopathy
Tachycardia mediated–cardiomyopathy
Nutritional deficiency: beriberi, selenium deficiency
Metabolic causes: hypocalcemia, hypophosphatemia
Endocrine disorders: hypo- and hyperthyroidism

change (mL/m²) of the LV end-systolic ventricular index (ESVI) was −14.5% for the 200 mg dose and −7.6% for the 50 mg dose (P<0.05 compared with placebo). The LV EF increased to +6% and 4%, respectively, from baseline.[11] *Practical Applications:* LV remodeling (dilation or hypertrophy) is considered detrimental and the precursor of future symptomatic HF. Reversal of LV dilation or hypertrophy is an ideal goal and concrete evidence of treatment success. The LV dilation can be transient or disappears after the causes are corrected. However, in many patients, there is a need to use BBs to reverse the dilating process, as proved by the RCT above. The list of conditions in which remodeling can be reversed is shown in Table 8-8.

Do Patients with Mild HF Benefit from CRT?

Can CRT (with or without an implantable cardioverter defibrillator [ICD]) in combination with optimal medical therapy (OMT) attenuate HF disease progression compared with OMT alone in patients with asymptomatic or mildly symptomatic HF and ventricular dyssynchrony? *Methodology:* The REVERSE (REsynchronization reVErses Remodeling in Systolic left vEntricular dysfunction) trial is a multicenter, randomized, double-blind, parallel-controlled trial that enrolled 610 patients. The patients were randomized in a 2:1 fashion to either CRT-on (n = 419) or CRT-off (n = 191). The selection criteria included NYHA Class II or previously symptomatic Class I HF patients with QRS duration ≥ 120 msec, LVEF ≤ 40%, and LV end diastolic diameter (LVEDD) ≥ 55 mm. The composite endpoints included all-cause mortality, HF hospitalizations, crossover due to worsening HF, NYHA class, and a patient global assessment. In addition, the prospectively powered secondary endpoint of LV end systolic volume index (LVESVi) assessed at baseline and 12-month follow-up was selected as the primary measure of LV remodeling. *Results:* There was a slight trend in the prespecified primary endpoint (clinical composite response) in favor of the CRT-on group, suggesting that fewer patients in the CRT-on group worsened than in the CRT-off group (16% vs. 21%, P = 0.10). More patients improved in the CRT-on group over the 12-month follow-up period (54% vs. 40%; P = 0.004). There was no difference in all-cause mortality between the two patient groups, with six deaths observed in each group (1%).

Significant differences were observed in several of the secondary endpoints. The prespecified secondary endpoint of LVESVi revealed a substantial decline in LV volume over the course of follow-up in the CRT-on versus CRT-off groups. Patients in the CRT-on group also demonstrated a highly significant reduction in LVESVi from baseline (-18.4 mL/m^2 vs. -1.3 mL/m^2; P<0.0001), suggesting that significant reverse LV remodeling occurred in the CRT-on group. CRT was shown to favorably delay the time to first HF-related hospitalization. The risk of an initial HF-related hospitalization over a 12-month follow-up period was significantly reduced by 53% in the CRT-on group, relative to CRT-off patients (hazard ratio 0.47, P = 0.03). *Harms:* In terms of safety, the overall implant success rate was 97%. LV-lead related complications occurred in 9.5% of patients. They included lead dislodgements, diaphragmatic stimulation, subclavian vein thrombosis, or similar problems (no lead infections were noted). *Practical Applications:* Although the primary endpoint of this study did not achieve statistical significance, the results nonetheless provide important information about the utility of CRT in patients with less severe HF. A significantly greater percentage of patients in the CRT-on group improved compared with the control group. In addition, secondary endpoints revealed positive changes in LV remodeling and significant improvement in LVEF as well as a significantly reduced risk of HF hospitalization.[12]

Do Patients with Mild HF Benefit from CRT and BiV?

Methods: During a 4.5-year period, 1820 patients with ischemic or nonischemic cardiomyopathy, an ejection fraction of 30% or less, a QRS duration of 130 msec or more, and New York Heart Association class I or II symptoms were randomly assigned in a 3:2 ratio to receive CRT plus an ICD (1089 patients) or an ICD alone (731 patients). The primary endpoint was death from any cause or a nonfatal HF event (whichever came first). *Results:* During an average follow-up of 2.4 years, the primary endpoint occurred in 187 of 1089 patients in the CRT–ICD group (17.2%) and 185 of 731 patients in the ICD-only group (25.3%) (hazard ratio in the CRT–ICD group,

0.66; 95% confidence interval [CI], 0.52 to 0.84; P=0.001). The benefit did not differ significantly between patients with ischemic cardiomyopathy and those with nonischemic cardiomyopathy. The superiority of CRT was driven by a 41% reduction in the risk of HF events, a finding that was evident primarily in a prespecified subgroup of patients with a QRS duration of 150 msec or more. CRT was associated with a significant reduction in left ventricular volumes and improvement in the ejection fraction. There was no significant difference between the two groups in the overall risk of death, with a 3% annual mortality rate in each treatment group. Serious adverse events were infrequent in the two groups. ***Practical Applications:*** CRT combined with ICD decreased the risk of heart-failure events in relatively asymptomatic patients with a low ejection fraction and wide QRS complex.[13]

TAKE-HOME MESSAGE

Data Collecting Collect all the data about the patient's history (smoking, high-sodium, high-cholesterol diet, alcohol abuse, lack of exercise, HTN, DM, and high cholesterol level), family history (early sudden death due to heart disease and history of early CAD), social history (work and behaviors), and perform a complete physical examination (signs of prior stroke, CAD, PAD, carotid murmur, weak peripheral pulses), all of which add weight to the clinical decision-making process.

Data Mining Recommend safe, appropriate, and efficacious investigation (including fasting lipid profile, fasting blood glucose, BUN and creatinine levels, weight, BMI, waist circumference), and especially echocardiography.

Management Recommend safe, appropriate, and efficacious therapy to maintain the stable health status of the patient over time (low-sodium, low-cholesterol diet, stopping smoking, losing weight, not drinking alcohol, exercising). For the Stage A HF patient, the main message is to change lifestyle and treat risk factors in order to prevent ventricular remodeling. For the Stage B HF patient, the main treatments emphasize primarily prevention with healthy lifestyle change (low-salt, low-cholesterol diet, fluid restriction, exercise, and medications [BBs and ACEIs]). Revascularization is indicated if there is reversible ischemia. Avoidance of all precipitating or aggravating factors is very important to prevent any clinical deterioration. Medications or any treatment to reverse the structural abnormality (LVH or dilation) should be pursued aggressively. CRT for Stage B patients is very promising.

Patient-Centered Care Get the patients involved in their own lifestyle modification to increase compliance with diet, exercise, medication, office visits, and testing in order to provide continuity of care.

References

1. Hess, O.M., Carroll J.D.: Clinical Assessment of Heart Failure, in Libby P., Bonow, R., Mann, D., Zipes, D., eds. Braunwald's Heart Disease: A Textbook of Cardiovascular Medicine. 8th edition, Philadelphia: W.B. Saunders Company, 2008, pp 561-582.

2. Harvey, W. P.: Cardiac pearls. Cedar Grove, New Jersey: Leannec Publishing, 1993, pp 43-112.

3. Francis, G. S., Wilson, T.: Clinical Diagnosis of heart failure. In Mann, D. L., ed: Heart Failure: A Companion to Braunwald's Heart Disease, Philadelphia: Elsevier, 2004, pp 506–526.

4. The Heart Outcomes Prevention Evaluation (HOPE) Investigators. Effects of an angiotensin-converting enzyme inhibitor, ramipril, on cardiovascular events in high-risk patients. N Engl J Med. 2000;342;145–153.

5. Flather, M. D., Yusuf, S., Kober, L., et al.: Long-term ACE-inhibitor therapy in patients with heart failure or left-ventricular dysfunction: a systematic overview of data from individual patients. ACE-Inhibitor Myocardial Infarction Collaborative Group. Lancet. 2000;6:355: 1575–1581.

6. SOLVD Investigators. Effect of enalapril on mortality and the development of heart failure in asymptomatic patients with reduced left ventricular ejection fractions. N Engl J Med. 1992;327:685–691.

7. Jong, P., Yusuf, S., Rousseau, M. F., et al. : Effect of enalapril on 12-year survival and life expectancy in patients with left ventricular systolic dysfunction: a follow-up study. Lancet. 2003;361:1843–1848.

8. Packer, M., Bristow, M.R., Cohn, J.N. et al., for the US Carvedilol Heart Failure Study Group. The effect of carvedilol on morbidity and mortality in patients with chronic heart failure. N Engl J Med. 1996; 334:1349–1355.

9. Keteyian, S., et al.: The Heart Failure and A Controlled Trial Investigating Outcomes of exercise traiNing (HF-ACTION) study. Presented at the American College of Cardiology's 58th Annual Scientific Session, Orlando, FL.

10. Jacobson, A.: Presented at the American College of Cardiology (ACC) 2009 Scientific Sessions. Orlando FL.

11. Colucci, W. A. S., Kolias, T. J., Adams, K. R., et al.: Metoprolol reverses LV remodeling in patients with asymptomatic systolic dysfunction: The REVERT trial. Recent and late breaking clinical trials. Program and abstracts from the 9th Annual Scientific Meeting of the Heart Failure Society of America, September 18-21, 2005, Boca Raton, FL.

12. Linde, C., Abraham, W. T., Gold, M. R., et al.: on Behalf of the REVERSE Investigators and Coordinators. REsynchronization reVErses Remodeling in Systolic left vEntricular dysfunction: Results of the REVERSE trial. Program and abstracts from the American College of Cardiology 2008 Scientific Sessions, March 29-April 1, 2008, Chicago, IL.

13. Moss, A.J., Hall, W.J., Cannom, D.S. et al., for the MADIT-CRT Trial Investigators Cardiac-Resynchronization Therapy for the Prevention of Heart-Failure Events. Published at www.nejm.org. September 1, 2009 (10.1056/NEJMoa0906431).

Severe Left Ventricular Dysfunction

Thach Nguyen, Pham Nguyen Vinh, William H. Wehrmacher, Dayi Hu, Do Doan Loi, and John O'Connell

Chapter Outline

DEFINITION

Heart failure (HF) is a clinical syndrome resulting from any structural and functional cardiac disorders that impair the capacity of the ventricle (LV) to fill or to eject the appropriate amount of blood.[1]

Patient Population in Focus

According to the ACC/AHA classification, in Stage C, a patient has all of the conventional signs and symptoms of HF. In Stage D, the patient has refractory end-stage HF. Patients in Stages C and D are the focus of this chapter.

Strategic Programming

The strategy is to identify early on the signs and symptoms of severe LV dysfunction through data collecting with a comprehensive history and physical examination. In patients in Stage D, the signs and symptoms of low cardiac output or hypoperfusion are prominent, especially in those who are well managed without excessive fluid retention. The next step is to perform data processing in order to formulate a preliminary diagnosis and a short list of differential diagnoses (COPD or pulmonary embolism). Then, using the method of data mining, tests may be ordered (BNP, stress testing, coronary angiography) in order to confirm (data converting) the main diagnosis of HF and to rule out (data filtering) the differential diagnoses.

DATA COLLECTING

Typical Symptoms

Dyspnea

Dyspnea is the main symptom of HF due to interstitial pulmonary edema.

Orthopnea

Orthopnea is dyspnea that occurs in the recumbent position; paroxysmal nocturnal dyspnea (PND) happens one to three hours after lying down, waking the patient up at night. The mechanism of PND is redistribution of fluid from the splanchnic circulation and the lower extremities while in the supine position. It takes one to three hours for the fluid to be absorbed from the extravascular space into the intravascular compartment, causing elevation of pulmonary capillary pressure and shortness of breath.[1]

DATA DECODING TIPS (CLINICAL PEARLS)
Orthopnea in Patients without HF

Orthopnea occurs not only in heart failure patients. Pulmonary patients with ascites or abdominal obesity, when lying down, can displace the internal organs, pushing the diaphragm upward. This will decrease the vital capacity of the lungs, causing orthopnea.

Fatigue

Inappropriate low cardiac output or hypoperfusion would manifest as decreased exercise tolerance, easy fatigue, lack of energy (no pep), or poor sense of well-being (not feeling well).

Nocturia

In the supine position, patients could have nocturia due to shifting of the extravascular fluid into the intravascular compartment. In an elderly patient, the concentrating function of the kidneys is decreased so there is no difference in the amount of urine produced during the day or at night. The patient needs to wake up twice or more at night to urinate, a phenomenon not seen in young patients.

Gastrointestinal Symptoms

Patients with HF could have a sense of fullness or pain in the right upper quadrant due to stretching of the liver capsule from congestion; fullness or pain in the left upper quadrant due to the splenic enlargement; or a bloating sensation due to mesenteric edema (which can also cause lower absorption of cardiac drugs, triggering acute heart failure). Nausea, anorexia, and early fullness (satiety) after a small meal may be caused by edema in the mesenteric area. A heavy feeling in the abdominal area may also result from the thickening of the abdominal wall by fluid infiltration.

The earliest symptoms of fluid retention can be elicited by asking the questions in Table 9-1.

Atypical Symptoms

Hypoperfusion can cause lightheadedness, disorientation, confusion, sleep and mood disturbances, presyncope, or syncope. However, drug reaction should always be the primary consideration for differential diagnosis, followed by hypothyroidism or depression.

Physical Examination

Typical Signs

General Inspection

Pallor or dusky discoloration of the skin suggests low cardiac output or peripheral vasoconstriction. Bilateral temporal wasting is the sign of cardiac cachexia in patients with severe LV dysfunction. Truncal obesity suggests the presence of sleep apnea or metabolic syndrome.

Vital Signs

Low-grade fever could be detected in chronic HF patients due to marked vasoconstriction or inflammation. The pulse pressure may diminish due to a lower cardiac output or peripheral vasoconstriction. A widened pulse pressure could represent high output failure, such as hyperthyroidism or anemia. Orthostatic hypotension can occur in patients with too much medication or excessive diuresis.

TABLE 9-1: Earliest Symptoms of Fluid Retention

Is the appetite bad?
If it is bad, then there is liver congestion (differential diagnoses: prerenal azotemia, renal failure)
Does the patient feel bloated or full quickly after a small meal?
Edema in the mesenteric area resulting in diminished absorption of foods and medication
Does the patient feel lack of energy?
Liver congestion (differential diagnoses: renal failure, hypothyroidism, low cardiac output, mental depression)
Is the patient aware that he or she has to make an effort to breathe?
The lungs are stiffer because the pulmonary veins are overfilled with blood

 DATA DECODING TIPS (CLINICAL PEARLS)
Bradycardia in Severe HF

Usually tachycardia accompanies severe HF. However, at the end stage, even with slight exercise or sympathetic stimulation, the heart rate does not increase because of complete beta-receptor blockage. This is a sign of end-stage LV failure and carries a bad prognosis.

Jugular Venous Pressure
The height of the internal and external jugular venous columns reflects the right atrial pressure. The most common cause of right HF is left HF induced pulmonary hypertension.

Pulmonary Examination
Crackles result from transudation of fluid from the intravascular space into the alveoli. They may be accompanied by expiratory wheezing.

 DATA DECODING TIPS (CLINICAL PEARLS)
Why Don't Patients with Severe LV Dysfunction Have Crackles?

Patients with well-compensated chronic HF may not have crackles even if the pulmonary capillary pressure is high (>24 mm Hg) because there is increased lymphatic drainage of the alveolar fluid.

Cardiac Examination
In cardiomegaly, the point of maximal impulse (PMI) can be felt over two interspaces and will displace below the fifth intercostal space, lateral to the midclavicular line. An S3 gallop may be heard in patients with severe LV decompensation.

JOB DESCRIPTION:

How to Listen to an S3 Gallop

The diastolic filling sound, S3, may be heard only when the patient is turned to the left lateral position, and one listens over the PMI with the bell of the stethoscope barely making a seal with the skin of the chest wall. As a rule, a ventricular (S3) diastolic gallop is not a loud sound. In fact, most gallops are faint, and one needs to listen very carefully and specifically for them. Most ventricular (S3) gallops are usually heard on every third or fourth beat rather than with every beat. On the other hand, an atrial (S4) gallop is more likely to be heard with almost every beat.[2] A faint ventricular gallop (S3) might be overlooked in a patient who has an emphysematous chest with an increase in anteroposterior (AP) diameter. However, by listening over the xiphoid or epigastric area, an S3 gallop might be easily detected.[2]

Examination of the Abdomen

If the jugular venous pressure is normal, hepatojugular reflux should be tested to confirm the presence of right HF. Hepatomegaly can be found in patients with HF and may regress with therapy. The dependent areas of the abdominal wall can become harder and have the sign of *peau d'orange* due to infiltration of fluid. Hemorrhoids, scrotal edema, or vulvar edema can also develop due to portal hypertension. At the end stage of HF, ascites can be found.

 JOB DESCRIPTION:

How to Do Percussion of the Abdomen if the Patient Is Ticklish

Occasionally a patient is hypersensitive (unusually ticklish) about having the examiner percuss (or palpate). To resolve this issue, the examiner can perform percussion over the patient's hand, which is placed over the abdomen.[2]

Examination of the Extremities

Patients with HF can have bilateral edema in the lower extremities. With recurrent edema from increased venous pressure, patients will have many pigmented spots on the shin secondary to recurrent infections (stasis dermatitis). In the bedridden patient, edema should be looked for diligently in the ankles, calves, thighs, presacral area, and back of the arms.

In a well-managed or early-stage HF patient, it is rare to see the conventional signs of HF—rales and leg edema. The patient needs to retain at least 5 liters of fluid in the abdominal area before the development of ankle edema. At any phase of HF, there is a need to evaluate the fluid status in different organs or areas in order to assess the extent of fluid retention or the success of fluid removal following treatment.

 DATA DECODING TIPS (CLINICAL PEARLS)
Guessing the Cardiac Output by Leg Examination

The cardiac output can be estimated from the temperature of the big toe. If the temperature is good, then the cardiac output is usually adequate. However, if the patient is on an intravenous pressor, there might be vasocontriction, which can lower the temperature of the big toe. As always, the temperature of the toes is compared to the temperature of the hands.[3]

DATA DECODING TIPS (CLINICAL PEARLS)
Why Doesn't a Patient with Bad LV Function No Longer Have Recurrent Left Heart Failure?

Dyspnea might become less frequent with the onset of right ventricular failure. There is less fluid going to the LV and therefore the preload is decreased. As a result, patients have fewer bouts of recurrent LV failure while having more symptoms and signs of right-sided heart failure.

DATA CONVERTING (FORMULATING THE MAIN DIAGNOSIS)

With the information from a detailed history and physical examination (H and P), a presumptive diagnosis can usually be made. What element in the H and P could help the physician formulate the diagnosis of HF? The sensitivity, specificity, and predictive accuracy of symptoms and signs for diagnosing heart failure are listed in Table 9-2.[4]

DATA MINING (WORK-UP)
Laboratory Testing

Laboratory tests include BUN, creatinine, Na, and K, as they can be affected by diuretics. A liver function test is important, as many medications are metabolized by the liver. Hemoglobin and hematocrit need to be followed, as hemodilution or anemia from chronic kidney disease is frequently found. Brain-type natriuretic peptide (BNP) is measured to differentiate HF from SOB due to pulmonary etiologies. High BNP level is also a bad prognostic factor.

TABLE 9-2: Sensitivity, Specificity, and Predictive Accuracy of Symptoms and Signs for Diagnosing Heart Failure

Symptoms or Signs	Sensitivity (%)	Specificity (%)	Predictive Accuracy (%)
Exertional dyspnea	66	52	23
Orthopnea	21	81	2
Paroxysmal nocturnal dyspnea	33	76	26
History of edema	23	80	22
Resting heart rate	7	99	6
Rales	13	91	21
Third heart sound	31	95	61
Jugular venous distention	10	97	2
Edema (on examination)	10	93	3

Chest X-Ray

In patients with HF, there are four abnormalities to be checked in an upright posteroanterior chest x-ray (CXR): (1) Cephalization of the pulmonary veins: Usually the apices of the lungs are clear because of lack of blood. In HF, the fluid has shifted up to the apex so there is increased vascular marking in the apices of the lungs. (2) Enlargement of the cardiac silhouette (half of the width of the thorax). (3) Pleural effusion with blunting of the costodiaphragmatic angle. (4) Interlobular effusions with horizontal lines at the two sides of the CXR (Kerley A and B lines)

Echocardiography

The echocardiography should show the chambers' size, type of remodeling (eccentric, concentric hypertrophy, or dilation), wall motion abnormalities, and LV and RV function. Valvular problems or pulmonary hypertension can easily be excluded by echocardiography.

Myocardial Perfusion Imaging

CAD as a cause of HF should be excluded by myocardial perfusion imaging (MPI). Exercise testing on a treadmill can provide information about the exercise capacity, reserve, and tolerance of the patient.

Left and Right Heart Catheterization

When right-sided heart failure is prominent or new, a right heart catheterization would determine the pulmonary artery pressure or the pulmonary artery wedge pressure for optimal fluid titration. The LV end diastolic pressure also helps to assess the fluid status and LV compliance. A coronary angiogram should be done if the MPI shows ischemia.

PROGRAMMED MANAGEMENT

Strategic Programming

The management plan for HF includes prevention and treatment of risk factors, administration of outcome-proven medications, and prevention of clinical deterioration as outlined in Table 9-3.

Therapeutic Lifestyle Changes

Risk factors and lifestyle modifications are the main treatment for all stages of HF, including no alcohol, no cigarettes, increased exercise, a low-sodium, low-cholesterol diet, fluid restriction, and a weight-loss program.

Exercise

Medically supervised programs (cardiac rehabilitation) are recommended during hospitalization. Physical activity of 30 to 60 minutes, seven days per week (minimum five days per week) is recommended. All

TABLE 9-3: Management Master Plan

Data Management (Standard Management)

Lifestyle modifications
Prevention of precipitating and aggravating factors
Standard pharmacologic management with BBs, ACEIs/ARBs
Optional use of diuretics
Percutaneous or surgical revascularization if indicated

Data Management (Advanced Management)

Optional use of arterial or venodilators
Reverse structural abnormalities (remodeling with hypertrophy or dilation)
Device therapy including implantable cardioverter defibrillators, biventricular pacing

System configuration correction	None
Root cause treatment	PCI, CABG
Work-around management	Destination therapy with LV assist device
System replacement	Cardiac transplant

ACEI: angiotensin-converting enzyme inhibitors, ARB: angiotensin receptor blocker, BB: beta blockers, CABG: coronary artery bypass graft surgery, PCI: percutaneous coronary intervention, LV: left ventricular.

patients should be encouraged to obtain 30 to 60 minutes of moderate-intensity aerobic activity, such as brisk walking, supplemented by an increase in daily activities (such as walking breaks at work, gardening, or household work).[5] All situations that can precipitate or aggravate HF should be clearly identified and prevented.

Diet

The patient should have a low-salt diet (no adding salt during cooking, no salt shaker on the table), and a 2000 cc fluid restriction a day (64 ounces = 8 cups). The visiting nurse from a home health program should come to the house and check the kitchen storage for foods with salt, especially the canned foods. The patient should be shown how to read the salt content on the label of canned or frozen foods.

Pharmacologic Treatment

Medications including beta blockers (BBs), ACEIs, or ARBs are absolutely essential. Other optional medications include diuretics, digoxin, aldosterone antagonists, and vasodilators (hydralazine and isosorbide) (Table 9-4).

As the disease progresses, more diuretics are required if the patients retain more fluid. BBs and ACEIs/ARBs are given for patients even with relative contraindications. Medications are increased to higher doses in an effort to control severe HF. Comorbidities and side effects, e.g., renal insufficiency, liver dysfunction, or orthostatic hypotension may occur. At this stage, an implantable cardioverter defibrillator (ICD) and chronic resynchronization therapy (CRT) are indicated. Finally, in the long-term strategic plan, any modality of treatment that can reverse the cardiac structural abnormality (dilated LV or LVH) should be pursued aggressively at the earliest possible opportunity.

TABLE 9-4: Management of Patients with Heart Failure

Medications to Prevent Functional Deterioration
ACEIs, BBs

Medications to Reduce Mortality
ACEIs, BBs, ARBs, hydralazine-ISDN, aldosterone antagonists

Medications to Control Symptoms
ACEIs, BBs, ARBs, digoxin, diuretics

Medications to Avoid
Most antiarrhythmic drugs, most calcium channel blockers, thiazolidinediones, nonsteroidal anti-inflammatory drugs, tricyclic antidepressants, antihistamines, and herbal medicine (ephedra, ma huang).

ACEI: angiotensin-converting enzyme inhibitors, ARB: angiotensin receptor blocker, BB: beta blockers, ISDN: isosorbide dinitrate.

TABLE 9-5: Dosage of Medications in Clinical Trials of Heart Failure

Drug	Starting Dose	Target Dose	Clinical Trial
Captopril	6.25 mg-12.5 tid	50 mg tid	SAVE[6]
Enalapril	2.5-5 mg bid	10-20 mg bid	CONSENSUS[7]
Ramipril	2.5 mg bid	5 mg bid	AIRE[8]
Trandolapril	1 mg/d	4 mg/d	TRACE[9]
Carvedilol	3.125 mg bid	25 mg bid 50 mg bid for >187 lb	COMET[10]
Metoprolol succinate	12.5-25 mg/d	200 mg/d	MERIT-HF[11]
Candesartan	4-8 mg/d	32 mg/d	CHARM-Altern[12]
Losartan	12.5 mg/d	50 mg/d	ELITE[13]
Valsartan	20 mg bid	160 mg bid	CHARM[14]
Spirinolactone	25 mg qd		RALES[15]
Isosorbide		120 mg	AHeft[16]
Hydralazine		225 mg	AHeft[16]

The major cause of acute decompensation is fluid overload. Fluid restriction and diuretics are the main treatments. There is no proof that these treatments prolong life, and they may cause complications. However, without judicious use of diuretics or without intelligent and disciplined fluid restriction, all patients with Stage C HF will relapse. As the reduction of mortality and morbidity from BBs or ACEIs is supported by numerous randomized clinical trials (RCTs), the patients should be given the same dosages at which the benefits were effective (Table 9-5).

Beta Blockers

BBs are one of the essential medications for severe LV dysfunction. The benefits, harms, and cost effectiveness were analyzed in the studies with BBs alone, BBs with ACE inhibition, or AR blockade.[11]

 EVIDENCE-BASED MEDICINE:

The MERITT-HF trial

Question: What is the role of beta blocker controlled-release/extended-release metoprolol succinate (metoprolol CR/XL) on mortality, hospitalization, symptoms, and quality of life in patients with HF? *Methodology:* This is a randomized, double-blind, controlled trial that enrolled 3991 chronic HF patients (NYHA II-IV, LVEF<0.4) who were stabilized with optimal standard therapy. Patients were randomized to metoprolol CR/XL, 25 mg once per day (NYHA class II) or 12.5 mg once per day (NYHA class III or IV), titrated for six to eight weeks up to a target dosage of 200 mg once per day (n = 1990) with matching placebo (n = 2001). **Results:** The incidences of all predefined endpoints were lower in the metoprolol CR/XL group than in the placebo group. These included total mortality or all-cause hospitalizations (641 vs. 767 events; risk reduction 19%, 95% CI, 10–27%, P<0.001), total mortality or hospitalizations due to worsening heart failure (311 vs. 439 events, risk reduction 31%, P<0.001), and number of hospitalizations due to worsening heart failure (317 vs. 451 events, P<0.001). **Evidence-Based Applications:** In this study of patients with symptomatic heart failure, metoprolol CR/XL improved survival, reduced heart failure hospitalizations, improved NYHA functional class, and had beneficial effects on patients' well-being.[11]

DATA MANAGEMENT TIPS (CLINICAL PEARLS)
BBs for Patients with COPD

In patients with COPD, use carvedilol with caution because it is nonselective, while metoprolol or atenolol are selective BBs. Carvedilol is better than metropolol succinate for increasing EF. Both decrease mortality. Metropolol succinate (long acting) is the type of metropolol best studied in CHF trials. Patients with low BP tolerated metoprolol better than carvedilol. Metoprolol worsens insulin resistance, while carvedilol has a neutral effect.[17]

How to know that the patient is doing well on beta blockers? The resting heart rate should be in the 60s. The heart rate should not increase to more than 100 with regular activities. The heart sounds are muffled, not crisp.

Angiotension-Converting Enzyme Inhibitor (ACEI)

ACEIs are one of the essential medications for severe LV dysfunction. The benefits, harms, and cost effectiveness of ACEIs alone and with BBs and patient subgroups are discussed below.

 EVIDENCE-BASED MEDICINE:

The CONSENSUS Trial

Question: What are the benefits of enalapril (2.5 to 40 mg per day) in the prognosis of severe CHF (NYHA functional class IV). **Methodology:** This is a double-blinded RCT, which randomly assigned 253 patients to receive either placebo (n = 126) or enalapril (n = 127). Conventional treatments for HF, including the use of other vasodilators, were continued in both groups. **Results:** The crude mortality at the end of six months (primary endpoint) was 26% in the enalapril group and 44% in the placebo group—a reduction of 40%

(P = 0.002). Mortality was reduced by 31% at one year (P = 0.001). The entire reduction in total mortality was found to be among patients with progressive HF (a reduction of 50%), whereas no difference was seen in the incidence of sudden cardiac death. A significant improvement in NYHA classification was observed in the enalapril group, together with a reduction in heart size and a reduced requirement for other medications for HF. *Harms:* The overall withdrawal rate was similar in both groups, but hypotension requiring withdrawal occurred in seven patients in the enalapril group; no patients in the placebo group withdrew. After the initial dose of enalapril was reduced to 2.5 mg daily in high-risk patients, this side effect became infrequent. *Evidence-Based Applications:* The addition of enalapril to conventional therapy in patients with severe CHF can reduce mortality and improve symptoms. The beneficial effect was due to a reduction in death from the progression of HF.

Angiotensin Receptor Blocker

Since they have a similar therapeutic mechanism to the ACEIs, the benefits, harms, and cost effectiveness of the ARBs, with or without BBs, in different dosages and patient subgroups are debated. A substantial proportion of patients, because of previous intolerance to ACE inhibitors, were studied in the CHARM-Alternative program.

 EVIDENCE-BASED MEDICINE:

The CHARM-Alternative Trial

Question: Does candesartan, an ARB, improve outcome in patients not taking an ACE inhibitor? *Methodology:* This is an RCT that enrolled 2028 patients with symptomatic HF and LVEF. Less than 40% of them were not receiving ACE inhibitors because of previous intolerance. Patients were randomly assigned candesartan (target dose 32 mg once daily) or matching placebo. The most common manifestation of ACE-inhibitor intolerance was cough (72%), followed by symptomatic hypotension (13%) and renal dysfunction (12%). *Results:* During a median follow-up of 33.7 months, 33% of patients in the candesartan group and 40% in the placebo group had cardiovascular death or hospital admission for CHF (unadjusted hazard ratio 0.77 [95% CI 0.67-0.89], P = 0.0004). Each component of the primary outcome was reduced, as was the total number of hospital admissions for CHF. *Harms:* Study-drug discontinuation rates were similar in the candesartan (30%) and placebo (29%) groups. *Evidence-Based Applications:* Candesartan was generally well tolerated and reduced cardiovascular mortality and morbidity in patients with symptomatic chronic HF who were intolerant to ACE inhibitors.[12]

Diuretics

Diuretics are not the first line of treatment in HF patients if there is no sign of fluid retention. A low-salt diet and fluid restrictions are the first preventive measures. If there is a sign of fluid overload, then diuretics should be prescribed. Once edema is controlled, low-dose diuretics can be used intermittently, as needed.

DATA MANAGEMENT TIPS (CLINICAL PEARLS)
Intelligent Use of Diuretics

Patients can develop clinical deterioration with diuresis if the patients are preload-dependent, such as in severe pulmonary hypertension, right ventricular failure, aortic stenosis, LV outflow tract obstruction, tamponade, constrictive pericarditis, or restrictive cardiomyopathy. Double the dose of oral diuretics when changing from IV to oral furosemide. Consider oral bumetanide, which is better absorbed in patients with HF, with a shorter half life. If a patient has problems with oral diuretics, twice weekly IV or IM furosemide at the office could keep the patient dry enough to be stable as an outpatient.

ADVANCED MANAGEMENT

Cardiac Resynchronization Therapy

LV failure can occur when the RV and LV fail to contract in a timely physiologic concordance due to conduction delays in the electrical activation of the ventricle (ventricular dyssynchrony). This phenomenon occurs in 15 to 30% of HF patients with dilated cardiomyopathy and bundle branch block (BBB).[18]

 EVIDENCE-BASED MEDICINE:

The MADITT Trial

Question: Do patients with severe cardiomyopathy and BBB benefit from CRT? *Methodology:* This is an RCT (813 people with NYHA class III–IV heart failure). *Results:* Standard care plus CRT significantly reduced the death and combined outcome (death from any cause or an unplanned hospitalization for a major cardiovascular event) when compared with standard care alone (combined outcome: 39% with CRT versus 55% with standard care alone, HR 0.63, 95% CI 0.51 to 0.77; death: 20% with CRT versus 30% with standard care alone, HR 0.64, 95% CI 0.48 to 0.85).[18] *Harms:* One RCT (409 people with CRT implant) showed that lead displacement occurred in 6%, coronary sinus dissection in 2%, pocket erosion in 2%, pneumothorax in 2%, and device-related infection in 1%.[19] *Practical*

Applications: People deriving benefit are those with severe symptoms of heart failure.[17] Since then, the recommendations of the ACC/AHA guidelines are for patients with LVEF ≤35%, wide QRS>120 ms, sinus rhythm, and NYHA functional class III or IV symptoms despite optimal medical treatment (OMT). The results of the MADITT trial above were reconfirmed by the Prevention of Sudden Cardiac Death II Registry (PreSCD Registry) which showed that patients at high risk for SCD who received an ICD one month or more after suffering an MI had a 44% lower mortality than their counterparts who did not get an ICD (P = 0.053). (Presented at the European Society of Cardiology September 2009 Congress in Barcelona Spain.)

Periodic Assessment

In patients with HF, symptomatic improvement can precede objective findings. The patient can feel better, breathe better even the if lungs still have rales and the chest x-ray still shows congestion. Daily weight checks can indentify how much fluid is removed.

DATA MANAGEMENT TIPS (CLINICAL PEARLS)
Evidence of Improvement of HF

Usually, the patient with HF develops decompensated HF because of decreased absorption of medication (especially diuretics) from the GI tract. So the physician should be sure of the following conditions:

- Normal oral medication absorption: No early stomach fullness (early satiety) due to mesenteric edema, which reduces absorption of the medications.
- The appetite is better (less right-sided heart failure with less liver congestion = less endotoxin) and there is less prerenal azotemia.
- Less shortness of breath (less pulmonary venous congestion) shows that fluid overload is reversed.
- The skin color looks pink (peripheral vasoconstriction was corrected). As abrupt and severe peripheral vasoconstriction (from any cause) can precipitate acute decompensated HF, reversal of peripheral vasoconstriction (by ACEIs or BBs) is a major component of treatment. If the patient still has vasoconstriction, he or she is still vulnerable for any relapse.

Complications

At this stage, a patient with HF takes an average of nine medications a day: a BB, an ACEI, a diuretic, digoxin, ASA, nitroglycerin, a statin, an aldosterone antagonist, and for African-American patients, hydralazine-ISDN (besides potassium, medication for diabetes, and for COPD). The occurrences of the side effects or patient noncompliance are due to multiple medications, complex multiple daily dosing, and the need for frequent adjustment with titration. These problems include increased BUN and creatinine, dizziness, and polypharmacy due to side effects of multiple drugs and interactions.

Increased BUN and Creatinine Levels

As more patients survive into advanced stages of HF, it is increasingly difficult to maintain optimal fluid balance with high doses of diuretics while preserving normal renal function. Usually creatinine increases 0.3 mg/dL or proportional rises of 25% following diuresis.[20] Worsening renal function limits neurohormonal therapy, leading to a longer hospital stay. This predicts a higher rate of early rehospitalization and most importantly, death.

⬭ DATA MANAGEMENT TIPS (CLINICAL PEARLS)
How to Manage Elevation of BUN and Creatinine

In many instances, the HF patients can stay asymptomatic with a slightly high level of BUN (25–30 mg). This implies that patients are dry enough, as they are at the optimal dosage of diuretics. If the BUN/creatinine ratio increases <50% and the patient is not congested, then the first therapeutic strategy is to hold the diuretics. Cut the dose of the ACEI in half if the BUN/creatinine ratio increases more than 50%. Stop the ACEI if the ratio increases more than 100%.

Dizziness

The patient on medication for HF can have dizziness from hypotension. The dose of BBs, ACEIs, or ARBs can be reduced. The medications can be taken separate from each other; the BB can be taken first thing in the morning with breakfast and then three hours later the ACEI or the ARB. This can reduce the chances for hypotension and dizziness. The patient should be instructed to stand up slowly from a lying or sitting position while holding on to something steady for one or two minutes before walking.

Comparison Between Beta Blocker Carvedilol and Metoprolol European (COMET) Trial

Methodology: This is an RCT trial of 3029 patients with ischemic (51%) or idiopathic cardiomyopathy (44%) comparing carvedilol (n = 1511) with metoprolol (n = 1518) in a follow-up period of 58 months. *Benefits:* MI was reported in 69 carvedilol and 94 metoprolol patients (hazard ratio [HR] 0.71, 95% CI 0.52 to 0.97, P = 0.03). Cardiovascular death or nonfatal MI was reduced by 19% in the carvedilol group (HR 0.81, 95% CI 0.72 to 0.92, P = 0.0009). Unstable angina was reported as an adverse event in 56 carvedilol and 77 metoprolol patients (HR 0.71, 95% CI 0.501 to 0.998, P = 0.049). Stroke occurred in 65 carvedilol and 80 metoprolol patients (HR 0.79, 95% CI 0.57 to 1.10). Stroke or MI occurred in 130 carvedilol and 168 metoprolol patients (HR 0.75, 95% CI 0.60 to 0.95, P = 0.015). Fatal MI or fatal stroke occurred in 34 carvedilol and 72 metoprolol patients (HR 0.46, 95% CI 0.31 to 0.69, P = 0.0002). *Practical Application:* According to the COMET trial, carvedilol improves vascular outcomes better than metoprolol.[10]

Indication of Digoxin in HF: The DIG Study

Methodology: This is a large RCT (6800 people, NYHA FC I–III, 94% on ACE inhibitors, 82% on diuretics) comparing digoxin and placebo for a mean follow-up period of 37 months. *Results:* It found no significant difference in all-cause mortality with digoxin [34.8%] versus placebo [35.1%]. Digoxin significantly reduced heart failure admissions and reduced the combined outcome of death or heart failure admissions (heart failure admissions: digoxin [27%] vs. placebo [35%]; RR 0.77, 95% CI 0.72 to 0.83; NNT 13). *Harms:* More patients had suspected digoxin toxicity (digoxin [12%] vs. placebo [8%]; RR 1.50, 95% CI 1.30 to 1.73). There were no significant differences between digoxin and placebo in the risk of ventricular fibrillation or tachycardia (digoxin [1.1%] vs. placebo [0.8%]). However, digoxin significantly increased rates of second- or third-degree atrioventricular block (digoxin [1.2%] vs. placebo [0.4%]). *Practical Applications:* Digoxin is best for patients with fast heart rate (sinus tachycardia, uncontrolled atrial fibrillation and atrial flutter). To avoid toxicity and advanced AV block, the digoxin level should be checked frequently and the dosage reduced when there are increased BUN and creatinine levels secondary to diuretics.[21]

DATA MANAGEMENT TIPS (CLINICAL PEARLS)
Avoiding Digoxin Toxicity

The physician must also carefully ensure that excessive dosage has been avoided by seeking evidence of toxicity. Although nausea and vomiting are clear evidence of toxicity, inquiry about whether the patient enjoyed breakfast (no anorexia) provides an earlier clue. Dysrhythmias of any sort require scrutiny because almost every known dysrhythmia has been reported to occur from digitalis intoxication. Since rhythms disturbance is a frequent occurrence observed during the course of clinical heart failure, expert evaluation must distinguish those incident to toxicity, when digoxin needs temporary withdrawal, from those incident to underlying causes of the heart failure, when continuation or even increased dosage may be necessary. Disturbances of vision, e.g., yellow vision, are also worth recognition although they are less frequent in patients receiving digoxin than among those receiving less purified preparations. Disturbances in the psyche (confusion, depression, hallucinations, bizarre mental symptoms) should not be overlooked because they occasionally provide evidence of toxicity. Reoccurrence of lethargy that had been relieved earlier in the treatment course is also worth consideration as an occasional sign of toxicity.[22]

Arterial and Venous Dilators: The AHeft Trial

Methodology: This is a large RCT (1050 African Americans with NYHA class 3 or 4 heart failure and dilated ventricles) comparing hydralazine plus isosorbide dinitrate with placebo.[5] *Benefits:* Hydralazine plus isosorbide dinitrate significantly improved the composite endpoint (weighted values for mortality from any cause, a first hospitalization for heart failure within 18 months, and change in quality of life at 6 months). The quality of life at 6 months was significantly improved compared with placebo (measured on a scale where lower scores indicate better quality of life: –5.6 with hydralazine-isorbide vs. –2.7 with placebo, P = 0.02). *Harms:* Headache and dizziness occurred significantly more often with hydralazine plus isosorbide dinitrate than with placebo (headache: 48% vs. 19%, P<0.001; dizziness: 29% vs. 12%, P<0.001, respectively).[16] *Caveats:* One systematic review has highlighted the potential risk of developing hydralazine-induced systemic lupus erythematous (SLE).[23] Although the risk is small because of lower doses used, people taking hydralazine should be monitored at each visit for signs and symptoms of SLE. A baseline antinuclear antibody level should be determined prior to initiating hydralazine. If any symptoms or signs of SLE develop, hydralazine therapy should be discontinued immediately. *Practical Applications:* This treatment could be used in combination with other medications for heart failure and in people who are intolerant to ACE inhibitors or angiotensin receptor blockers. With the results of the A-Heft trial, the ACC and AHA guidelines suggest the use of ISDN plus hydralazine in African-Americans patients and non-African Americans who remain symptomatic despite maximal therapy with BBs and ACEIs. The combination of hydralazine and isosorbide dinitrate would not be considered first-line therapy for the treatment of heart failure.[5]

Aldosterone Receptor Antagonist for HF

This is a large RCT (1663 people with heart failure, NYHA FC 3 and 4, LV EF < 0.35, all taking ACE inhibitors, loop diuretics, and most taking digoxin) comparing spironolactone 25 mg daily versus placebo.[15] *Benefits:* Spironolactone significantly reduced all-cause mortality compared with placebo after two years (mortality: spironolactone [35%] versus placebo [46%]; RR 0.75, 95% CI 0.66 to 0.85; NNT 9).

Harms: There was no evidence that adding spironolactone to an ACE inhibitor increased the risk of clinically important hyperkalemia.[15] Gynecomastia, or breast pain, was reported in 10% of men given spironolactone and 1% of men given placebo (P<0.001). The rate of hospitalization for hyperkalemia increased from 2.4/1000 people to 11.0/1000 people (P<0.001). *Practical Applications:* Aldosterone antagonist is recommended for patients with NYHA class IV or class III, LVEF ≤35% while receiving standard therapy, including diuretics. The low dose of 25 mg/daily is for HF, while the higher dose of 50 mg/tid is for patients with ascites.[19] It is not recommended when creatinine is >2.5 mg/dL (or creatinine clearance is <30 mL/min), serum potassium is >5.0 mmol/L, or in conjunction with other potassium-sparing diuretics. Serum potassium concentration should be monitored frequently following initiation or change in doses of aldosterone antagonist.[15]

Prevention of Relapse

The compensated condition in Stage B or C can change quickly when any precipitating factor tips over the precarious clinical balance (Table 9-6). This is why prevention of any precipitating or aggravating factor is the second most important strategy in this group of patients.

Prevention of Recurrent Heart Failure

The first tactic is removal of excess fluid with an IV diuretic and fluid restriction. Frequent checks of K level, BUN, and creatinine are needed. Digoxin is indicated, especially if there is atrial arrhythmia; however, these patients carry a higher risk for toxicity. In this phase, the second tactic is to give more medications or to optimize the dose of existing ones while at the same time fending off more frequent and severe side effects. The complete management of these patients is listed in Table 9-7.

DM should be well controlled and HbA1c should be less than 7%. Thiazolidinediones should be avoided if there is any sign of congestion.

TABLE 9-6: Precipitating Factors of Heart Failure

Fluid and sodium impropriety
Infection
Brady- or tachyarrhythmia
Myocardial ischemia or myocardial infarction
Physical (doing too much at home) or emotional stress
Pulmonary embolism
High-output states such as anemia, thyrotoxicosis, Paget's disease, pregnancy, beriberi, and arteriovenous fistula
Cardiac infection and inflammation (myocarditis, infective endocarditis)
Comorbidities (renal, liver, thyroid, respiratory insufficiency)
Cardiac toxin (chemotherapy, cocaine, alcohol)

TABLE 9-7: Management of Severe and Recurrent Heart Failure

Elimination of all medications that can aggravate HF (with emphasis on NSAIDs, thiazolidinediones)
IV diuretics with daily check of electrolytes, BUN, creatinine levels
IV vasodilator including nitroglycerin or nitroprusside
Exercise
New medications on top of BBs, ACEIs, CRT: hydralazine-ISDN, aldosterone antagonists
CRT and ICD
Enrollment in a HF clinic for daily follow-up after discharge
Nursing-home care
Referral to a cardiac transplant program
Ultrafiltration (investigational)

ACEI: angiotensin-converting enzyme inhibitors, BB: beta blockers, BUN: blood urea nitrogen, CRT: cardiac resynchronization therapy, HF: heart failure, ICD: implantable cardioverter defibrillator, ISDN: isosorbide dinitrate, IV: intravenous.

Body weight should be around 15% of ideal. Hypo- or hyperthyroidism should also be treated.

For patients with HF and COPD, the patient should live in a smoke-free environment and practice aggressive infection prevention with influenza/pneumonia vaccine, early treatment of upper respiratory infections, sleep apnea therapy, use of bronchodilators, and 24-hour oxygen if needed.

Patients with arthritis should avoid nonsteroidal anti-inflammatory drugs, keep weight at 15% of the ideal, and exercise regularly. For patients with atrial fibrillation, the ventricular response has to be controlled. We should try to convert the AF to regular sinus rhythm as early as possible.

DATA MANAGEMENT TIPS (CLINICAL PEARLS)
Proof of Clinical Improvement

Watching carefully for subsidence of distention of the neck veins, improvement in breathing, ability to recline fully, improvement from the weakness and fatigue produced by digitalis therapy along with a reduction in right upper abdominal discomfort and fullness, a reduction in edema (*weighing should be done frequently*), and an improvement in skin color will provide evidence of the improvement in cardiac contraction. These guidelines not only provide an index for therapeutic management but also proof of clinical benefits.[22]

TABLE 9-8: Performance Indicators of Comprehensive Care in the Office Setting

LV systolic function assessment and documentation in chart
Change of body weight at each visit
Blood pressure measurement at each visit
Completion of a physical examination pertaining to volume status
Assessment of functional capacity and activity level
Presence or absence of exacerbating factors: unstable CAD, uncontrolled HTN, new or worsening valvular disease
Patient understanding of and compliance with sodium restrictions
Patient understanding of and compliance with medical regimen
History of arrhythmia, syncope, presyncope, or palpitation
Beta blockers
Angiotensin converting enzyme inhibitor or angiotensin receptor blocker
Implantable cardioverter defibrillator if EF<35% or indicated when symptomatic
CRT in patients with ventricular dsysynchrony
Warfarin for atrial fibrillation

CAD: coronary artery disease, CRT: cardiac resynchronization therapy, EF: ejection fraction, HTN: hypertension, LV: left ventricular.

Performance Assessment

Since HF is the manifestation of a long and complex process, the management of these patients also needs to be comprehensive. In order to guarantee the best care for these HF patients, the American College of Cardiology (ACC) and the Heart Failure Society of America (HFSA) guidelines suggested a checklist of essential steps assuring the completeness of treatment. It is shown in Table 9-8.[5]

Social Support

As the patient becomes stable and is mentally capable of understanding and complying with medical treatment, diet, fluid restriction, and exercise (activity restriction), then the chance for being asymptomatic for a long time is reasonably good. The social support from the family is critical to set up a routine program for medication, exercise, meals, bowel movements, and personal hygiene. Any problem with depression should be addressed because it can cause noncompliance with medication and diet. If the patient lives alone, anxiety attacks are a common reason for decompensation and hospitalization. Without support of a family, the patient will return to the hospital and end up in a nursing home. This could be a blessing because now the patient is forced to be on a low-salt diet with fluid restrictions and without heavy domestic chores.

TROUBLE-SHOOTING AND DEBUGGING

Treatment is standard for any physician caring for a patient with severe HF. When the problems are not controlled as expected, management requires the expertise and experience of a consultant cardiologist. The common questions from the referral physicians to the consultant cardiologist in the management of severe HF are discussed below.

Should BNP Be Measured More Frequently as a Guide? The STARS-BNP Multicenter Study

Methodology: This is a multicenter study to evaluate the prognostic impact of a therapeutic strategy using BNP levels. Two hundard twenty NYHA FC II to III patients considered to have been optimally treated with ACEIs, beta blockers, and diuretics by CHF specialists were randomized to medical treatment according to either current guidelines (clinical group) or a goal of decreasing BNP levels <100 pg/mL (BNP group). *Benefits:* Mean dosages of ACEIs and beta blockers were significantly higher in the BNP group (P<0.05), whereas the mean increase in furosemide dosages was similar in both groups. During follow-up (median 15 months), significantly fewer patients reached the combined endpoint in the BNP group (24 vs. 52%, P<0.001).[24]

However, using individualized levels of the biomarker NT-proBNP to guide the treatment of patients with chronic heart failure did not improve their morbidity or mortality over standard clinical management, according to results of the Can Pro-Brain-Natriuretic Peptide Guided Therapy of Chronic Heart Failure Improve Heart Failure Morbidity and Mortality? (PRIMA) study.[25] *Practical Applications:* In optimally treated CHF patients, a BNP-guided strategy reduced the risk of CHF-related death or hospital stay for CHF. The result was mainly obtained through an increase in ACEI and beta blocker dosages.[24.]

What is the Significance of Anemia in HF Patients?

Anemia is prevalent in heart failure and may portend poor outcomes. There is a need to determine the characteristics and long-term prognosis of anemia in ambulatory patients with chronic heart failure. *Methods:* Data from 6159 consecutive outpatients with chronic, stable heart failure were reviewed at baseline, short-term (3-month) follow-up, and long-term (6-month) follow-up between 2001 and 2006. Mortality rates were determined from 6-month follow-up to end of study period. *Results:* Prevalence of anemia (hemoglobin [Hb] <12 g/dL for men, <11 g/dL for women) was 17.2% in our cohort. Diabetes, B-natriuretic peptide, left ventricular ejection fraction, and estimated glomerular filtration rate were independent predictors of baseline anemia. Documented evaluation of anemia was found in only 3% of all anemic patients and was better in internal medicine than in cardiology clinics. At 6-month follow-up, new-onset anemia developed in 16% of patients, whereas 43% patients with anemia at baseline had resolution of their hemoglobin levels. Higher total mortality rates were evident in patients with persistent anemia (58% vs. 31%, P<0.0001) or with incident anemia (45% vs. 31%, P<0.0001) compared with those without anemia at 6 months. *Practical Applications:* These observations in a broad unselected outpatient cohort suggest that anemia in patients with heart failure is under-recognized and underevaluated. However, resolution of anemia was evident in up to 43% of patients who presented initially with the disease and did not pose a greater long-term risk for all-cause mortality. However, the presence of persistent anemia conferred poorest survival in patients with heart failure when compared with that of incident, resolved, or no anemia.[26]

How to Predict Deterioration of HF

In the follow-up stable patients with severe dilated cardiomyopathy, many patients could have relapse of HF at any time. How can the appearance of decompensated HF be predicted? Do intrathoracic impedance data predict heart-failure events? Or is it a high tech toy? The Chronicle Offers Management to Patients with Advanced Signs and Symptoms of Heart Failure (COMPASS-HF) tried to answer these questions.

Does a HF management strategy using continuous intracardiac pressure monitoring decrease HF morbidity? *Methods:* The study was a prospective, multicenter, randomized, single-blinded, parallel-controlled trial of 274 New York Heart Association functional class III or IV HF patients who received an implantable continuous hemodynamic monitor. Patients were randomized to a Chronicle (Medtronic Inc., Minneapolis, Minnesota) (n = 134) or control (n = 140) group. All patients received optimal medical therapy, but the hemodynamic information from the monitor was used to guide patient management only in the Chronicle group. Primary endpoints included freedom from system-related complications, freedom from pressure-sensor failure, and reduction in the rate of HF-related events (hospitalizations and emergency or urgent care visits requiring intravenous therapy). *Results:* The two safety endpoints were met with no pressure-sensor failures and system-related complications in only 8% of the 277 patients who underwent implantation (all but four complications were successfully resolved). The primary efficacy endpoint was not met because the Chronicle group had a nonsignificant 21% lower rate of all HF-related events compared with the control group (P = 0.33). A retrospective analysis of the time to first HF hospitalization showed a 36% reduction (P = 0.03) in the relative risk of a HF-related hospitalization in the Chronicle group. *Practical Applications:* The implantable continuous hemodynamic monitor-guided care did not significantly reduce total HF-related events compared with optimal medical management. Additional trials will be necessary to establish the clinical benefit of implantable continuous hemodynamic monitor-guided care in patients with advanced HF.[27]

What is the Significance of Severe Weight Loss in HF Patients?

Is weight loss an important predictor of poor prognosis in patients with chronic heart failure? *Methodology:* In the current study, the researchers examined the effect of weight loss on mortality in a large sample of patients enrolled in the CHARM (Candesartan in Heart failure: Reduction in Mortality and morbidity) program. The subjects represented a broad spectrum of HF, including both reduced and preserved left ventricular (LV) systolic function. The change in weight over 6 months in 6933 patients and its association with subsequent mortality (1435 deaths) over a median of 32.9 months were assessed. *Results:* A significant monotonically increasing association was observed between the percentage of weight loss over six months and excess mortality for cardiovascular and other causes of death. Compared with patients with less than 1% weight change, patients with 5% to 7% weight loss had a 50% increase in mortality hazard, and those with over 7% weight loss had a 62% increase in hazard. The risk associated with weight loss was especially high among subjects who were already thin at study entry. Results of the time-updated analyses showed an even stronger association between weight loss and short-term mortality risk. Patients with a last recorded weight loss over 10% had a four-fold increased risk (hazard ratio 4.4) compared to those with currently stable weight. *Practical Applications:* Good patient management requires ongoing monitoring of weight changes over time, calling for increased vigilance, particularly when weight loss > 5% is detected, as this indicates the presence of cachexia in a short period of time.[28]

TAKE-HOME MESSAGE

Data Collecting Collect all the data about the patient's history (of smoking, high-salt, high-cholesterol diet, alcohol abuse, lack of exercise, HTN, DM, high cholesterol level), family history (of early sudden death due to heart disease, history of early CAD), social history (work and behaviors) and from a complete physical examination (signs of prior stroke, CAD, PAD, carotid murmur, weak peripheral pulses), all of which add weight to the clinical decision-making process.

Data Mining Recommend safe, appropriate, and efficacious investigation (including fasting lipid profile, fasting blood glucose, BUN and creatinine levels, weight, BMI, waist circumference) BNP, echocardiography.

Management Recommend safe, appropriate, and efficacious therapy to maintain the stable health status of the patient over time (low-salt, low-cholesterol diet, stopping smoking, losing weight, no drinking alcohol, exercise). The main treatments of Stage C asymptomatic HF patients with abnormal structural changes emphasize prevention with healthy lifestyle changes (low-salt, low-cholesterol diet, fluid restrictions, exercise, and medications [BBs and ACEIs]). Revascularization is indicated if there is reversible ischemia. Avoidance of all precipitating or aggravating factors is very important to prevent any clinical deterioration. CRT is indicated if there is wide QRS complex and if the EF is still <35% after a few months of optimal medical treatment (including BB and ACEI).

Patient-Centered Care Get the patients involved in their own lifestyle modification to increase compliance with diet, exercise, medication, office visits, and testing in order to provide continuity of care.

References

1. Hess, O.M., Carroll, J.D.: Clinical Assessment of Heart Failure, in Libby, P., Bonow, R., Mann, D., Zipes, D., eds.: Braunwald's Heart Disease: A Textbook of Cardiovascular Medicine 8th edition, Philadelphia: W.B.Saunders, 2008, pp 561-582.
2. Harvey, W. P.: Cardiac pearls. Cedar Grove, NJ: Leannec Publishing, 1993, pp 43-112.
3. Perloff, J. K.: Physical Examination of the Heart and Circulation. Shelton, CT.: People's Medical Publishing House, 2009.
4. Harlan, W. R., Oberman, A., Grimm, R., et al.: Chronic congestive heart failure in coronary artery disease: Clinical criteria. Ann Intern Med. 1977;86:133.
5. Hunt, S.A., Abraham, W.T., Chin, M.H., et al.: The ACC/AHA Guideline Update for the Diagnosis and Management of Chronic Heart Failure in the Adult. JACC. 2005;46: 1116–1143.
6. Packer, M., Coats, A. J., Fowler, M. B., et al.: Effect of carvedilol on survival in severe chronic heart failure. N Engl J Med. 2001;344:1651–1658.
7. The CONSENSUS Trial Study Group. Effects of enalapril on mortality in severe congestive heart failure. Results of the Cooperative North Scandinavian Enalapril Survival Study (CONSENSUS). N Engl J Med. 1987;316:1429–1435.
8. The Acute Infarction Ramipril Efficacy (AIRE) Study Investigators. Effect of ramipril on mortality and morbidity of survivors of acute

myocardial infarction with clinical evidence of heart failure. Lancet. 1993;342:821–828.

9. Kober, L., Torp-Pedersen, C., Carlsen, J. E., et al.: A clinical trial of the angiotensin-converting enzyme inhibitor trandolapril in patients with left ventricular dysfunction after myocardial infarction. Trandolapril Cardiac Evaluation (TRACE) Study Group. N Engl J Med. 1995; 333(25):1670–1676.

10. Remme, W. J., Torp-Pedersen, C., Cleland, J. G.: Carvedilol protects better against vascular events than metoprolol in heart failure: results from COMET. J Am Coll Cardiol. 2007;49(9):963–967.

11. Hjalmarson, A., Goldstein, S., Fagerberg, B., et al.: for the MERIT-HF Study Group: Effects of Controlled-Release Metoprolol on Total Mortality, Hospitalizations, and Well-Being in Patients With Heart Failure. The Metoprolol CR/XL Randomized Intervention Trial in Congestive Heart Failure (MERIT-HF) JAMA. 2000;283:1295–1302.

12. Granger, C. B., McMurray, J. J., Yusuf, S., et al.: CHARM Investigators and Committees. Effects of candesartan in patients with chronic heart failure and reduced left-ventricular systolic function intolerant to angiotensin-converting-enzyme inhibitors: the CHARM-Alternative trial. Lancet. 2003;362:772–776.

13. Pitt, B., Poole-Wilson, P. A., Segal, R., et al.: Effect of losartan compared with captopril on mortality in patients with symptomatic heart failure: Randomised trial – the losartan heart failure survival study ELITE II. Lancet. 2000;355:1582–1587.

14. Cohn, J. N., Tognoni, G.: A randomized trial of the angiotensin-receptor blocker valsartan in chronic heart failure. The Valsartan Heart Failure Trial Investigators. N Engl J Med. 2001;345:1667–1675.

15. Pitt, B., Zannad, F., Remme, W. J., et al.: for the Randomized Aldactone Evaluation Study Investigators. The effects of spironolactone on morbidity and mortality in patients with severe heart failure. N Engl J Med. 1999;341:709–717.

16. Taylor, A. L., Ziesche, S., Yancy, C., et al.: Combination of isosorbide dinitrate and hydralazine in blacks with heart failure. [erratum appears in N Engl J Med. 2005;352:1276]. N Engl J Med. 2004;351:2049–2057.

17. Bakris, G. et al.: Metabolic effects of carvedilol vs metoprolol in patients with type 2 diabetes mellitus and hypertension. JAMA. 2004; 292;227–236.

18. Cleland, J. G. F., Daubert, J. C., Erdmann, E., et al.: The effect of cardiac resynchronization on morbidity and mortality in heart failure. N Engl J Med. 2005;352:1539–1549.

19. Gold, M., Higgins, S., Daoud, E., et al.: Comparison of complication-free rate between ICD and CRT-D trials Heart Rhythm, 2007;2: S204-S204.

20. Weinfeld, M.S., Chertow, G.M., Warner Stevenson, L.: Aggravated renal dysfunction during intensive therapy for advanced chronic heart failure. Am Heart J. 1999;138:285–290.

21. Digitalis Investigation Group. The effect of digoxin on mortality and morbidity in patients with heart failure. N Engl J Med. 1997;336: 525–533.

22. Hussain, Z., Sindle, J., Hauptman, P.J.: Digoxin use and digoxin toxicity in the Post-DIG Trial Era J Cardiac Failure. 12:343-6, 2006.
23. Finks, S. W., Finks, A. L., Self, T. H., et al.: Hydralazine-induced lupus: maintaining vigilance with increased use in patients with heart failure. South Med J. 2006;99:18–22.
24. Jourdain, P., Jondeau, G., Funck, F., et al. : Plasma brain natriuretic peptide-guided therapy to improve outcome in heart failure: the STARS-BNP Multicenter Study. J Am Coll Cardiol. 2007;49:1733–1739.
25. Can Pro-Brain-Natriuretic Peptide Guided Therapy of Chronic Heart Failure Improve Heart Failure Morbidity and Mortality? (PRIMA) Study presented at the American College of Cardiology, 2009 Scientific Sessions. Orlando FL.
26. Tang, W., Tong, W., Jain, A., et al.: Evaluation and Long-Term Prognosis of New-Onset, Transient, and Persistent Anemia in Ambulatory Patients With Chronic Heart Failure. J Am Coll Cardiol. 2008;51:569–576.
27. Bourge, R. C., Abraham, W. T., Adamson, P. B., on behalf of the COMPASS-HF Study Group. Randomized Controlled Trial of an Implantable Continuous Hemodynamic Monitor in Patients With Advanced Heart Failure. The COMPASS-HF Study. J Am Coll Cardiol. 2008;51:1073–1079.
28. Pocock, S.J., McMurray, J.J., Dobson, J.: Weight loss and mortality risk in patients with chronic heart failure in the candesartan in heart failure: assessment of reduction in mortality and morbidity (CHARM) programme. Eur Heart J. 2008;29:2641–2650.

Advanced Heart Failure and Heart Transplant

CHAPTER

10

Krishna K. Gaddam, Pridhvi Yelamanchili, and Hector Ventura

Chapter Outline

INTRODUCTION

Recent advances in heart failure (HF) therapy have resulted in considerable improvements in quality of life and survival of patients with HF. As a consequence of improvements in treatment and increasing life expectancy, overall prevalence of HF and the proportion of patients with advanced HF are increasing. In spite of the recent advances, HF-related mortality remains high and continues to rise. Eighty percent of men and 70% of women <65 years of age diagnosed with HF will die within 8 years.[1]

Patient Population in Focus

There are four stages of HF.[2] In Stage C, the patient has structural heart disease with prior or current symptoms of HF. Patients with Stage C HF could be well compensated and minimally symptomatic, hospitalized with decompensated HF, or have recurrent decompensations followed by compensation with treatment. Stage D HF includes patients with refractory HF requiring specialized interventions (Figure 10-1). In this chapter we will discuss the presentation, risk stratification, and management of patients with advanced heart failure, which includes patients in Stage C requiring frequent hospitalizations and those in Stage D HF.

DATA COLLECTING

Fluid retention, dyspnea, and exercise intolerance are the cardinal symptoms of HF. Dyspnea and exercise intolerance are mostly experienced on exertion in the initial stages of HF. Patients with advanced HF often present with manifestations of low cardiac output such as renal insufficiency, early satiety, poor appetite, abdominal pains, nausea, decreased mentation, memory problems, and cognitive impairment which are often reversible with the treatment of HF.

PROGRAMMED MANAGEMENT

Strategic Programming

Every attempt should be made to identify and correct reversible causes of HF, such as poor compliance with diet and medications, myocardial ischemia, tachy-or bradyarrhythmias, and valvular disease in patients presenting with worsening HF in spite of optimal medical treatment (Table 10-1).

Pharmacologic Therapy

As outlined in the previous chapters, regular exercise, salt and fluid restrictions, diuretics, angiotensin-converting enzyme inhibitors (ACEIs) or angiotensin receptor blockers (ARBs) in patients who are intolerant of ACEIs and beta blockers constitute the mainstay of therapy for patients

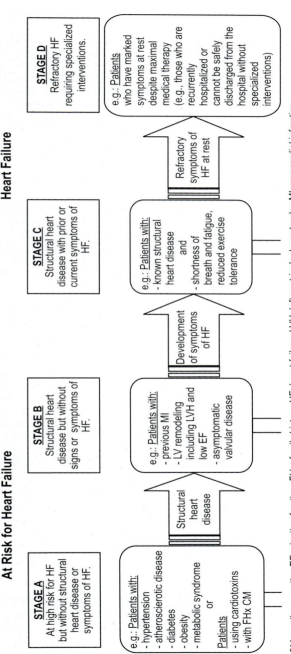

Figure 10-1 Stages in the development of heart failure. FHx CM indicates family history of cardiomyopathy. (Modified and reprinted with permission from Hunt SA, Abraham WT, Casey Jr. DE, et al. ACC/AHA 2005 guideline update for the diagnosis and management of chronic heart failure in the adult: a report of the American College of Cardiology/American Heart Association J Am Coll Cardiol. 2005;46:e1-e82).

CM: cardiomyopathy, EF: ejection fraction, FHx: family history, HF: heart failure, LVH: left ventricular hypertrophy, MI: myocardial infarction.

TABLE 10-1: Management Master Plan

	Mechanism of Disease	Direct Treatment	General Treatment
Index Problem: Severe Dilated LV	Severely depressed EF	Surgical restoration of LV geometry, passive ventricular constraint devices, mitral valve annuloplasty	Positive inotropic therapy, treatment of ischemia: CABG, TMR
Upstream of Index Problem	Pulmonary venous (capacitance) system overloaded	Judicious use of diuretic, CRT (software correction for synchronous contraction of LV and RV)	Beta blockade to decrease HR so O_2 demand
Downstream of Index Problem	Distal peripheral arteries: vasoconstriction	Intra-aortic balloon pump (IABP)	ACEIs/ARBs to reverse vasoconstriction
Work-around Configuration		LVAD	
System Recovery	Prone for VT or VF = SCD	ICD	
System Replacement	ESHF	Heart transplant	

LV: left ventricle, EF: ejection fraction, CABG: coronary arterial bypass grafts, CRT: cardiac resynchronization therapy, ACEI: angiotensin converting enzyme inhibitor, IABP: intra aortic balloon pump, LVAD: left ventricular assist device, VT: ventricular tachycardia, VF: ventricular fibrillation; SCD: sudden cardiac death, ICD: implantable cardioverter defibrillator, ARB: angiotensin receptor blocker, ESHF: end stage heart failure, HR: heart rate, RV: right ventricle, TMR: transmyocardial laser revascularization.

with HF. Several large placebo controlled trials have clearly shown that ACEIs, ARBs, and beta blockers improve symptoms and decrease morbidity and mortality in patients with reduced left ventricular systolic function. Diuretics, particularly loop diuretics, are used for symptomatic treatment (fluid retention) but have not proved to improve mortality.

The Randomized Aldactone Evaluation Study (RALES)[3] and Eplerenone Post Acute Myocardial Infarction Heart Failure Efficacy and Survival Study (EPHESUS)[4] trials showed that, in addition to treatment with ACEIs, beta blockers, and diuretics, addition of spironolactone (a nonselective aldosterone antagonist) or eplerenone (a selective aldosterone antagonist) improves survival and decreases the frequency of hospitalizations in patients with NYHA class III-IV symptoms.

Vasodilators, such as hydralazine and nitrates, should be considered in patients intolerant to ACEIs or ARBs due to poor renal function or hyperkalemia or in patients with persistent symptoms despite treatment with renin angiotensin aldosterone antagonists and beta blockers, particularly African Americans.[5] Digoxin therapy may be considered for heart rate control in the setting of atrial fibrillation. In patients with severe systolic heart failure with persistence of symptoms in spite of maximal therapy with ACEIs, beta blockers, and diuretics, digoxin has been shown to reduce symptoms and decrease hospitalizations.[6]

Implantable Cardioverter Defibrillator and Cardiac Resynchronization Therapy

Patients with HF and left ventricular dilation have a high risk of sudden death most commonly due to ventricular arrhythmias besides other causes such as ischemic events, electrolyte disturbances and thromboembolic events. MADIT II[7], SCD-HeFT,[8] and COMPANION[9] trials have clearly proved the mortality benefit of an ICD in addition to conventional medical therapy in patients with ischemic and nonischemic dilated cardiomyopathy with LVEF <35%. The American and European HF guidelines recommend an ICD implantation in all patients with ischemic and nonischemic dilated cardiomyopathy with LVEF <35% and in whom survival with good functional capacity is otherwise anticipated to extend beyond 1 year. All patients with NYHA class III-IV HF with evidence of atrioventricular dysynchrony by electrocardiogram (QRS duration > 120 ms) should be considered for cardiac resynchronization therapy (CRT).[9-10]

Intravenous Inotropic Therapy

Positive inotropic agents are indicated in patients with acute decompensated heart failure with pulmonary congestion and signs of hypoperfusion (cardiogenic shock). Dobutamine (a beta-adrenergic agonist) is recommended for treatment of patients with low cardiac output and reduced blood pressure. Concomitant use of beta blockers with dobutamine may attenuate the benefit of either agent. Milrinone (a phosphodiesterase inhibitor) is preferred over dobutamine in patients without hypotension but with low cardiac output and symptoms of hypoperfusion. Milrinone is a phosphodiesterase enzyme (which is an enzyme that breaks down cyclic adenosine monophosphate [cAMP], inhibitor, resulting in a net increase in cAMP levels, which in turn results in the inotropic effects. Thus the effects of milrinone are independent of those of beta-adrenergic receptors. Hence, beta blocker usage is not contraindicated with milrinone. Both these agents can only be administered intravenously and are proarrhythmic. Positive ionotropes have been shown to improve hemodynamics and bring about rapid relief of symptoms.[11-12] Concerns have been raised about the use of these agents, particularly in the long term on a continuous basis due to increased mortality.[13-14] Continuous or long-term intermittent infusion of ionotropes is only recommended as a bridge to heart transplantation or may also be considered for palliation of symptoms in patients with refractory heart failure who are not eligible for a more definitive therapy, such as heart transplantation.

ADVANCED MANAGEMENT
Nontransplant Surgical Options
Coronary Artery Bypass Grafting (CABG)
Ischemic heart disease is the most common cause of heart failure. Coronary artery bypass grafting (CABG) should be considered for patients with three-vessel coronary artery disease and demonstrable myocardial viability.

 EVIDENCE–BASED MEDICINE:

CABG Versus Medical Therapy: The Duke Databank

In a single center observational study,[15] patients who underwent cardiac catheterization for the first time and were noted to have ≥ 75% stenosis in one of the three major epicardial vessels and an ejection fraction ≤ 40% with NYHA class II or greater symptoms were classified into medical therapy group (n = 1052) or CABG group (n = 339), depending on which therapy they received within 30 days of catheterization. Within the first 30 days, medical treatment had a survival benefit over CABG for one-($P = 0.01$) and three-($P = 0.03$) vessel disease. For two-vessel disease, there was no significant difference between medicine and CABG ($P = 0.36$). In the follow-up period > 30 days from baseline, the adjusted overall survival at 1 (83% vs. 74%), 5 (61% vs. 37%), and 10 (42% vs. 13%) years strongly favored CABG over medical treatment ($P<0.0001$).

Myocardial Viability
Myocardial viability can be assessed using various modalities, such as positron emission tomography (PET) with fluorodeoxyglucose (FDG) imaging, single photon emission tomography (SPECT) with thallium-201, technetium-99m sestamibi or technetium-99m tetrofosmin imaging, dobutamine stress echocardiography (DSE), and magnetic resonance imaging (MRI) with gadolinium. There is a strong association between myocardial viability on noninvasive testing and improved survival after revascularization in patients with chronic CAD and LV dysfunction.[16]

For patients with defined myocardial viability, revascularization resulted in a 79.6% relative reduction in risk of death compared to medical treatment. For patients without viability, annual mortality was not significantly different according to treatment method: 7.7% with revascularization versus 6.2% with medical therapy (P = ns).[16] Recent advances of MRI late hyper-enhancement show that it is highly specific and sensitive but not yet readily available.

Transmyocardial Laser Revascularization
Other novel techniques, such as transmyocardial laser revascularization and percutaneous intramyocardial autologous bone marrow cell implantation, are being investigated in the treatment of patients with refractory or end-stage coronary artery disease not amenable to percutaneous coronary intervention or coronary artery bypass graft surgery. Early studies have shown improvement in angina and exercise capacity in patients with severe angina.[17-18] Larger randomized, controlled-outcome trials are required to establish the clinical utility of these techniques in the treatment of coronary artery disease.

Surgical Restoration of Left Ventricular Geometry
Operative methods that reduce left ventricular volume and "restore" ventricular elliptical shape are being evaluated. The International Reconstructive Endoventricular Surgery returning Torsion Original Radius Elliptical shape to the left ventricle (RESTORE) showed that surgical ventricular restoration is highly effective in improving LV systolic function, NYHA functional class, and decreasing hospitalizations for heart failure in patients with ischemic cardiomyopathy.[19] However, the Surgical Treatment for Ischemic Heart Failure (STITCH TRIAL) did not show a difference in symptoms, rate of death, or hospitalization between patients who were treated with CABG alone versus those treated with CABG together with ventricular reconstruction.[20] Routine surgical restorations are not recommended at present.

Mitral Annuloplasty
Mitral annuloplasty in patients with significant mitral regurgitation helps reverse adverse remodeling and has been shown to improve symptoms in patients with end-stage dilated cardiomyopathy.[21] A recent retrospective analysis, however, did not show any long-term mortality benefit conferred by mitral valve annuloplasty for significant mitral regurgitation with severe left ventricular dysfunction.[22] Isolated mitral valve repair is not routinely recommended for patients with advanced heart failure.

Mechanical Support Devices
Severely decompensated heart failure is characterized by fluid overload, low cardiac output, hypotension, and diuretic resistance. Mechanical circulatory support devices, such as the intra-aortic balloon pump

(IABP) or ventricular assist devices (VAD), are increasingly used in such situations. IABP has emerged as the single most effective and widely used circulatory assist device. It is indicated in a low cardiac output state in patients with advanced HF as a bridge to transplantation or in acute decompensated HF. The use of IABP is limited by the invasive nature of the procedure, restriction of patient mobility, risks of thromboembolism, bleeding, and infection. VADs are mechanical pumps that assist the failing ventricle (left or right) in maintaining adequate circulation (Figure 10-2). They are defined as pulsatile or continuous flow, based on their flow and as extracorporeal, paracorporeal, or intracorporeal according to the implantation site (Table 10-2). Left ventricular assist devices (LVADs) are more commonly used than right ventricular assist devices.

When is a ventricular assist device indicated and which type? LVADs are currently used (1) as a "bridge" to heart transplantation in patients listed for transplantation but who are clinically deteriorating before a donor heart is available, or (2) as replacement (destination) therapy for failing hearts in patients who are not candidates for heart transplantation. At the present time, the Thoratec implantable VAD, HeartMate XVE, HeartMate II, and Novacor LVAD are the approved devices for bridging to transplant, whereas HeartMate XVE is the only device approved for destination therapy. Major complications associated with

TABLE 10-2: Different Types of Ventricular Assist Devices

Device	Site	Mechanism of Action	Configuration
IABP	Extracorporeal	Pulsatile	LVAD
Impella	Extracorporeal	Continuous flow	LVAD
ABIOMED BVS	Extracorporeal	Pulsatile	LVAD/RVAD/ BiVAD
JARVIK 2000	Intracorporeal	Continuous flow	LVAD
DeBakey VAD	Intracorporeal	Continuous flow	LVAD
Novacor LVAS	Intracorporeal	Pulsatile	LVAD
Thoratec	Intracorporeal	Pulsatile	LVAD/RVAD/ BiVAD
Heart Mate XVE	Intracorporeal	Pulsatile	LVAD
Heart Mate II	Intracorporeal	Continuous flow	LVAD

IABP: intra aortic balloon pump, LVAD: left ventricular assist device, RVAD: right ventricular assist device, BiVAD: biventricular assist device.

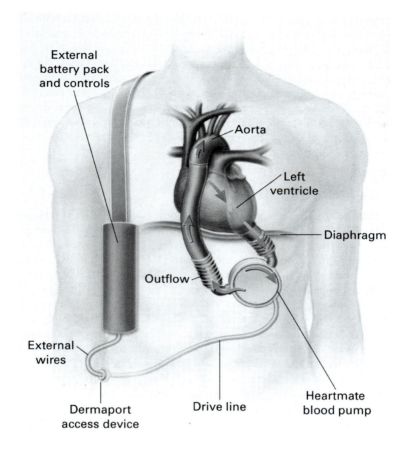

External
battery pack
and controls

Aorta

Left
ventricle

Diaphragm

Outflow

External
wires

Dermaport
access device

Drive line

Heartmate
blood pump

Figure 10-2 An intracorporeal left ventricular assist device and its components. The inflow cannula is inserted into the apex of the left ventricle, and the outflow cannula is anastomosed to the ascending aorta. Blood returns from the lungs to the left side of the heart and exits through the left ventricular apex and across an inflow valve into the pumping chamber. Blood is then actively pumped through an outflow valve into the ascending aorta. The pumping chamber is placed within the abdominal wall. One transcutaneous line carries the electrical cable and air vent to the battery pack and electronic controls, which are worn on a shoulder holster or belt. (Reprinted with permission from Goldstein DJ et al NEJM. 1998;339:1522–1533).

LVADs include bleeding, infection, and device malfunction. Temporary right ventricular failure immediately following an LVAD placement can occur in 30% of patients requiring ionotropes or RVADs.

Smaller size, greater durability, and lower risk of infection with the newer continuous flow devices (DeBakey VAD, HeartMate II, and Jarvik 2000) offer an advantage over the pulsatile flow devices, which are limited by their large size, risk of disk failure, and infection. Jarvik 2000, a newer, axial-flow impeller pump that is currently under investigation is smaller, totally implantable, and silent with a potentially lower risk of infections, thrombosis, and hemolysis, thus promising to be a better device. The results of the Randomized Evaluation of Mechanical Assistance for the Treatment of Congestive Heart Failure (REMATCH) trial follow.

 EVIDENCE-BASED MEDICINE:

The REMATCH Trial

Methodology: This is a randomized trial comparing LVAD (Heart-Mate XVE) with medical therapy.[23] REMATCH randomized 129 patients with NYHA class IV HF symptoms who were deemed ineligible for cardiac transplantation to LVAD implantation (n = 68) or standard medical management (n = 61). ***Results:*** There was a 48% significant reduction in mortality from any cause in the LVAD group when compared with the medical therapy group (relative risk, 0.52; 95% confidence interval [CI], 0.34-0.78; P = 0.001). Quality of life was significantly improved at one year in the device group. The one-year survival rate was significantly higher in the LVAD group than in the medical therapy group at 52% and 25%, respectively (P = 0.002). The two-year survival rates were not significantly different at 23% and 8%, respectively. ***Harms:*** Infection, bleeding, and device malfunction were 2.4 times more likely to occur in the LVAD group than in the medical therapy group. ***Evidence-Based Applications:*** Which is a better bridge to heart transplantation—ionotropes or ventricular assist devices? Patients who receive the HeartMate as a bridge to transplantation may have a better outcome compared to patients treated with an intravenous ionotrope.[24–25] Despite the improved outcome with HeartMate, the potential risk versus benefit compared with ionotropic support needs to be considered in the individual patient.

Passive Ventricular Constraint Devices

Less popular devices currently under investigation include the Acorn cardiac support device (a biocompatible polyester mesh designed to wrap around both ventricles which provides end diastolic support to reduce myocardial stretch and ventricular wall stress) and Myosplint (which consists of three myosplints placed perpendicular to the long axis of the left ventricle drawing the ventricular walls inward and designed to reduce myocardial wall stress). The Acorn device has been shown to improve left ventricular chamber size and function and to reverse cellular remodeling and hypertrophy in preclinical studies.[26–27] Myosplint implantation has been shown to decrease myocardial stress, and improvement in ejection fraction has been shown in a canine model.[28] Their safety and utility in humans are being evaluated.

A More User Friendly LVAD

Weighing 25 g and smaller than a man's thumb, a rotor-based pump (Synergy; CircuLite, Saddle Brook, NJ) provided "partial ventricular support," boosting hemodynamics rather than taking it over, in a 16-patient "first-in-human" experience. Implanted in men and women with recurrent advanced heart failure (INTERMACS level 4), who were ambulatory and not on inotropic therapy and either listed or otherwise suitable for a heart transplant, the Synergy pump made the patients feel markedly better, improved their mean arterial and capillary-wedge pressures and cardiac index the first day of implantation, and sustained the benefits over an average of about 11 weeks. Measured prior to surgery and during the 24-hour postoperative period, the group averages for mean artery pressure went up 5 mm Hg ($P = 0.02$) and cardiac index climbed by 1.3 L/min/m^2 ($P<0.001$). The average pulmonary artery diastolic pressure fell by 9 mm Hg ($P = 0.01$). Mean peak VO_2 increased from 9.6 mL/kg/min to 14.1 mL/kg/min ($P = 0.01$).[29]

HEART TRANSPLANTATION

Heart transplantation is the treatment of choice for patients with heart failure refractory to medical therapy. Data from the 2008 report from the registry of the International Society for Heart and Lung Transplant (ISHLT) showed that patient survival at one and three years for patients who received cardiac transplantation was approximately 85 and 79%, respectively (Figure 10-3).[30] Recent advances in medical and device therapies have also improved the survival of heart failure patients comparable to that of post–heart transplant patients.[31] There are more patients who need heart transplantation than there are donor hearts available. Heart transplantation should be limited to patients who are most likely to benefit from it with a significant improvement in symptoms and life expectancy. The ISHLT has published listing criteria to guide transplant centers to risk stratify and select patients for heart transplantation. Nonischemic cardiomyopathy and coronary artery disease are the most common indications for heart transplantation. The indications and contraindications for heart transplantation and the recommended schedule for heart transplant evaluation are detailed in Table 10-3 and Table 10-4.

(text continued on page 269)

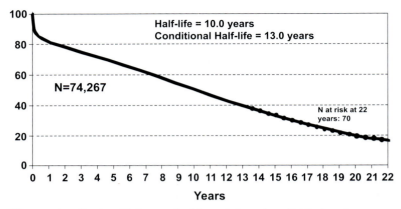

Figure 10-3 Kaplan-Meier survival for adult and pediatric heart transplants performed between January 1982 and June 2006. Conditional half-life = time to 50% survival for those recipients surviving the first year post-transplantation. (Reprinted with permission from Taylor, D.O., et al., J Heart Lung Transplant. 2008;27:943–956.)

TABLE 10-3: Selection Criteria for Heart Transplantation

Cardiomyopathy – Patients with cardiac conditions not responding to maximal medical therapy (e.g., ischemic cardiomyopathy, intractable angina in spite of maximal tolerated medical therapy, not amenable to CABG/PTCA), dilated cardiomyopathy, valvular heart disease, hypertensive heart disease, hypertrophic cardiomyopathy (persistent heart failure despite maximal medical therapy including alcohol ablation, myomectomy, mitral valve replacement, and pacemaker therapy), congenital heart disease (not amenable to surgical correction and in which fixed pulmonary hypertension is not a complication) should be considered for heart transplantation.

Intractable Arrhythmias – Uncontrolled with ICD, not amenable to electrophysiologic-guided single or combination), medical therapy, not a candidate for ablative therapy

Age Limit – Patients ≤70 years of age should be considered for cardiac transplantation. Carefully selected patients >70 years of age may be considered for cardiac transplantation. There is an increasing tendency to perform transplantation in older patients. It has been proposed to use an alternate list or strategy of allocating organs from older donors (that would otherwise be unused) to older recepients.

(continued)

TABLE 10-3: Selection Criteria for Heart Transplantation *(continued)*

Weight Limit – It is recommended that a body mass index (BMI) of <30 kg/m^2 or percent ideal body weight (PIBW) <140% is preferred for listing for cardiac transplantation. Obese patients are at an increased risk for poor wound healing, infection, lower extremity thrombus, and pulmonary complications.

Diabetes – Diabetes with end-organ damage other than nonproliferative retinopathy or poor glycemic control (hemoglobin A$_{1C}$ >7.5) despite optimal effort is a relative contraindication.

Renal Dysfunction – Presence of irreversible renal dysfunction (estimated GFR <40 mL/min) is a relative contraindication. Combined heart-kidney transplantation may be considered in patients with irreversible renal failure.

Cerebrovascular Disease/Peripheral Vascular Disease – Clinically severe symptomatic cerebrovascular disease, which is not amenable to revascularization, may be considered a contraindication. Peripheral vascular disease may be considered a relative contraindication when its presence limits rehabilitation and revascularization is not a viable option.

Neoplasms – Active neoplasms from origins other than the skin are an absolute contraindication to cardiac transplantation. Depending on tumor type and response to therapy, if tumor recurrence is low and metastatic work-up is negative, then cardiac transplantation can be considered. Cancers that have been in remission for 5 years or longer may be acceptable for transplant evaluation. All patients should be screened as per American Cancer Society guidelines for malignancies.

Other Comorbidities – Such as amyloidosis, any active infections including human immunodeficiency virus infection and sarcoidosis, are exclusions for cardiac transplantation

Psychosocial Conditions – All patients being considered for transplantation should be assessed for ability to give informed consent and comply with instructions and support systems conditions. Mental retardation or dementia is a relative contraindication.

Tobacco and Substance Abuse – Active tobacco smoking is a relative contraindication. Active tobacco smoking during the previous six months is a risk factor for poor outcome after transplantation. Patients who remain active substance abusers (including alcohol) should not receive heart transplantation.

TABLE 10-4: Recommended Schedule for Heart Transplant Evaluation

Test	Baseline	Repeat 3 Months	6 Months	9 Months	12 Months (and Yearly)
Complete H & P	X				
Follow-up assessment		X	X	X	X
Weight/BMI	X	X	X	X	X
Immunocompatibility					
ABO	X				
Repeat ABO	X				
HLA tissue typing	Only at transplant				
PRA and flow cytometry	X				
• >10%	Every 1-2 months				
• VAD	Every 1-2 months				
• Transfusion	2 weeks after transfusion and then 9 months × 6 months				
Assessment of heart failure severity					
Cardiopulmonary exercise test with RER	X				
Echocardiogram	X		X		X
Right-sided heart catheterization (vasodilator challenge as indicated)	X				X
ECG	X				X

Evaluation of multiorgan function					
Routine lab work (BMP, CBC, LFT)	X	X	X	X	X
PT/INR More frequent per protocol if on VAD or coumadin	X				
Urinalysis	X	X	X	X	X
GFR (MDRD quadratic equation)	X	X	X	X	X
Unlimed urine sample for protein excretion	X	X	X	X	X
PFT with arterial blood gases	X				
CXR (PA and lateral)	X				X
Abdominal ultrasound	X				
Carotid Doppler (if indicated or >50 y)	X				
ABI (if indicated or >50 y)	X				
DEXA scan (if indicated or >50 y)	X				
Dental examination	X				X
Ophthalmologic examination (if diabetic)	X				X
Infectious serology and vaccination					
Hep B surface Ag	X				
Hep B surface Ab	X				
Hep B core Ab	X				
Hep C Ab	X				
HIV	X				
RPR	X				
HSV IgG	X				
CMV IgG	X				
Toxoplasmosis IgG	X				

(continued)

TABLE 10-4: Recommended Schedule for Heart Transplant Evaluation *(continued)*

Test	Baseline	3 Months	6 Months	9 Months	12 Months (and Yearly)
EBV IgG	X				
Varicella IgG	X				
PPD	X				
Flu shot (q 1 year)	X				
Pneumovax (q 5 years)	X				
Hep B immunizations: 1_2_3_	X				
Hep B surface Ab (immunity)	6 weeks after third immunization				
Preventive and malignancy					
Stool for occult blood × 3	X				X
Colonoscopy (if indicated or >50 y)	X				
Mammography (if indicated or >40 y)	X				X
Gyn/Pap (if indicated ≥18 y sexually active)	X				X
PSA and digital rectal exam (men >50 y)	X				X
General consultations					
Social work	X				
Psychiatry	X				
Financial	X				
Neuro/psych (if applicable)	X				

DATA MINING
Cardiopulmonary Exercise Testing (CPX)

Exercise intolerance is one of the hallmarks of disease severity in patients with chronic heart failure. CPX is a well-established prognostic test in patients with chronic heart failure and is routinely used in determining the candidacy for cardiac transplantation. Exercise capacity can be quantitated clinically by measuring oxygen uptake (VO_2), carbon dioxide production (VCO_2) and minute ventilation during exercise with rapidly responding gas analyzers. Directly measured VO_2 has been shown to be a reproducible marker of exercise tolerance in chronic heart failure and to provide objective and additional information regarding the patient's clinical status and factors that limit exercise performance. Despite increasing workload, the maximal oxygen uptake (VO_2 max) eventually reaches a plateau in normal individuals. Patients with heart failure rarely reach a true plateau of oxygen consumption with increasing workloads, and hence the term "peak VO_2" is used instead of the VO_2 max. A peak VO_2 of 20 mL/kg/min is considered normal.

 EVIDENCE-BASED MEDICINE:

Peak VO_2 and Survival After Cardiac Transplant

In a study including 114 consecutive subjects referred for cardiac transplantation, patients were divided into three groups based on exercise data: Group 1 included patients with peak $VO_2 \leq 14$ mL/kg/min who were accepted as transplant candidates; Group 2 included patients with peak $VO_2 > 14$ mL/kg/min who were considered too well for transplantation; and Group 3 included patients with peak $VO_2 \leq 14$ mL/kg/min who were rejected for transplantation because of noncardiac reasons, such as malignancy or advanced lung disease; they served as the control group. Patients with a peak $VO_2 > 14$ mL/kg/min (Group 2) had a cumulative one-and two-year survival rate of 94% and 84%, respectively, which were equal to survival levels after transplantation. However, patients in Group 1 had a one-year survival rate of 70% and those in Group 3 had survival rates of only 47% and 32% at one and two years, respectively. In Group 3, patients with peak $VO_2 \leq 10$ mL/kg/min had the lowest survival, while those between 10 and 14 mL/kg/min had an outcome that was only slightly worse than patients in Group 1.[32]

Peak VO_2 varies by gender, age, and lean body weight. Peak VO_2 corrected for these factors has been suggested to be a more accurate determinant of prognosis.[33–34] In HF patients, measurement of peak VO_2 is often limited by deconditioning, lack of motivation, difficulty exercising with measurement apparatus, and body composition. Factors such as severe muscular deconditioning, peripheral arterial disease, arthritis, angina pectoris, or low patient motivation should be excluded in order to accurately interpret a CPX. Additional measures of CPX, such as respiratory exchange ratio (RER) (VCO$_2$/VO$_2$) and ventilation to carbon dioxide slope (VE/VCO$_2$) may be helpful and are better prognostic indicators in patients with submaximal exercise testing. Current recommendations for using CPX parameters to guide transplant listing are included in Table 10-5. Patients should not be listed solely on the criterion of a peak VO$_2$ measurement.

Heart Failure Survival Scores

Various models have been developed to predict survival in patients with heart failure. The Heart Failure Survival Score (HFSS) (Table 10-6)[35]

TABLE 10-5: Recommendations for Cardiopulmonary Exercise Testing to Guide Transplant Listing:

Class I

A maximal CPX is defined as one with respiratory exchange ratio (RER) > 1.05 and achievement of an anaerobic threshold on optimal pharmacologic therapy (*Level of Evidence: B*).
In patients intolerant of a beta blocker, a cutoff for peak VO$_2$ of ≤ 14 mL/kg/min should be used (*Level of Evidence: B*).
In the presence of a beta blocker, a cutoff for peak VO$_2$ of ≤ 12 mL/kg/min should be used (*Level of Evidence: B*).

Class IIa

In young patients (<50 years) and women, it is reasonable to consider using alternative standards in conjunction with peak VO$_2$ to guide listing, including percent of predicted (≤50%) peak VO$_2$ (*Level of Evidence: B*).

Class IIb

In the presence of a submaximal CPX test (RER <1.05), use of ventilation equivalent to a carbon dioxide (VE/VCO$_2$) slope of >35 as a determinant in listing for transplantation may be considered (*Level of Evidence: B*).
In obese (body mass index > 30 kg/m^2) patients, a lean body mass-adjusted peak VO$_2$ (lean peak VO$_2$) of <19 mL/kg/min can serve as an optimal threshold to guide prognosis (*Level of Evidence: B*).

Class III

Listing patients based solely on the criterion of a peak VO$_2$ measurement should not be performed (*Level of Evidence: C*).

TABLE 10-6: Calculation of Heart Failure Survival Score

Clinical Characteristic	Value (χ)	Coefficient (β)	Product
Ischemic cardiomyopathy	1	+0.6931	+0.6931
Resting heart rate	90	+0.0216	+1.9440
Left ventricular ejection fraction	17	−0.0464	−0.7888
Mean BP	80	−0.0255	−2.0400
IVCD	0	+0.6083	0
Peak VO$_2$	16.2	−0.0546	−0.8845
Serum sodium level	132	−0.0470	−6.2040

HFSS is a composite score calculated using seven separate variables that have been separately identified and validated as prognostic measures. Each of the component variables is assigned a model coefficient based on regression models. It is calculated by taking the absolute value of the sums of the products of each component variable's value and its model coefficient. Patients are stratified into low (≥ 8.10), medium (7.20 to 8.09), and high risk (<7.20). Among the patients in the validation sample, one-year survival rates without transplant for these three strata were 88, 60, and 35%, respectively.

and The Seattle Heart Failure Model[36] (an interactive program that helps estimate the one-, two-, and five-year survival rates and the benefit of adding medications and/or devices for an individual patient is available at www.SeattleHeartFailureModel.org) are the most widely used models for predicting survival in ambulatory patients. The Enhanced Feedback for Effective Cardiac Treatment (EFFECT) (available at http://www.ccort.ca/CHFriskmodel.asp) and Acute Decompensated Heart Failure National Registry (ADHERE) risk tree models were developed to predict 30-year and one-year mortality in patients hospitalized with acute decompensated HF.

Which is a better predictive model for mortality in heart failure patients? ISHLT recommends using the Heart Failure Survival Score (HFSS) to determine prognosis and guide the listing for transplantation for ambulatory heart failure patients, particularly in ambiguous patients (those with peak VO$_2$ > 12 and <14 mL/kg/min). However, HFSS was developed from a subset of patients treated only with ACE inhibitors, digoxin, and diuretics. In the present era of beta blockers, CRT, and ICDs, the validity of HFSS has been questioned. An alternative model, The Seattle Heart Failure Model derived from a cohort of 1125 heart failure patients using some commonly obtained clinical, pharmacologic, device, and laboratory characteristics and further validated in five additional cohorts including ~10,000 patients and about 17,300 person-years of follow-up, has been shown to provide an accurate estimate of one-, two-, and three-year survival rates (r = 0.97–0.99).[36]

Right Heart Catheterization and Hemodynamics

Routine right heart catheterization to assess the severity of heart failure is not recommended. Right heart catheterization and hemodynamic assessment are useful in tailoring therapy in advanced heart failure and in acute settings.[37] In preparation for listing for cardiac transplantation, a right heart catheterization should be performed on all candidates to assess for pulmonary hypertension and cardiac output. A pulmonary artery systolic pressure (PASP) > 50 mm Hg or transpulmonary gradient (TPG) > 15 or the pulmonary vascular resistance (PVR) > 3 warrants a vasodilator challenge with inhaled nitric oxide or intravenous nitrates to determine reactivity. If unsuccessful, hospitalization with continuous hemodynamic monitoring should be performed, as often the PVR will decline after 24 to 48 hours of treatment. Irreversible pulmonary hypertension despite adequate therapy with diuretics, vasodilators, and/or mechanical cardiac support devices (IABP, LVAD) is a poor prognosticator in patients with advanced heart failure and is a relative contraindication for listing for heart transplantation.

DATA MANAGEMENT

United Network for Organ Sharing (UNOS) Listing for Cardiac Transplantation

Once evaluation is completed, appropriate patients are listed for cardiac transplantation. The donor organ procurement and distribution are regulated by the UNOS in the United States.[37] There are typically four UNOS listing categories based on the severity of cardiac illness.

UNOS Status 1A: This is the highest priority category. Patients on mechanical ventilation (for no more than 30 days) or mechanical cardiac support such as IABP or ventricular assist devices, high-dose inotropic agents, and continuous hemodynamic monitoring are included in this category.

UNOS Status 1B: Patients with a ventricular assist device implanted for >30 days, inpatient or outpatient continuous inotropic agent infusion at a low dose.

UNOS Status 2: All others active on the transplant list.

UNOS Status 7: Temporarily inactive.

All listed patients should be reevaluated at three-to six-month intervals for improvement or deterioration and their status adjusted accordingly.

ADVANCED MANAGEMENT

Transplantation Surgery and Postoperative Care

Patients <50 years of age who are brain dead are usually potential cardiac donors. Contraindications for heart donation include significant heart dysfunction, congenital heart disease, malignancies (except basal cell and squamous cell carcinomas of the skin and primary tumors of the central nervous system with low metastatic potential), or transmissible diseases. Once brain death is declared, the organ procurement organization (OPO) should be involved for further donor management, whose main focus is to maintain the function of the organs to be transplanted. The most suitable recipient based on ABO compatibility, body size compatibility (within 20% difference of height and weight) and within 2 to 4 hours of reach of the hospital where the donor is available is identified and matched to receive the heart. Longer ischemic time of the donor heart is associated with a higher risk of death after transplantation. Hence every effort is made to limit the ischemic time to a maximum of 4 to 5 hours.

The donor heart is then transplanted in a matching recipient by one of three surgical approaches—orthotopic (donor heart implanted in place of the native heart by classic Shumway-Lower biatrial anastomoses or bicaval anastomoses) or heterotropic (donor heart piggy-backed beside the native heart). The bicaval anastomoses is the most commonly used technique and it preserves the donor atria. It is associated with reduced postoperative epinephrine requirement, tricuspid regurgitation (which is more common with the biatrial technique), temporary pacing requirements, and fewer arrhythmias. Disadvantages include prolonged ischemic time and a rare potential to develop stenosis at the superior vena caval and inferior vena caval anastomoses. Heterotropic transplantation is rarely performed today but may be particularly indicated in patients with severe fixed pulmonary hypertension in order to prevent right heart failure of the naïve donor heart or in case of a significant size mismatch (donor-to-recepient weight ratio <75%).

During the immediate postoperative period (often up to 48 hours), vasoconstrictors to maintain adequate blood pressure and support with inotropes and occasionally an IABP may be required. Temporary epicardial (atrial and ventricular) pacing is maintained until the intrinsic allograft heart rates start picking up. The inherent intrinsic allograft heart rate should be checked every day by turning the epicardial pacer off. It typically takes 48 to 72 hours for the intrinsic rate to start picking up. In case of insufficient intrinsic rates, chronotropic stimulants, such as isoproterenol or theophylline, may be indicated to help maintain adequate heart rates. A few transplant recipients may require a permanent pacemaker due to sinus node or atrioventricular node dysfunction.

A first-generation cephalosporin or vancomycin in penicillin-sensitive patients is advised for the first 24 hours.

Acute allograft dysfunction, right heart failure (commonly occurring in patients with pulmonary hypertension, donor-recipient size mismatch-or those receiving multiple blood product infusions), atrial flutter/fibrillation (often signs of allograft rejection), ventricular tachyarrhythmias (most likely suggestive of myocardial ischemia), renal failure (secondary to ischemic injury from aortic cross-clamping, postoperative hypotension, or medication-induced after initiating calcineurin inhibitors) may complicate the immediate postoperative period, warranting support with ionotropes, mechanical circulatory support devices, and temporary renal replacement therapies.

Immunosuppression

High-dose steroids, azathioprine, and thymoglobulin were the mainstays of immunosppresive therapy in the early days of transplantation. The introduction of the calcineurin inhibitor cyclosporine has revolutionized immunosppressive therapy and markedly improved post-transplant survival. Current practice is to use a triple drug regimen, including a calcineurin inhibitor (cyclosporine or tacrolimus/FK506), steroids (usually prednisone), and an antiproliferative agent (azathioprine, mycophenolate mofetil or MMF). High-dose corticosteroids (most often methylprednisolone) are started intraoperatively. The calcineurin inhibitor (usually tacrolimus) and antiproliferative agents (commonly mycophenolate mofetil) are started 12 to 24 hours postsurgery. Initiation of calcineurin inhibitors may be delayed if renal function is impaired perioperatively. Although it is controversial, some transplant centers may use induction therapy with anti–T-cell monoclonal antibodies (OKT3), anti–thymocyte globulin (thymoglobulin), daclizumab (Zenapax), or basiliximab (Simulect) in the first 5 to 14 days postoperatively in patients at high risk for early rejection or to delay calcineurin inhibitor initiation for renal sparing. Higher incidence of infections (specifically cytomegalovirus infections), rebound rejection, and lymphoproliferative disorders are a concern with the use of induction therapy.

Allograft Rejection

The recipient's immune system recognizes the alloantigens as foreign and constantly tries to rid the body of the foreign tissue, which is kept in check by immunosuppression therapy. Allograft rejection may occur at any point post-transplant and could be a result of one of three mechanisms—hyperacute (occurs within minutes to hours and is caused by preformed antibodies in the recipient and can be avoided by carefully screening for possible donor-specific antibodies using a panel reactive antibody [PRA]), humoral (antibody-mediated), or cell-mediated. Acute cellular rejection is the most common form of rejection and occurs in one-third to one-half of heart transplant recipients, who can be diagnosed by endomyocardial biopsy and graded by the ISHLT grading system as follows:

Grade 0 R: no rejection; Grade 1 R: mild rejection (interstitial and/or perivascular infiltrate with up to one focus of myocyte damage; Grade 2 R: moderate rejection (two or more foci of infiltrate with associated myocyte damage; Grade 3 R: severe rejection (diffuse infiltrate with multifocal myocyte damage, with or without edema, hemorrhage, or vasculitis).[38] Hyperacute rejection is often fatal and requires repeat transplantation or use of artificial heart support. In case of humoral or cellular rejection, mild rejection with no significant clinical deterioration requires no changes in therapy, whereas moderate to severe rejection warrants treatment irrespective of clinical changes. Treatment is usually with high dose steroids or in the case of rejection with hemodynamic compromise, antilymphocyte therapy (OKT3, lymphocyte immunoglobulin [ATGAM], rabbit antithymocyte globulins [RATG[]) and/or high dose intravenous steroids are used. The incidence of rejection is highest in the first month post-transplantation and then subsequently decreases to a low but constant rate. During the first year, routine surveillance biopsies are performed at regular intervals which vary at different transplant centers.

Post-Transplant Infections

Immunosuppressants, while decreasing the incidence of rejection, increase the risk of opportunistic infections. Cytomegalovirus (CMV), *Pneumocystis carinii*, and fungal infections are common in post solid-organ transplant patients; hence prophylactic agents to prevent these infections should be considered and initiated in all patients post-transplant. Trimethoprim-sulfamethoxazole is given universally to all transplant recipients who do not have sulfa allergies and is particularly effective in preventing *Pneumocystis carinii* infections and also listeriosis, toxoplasmosis, and nocardiosis. Routine prophylaxis with antifungal agents has not been shown to improve mortality in solid-organ transplant patients, but given the high incidence of and mortality associated with invasive mycoses in the solid-organ transplant population, targeted prophylaxis for fungal infections in patients at highest risk for such infections is reasonable. Ganciclovir and valganciclovir are preferred agents for CMV prophylaxis. Acyclovir and valacyclovir are also effective and may be used in low-risk patients.

Infections are very common following solid-organ transplantation, particularly in the first year. It is advised to aggressively investigate even a low-grade fever in post-transplant patients, especially during the first

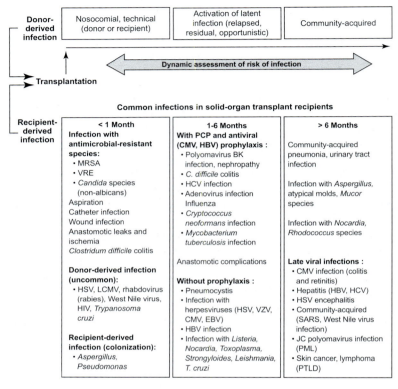

Figure 10-4 Changing timeline of infection after organ transplantation. MRSA, methicillin-resistant *Staphylococcus aureus*; VRE, vancomycin-resistant *Enterococcus faecalis*; HSV, herpes simplex virus; LCMV, lymphocytic choriomeningitis virus; HIV, human immunodeficiency virus; PCP, *Pneumocystis carinii*; HBV, hepatitis B virus; VZV, varicella zoster virus; SARS, severe acute respiratory syndrome; PML, progressive multifocal leukoencephalopathy; PTLD, post-transplantation lymphoproliferative disorder. (Reproduced with permission from Fishman JA et al. N Engl J Med. 2007;357:2601–2614.)

30 days, as these patients don't necessarily mount a sufficient immune response to develop the clinical signs and symptoms of infection due to the chronic immunosuppression. The most common infections, depending on the time after transplantation, are shown in Figure 10-4. Patients should be treated with appropriate antimicrobials chosen based upon the clinical suspicion and tailored according to the microbiological and serological studies.

Long-Term Complications of Cardiac Transplantation

Allograft coronary artery disease or allograft vasculopathy, which is diffuse obliterative coronary artery disease, is the major long-term complication of cardiac transplantation. As with any other solid-organ transplantation, hypertension, diabetes, and osteoporosis are commonly attributable to the long-term steroid use. Chronic immunosuppression also increases the risk of malignancies (most commonly lymphoproliferative disorders).

END-OF-LIFE CARE (PALLIATIVE THERAPY)

All patients with heart failure should be approached regarding wishes for resuscitative care and their wishes should be documented in a living will or other advanced medical directive. Palliative measures including inotropes should be considered and offered to patients with advanced heart failure who do not qualify for heart transplantation and are unresponsive to medical therapy. Hospice care at home, in a hospital, or at specialized centers may be considered for patients with NYHA class IV symptoms, those with a life expectancy of six months or less, and those with refractory heart failure after exhausting all the options of standard of care. Hospices generally provide oral medications and symptomatic management. Some hospices may provide complex treatments, such as intravenous inotropes or continuous positive airway pressure (CPAP). Continued participation of the clinician and meticulous management of fluid status are essential to maximize quality of life even after the patient enrolls in hospice.[39]

TAKE-HOME MESSAGE

Data Collecting Patients with advanced heart failure may present with symptoms of hypoperfusion, including exercise intolerance, fatigue, decreased appetite, abdominal cramps, anorexia, renal failure, liver failure, memory problems, and cognitive impairment predominantly, even in the absence of fluid retention or shortness of breath.

Data Mining Patients presenting with worsening heart failure despite optimal medical treatment should be carefully and repeatedly assessed to identify and correct reversible causes such as noncompliance with diet and medications, myocardial ischemia, tachy-or bradyarrhythmias, and valvular disease.

Management Heart transplantation improves quality of life and survival in patients with advanced heart failure and is the treatment of choice for patients with heart failure refractory to medical therapy. However, there are more patients who need heart transplantation than there are donor hearts available, and transplantation is associated with a commitment to lifelong immunosuppression and related long-term complications. If, despite all of the above efforts, patients continue to deteriorate, they may be considered for cardiac transplantation. Ionotropes and cardiac mechanical assist devices (IABP, LVADs) may be considered as a bridge to transplant or destination therapies. Patients with NYHA class IV symptoms and life expectancy of six months or less, if not candidates for any of the definitive therapies such as heart transplantation or a VAD as a destination therapy, should be considered and referred to hospice care.

Patient-Centered Care Get the patients involved in their own lifestyle modification to increase compliance with diet, exercise, medication, office visits, and testing in order to provide continuity of care.

References

1. Rosamond, W., Flegal, K., Furie, K., et al.: Heart disease and stroke statistics – 2008 update: A report from the American Heart Association Statistics Committee and Stroke Statistics Subcommittee. Circulation. 2008; 117:e25–146.
2. Hunt, S. A., Abraham, W. T., Chin, M. H., et al.: ACC/AHA 2005 guideline update for the diagnosis and management of chronic heart failure in the adult: A report of the American College of Cardiology/American Heart Association Task Force on Practice Guidelines (Writing Committee to Update the 2001 Guidelines for the Evaluation and Management of Heart Failure). J Am Coll Cardiol. 2005; 46:e1–82.
3. Pitt, B., Zannad, F., Remme, W. J., et al.: The effect of spironolactone on morbidity and mortality in patients with severe heart failure. Randomized Aldactone Evaluation Study Investigators. N Engl J Med. 1999; 341:709–717.
4. Pitt, B., Remme, W., Zannad, F., et al.: Eplerenone, a selective aldosterone blocker, in patients with left ventricular dysfunction after myocardial infarction. N Engl J Med. 2003;348:1309–1321.
5. Taylor, A. L., Ziesche, S., Yancy, C., et al.: Combination of isosorbide dinitrate and hydralazine in blacks with heart failure. N Engl J Med. 2004;351:2049–2057.
6. The effect of digoxin on mortality and morbidity in patients with heart failure. The Digitalis Investigation Group. N Engl J Med. 1997;336: 525–533.
7. Moss, A. J., Zareba, W., Hall, W. J., et al.: Prophylactic implantation of a defibrillator in patients with myocardial infarction and reduced ejection fraction. N Engl J Med. 2002;346:877–883.
8. Bardy, G.H., Lee, K.L., Mark, D.B., et al. Amiodarone or an implantable cardioverter-defibrillator for congestive heart failure. N Engl J Med. 2005;352:225–37.
9. Bristow, M. R., Saxon, L. A., Boehmer, J., et al.: Cardiac resynchronization therapy with or without an implantable defibrillatorin advanced chronic heart failure. N Engl J Med. 2004;350:2140–2150.

10. Cleland, J. G. F., Daubert, J., Erdmann, E., et al.: The effect of cardiac resynchronization on mortality and morbidity in heart failure. N Engl J Med. 2005;352:1539–1549.
11. Anderson, J. L.: Hemodynamic and clinical benefits with intravenous milrinone in severe chronic heart failure: results of a multi-center study in the United States. Am Heart J. 1991;121:1956–1964.
12. Mehra, M. R., Ventura, H. O., Kapoor, C., et al.: Safety and clinical utility of long-term intravenous milrinone in advanced heart failure. Am J Cardiol. 1997;80:61–64.
13. Cuffe, M. S., Califf, R. M., Adams, K. F., et al.: Short-term intravenous milrinone for acute exacerbation of chronic heart failure: A randomized controlled trial. JAMA. 2002;287:1541–1547.
14. Upadya, S., Lee, F. A., Saldarriaga, C., et al.: Home continuous positive ionotropic infusion as a bridge to cardiac transplantation in patients with end-stage heart failure. J Heart Lung Transplant. 2004;23:466–472.
15. O'Connor, M. C., Velazquez, E. J., Gardner, L. H., et al.: Comparison of coronary artery bypass grafting versus medical therapy on long-term outcome in patients with ischemic cardiomyopathy (a 25 year experience from Duke cardiovascular disease databank). Am J Cardiol. 2002;90:101–107.
16. Pagano, D., Townend, J. N., Littler, W. A., et al.: Coronary artery bypass surgery as treatment for ischemic heart failure: the predictive value of viability assessment with quantitative positron emission tomography for symptomatic and functional outcome. J Thorac Cardiovasc Surg. 1998;115:791–799.
17. Oesterle, S. N., Sanborn, T. A., Ali, N., et al.: Percutaneous transmyocardial laser revascularization for severe angina: the PACIFIC randomized trial. Potential Class Improvement From Intramyocardial Channels. Lancet 2000;356:1705–1710.
18. Tse, H. F., Thambar, S., Kwong, Y. L., et al.: Comparative evaluation of long-term clinical efficacy with catheter-based percutaneous intramyocardial autologous bone marrow cell implantation versus laser myocardial revascularization in patients with severe coronary artery disease. Am Heart J. 2007;154:982.e1–6.
19. Athanasuleas, C. L., Buckberg, G. D., Stanley, A. W. H., et al.: Surgical ventricular restoration in the treatment of congestive heart failure due to post-infarction ventricular dilation. J Am Coll Cardiol, 2004;44:1439–1445.
20. Jones, R.H., Velazquez, E.J., Michler, R.E., et al.: Coronary bypass surgery with or without surgical ventricular reconstruction. N Engl J Med. 2009;360:1705–17.
21. Smolens, I.A., Pagani, F.D., Bolling, S.F.: Mitral valve repair in heart failure. Eur J Heart Fail. 2000;2:365–71.
22. Wu, A.H., Aaronson, K.D., Bolling, S.F., et al.: Impact of mitral valve annuloplasty on mortality risk in patients with mitral regurgitation and left ventricular systolic dysfunction. J Am Coll Cardiol. 2005;45:381–7.

23. Rose, E.A., Gelijns, A.C., Moskowitz, A.J., et al.: Long-term use of a left ventricular assist device for end-stage heart failure. N Engl J Med. 2001;345:1435–43.
24. Bank, A.J., Mir, S.H., Nguyen, D.Q., et al.: Effects of left ventricular assist devices on outcomes in patients undergoing heart transplantation. Ann Thorac Surg. 2000;69:1369–74.
25. Aaronson, K.D., Eppinger, M.J., Dyke, D.B., et al.: Left ventricular assist device therapy improves utilization of donor hearts. J Am Coll Cardiol. 2002;39:1247–54.
26. Blom, A.S., Mukherjee, R., Pilla, J.J., et al.: Cardiac support device modifies left ventricular geometry and myocardial structure after myocardial infarction. Circulation. 2005;112:1274–83.
27. Cheng, A., Nguyen, T.C., Malinowski, M., et al.: Passive ventricular constraint prevents transmural shear strain progression in left ventricular remodeling. Circulation. 2006;114(1 Suppl):I–79–86.
28. Takagaki, M., Rottenberg, D., McCarthy, P.M., et al.: A novel miniature ventricular assist device for hemodynamic support. ASAIO. 2001;47:412–6.
29. Meyns, B., Klotz, S., Simon, A., et al.: Proof of concept: hemodynamic response to long-term partial ventricular support with the synergy pocket micro-pump. J Am Coll Cardiol. 2009;54:87–8.
30. Taylor, D.O., Edwards, L.B., Aurora, P., et al.: Registry of the International Society for Heart and Lung Transplantation: twenty-fifth official adult heart transplant report-2008. J Heart Lung Transplant. 2008;27:943–56.
31. Butler, J., Khadim, G., Paul, K.M., et al.: Selection of patients for heart transplantation in the current era of heart failure therapy. J Am Coll Cardiol. 2004;43:787–93.
32. Mancini, D.M., Eisen, H., Kussmaul, W., et al.: Value of peak exercise oxygen consumption for optimal timing of cardiac transplantation in ambulatory patients with heart failure. Circulation. 1991;83:778–86.
33. Stelken, A.M., Younis, L.T., Jennison, S.H., et al.: Prognostic value of cardiopulmonary exercise testing using percent achieved or predicted peak oxygen uptake for patients with ischemic and dilated cardiomyopathy. J Am Coll Cardiol. 1996;27:345–52.
34. Osman, A.F., Mehra, M.R., Lavie, C.J., et al.: The incremental prognostic importance of body fat adjusted peak oxygen consumption in chronic heart failure. J Am Coll Cardiol. 2000;36:2126–31.
35. Aaronson, K.D., Schwartz, J.S., Chen, T.M., et al.: Development and prospective validation of a clinical index to predict survival in ambulatory patients referred for cardiac transplant evaluation. Circulation. 1997;95:2660–7.
36. Levy, W.C., Mozaffarian, D., Linker, D.T., et al.: The Seattle Heart Failure model: prediction of survival in heart failure. Circulation. 2006;113:1424–33.
37. Mehra, M., Kobashigawa, J., Starling, R., et al.: Listing criteria for heart transplantation: International Society for Heart and Lung Transplantation guidelines for the care of transplant candidates — 2006. J Heart Lung Transplant. 2006;25:1024–42.

38. Stewart, S., Winters, G.L., Fishbein, M.C., et al.: Revison of the 1990 working formulation for the standardization of nomenclature in the diagnosis of heart rejection. J Heart Lung Transplant. 2005;24:1710–20.
39. Goodlin, S.J., Hauptman, P.J., Arnold, R., et al.: Consensus statement: Palliative and supportive care in advanced heart failure. J Card Fail. 2004;10:200–9.

Aortic Stenosis

Stilianos Efstratiadis, Andrew D. Michaels,
Lefeng Wang, Zhang Shuang Chuan,
Joel Mulungu, Navin Nanda,
and Nguyen Quang Tuan

Chapter Outline

DEFINITION

Obstruction of the left ventricular (LV) outflow is localized most commonly at the level of the aortic valve. Valvular aortic stenosis (AS) has the following three major causes: (1) congenital unicuspid or bicuspid valve, (2) rheumatic valvular degeneration, and (3) degenerative senile calcific changes. Subvalvular or supravalvular AS is much less common.

Population in Focus

The incidence of bicuspid aortic valve disease is between 0.5% and 2% of the population. Calcification of the bicuspid aortic valve is the most common cause of AS in patients between 40 and 60 years of age. While rheumatic AS is very rare in the absence of rheumatic mitral valve disease, the aortic valve is the second-most commonly involved valve in rheumatic heart disease. Degenerative senile calcific AS is present in approximately 2% of people older than 65, 3% of people older than 75, and 5% of people older than 85. Degenerative calcification of the aortic valve accounts for 90% of aortic valve replacements in patients older than 70.

Strategic Programming

Based on a computational cardiac model, the index problem of AS is the obstruction of the cardiovascular system at the level of the aortic valve. This is a hardware problem. The upstream area is the left ventricle, pulmonary vascular system, and the right side of the heart. The downstream area is the aorta and the peripheral vasculature. In the investigation of patients with AS, the strategy is to identify patients with AS through data collecting with a comprehensive history (complaint of chest pain, shortness of breath, dizziness, syncope, or no symptoms) and physical examination (e.g., systolic murmur at the second right intercostal space (ICS), slow rate of rise on the carotid pulse). The next step is to perform data processing in order to formulate a preliminary diagnosis and a short list of differential diagnoses (e.g., hypertrophic cardiomyopathy) Then, using the method of data mining, tests may be selectively performed (echocardiography, exercise stress test, low-dose dobutamine stress test, left heart catheterization, coronary angiography) in order to confirm (data converting) the main diagnosis of AS and to rule out (data filtering) the differential diagnoses.

DATA COLLECTING

Investigation Master Plan

When a physician sees a patient suspected of having AS, there are seven main areas of interest for data collecting (history and physical examination) based on a computational cardiac model.

The main area of interest: Aortic valve. In general, a patient with AS is asymptomatic at early stages. There are no subjective symptoms. The main physical finding related directly to AS is a systolic murmur at the second right ICS. AS is a hardware problem (zone A).

The upstream area of AS is the left ventricle, the pulmonary vasculature, and the right side of the heart (zone B).

The downstream area is the aorta and the peripheral arteries. There could be dilation of the ascending aorta (zone C).

The system configuration: There is no problem with the configuration; there is obstruction at the aortic valve (zone E).

The work-around configuration: No work-around is available here (zone D).

The cardiovascular system: If there is longstanding AS, the cardiovascular system bears the effect of high LV pressure due to AS, causing left ventricular hypertrophy (LVH) and heart failure (HF). The symptoms and signs are of upstream end-organ damage or failure and not due to AS per se. The patient can have chest pain due to increased oxygen demand from the LVH with a patent coronary artery.

The network (the whole body): Longstanding AS can cause syncope because of transient hypotension, sudden death due to left and right HF, and renal failure due to poor renal perfusion (zone F).

History

A long asymptomatic period exists in patients with AS. There is gradual worsening of the outflow obstruction and an increase of the pressure overload on the LV.

Typical Symptoms

The typical symptoms of AS include angina pectoris, syncope, and heart failure. Angina occurs in approximately two-thirds of patients with severe AS. Syncope can result from arrhythmias or exercise-induced reflex vasodilation. Dyspnea usually indicates congestive heart failure. These symptoms appear most commonly in the fifth or sixth decade of life in patients with congenital or rheumatic AS, and in the seventh to ninth decade for those with degenerative AS.

Physical Examination

Arterial Pulse

The intensity and upslope of the arterial pulse diminish as the severity of AS increases. The carotid pulse has a slow upstroke, a delayed peak, and reduced amplitude. In advanced stages of AS, systolic and pulse pressures may appear decreased, reflecting low stroke volume. The anacrotic notch and coarse systolic vibration are better appreciated in the carotid arterial pulse, producing the carotid shudder.

Venous Pulse

The jugular venous pulse may show a prominent wave, reflecting reduced right ventricular compliance due to pulmonary hypertension or right ventricular hypertrophy. In advanced stages of AS when the pulmonary hypertension causes secondary right ventricular failure and tricuspid regurgitation, the waves can become prominent.

Cardiac Examination

On palpation, the cardiac impulse may become sustained and displaced inferiorly and laterally. Palpation of a systolic thrill is usually best appreciated in the second left intercostal space, is frequently transmitted to the carotid arteries, and is highly specific for severe AS.

On auscultation, the second heart sound intensity may be soft due to calcification and immobility of the aortic valve's making the aortic component of the second heart sound inaudible. An aortic systolic ejection sound occurs simultaneously with the halting upward movement of the aortic valve and suggests a bicuspid aortic valve.

The harsh crescendo-decrescendo systolic murmur of AS is heard best at the base of the heart and radiates to the carotid arteries. As the severity of AS increases, the peak of this murmur occurs later in systole. In the late stages of AS, when the LV systolic dysfunction ensues, the systolic murmur becomes softer and may disappear.

Additional findings seen with severe AS include paradoxical splitting of the second heart sound (the normal splitting of the second heart sound is reversed: aortic valve closure [A2] occurs after the pulmonic valve closure [P2], and a prominent fourth heart sound [S4] due to ventricular hypertrophy is heard).

DATA DECODING TIPS (CLINICAL PEARLS)
Differentiating Between Aortic Stenosis and Pulmonic Stenosis

The ejection sound of a bicuspid aortic valve is generally well heard at the apex as well as over the aortic area. It does not alter with respiration. On the other hand, a pulmonic ejection sound from a congenital pulmonic valve stenosis usually localizes over the second or third intercostal space of the left sternal border and characteristically has an ejection sound that may decrease or even disappear coincident with inspiration. It is generally not heard at the apex, as is the rule with a bicuspid aortic stenosis.

DATA DECODING TIPS (CLINICAL PEARLS)
Differentiating Between Systolic Murmur of Aortic Stenosis and Mitral Regurgitation

To differentiate between the systolic murmur of AS and that of MR, concentrate on the murmur after a post-extra systolic pause. For AS, the murmur increases in intensity after the pause; with MR, the murmur remains essentially unchanged. If one hears a high frequency, musical diamond-shaped systolic murmur only at the apex, immediately think of and rule out AS.

DATA MINING (WORK-UP)
Electrocardiography (ECG)

The main ECG finding is LV hypertrophy, which is present in 85% of patients with severe AS. Conduction disease, including left bundle branch block, may develop in patients with AS with ventricular dysfunction. The extensive calcific changes may cause various forms of atrioventricular or intraventricular block in a small percentage of patients. There is occasionally a "pseudoinfarction" pattern, manifested by a loss of R waves in the right precordial leads. Left atrial enlargement is present in more than 80% of patients with severe AS.

Chest X-Ray

Although the cardiac silhouette is usually normal, cardiomegaly will be evident in those with LV dilation and failure. Poststenotic dilation of the ascending aorta is a common finding; marked dilation may be seen in bicuspid aortic valve disease. Calcification of the aortic valve is present in nearly all adults with severe AS but is more easily detected on fluoroscopy as compared to chest radiography.

Echocardiography

Echocardiography is the most important imaging technique for evaluating and following patients with AS. Two-dimensional transthoracic-echocardiography (TTE) can detect valvular calcification; determine the number of aortic cusps; identify commissural fusion; determine the severity of the stenosis and insufficiency; and assess biventricular size, function, and hypertrophy. Rheumatic AS is characterized by fusion of the commissures. The aortic valve anatomy can be better defined by TEE, particularly using the short axis view of the aortic valve. Echocardiography can assess the aortic root diameter in patients with bicuspid aortic valve. Three-dimensional echocardiographic methods hold promise for better assessment of the severity of AS.

Doppler echocardiography is used to calculate the LV-aortic pressure gradient from the systolic aortic valve velocity signal using a modified Bernoulli (continuity) equation. Doppler flow assessment is typically more accurate using TTE rather than TEE. The mean gradients determined by this method correlate well with those obtained from left heart catheterization. It is important to recognize that the peak instantaneous aortic valve gradient is typically much higher than the peak-to-peak gradient assessed by cardiac catheterization.

Color-flow Doppler can detect and determine the severity of aortic insufficiency, which coexists in 75% of AS patients. In patients with severe LV dysfunction and low cardiac output, assessing the severity of AS can be enhanced by low-dose dobutamine infusion to assess valve hemodynamics at a higher cardiac output.

 SMART THINKING:

Which Patients with Bicuspid Valve Will Develop Severe AS?

Analysis of bicuspid aortic valve (BAV) morphology is of prognostic relevance, as the fusion of the right- and noncoronary leaflets (R-N) is associated with a greater degree of valve dysfunction compared with fusion by other leaflets (L-R or L-N). ***Methodology:*** A nested cohort study of young patients (mean age, 16 years) was conducted on 310 patients with right- and left-coronary leaflet (R-L) and R-N fusion who were selected randomly from an inception cohort of 1192 patients with BAV. ***Results:*** The R-N fusion (n = 108) was strongly predictive of valve intervention when compared with the R-L fusion (n = 202; hazard ratio 4.5, 95% confidence interval [CI] 2.5 to 8.1; P < 0.0001). In a longitudinal analysis of 799 echocardiograms, R-N fusion also was associated with a greater progression of valve dysfunction. This was true for both increasing aortic valve gradient (generalized estimating equations [GEE] risk ratio 27.2, 95% CI 1.2 to 619.6, P = 0.0386) and aortic regurgitation (GEE risk ratio 2.4, 95% CI 1.3 to 4.3, P = 0.0029). ***Practical Applications:*** Therefore the R-N fusion is associated with a more rapid progression of aortic stenosis and regurgitation and a shorter time to valve intervention.[1]

Cardiac Catheterization

As echocardiography provides information regarding LV function, aortic valve morphology and mobility, and the hemodynamic severity of AS, the principal role of the cardiac catheterization laboratory is to provide coronary artery imaging prior to valve surgery. Coronary angiography is generally indicated in men older than 40 and women older than

TABLE 11-1: Severity of Aortic Stenosis

Severity	Mean Gradient	Aortic Valve Area	Indexed Valve Area
	(mm Hg)	(cm^2)	(cm^2/m^2)
Mild	<25	1.5-2.0	0.9-1.2
Moderate	25-40	1.0-1.5	0.6-0.9
Severe	41-50	0.8-0.9	0.5-0.6
Critical	>50	<0.8	<0.5

50 to determine whether coronary artery revascularization would be needed at the time of aortic valve replacement.

Invasive hemodynamic assessment of the aortic valve is indicated only when echocardiographic data are equivocal or suboptimal or when there is a discrepancy between the clinical and echocardiographic findings. As there is an increased risk of stroke in patients with AS undergoing retrograde left heart catheterization, this procedure should be done only when invasive hemodynamics are required for patient assessment.

Using either echocardiography and/or left heart catheterization, the definitions for AS severity are based on the mean aortic valve area and the calculated aortic valve area (Table 11-1). For comparison, the normal aortic valve has an area of 3-4 cm,^{2} with no systolic pressure gradient. Further refinement of these definitions is appropriate for small or large patients, as the valve area may be indexed to body surface size.

PROGRAMMED MANAGEMENT
Strategic Programming

There is no effective medical therapy for severe AS; AS is a mechanical obstruction to blood flow that requires mechanical correction. In children with congenital AS, the fused valve leaflets are merely fused and therefore respond exceptionally well to percutaneous balloon valvotomy. In adults with calcific valvular disease, however, balloon valvotomy only temporarily relieves symptoms, does not prolong survival, and therefore does not offer definitive durable therapy. Thus, adults with significant AS require replacement of the valve (Table 11-2).

The risks of replacing that valve must be weighed against the risks of delaying surgery. Natural history studies uniformly demonstrate that once angina, syncope, or symptoms of heart failure develop in patients with severe AS, the patient's life span is drastically shortened unless the valve is replaced. Of the AS patients who present with angina, half will

TABLE 11-2: Management Master Plan

Data Management	Carefully controlled BP
	Low-sodium diet
	Preventive measures
System Configuration Correction	Aortic valve replacement
	Percutaneous aortic valve stenting
Work-Around Management	None
System Replacement	None

die within five years without aortic valve replacement. Of the 15% of patients who present with syncope, half will die within three years. Of the 50% who present with heart failure symptoms, half will die within two years unless the aortic valve is replaced. In contrast, 10-year age-corrected rates of survival among patients who have undergone aortic valve replacement approach the rates in the normal population.

Asymptomatic Patients

Asymptomatic patients with severe AS have outcomes similar to age-matched adults without valvular heart disease; however, disease progression with symptom onset is common. In a prospective study of 123 asymptomatic adults with an initial jet velocity of at least 2.6 m/second, the rate of symptom development was 38% at three years. However, clinical outcome was strongly dependent on AS severity, with an event-free survival of 84% at two years in those with a jet velocity less than 3 m/second compared with only 21% in those with a jet velocity greater than 4 m/second. Therefore, patients with asymptomatic severe AS require frequent monitoring for development of symptoms and progression of the disease.

Supervised exercise echocardiographic testing of "asymptomatic" patients with severe AS can often elicit symptoms and/or ventricular dysfunction. In these patients with poor exercise tolerance due to severe AS, aortic valve replacement is recommended. Electrocardiographic ST depression during exercise occurs in 80% of adults with asymptomatic AS and has no known prognostic significance. Echocardiographic imaging is often helpful to identify subclinical exercise-induced ventricular dysfunction. When the medical history is unclear, exercise testing can identify a limited exercise capacity, an abnormal blood pressure response, or even exercise-induced symptoms. Exercise testing in asymptomatic patients should be performed under the supervision of an experienced physician with close monitoring of blood pressure and the ECG.

Medical Therapy for Asymptomatic Patients

Antibiotic prophylaxis is no longer indicated for patients with asymptomatic AS for the prevention of infective endocarditis. For those with rheumatic AS, antibiotics are recommended for the secondary prevention of recurrent acute rheumatic fever until at least the age of 40. Patients with associated systemic hypertension should be treated cautiously with antihypertensive agents, avoiding hypotension.

Symptomatic Patients

Although there are no prospective randomized trials comparing surgical aortic valve replacement with medical management, retrospective observational studies have shown that surgical repair is associated with significantly higher survival rates and is usually accompanied by symptom improvement. The 10-year survival rate in Medicare patients after aortic valve replacement is comparable to that observed for those who do not have AS. Although these observational studies may have limitations, such as selection bias, a greater than four-fold difference in survival between surgically and medically treated patients supports the well-accepted recommendation that aortic valve replacement should be performed promptly in symptomatic patients.

ADVANCED MANAGEMENT

Treatment to Prevent Worsening of AS

There are no medical treatments proven to prevent or delay the disease process involving aortic leaflet sclerosis or stenosis. The association of AS with clinical and pathophysiologic factors similar to atherosclerosis has led to the hypothesis that intervention may be possible to slow or prevent disease progression in the valve leaflets.[2-5] Specifically, the effect of lipid-lowering therapy on the progression of calcific AS has been examined in several studies using echocardiography or cardiac computed tomography to measure disease severity. While several small, retrospective studies suggested a possible benefit with statins, a prospective, randomized, placebo-controlled trial in patients with calcific aortic valve disease failed to demonstrate a benefit with atorvastatin in reducing the progression of aortic valve stenosis over a 3-year period.[6] In another study, administration of simvastatin and ezetimibe resulted in no reduction in clinical events related to aortic stenosis.[7] A long-term study of AS patients treated with rosuvastatin is under way.

AS with Low Cardiac Output/ Low Gradient Aortic Stenosis

Patients with severe AS and low cardiac output may have a relatively low transvalvular mean pressure gradient <30 mm Hg. Such patients can be difficult to distinguish from those with low cardiac output due to heart failure but with only mild-to-moderate AS. In those with anatomically severe AS, the stenotic valvular lesion contributes to an elevated afterload, decreased ejection fraction, and low stroke volume. In those with a small calculated aortic valve area due to heart failure, primary contractile dysfunction is responsible for the decreased ejection fraction and low stroke volume; the problem is further complicated by reduced valve opening forces that contribute to limited valve mobility and apparent valvular stenosis. In both situations, the low-flow state and low pressure gradient contribute to a calculated effective valve area that meets the criteria for severe AS.

In patients with low cardiac output who have a mean aortic valve gradient of less than 30 mm Hg and a calculated aortic valve area of less than 0.8 cm², it may be useful to determine the transvalvular pressure gradient and aortic valve area at baseline and again during low-dose dobutamine infusion. Such studies can be performed in the echocardiography or cardiac catheterization laboratory. If the dobutamine infusion produces an increase in stroke volume and an increase in the aortic valve area greater than 0.2 cm² with little change in the gradient, it is likely that baseline evaluation overestimated the severity of stenosis. In contrast, patients with anatomically severe AS have no change in the calculated valve area, with an increase in stroke volume, cardiac output, and the aortic valve gradient. These patients are likely to respond favorably to surgery.

Patients who fail to show an increase in stroke volume with dobutamine, referred to as "lack of contractile reserve," appear to have a very poor prognosis with either medical or surgical therapy. Dobutamine stress testing in patients with AS should be performed only in centers with experience in pharmacologic stress testing and should be closely supervised by a cardiologist.

 EVIDENCE-BASED MEDICINE:

Surgical Outcome in Patients with Low-Gradient AS

A large multicenter series of patients operated on for low-flow/low-gradient aortic stenosis (LF/LGAS) were evaluated to stratify the operative risk, assess whether perioperative mortality had decreased over recent years, and to analyze the postoperative outcome.[8] *Methodology:* A total of 217 consecutive patients (168 men, 77%) with severe aortic stenosis (area <1 cm²), low ejection fraction (EF) (≤35%), and low mean gradient (MG) (=30 mm Hg) who underwent aortic valve replacement (AVR) between 1990 and 2005 were included. *Results:* Perioperative mortality was 16% and decreased dramatically from 20% in the 1990 to 1999 period to 10% in the 2000 to 2005 period. Higher European System for Cardiac Operative Risk Evaluation score (EuroSCORE), very low MG and EF, New York Heart Association functional Class III or IV, history of congestive heart failure, and multivessel coronary artery disease (MVD) were associated with perioperative mortality. On multivariate analysis, very low preoperative MG and MVD were predictors of excess perioperative mortality. In the subgroup of patients with dobutamine stress echocardiography, the absence of contractile reserve was a strong predictor of perioperative mortality. Overall five-year survival rate was 49 ± 4%. Lower MG, higher EuroSCORE, prior atrial fibrillation, and MVD were identified as independent predictors of overall long-term mortality. *Practical Applications:* In view of the very poor prognosis of unoperated patients, the current operative risk, and the long-term outcome after surgery, AVR is the treatment of choice in the majority of cases of LF/LGAS.

Predictors of Mortality Before AVR: EuroScore Versus BNP

The accuracy of the logistic EuroSCORE (logES), a widely used risk prediction algorithm for cardiac surgery including aortic valve surgery, usually overestimates observed perioperative mortality. Elevated brain natriuretic peptide (BNP) in symptomatic patients with AS is associated with poor short-term outcomes after AVR. A study compared BNP with logES for predicting short- and long-term outcomes in symptomatic patients with severe AS undergoing aortic valve replacement.[9] A group of 144 consecutive patients referred for AV replacement (42% women, 73 ± 9 years, mean aortic gradient 51 ± 18 mm Hg and LV ejection fraction 61 ± 11%) underwent either isolated aortic valve replacement (58%) or combined with bypass grafting. Preoperative median BNP plasma levels and logES were 157 pg/mL (interquartile range [IQR] 61 to 440) and 6.6% (IQR 4.2 to 12.2), respectively. The perioperative mortality was 6% and the overall mortality by the end of the study was 13%. Patients with logES >10.1% (upper tertile) had a higher risk of dying over time (hazard ratio [HR] 2.86; P = 0.037), as had patients with BNP >312 pg/ml (HR 9.01; P<0.001). Discrimination (based on C statistic) and model performance was superior for BNP compared to logES. At the bivariable analysis, only BNP was an independent predictor of death (HR 8.2; P = 0.002). Preoperative BNP was even more accurate than logES in predicting outcome. In conclusion, in symptomatic patients with severe AS, high preoperative BNP plasma level and high logES confirm their predictive value for short- and long-term outcome.

BENEFITS, HARMS, AND COST-EFFECTIVENESS:

Aortic Valvular Surgery

The clinical benefit of heart valve replacement surgery has been well-documented. In a study examining AVR's cost-effectiveness, it was found to be very cost-effective for patients at all ages, even elderly patients.[13] From 1961 through 2003, 4617 patients older than 20 years underwent AVR at three hospitals in Portland, Oregon. Of those, 502 (10.9%) were octogenarians and 23 (0.5%) were nonagenarians. The total follow-up was 31,671 patient-years, with a maximum of 41 years. Survival (mean $\pm$ SE) after AVR was $50 \pm 0.9\%$, $20 \pm 1.0\%$, $6.8 \pm 0.8\%$, and $3.9 \pm 0.8\%$ at 10, 20, 30, and 40 years, respectively. The total life-years after AVR were 53,323. The total expected life-years without surgery were 10,157. The total value of the life-years after AVR was $14.6 billion; the total value of the expected life-years without surgery was $3.0 billion. Thus the value of life-years gained by AVR was $11.6 billion. After deduction of the lifetime cost of $451 million, the net value of AVR was $11.2 billion. The mean net value decreases according to age at surgery but is still worth $600,000 for octogenarians and $200,000 for nonagenarians. The value of AVR considered only the extended life-years of our patients relative to their expected lifetimes if not operated on. These extra years also had a higher quality of life than exists with the natural history of the disease. A monetary value could also be attached to this improvement in quality of life.

Aortic Valve Surgery for Elderly Patients

The outcomes of patients older than 80 undergoing cardiac surgery reporting in-hospital morbidity and mortality were evaluated in 67,764 patients (4743 octogenarians) undergoing cardiac surgery at 22 centers in Canada examining the predictors of in-hospital mortality in octogenarians compared with those predictors in younger patients.[14] Octogenarians undergoing cardiac surgery had fewer comorbid illnesses but higher disease severity and surgical urgency than younger patients and had significantly higher in-hospital mortality rates after cardiac surgery than younger patients: coronary artery bypass grafting (CABG) only (8.1% vs. 3.0%), CABG/aortic valve (10.1% vs. 7.9%), and CABG/mitral valve (19.6% vs. 12.2%). In addition, they had twice the incidence of postoperative stroke and renal failure. The preoperative clinical factors predicting CABG mortality in the very elderly were quite similar to those for younger patients, with age, emergency surgery, and prior CABG being the powerful predictors of outcome in both age categories. Of note, elderly patients without significant comorbidity had in-hospital mortality rates of 4% after CABG, 7% after CABG with aortic valve replacement (CABG/AVR), and 18% after CABG with mitral valve replacement (CABG/MVR). Therefore, risks for octogenarians undergoing cardiac surgery are less than previously reported, especially for CABG only or CABG/AVR. In selected octogenarians without significant comorbidity, mortality approaches that seen in younger patients.[14]

Update on Prosthetic Valve Disease

More than 80 models of artificial valves have been introduced since 1950. Prosthetic valves are either created from synthetic material (mechanical prosthesis) or fashioned from biological tissue (bioprosthesis). The following three main designs of mechanical valves exist: the caged ball valve, the tilting disk (single leaflet) valve, and the bileaflet valve. The only Food and Drug Administration (FDA)-approved caged ball valve is the Starr-Edwards valve. Tilting disk valve models include the Medtronic Hall valve, Omnicarbon (Medical CV) valves, Monostrut (Alliance Medical Technologies), and the discontinued Bjork-Shiley valves. Bileaflet valves include the St. Jude (St. Jude Medical), which is the most commonly implanted valve in the United States; CarboMedics valves (Sulzer CarboMedics); ATS Open Pivot valves (ATS Medical); and On-X and Conform-X valves (MCRI). Bioprosthetic (xenograft) valves are made from porcine valves or bovine pericardium. Porcine models include the Carpentier-Edwards valves (Edwards Lifesciences) and Hancock II and Mosaic valves (Medtronic). Pericardial valves include the Perimount series valves (Edwards LifeSciences). Ionescu-Shiley pericardial valves have been discontinued. More recently, stentless porcine valves have been used. They offer improved hemodynamics with a decreased transvalvular pressure gradient when compared with older stented models. These models include the Edwards Prima Plus, Medtronic Freestyle, and Toronto SPV valve (St. Jude Medical). Homografts or preserved human aortic valves are used in a minority of patients.

Malfunctioning Prosthetic Valves

In patients with malfunctioning prosthetic valves, symptoms are dependent on the type of valve, its location, and the nature of the complication. With valvular breakage or dehiscence, failure occurs acutely with rapid hemodynamic deterioration. Failure occurs more gradually with valve thrombosis, calcification, or degeneration.

Because of their smaller orifice size, all aortic valves produce some degree of outflow obstruction with a resultant systolic ejection murmur. Caged ball and small porcine valves produce the loudest murmurs. The intensity of the murmur increases with rising cardiac output. Tilting disk valves and bileaflet valves do not occlude their outflow tract completely when closed, allowing some back flow. This causes a low-intensity diastolic murmur. One should suspect prosthetic aortic valve failure in any patient with a greater than 2/6 diastolic murmur. Caged ball and tissue valves cause no diastolic murmur because they completely occlude their outflow tracts in the closed position. Consider any degree of diastolic murmur in these patients pathologic until proven otherwise. Patients with acute valvular failure present with cardiogenic shock and severe hypotension. Evidence of poor tissue perfusion is present, including diminished peripheral pulses, cool or mottled extremities, confusion or unresponsiveness, and decreased urine output. A hyperdynamic precordium and right ventricular impulse is present in 50% of patients with acute valvular failure. Absence of a normal valve closure sound or presence of an abnormal regurgitant murmur is an important clue to the presence of prosthetic valvular failure. Patients with subacute valvular failure often present with signs of gradually worsening left-sided congestive heart failure. Rales and jugular venous distention may be present. Patients with subacute valvular failure may present with a new regurgitant murmur or absence of normal closing sounds. A new or worsening hemolytic anemia may be the only presenting abnormality in patients with subacute valvular failure.

Prosthetic Valve Endocarditis

The clinical manifestations of prosthetic valve endocarditis (PVE) are often obscure. Fever occurs in 97% of patients with PVE. A new or changing murmur is present in 56% of patients. Absence of a murmur does not exclude the diagnosis. Valvular dehiscence, stenosis, or perforation causes the murmur. They may not occur early in the course of the illness. Signs considered classic for native valve endocarditis, including petechiae, Roth spots, Osler nodes, and Janeway lesions, often are absent in PVE. Splenomegaly supports the diagnosis but is present in only 26% of early PVE cases and in 44% of late PVE cases. PVE may present as congestive heart failure, septic shock, or primary valvular failure. Systemic emboli may be the presenting symptom in 7 to 33% of cases of PVE. This is more common with fungal etiologies.

Patients with complications related to embolization present with signs related to the site of embolization. Stroke syndromes are the most common; however, patients may present with MI, sudden death, or visceral or peripheral embolization. Systemic embolization should alert the physician to suspect valve thrombosis or PVE. Signs due to anticoagulant-related hemorrhage depend on the site of hemorrhage.

TROUBLE-SHOOTING AND DEBUGGING

Treatment of AS can be provided by any physician. When the results are not achieved as expected, management requires the expertise of a consultant cardiologist. The common questions from the referral physicians to the consultant cardiologist in the management of AS are as follows.

What is the Role of Percutaneous Aortic Balloon Valvuloplasty?

Surgical valve replacement should be considered the treatment of choice for severe AS patients regardless of age. Increasing numbers of octogenarians and nonagenarians with severe symptomatic AS are considered for open heart surgery. It has been difficult to weigh the risks of surgery in older patients and the risks of the natural history of severe symptomatic AS treated medically. Surgical success rates for these very elderly patients are improving but remain suboptimal. In-hospital death and stroke rates may be as high as 15%. Moreover, if coronary artery bypass graft surgery and aortic valve replacement are required in older patients with comorbidities, surgical mortality rates approach 20%. Mean duration of postoperative hospital stay in most reports is two weeks for elderly patients. More than half of all octogenarians are discharged to rehabilitation facilities, even after minimally invasive surgical approaches are used, and 20% are rehospitalized within one month. Furthermore, many elderly patients refuse surgery despite favorable outcomes. For these reasons, less invasive, percutaneous therapy has become an attractive option for treating patients with AS (Table 11-3).

The valvuloplasty balloon crosses the aortic valve in a retrograde fashion and is inflated briefly during rapid ventricular pacing at 200 bpm to preserve balloon stability across the aortic valve during inflation. Valvuloplasty immediately increases the aortic valve area and reduces the transvalvular gradient. A consistent limitation of percutaneous balloon valvuloplasty has been the high restenosis rate and the need for reintervention.[10.] While prior valvuloplasty registries have reported very high morbidity rates due to vascular injury, newer techniques using suture-mediated vascular closure have reduced the vascular complications associated with balloon

---

TABLE 11-3: Patients with Severe AS in Whom Percutaneous Balloon Aortic Valvuloplasty May Be Considered

- Bridge to surgical aortic valve replacement in hemodynamically unstable patients
- Increased perioperative risk, Society of Thoracic Surgeons (STS) risk score >15% for operative mortality
- Severe comorbidities such as porcelain aorta, severe lung disease, hepatic failure
- Severe and/or disabling neuromuscular or arthritic conditions that would limit the ability to undergo postoperative rehabilitation

valvuloplasty. Investigations suggest that repeat balloon valvulo-plasty in AS patients across a wide age range (59 to 104 years) may improve three-year survival rates over outcomes after a single di-latation. Repeat balloon aortic valvuloplasty typically can be per-formed. Most patients have symptomatic relief for up to one year.

What Is the Present Status of Percutaneous Aortic Valve Replacement?

The need for alternative, durable treatment options for high-risk patients with severe AS is justified by the fact that as many as one-third of elderly patients with comorbidities and symptomatic severe AS are denied surgery. A less invasive procedure to minimize cardio-vascular complications associated with general anesthesia, thoraco-tomy, and heart-lung machine is sought.

After the evaluation of a percutaneous valve replacement strategy in animal models, Cribier and colleagues performed the first human implantation of a balloon-expandable aortic valve prosthesis. By 2009, more than 1000 high-risk patients had undergone percuta-neous aortic valve replacement within clinical trials. Improvements in catheter and valve design are currently under way, enrolling pa-tients in randomized clinical trials assessing the safety and efficacy of percutaneous retrograde and minimally-invasive transapical ante-grade aortic valve replacement. Balloon-expandable and self-ex-pandable percutaneously delivered aortic valves are in clinical development. *Aortic Valve Stenting:* This study was designed to study the behavior of a stent deployed inside human stenotic aortic valves.[12] *Methodology:* Thirty-five patients with severe AS were in-cluded in the study. Sixteen patients (46%) had bicuspid aortic valves. A self-expandable stent specifically designed for VS implan-tation was deployed intraoperatively inside the aortic valve before surgical aortic valve replacement. *Results:* In tricuspid aortic valves, the shape of stent deployment was circular, triangular, or elliptic in 68%, 21%, or 11%, respectively. Noncircular stent deployment was frequent in bicuspid aortic valves (the elliptic deployment being the rule [79%]), and stent underdeployment was constant. The incidence of gaps between the stent external surface and the aortic valve did not differ between tricuspid and bicuspid valves (58% vs. 43%; P = 0.49). Sharp calcific excrescences protruding inside the stent lumen were present in three cases (9%). Ex vivo study of a VS confirmed that the regularity of the coaptation line of the leaflets was critically dependent on the presence or the absence of stent misdeployment. *Practical Applications:* Stent misdeployment was constant in bicus-pid valves and occurred in one-third of cases of tricuspid valves. Pre-mature failure of implanted VS (secondary to valve distortion or traumatic injury to the leaflets by calcific excrescences) might be an important concern in AV stenting.

How to Evaluate the Severity in a Patient with AS and MS?

Coexisting aortic and mitral valve stenosis is most commonly due to rheumatic heart disease. Echocardiography is the most important noninvasive imaging test to assess the severity of valvular disease in addition to examining valve morphology, calcification, and insufficiency. Invasive cardiac catheterization may be useful to assess the mitral and aortic valve gradients and valve area in those with inconclusive data from echocardiography. Left heart catheterization is required, with simultaneous left ventricular and pulmonary capillary wedge pressure for mitral valve gradient and simultaneous left ventricular and ascending aortic pressure for aortic valve gradient. In younger patients without significant aortic valve calcification, mitral and aortic valvuloplasty may be a good option for those with severe left-sided valvular heart disease. The majority of patients with severe aortic and mitral valve stenosis are treated with surgical valve repair and/or replacement. In those with severe mitral valve disease, an aortic valve area <1.5 cm^2 usually warrants simultaneous treatment for aortic stenosis.

Should Patients with Moderate AS and Severe LV Function Have CRT and ICD Before Valvular Replacement?

As discussed, there are some patients with severe AS who are not candidates for surgical or percutaneous AVR. There have been several case reports of inoperable patients with severe AS who received clinical benefit from cardiac resynchronization therapy (CRT).[17-18] Patients with severe AS may have ventricular dyssynchrony, evidenced by a prolonged QRS complex or abnormal tissue Doppler echocardiography. CRT may improve ventricular dyssynchrony, resulting in an increased contractile state. Addition of an implantable cardiac defibrillator (ICD) may reduce the risk of sudden death in patients with severe AS who are not candidates for AVR. Further research is under way to evaluate the efficacy of CRT/ICD in inoperable patients with severe, symptomatic AS.

TAKE-HOME MESSAGE

Data Collecting Collect all the data about the patient's history (of smoking, high-sodium, high-cholesterol diet, alcohol abuse, lack of exercise, HTN, DM, high cholesterol level), family history (of early sudden death due to heart disease, history of early CAD) social history (work and behaviors), and from a complete physical examination (signs of prior stroke, CAD, PAD, systolic murmur at the second right ICS, intensity of S2, weak peripheral pulses), all of which add weight to the clinical decision-making process.

Data Mining Recommend safe, appropriate, and efficacious investigation (echocardiography or left heart catheterization, including fasting lipid profile, fasting blood glucose, BUN and creatinine levels, weight, BMI, and waist circumference). Test to confirm: Echocardiography is the most important noninvasive imaging technique for evaluating AS patients and guiding the selection for valve replacement. Supervised exercise echocardiographic stress testing can often elicit symptoms in patients with severe AS who feel they are asymptomatic.

Management Recommend safe, appropriate, and efficacious therapy to maintain the stable health status of the patient over time (e.g., surgery or stenting of the AV and low-sodium, low-cholesterol diet, stopping smoking, losing weight, not drinking alcohol, exercising). Identifying symptomatic patients: Mortality dramatically increases after AS becomes symptomatic from angina pectoris, syncope, or exertional dyspnea. The average overall survival rate is two to three years in symptomatic patients without surgical treatment. Standard treatment: Surgical valve replacement is the treatment of choice for symptomatic patients with severe AS. Alternative treatments: Many elderly patients with severe AS may not be optimal surgical candidates due to hemodynamic instability or comorbidities that increase surgical risk. Current options include percutaneous balloon aortic valvuloplasty, which is limited by a high restenosis rate and the need for reintervention. Current studies are evaluating percutaneous aortic valve replacement as a less invasive alternative to surgical aortic valve replacement.

Patient-Centered Education and Care Get the patients involved in their own lifestyle modifications to increase compliance with diet, exercise, medication, office visits, and testing in order to provide continuity of care.

References

1. Fernandes, S. M., Khairy, P., Sanders, S. P., et al.: Bicuspid aortic valve morphology and interventions in the young. J Am Coll Cardiol. 2007;49: 2211–2214.
2. Otto, C. M., Burwash, I. G., Legget, M. E., et al.: Prospective study of asymptomatic valvular aortic stenosis. Clinical, echocardiographic, and exercise predictors of outcome. Circulation. 1997;95:2262–2270.
3. Pohle, K., Maffert, R., Ropers, D., et al.: Progression of aortic valve calcification: association with coronary atherosclerosis and cardiovascular risk factors. Circulation. 2001;104:1927–1932.
4. Bellamy, M. F., Pellikka, P. A., Klarich, K. W., et al.: Association of cholesterol levels, hydroxymethylglutaryl coenzyme-A reductase inhibitor treatment, and progression of aortic stenosis in the community. J Am Coll Cardiol. 2002;40:1723–1730.
5. Rosenhek, R., Rader, F., Loho, N., et al.: Statins but not angiotensin-converting enzyme inhibitors delay progression of aortic stenosis. Circulation. 2004;110:1291–1295.
6. Cowell, S. J., Newby, D. E., Prescott, R. J., et al.: A randomized trial of intensive lipid-lowering therapy in calcific aortic stenosis. N Engl J Med. 2005;352:2389–2397.

7. Rossebo, A. B., Pedersen, T. R., Boman, K., et al: for the SEAS Investigators. Intensive lipid lowering with simvastatin and ezetimibe in aortic stenosis. N Engl J Med. 2008;25;359:1343–1356.
8. Levy, F., Laurent, M., Monin, J. L., et al.: Aortic valve replacement for low-flow/low-gradient aortic stenosis operative risk stratification and long-term outcome: a European multicenter study. J Am Coll Cardiol. 2008;51:1466–1472.
9. Pedrazzini, G. B., Masson, S., Latini, R., et al.: Comparison of brain natriuretic peptide plasma levels versus logistic EuroSCORE in predicting in-hospital and late postoperative mortality in patients undergoing aortic valve replacement for symptomatic aortic stenosis. Am J Cardiol. 2008;102:749–754.
10. Otto, C. M., Mickel, M. C., Kennedy, J. W., et al.: Three-year outcome after balloon aortic valvuloplasty. Insights into prognosis of valvular aortic stenosis. Circulation. 1994;89:642–650.
11. Bonow, R. O., Carabello, B. A., Chatterjee, K., et al.: 2008 focused update incorporated into the ACC/AHA 2006 guidelines for the management of patients with valvular heart disease. A report of the American College of Cardiology/American Heart Association Task Force on Practice Guidelines (Writing Committee to Revise the 1998 Guidelines for the Management of Patients with Valvular Heart Disease). J Am Coll Cardiol. 2008;52:1–142.
12. Zegdi, R., Ciobotaru, V., Noghin, M., et al.: Is it reasonable to treat all calcified stenotic aortic valves with a valved stent? Results from a human anatomic study in adults. J Am Coll Cardiology. 2008;51:79–584.
13. Wu, Y., Jin, R., Gao, G., et al.: Cost-effectiveness of aortic valve replacement in the elderly: an introductory study. J Thorac Cardiovasc Surg. 2007;133:608–613.
14. Alexander, K. P., Anstrom, K. J., Muhlbaier, L. H., et al.: Outcomes of cardiac surgery in patients > or = 80 years: results from the National Cardiovascular Network. J Am Coll Cardiol. 2000;35:731–738.
15. Craver, J. M., Goldstein, J., Jones, E. L., et al.: Clinical, hemodynamic, and operative descriptors affecting outcome of aortic valve replacement in elderly versus young patients. Ann Surg. 1984;199:733–741.
16. Thourani, V. H., Myung, R., Kilgo, P., et al.: Long-term outcomes after isolated aortic valve replacement in octogenarians: a modern perspective. Ann Thorac Surg. 2008;86:1458–1464.
17. Antonini-Canterin, F., Baldessin, F., Brieda, M., et al.: Cardiac resynchronization therapy as an 'alternative' approach to a non-operable severe aortic stenosis with left ventricular dysfunction. J Heart Valve Dis. 2006;15:206–208.
18. Horstkotte, D., Piper, C., Vogt, J., et al.: Cardiac resynchronization therapy as an alternative to valve replacement in high-risk patients with a chronically decompensated aortic stenosis? J Heart Valve Dis. 2006;15:203–205.

Venous Disease

*Theodore Conrad Tan, Aravinda
Nanjundappa, Pham Manh Hung,
and Ho Thuong Dung*

Chapter Outline

SUPERFICIAL VEIN THROMBOPHLEBITIS

Definition

Superficial vein thrombophlebitis may occur spontaneously or as a complication of medical or surgical interventions. Superficial phlebitis with infection, such as phlebitis originating at an intravenous catheter site, is referred to as septic thrombophlebitis.

Strategic Programming

The first step is to identify patients through data collecting with a comprehensive history and physical examination. Superficial thrombophlebitis often progresses through perforating veins to involve the adjacent deep veins. In the case of spontaneous thrombophlebitis, a superficial phlebitis at one location may be accompanied by occult deep vein thrombosis in noncontiguous veins in the same leg or even in the contralateral leg. This occurs because hypercoagulable states tend to produce thrombosis simultaneously at multiple sites in both the superficial and deep venous systems. Phlebitis should be assumed to involve the deep veins until proven otherwise because superficial vein thrombophlebitis and deep vein thrombophlebitis share the same pathophysiology, pathogenesis, and risk factors.

The next step is to perform data processing in order to formulate a preliminary diagnosis and a short list of differential diagnoses (e.g., deep vein thrombosis, varicose veins). Then, using the method of data mining, tests could be ordered (Doppler ultrasound, venography) in order to confirm (data converting) the main diagnosis of superficial vein thromboplebitis and to rule out (data filtering) the differential diagnoses.

Every effort should be made to prevent superficial phlebitis from progressing to involve the deep veins because damage to deep vein valves leads to chronic deep venous insufficiency (often referred to as post-phlebitic syndrome) as well as to recurrent PE and a risk of death.

DATA COLLECTING

History

Patients with superficial thrombophlebitis often give a history of a gradual onset of localized tenderness, followed by the appearance of an area of erythema along the path of a superficial vein. There may be a history of local trauma, prior similar episodes, varicose veins, prolonged travel, or enforced stasis. The patient should be asked about risk factors for hypercoagulability, but the absence of identifiable risk factors has no prognostic value. Occasionally, there is a spurious history of sudden onset of pain. A true sudden onset of pain suggests some other etiology for the symptoms. Similarly, patients occasionally report the recent, sudden development of venous ulcers, stasis changes, and other conditions that, upon inspection, obviously have been present for many months or years.

Physical Examination

Swelling may result from acute venous obstruction (as in deep vein thrombosis) or from deep or superficial venous reflux, or it may be caused by an unrelated condition, such as hepatic insufficiency, renal failure, cardiac decompensation, infection, trauma, or environmental effects. Lymphedema may be primary or it may be secondary to overproduction of lymph due to severe venous hypertension.

Normal veins are distended visibly at the foot, ankle, and occasionally in the popliteal fossa but not in the rest of the leg. Normal veins may be visible as a blue subdermal reticular pattern, but dilated superficial leg veins above the ankle are usually evidence of venous pathology. Darkened, discolored, stained skin or nonhealing ulcers are typical signs of chronic venous stasis, particularly along the medial ankle and the medial lower leg. Chronic varicosities or telangiectasias may also be observed. Acute deep venous obstruction may cause the sudden appearance of new vessels, large or small, that have become dilated to serve as a bypass pathway. New varices and telangiectasias often appear during pregnancy, principally due to hormonal changes that make the vein wall and valves more pliable. Although hormonally mediated varicosities of pregnancy are common, the sudden appearance of dilated varicosities during pregnancy still warrants evaluation for acute deep vein thrombosis, which is also common in pregnancy.

DATA DECODING TIPS (CLINICAL PEARLS)
How to Examine a Patient for Superficial Thrombophlebitis and Deep Vein Thrombosis

The common sites are the saphenous veins and their tributaries. During the acute state, an indurated, tender cord of varying length is not only palpable but also visible as a red line along the course of the inflamed vessel. Importantly, edema of the extremities is virtually never present. As acute inflammation subsides, a nontender cord sometimes remains palpable for weeks. With the patient supine and the knee flexed, the examiner systematically and gently uses the fingertips to compress the relaxed calf muscles against the tibia. It should be underscored that gentle compression with the fingertips is the appropriate technique. Squeezing the calf should be avoided, because this maneuver elicits pain in normal subjects. The response to dorsiflexion of the foot (Homans' sign) is far less sensitive than systematic compression of the calf as described above.[1]

It is true that in the presence of calf vein thrombophlebitis, there may be resistance to dorsiflexion of the foot with or without accompanying pain. However, a positive Homans' sign is present in only about 50% of patients with documented calf thrombophlebitis, and the sign is sometimes elicited in the absence of venous thrombosis.[1]

Palpation of a painful or tender area may reveal a firm, thickened, thrombosed vein. Palpable thrombosed vessels are virtually always superficial, but combined deep and superficial venous thrombosis is very common. A thrombosed popliteal vein sometimes may be palpated in the popliteal fossa and a thrombosed common femoral vein sometimes may be palpated at the groin.

Risk Factors

Pregnancy and the puerperium are recognized risk factors for phlebitis. High-dose estrogen therapy is also a risk factor, but no intrinsic sex-linked preferential risk exists for the disease. The likelihood of thrombophlebitis is increased through most of pregnancy and for approximately six weeks after delivery. This is partly due to increased platelet stickiness and partly due to reduced fibrinolytic activity.

The most important clinically identifiable risk factors for thrombophlebitis are a prior history of superficial phlebitis, deep vein thrombosis, or pulmonary embolism. Other extremely common risk markers include recent surgery or pregnancy, prolonged immobilization, or underlying malignancy.

DATA MINING

Most patients with thrombophlebitis have a normal PT and PTT, and active thrombophlebitis is not uncommon in patients with a therapeutically elevated INR due to warfarin therapy. A low white blood cell (WBC) count lowers the likelihood of an infectious process and raises the likelihood of phlebitis. An elevated WBC count is nonspecific because both normal and elevated WBC counts are common in patients with thrombophlebitis. Chronic venous insufficiency (venous congestion due to reflux) and superficial or deep vein thrombosis can mimic leg cellulitis very closely, and true cellulitis (with an elevated WBC count) is a frequent complication of both diseases.

The latex agglutination test (known by various trade names) is completely unreliable, with a sensitivity of only 50 to 60% for DVT and PE. Tests for causes of hypercoagulable states can be identified through laboratory studies, including tests for factor V, protein C deficiency, protein S deficiency, and antithrombin III deficiency, antiphospholipid antibodies, and lupus anticoagulant. All patients with sterile superficial phlebitis must undergo a complete workup, including an anatomic imaging test to rule out DVT, because it is impossible to determine from clinical examination whether the process has spread to involve the deep veins. Anatomic imaging is performed using contrast venography, B-mode ultrasound, or MRI to produce an actual picture of the deep vessels and their contents.

 DATA MINING TIPS (CLINICAL PEARLS)
Duplex Ultrasound

Duplex ultrasound is the initial diagnostic study of choice for most patients with signs and symptoms of phlebitis. When phlebitis reflects an underlying hypercoagulable state, superficial phlebitis in one area may accompany deep vein thrombosis in another area or even in the other leg. For this reason, duplex examination should not be limited to just one leg or to just one area of one leg. Unfortunately, duplex ultrasound is not perfectly sensitive, and it fails to detect DVT in many patients who are ultimately proven to have had a DVT.

Magnetic Resonance Venography (MRV)

This noninvasive test is probably more sensitive and more specific than ultrasound in the detection of deep venous thrombophlebitis. Unfortunately, MRV is not readily available at many institutions, and many radiologists are inexperienced at reading MRV studies. MRV has a great advantage in the assessment of symptoms attributed to venous disease because it can reveal an alternate diagnosis in 60% of the cases in which primary venous disease is not the culprit.

Invasive Contrast Venography

This has long been the standard for evaluation of the venous system. It is used to guide direct transcatheter infusion of fibrinolytic agents in an increasing number of patients with deep venous thrombosis.

Physiologic Tests of Venous Function

These tests are used to assess venous function in both the deep and the superficial venous systems, but they are of secondary importance in patients with active phlebitis. These tests can sometimes detect deep system thrombophlebitis, but only when significant obstruction to outflow has produced significant venous congestion. The criterion for functional testing of the lower extremity venous system is invasive ambulatory venous pressure (AVP) monitoring. The most common noninvasive tests are impedance plethysmography, photoplethysmography (including light reflection rheography and digital techniques), and pneumoplethysmography (including quantitative air plethysmography). All of these tests address the same physiologic functional measures. The physiologic parameters that are measured include the maximum venous outflow (MVO), calf muscle pump expulsion fraction (MPEF), and venous refilling time (VRT) of the extremity. The MVO and MPEF are decreased when the deep veins are occluded significantly. The MPEF also is decreased when primary failure of the calf muscle pump mechanism occurs. The VRT is shortened when valvular damage in the deep or superficial veins allows venous blood to reflux downward into the extremity.

PROGRAMMED MANAGEMENT

Strategic Programming

If diagnostic tests show that the deep system is not involved, a rational approach to the initial treatment of superficial phlebitis can be based upon the patient's history and risk factors, together with the results of a detailed ultrasound examination. Recognized causes of venous stasis, such as air travel or extended bed rest, are strongly contraindicated in all patients with phlebitis of any type. The goals of therapy for superficial phlebitis are to prevent progression into the deep venous system and to hasten the resolution of the inflammatory and thrombotic processes in areas already involved. The most easily treated patients are those with superficial phlebitis not involving the greater saphenous vein above the knee, without known risk factors and with no prior thromboembolic history. Such patients most often respond to the combination of nonsteroidal anti-inflammatory agents, gradient compression hose, increased ambulation, and early repeat examination. The most aggressive treatment is necessary for patients with superficial phlebitis involving the greater saphenous vein above the knee because greater saphenous phlebitis often ascends to pass through the saphenofemoral junction at the groin and into the deep venous system.

Pharmacologic Therapy

Nonsteroidal anti-inflammatory agents are useful in reducing pain and in limiting the contribution of local inflammation. Anticoagulation with heparin is useful in preventing the progression of thrombosis. Local fibrinolysis is useful when the deep system is involved or threatened as well as when preserving the patency of a superficial vessel is important. Increased ambulation is important to avoid venous stasis that can contribute to the progression of thrombosis.

More aggressive treatment is indicated for patients who have a prior history of deep thrombophlebitis, for those with known irreversible risk factors for venous thrombosis, and for those with decreased mobility. These patients are treated as outpatients with full-dose anticoagulation using subcutaneous low-molecular-weight heparin (LMWH). Nonsteroidal anti-inflammatory agents, gradient compression hose, increased ambulation, and early repeat examination are also essential. Antibiotics should be used in any patients in whom the phlebitis may be septic.

Gradient Compression

Gradient compression stockings are an often-overlooked adjunctive therapy that is both benign and effective. Gradient compression hose are highly elastic stockings providing a gradient of compression that is highest at the toes (at least 30 to 40 mm Hg) and gradually decreases to the level of the thigh. This amount of compression reduces capacitive venous volume by approximately 70% and increases the measured velocity of blood flow in the deep veins by a factor of five or more. Gradient compression hose also have been shown to increase local and regional intrinsic fibrinolytic activity.

ADVANCED MANAGEMENT

Surgical Evacuation

A painful section of a superficial vein containing a palpable intravascular coagulum may be treated by puncture incision and evacuation of the clot. This procedure often produces marked rapid relief and rapid resolution of the inflammation.

Indication for Thrombolytic Therapy

Local transcatheter fibrinolytic therapy can arrest the progression of disease in most cases, and it is now the treatment of choice when greater saphenous phlebitis approaches the saphenofemoral junction.

Treatment of Deep Vein Thrombophlebitis

Phlebitis that has progressed to involve any other deep veins (anterior or posterior tibial veins, proximal peroneal vein, popliteal vein, or femoral vein at any level) is a serious and life-threatening condition that must not be confused with superficial venous thrombophlebitis. Contrary to popular belief, deep tibial vein thrombophlebitis carries nearly the same risk of fatal PE as thrombus in the more proximal deep veins of the thighs. Deep vein thrombophlebitis mandates immediate full-dose anticoagulation and an evaluation for possible occult PE (seen in 60% of asymptomatic patients). Strict gradient compression therapy is essential. Maintenance of ambulation is routine in Europe but only recently has begun to be adopted in the United States. Patients with DVT always should be considered as potential candidates for transcatheter fibrinolytic therapy, which can reduce the incidence of chronic postphlebitic syndrome by at least 50% and also can reduce the risk of recurrence and of progression to PE.

CHRONIC VENOUS INSUFFICIENCY

DATA COLLECTING

History

The clinical presentation of chronic venous insufficiency spans a spectrum from asymptomatic but cosmetically troublesome small blue ectatic veins and varicosities to severe fibrosing panniculitis, dermatitis, edema, and ulceration. Patients may have no symptoms or may complain of leg fullness, aching discomfort, heaviness, nocturnal leg cramps, or bursting pain upon standing. The pain may be worse during the menstrual cycle or pregnancy due to increased fluid volume and/or higher circulating levels of estrogen. Pain may be severe enough to make ambulation difficult or even impossible.

DATA DECODING TIPS (CLINICAL PEARLS)
Chronic Venous Insufficiency

Chronic venous insufficiency is a sequel to incompetence of the valves of superficial (saphenous) and deep (iliofemoral) veins. The physical signs are characteristic. Involvement is asymmetric, sometimes unilateral. The leg is chronically swollen and the skin and subcutaneous tissues indurated and discolored by brownish pigmentation, chiefly around the malleoli but often extending proximally to the contiguous anterior aspect of the leg.[1]

Cellulitis is common, and ulcers tend to be chronic, recalcitrant, and recurrent. The edema and ulceration associated with chronic venous insufficiency is usually distinguishable from other entities producing similar findings on the physical examination.

Guidelines have been published for the classification and grading of the chronic venous disease. Staging is based on the clinical, etiologic, anatomic, and pathophysiologic (CEAP) classification from the American Venous Forum, 2004. The CEAP system classifies limbs according to Clinical signs, Etiology, Anatomic distribution, and Pathophysiologic condition. The CEAP classification is helpful in documenting the severity of changes over time and for standardized reporting[2] (Table 12-1).

Physical Examination

The most frequently encountered manifestation of venous insufficiency is venous dilation. The size of the dilated vein may range from blue, ectatic, submalleolar flairs no larger than 1 mm in diameter to various degrees of vessel dilation and tortuosity that are apparent on observation and palpation. Of the latter, reticular veins are dilated but nonpalpable subdermal veins up to 4 mm in diameter, while varicose veins are palpable, subcutaneous veins usually larger than 4 mm in diameter.[3]

Venous flairs, reticular veins, and small varicose veins are typically asymptomatic, although occasionally they may itch or bleed profusely if accidentally injured. Some patients may seek consultation at this stage because of a prolonged episode of venous bleeding, superficial thrombophlebitis due to sluggish venous flow, or the unsightly nature of the venous flairs and varicosities.

TABLE 12-1: Clinical Signs, Etiology, Anatomic Distribution, and Pathophysiology (CEAP)

Clinical Signs

- C_0 No visible or palpable signs of venous disease
- C_1 Telangiectases or reticular veins
- C_2 Varicose veins
- C_3 Edema
- C_{4a} Pigmentation or eczema
- C_{4b} Lipodermatosclerosis or atrophie blanche
- C_5 Healed venous ulcer
- C_6 Active venous ulcer
- S Symptomatic, includes: ache, pain, tightness, skin irritation, heaviness, muscle cramps, and other complaints attributable to venous dysfunction
- A Asymptomatic

Etiologic Classification

- Ec Congenital
- Ep Primary
- Es Secondary (post-thrombotic)
- En No venous cause identified

Anatomic Classification

- As Superficial veins
- Ap Perforator veins
- Ad Deep veins
- An No venous location identified

Pathophysiologic Classification

- Basic CEAP
  - Pr Reflux
  - Po Obstruction
  - Pr,o Reflux and obstruction
  - Pn No venous pathophysiology identifiable

Edema

Edema formation is the hallmark of chronic venous insufficiency; it is present in all but the earliest stages. Long-standing venous insufficiency is characterized by the development of dependent ankle edema, followed by edema in the calf region. Mild edema may only be found at the end of the day, although it can become persistent and massive. In venous insufficiency, the edema is limited to the lower extremities and is often unilateral (particularly early on). It often subsides with recumbency and is often accompanied by varicosities, hyperpigmentation, and the other signs of venous disease. There is a poor response to diuretics, with some patients developing signs of hypoperfusion. The development of edema may be associated with a tan or reddish-brown hue to the skin. The skin changes are initially most prominent at the medial ankle from the break-down of red blood cells that have extravasated through damaged cap-illaries and smaller vessels. The skin becomes prone to venous stasis dermatitis following the onset of hyperpigmentation. The dermatitis is characterized by itching, weeping, scaling, erosions, and crusting. The dry, irritated, and heavily crusted skin causes pruritus, which can be dif-ficult to relieve, and excoriations due to scratching are often present.[3.]

Lipodermatosclerosis

Severe, chronic venous insufficiency may lead to the development of lipo-dermatosclerosis, a fibrosing panniculitis of the subcutaneous tissue char-acterized by a firm area of induration, that is located at the medial ankle initially and extends circumferentially around the entire leg, up to the midleg in more advanced cases. The skin overlying the panniculitis is typically heavily pigmented and bound down to the subcutaneous tis-sues. The fibrosis may be so extensive and constrictive as to girdle and strangle the lower leg, further impeding lymphatic and venous flow. These changes are associated with a brawny edema above the fibrosis and on the foot below. Thus, an advanced case of lipodermatosclerosis may resemble an inverted champagne bottle. Patients with lipoder-matosclerosis are particularly prone to repeated bouts of cellulitis, usu-ally caused by staphylococcal or streptococcal organisms. In addition, atrophie blanche (a cutaneous manifestation of livedoid vasculopathy), 2-to 5-mm macules of depigmentation corresponding to areas of avas-cular fibrotic skin, may develop within the areas of heavy pigmentation over the lipodermatosclerosis.[4.]

Venous Ulcers

Venous ulcers may be seen and are located low on the medial ankle over a perforating vein or along the line of the long or short saphenous veins. They can, however, occur higher on the leg if precipitated by trauma, but never higher than the knee or on the forefoot. The ulcers may be multiple or single and are typically tender, shallow, red-based, or occa-sionally exudative.

Risk Factors

The incidence of venous insufficiency and ulceration increases with age, obesity, a history of phlebitis or venous thrombosis, and serious leg trauma. Other risk factors include a family history of venous disease, evidence of ligamentous laxity, prolonged standing, and childbirth. Men who worked as laborers had higher rates of severe disease than nonlaborers. Despite the well-known association, a history of deep venous thrombosis is obtained in less than one-third of all patients with chronic venous insufficiency; less than one-half have post-thrombotic changes noted on venography. Other conditions that might be important in the development of chronic venous insufficiency include previous leg injury or surgery, primary valve or venous wall degeneration, congenital absence of valves, and arteriovenous shunts.

DATA MINING
Duplex Ultrasound

Lower-extremity duplex ultrasonography helps exclude DVT. Absence of edema and a reduced ankle-brachial index suggest peripheral arterial disease rather than chronic venous insufficiency and postphlebitic syndrome. Doppler bidirectional flow studies and Doppler color-flow studies are used to assess venous flow, its direction, and the presence of thrombus.

Photoplethysmography

Photoplethysmography uses infrared light to assess capillary filling during exercise. Increased capillary filling is indicative of venous reflux and, consequently, incompetent veins. Outflow plethysmography should be done to show that the veins should quickly return to baseline pressures. Failure to do so indicates reflux.

DATA CONVERTING

Diagnosis is usually based on history and physical examination. A clinical scoring system that ranks five symptoms (pain, cramps, heaviness, pruritus, and paresthesia) and six signs (edema, hyperpigmentation, induration, venous ectasia, blanching hyperemia, and pain with calf compression) on a scale of 0 (absent or minimal) to 3 (severe) is increasingly recognized as a standard diagnostic tool of disease severity. Scores of 5 to 14 on two visits separated by more than 6 months indicate mild-to-moderate disease, and scores of higher than 15 indicate severe disease.

MANAGEMENT

Nonsurgical treatments for CVI include leg elevation, compression stockings, Unna boots, and injection sclerotherapy.

Surgical Therapy

Approximately 8% of patients require surgical intervention for CVI. Surgical treatment is reserved for those with discomfort or ulcers refractory to medical management. Vein ligation is the treatment of choice for superficial vein disorders, often using the stab evulsion technique. Typically, stab evulsion is limited to areas above the knee in the greater saphenous system to avoid damage to the saphenous nerve or sural nerve. This technique is reserved for CVI in which reflux in the saphenous system occurs and causes severe symptoms. For this reason, a diagnosis (usually accomplished with photoplethysmography or duplex imaging of reflux) must be established preoperatively. Hematoma, sural or saphenous nerve damage, and infection are possible complications of vein ligation.

The decision to operate on a patient with venous obstruction in the deep veins should be made only after a careful assessment of symptom severity and direct measurement of both arm and foot venous pressures. Venography alone is not sufficient because many patients with occlusive disease have extensive collateral circulation, rendering them less symptomatic. Clot lysis (tissue plasminogen activator [TPA], urokinase) and thrombectomy have been tried but have largely been abandoned owing to extremely high recurrence rates.

For iliofemoral disease, the operation of choice is a saphenous vein crossover graft resulting in the diversion of venous blood through the graft and into the intact contralateral venous system.

Valvuloplasty is reserved for patients with a congenital absence of functional valves. When combined with the ligation of perforating veins, valvuloplasty has a superior outcome in 80% of cases after five years.

DEEP VEIN THROMBOSIS

Definition

Deep vein thrombosis (DVT) and pulmonary embolism (PE) are major public health problems in the United States. Estimates suggest that 350,000 to 600,000 Americans have a DVT or PE each year and that at least 100,000 people die as a result. Based on the Longitudinal Investigation of Thromboembolism Etiology (LITE) study, the Atherosclerosis Risk in Communities (ARIC), and the Cardiovascular Health Study (CHS), it was noted that the rates were higher in men than women and increased with age in both sexes.[5]

DATA COLLECTING

Risk Factors

The MEDENOX study had shown that the presence of an acute infectious disease, age of more than 75 years, cancer, and a history of prior VTE were factors for increased risk for venous thromboembolism (VTE). Other risk factors include a history of immobilization or prolonged hospitalization/bed rest, recent surgery, obesity, prior episodes of venous thromboembolism, lower extremity trauma, malignancy, oral contraceptive use, hormone replacement therapy, pregnancy or postpartum status, history of stroke, MI, DM, or atrial fibrillation and a history of varicosities.[6-7]

History

Classic symptoms of DVT include swelling, pain, and discoloration in the involved extremity. There is not necessarily a correlation between the location of symptoms and the site of thrombosis. Symptoms in the calf alone are often the presenting manifestation of significant proximal vein involvement, while some patients with whole leg symptoms are found to have isolated calf vein DVT. A complete thrombosis history includes the age of onset, location of prior thromboses, and results of objective diagnostic studies documenting thrombotic episodes in the patient as well as in any family members. A positive family history is particularly important because a well-documented history of venous thrombosis in one or more first-degree relatives strongly suggests the presence of a hereditary defect.

Physical Examination

Physical examination may reveal a palpable cord (reflecting a thrombosed vein), calf pain, ipsilateral edema, or swelling with a difference in calf diameters, warmth, tenderness, erythema, and/or superficial venous dilation. There may be pain and tenderness in the thigh along the course of the major veins. Tenderness on deep palpation of the calf muscles is suggestive but not diagnostic. Homans' sign is also unreliable.

The physical examination may also reveal signs of hepatic vein thrombosis (Budd-Chiari syndrome) such as ascites and hepatomegaly or edema due to the nephrotic syndrome. The hypercoagulable state associated with the nephrotic syndrome may manifest as renal vein thrombosis, which is usually asymptomatic unless associated with pulmonary embolism.

DATA DECODING TIPS (CLINICAL PEARLS)
Sensitivity and Specificity in the History and Physical Examination for DVT

History and physical examination (H and P) alone are limited in making the diagnosis of DVT. In fact, only 50% of patients who are initially thought to have DVT by H and P will have an abnormal duplex ultrasound. Some cases of lower extremity DVT, especially those in the tibial and distal popliteal veins, may be silent or nearly asymptomatic, presenting with only subtle leg swelling. Although there is a risk of pulmonary embolus and postphlebitic syndrome in these cases, the risk is low given the distal location and limited extent of thrombosis. In rare instances, the first sign of lower-extremity DVT can be pulmonary embolus. The complexity of lower-extremity venous disorders emphasizes the need for a careful and complete history and physical exam as well as the liberal use of the duplex ultrasound as a diagnostic adjunct.

Phlegmasia Cerulea Dolens

Phlegmasia cerulea dolens is an uncommon form of massive proximal iliofemoral venous thrombosis of the lower extremities associated with a high degree of morbidity, including sudden severe leg pain with swelling, cyanosis, edema, venous gangrene, compartment syndrome, and arterial compromise, often followed by circulatory collapse and shock. Delay in treatment may result in death or loss of the patient's limb.

DATA DECODING TIPS (CLINICAL PEARLS)
Checking the Lower Legs for DVT

Calf tenderness may be present in acute deep venous thrombosis but is not specific. Such tenderness may occur with muscle strain, contusion, or hematoma. Forceful dorsiflexion of the foot elicits calf pain in 35% of patients with acute deep venous thrombosis (Homans' sign). However, this test is also positive with muscular strains and lumbosacral disorders. While the patient is talking and answering the question, the physician's fingers are palpating the calf of both extremities. If the patient stops in the middle of answering a question and says, "Oh, that hurts," this is consistent with the diagnosis of thrombophlebitis.[8]

Because venous thromboembolism may be the first manifestation of an underlying malignancy, rectal examination and stool testing for occult blood should be performed, and women should undergo a pelvic examination to rule out the presence of a previously unsuspected pelvic mass or malignancy.

DATA FILTERING

The differential diagnosis in patients with suspected DVT includes a variety of disorders, including musculoskeletal injury and venous insufficiency. Other problems that may mimic the signs and symptoms of DVT include muscle strain or tear, lymphangitis or lymph obstruction, leg swelling in a paralyzed limb, venous insufficiency, popliteal cyst, cellulitis, knee pathologies, drug-induced edema, and calf muscle injury or tear.

DATA MINING

When approaching a patient with suspected DVT of the lower extremity, it is important to appreciate that only a minority of patients actually have the disease and will require anticoagulation. This illustrates the importance of using validated algorithms to evaluate patients with suspected DVT, along with objective testing to establish the diagnosis. Given the potential risks associated with proximal lower extremity DVT that is not treated (fatal pulmonary emboli) and the potential risk of anticoagulating a patient who does not have a DVT (fatal bleeding), accurate diagnosis is essential.

The initial laboratory evaluation in patients with venous thrombosis should include a complete blood count and platelet count, coagulation studies (prothrombin time, activated partial thromboplastin time), renal function tests, and urinalysis. A negative D-dimer assay may be insufficient to rule out DVT as a stand-alone test in patient populations with a high prevalence of venous thromboembolism.

A number of invasive and noninvasive approaches are possible, including contrast venography, impedance plethysmography, compression ultrasonography, and D-dimer testing. In most circumstances, compression ultrasonography is the noninvasive approach of choice for the diagnosis of symptomatic patients with a first episode of suspected DVT. A positive noninvasive study in patients with a first episode of DVT usually establishes the diagnosis. If the initial study is negative and the clinical suspicion of DVT is high, a repeat study should be obtained on days 5 to 7. Use of a single study via extended (complete) lower extremity ultrasonography may obviate the need for repeat testing. However, this technique requires specialized instrumentation and is highly dependent on user expertise.

Venography is currently used only when noninvasive testing is not clinically feasible or the results are equivocal.

DATA CONVERTING (MAKING A DIAGNOSIS)

Once the DVT is confirmed by the conventional tests, a search for causes of DVT is indicated. The conditions that predispose and cause DVT are listed in Table 12-2.

PROGRAMMED MANAGEMENT

The main objectives of treatment of DVT are to prevent further clot extension, acute pulmonary embolism, and reduce the risk of recurrent thrombosis. It may be necessary to treat the thrombosis if it is massive iliofemoral thrombosis with acute lower limb ischemia and/or venous

TABLE 12-2: Causes of Venous Thrombosis

Inherited Thrombophilia

Factor V Leiden mutation
Prothrombin gene mutation
Protein S deficiency
Protein C deficiency
Antithrombin (AT) deficiency
Dysfibrinogenemia

Acquired Disorders

Malignancy
Presence of a central venous catheter
Surgery, especially orthopedic
Trauma
Pregnancy
Oral contraceptives
Hormone replacement therapy
Tamoxifen
Immobilization
Congestive failure
Antiphospholipid antibody syndrome
Myeloproliferative disorders
Polycythemia vera
Essential thrombocythemia
Paroxysmal nocturnal hemoglobinuria
Inflammatory bowel disease
Nephrotic syndrome
Hyperviscosity
Waldenström's macroglobulinemia
Multiple myeloma
Marked leukocytosis in acute leukemia
Sickle cell anemia

gangrene (phlegmasia cerulea dolens). We also want to limit the development of late complications, such as the postphlebitic syndrome, chronic venous insufficiency, and chronic thromboembolic pulmonary hypertension.

Anticoagulant Therapy

Anticoagulant therapy is indicated for patients with symptomatic proximal DVT because pulmonary embolism will occur in approximately 50 % of untreated individuals, most often within days or weeks of the event. Based on the recommendations of the 2008 ACCP evidence-based clinical practice guidelines for antithrombotic and thrombolytic therapy, the British Committee for Standards in Haematology, the joint guidelines of the American College of Physicians and the American Academy of Family Physicians, and the American Heart Association/American College of Cardiology, patients with DVT or pulmonary embolism should be treated acutely with LMW heparin, fondaparinux, unfractionated intravenous heparin, or adjusted-dose subcutaneous heparin. Treatment with LMW heparin, fondaparinux, or unfractionated heparin should be continued for at least five days, and oral anticoagulation should be overlapped with LMW heparin, fondaparinux, or unfractionated heparin for at least four to five days.

The ACCP Guidelines suggest that platelet counts be obtained regularly to monitor for the development of thrombocytopenia, and the heparin should be stopped if any one of the following occurs: a precipitous or sustained fall in the platelet count or a platelet count less than $100,000/\mu L$. The use of thrombolytic agents, surgical thrombectomy, or percutaneous mechanical thrombectomy in the treatment of venous thromboembolism must be individualized. Patients with hemodynamically unstable PE or massive iliofemoral thrombosis (phlegmasia cerulea dolens) and who are also at low risk to bleed are the most appropriate candidates for such treatment.

Inferior Vena Caval Filter Placement

Inferior vena caval filter placement is recommended when there is a contraindication to, or a failure of, anticoagulant therapy in an individual with or at high risk for proximal vein thrombosis or PE. It is also recommended in patients with recurrent thromboembolism despite adequate anticoagulation, for chronic recurrent embolism with pulmonary hypertension, and with the concurrent performance of surgical pulmonary embolectomy or pulmonary thromboendarterectomy.

Anticoagulation

Oral anticoagulation with warfarin should prolong the INR to a target of 2.5 (range: 2.0 to 3.0). If oral anticoagulants are contraindicated or inconvenient, long-term therapy can be undertaken with adjusted-dose unfractionated heparin, low molecular weight heparin, or fondaparinux. Because of ease of use, especially in the outpatient setting, LMW heparin or fondaparinux is preferred to unfractionated heparin. Patients with a first thromboembolic event in the context of a reversible or time-limited risk factor (trauma or surgery) should be treated for at least three months. Patients with a first idiopathic thromboembolic event should be treated for a minimum of three months. Following this, all patients should be evaluated for the risk/benefit ratio of long-term therapy. Indefinite therapy is preferred in patients with a first unprovoked episode of proximal DVT who have a greater concern about recurrent VTE and a relatively lower concern about the burdens of long-term anticoagulant therapy. In patients with a first isolated unprovoked episode of distal DVT, three months of anticoagulant therapy should be given rather than indefinite therapy. Most patients with advanced malignancy should be treated indefinitely or until the cancer resolves. The general medical management of the acute episode of DVT is individualized. Once anticoagulation has been started and the patient's symptoms (pain, swelling) are under control, early ambulation is advised.

During initial ambulation and for the first two years following an episode of VTE, use of an elastic compression stocking has been recommended to prevent the postphlebitic syndrome.

LYMPHEDEMA
Definition

Lymphedema refers to the pathologic accumulation of protein-rich fluid in the interstitium due to a lymphatic drainage defect. It often affects the extremities, but it can involve the face, genitalia, or trunk.

Causes

The primary causes include congenital lymphedema, lymphedema praecox, and lymphedema tarda. Congenital lymphedema, also known as Milroy disease, is an autosomal dominant familial disorder of the lymphatic system that manifests at birth to 1 year and is linked to a mutation that inactivates VEGFR3.[9-10] It is often due to anaplastic lymphatic channels. The lower extremity edema is most commonly bilateral, pitting, and nonpainful. It has been associated with cellulitis, prominent veins, intestinal lymphangiectasias, upturned toenails, and hydrocele. Lymphedema praecox, also known as Meige disease, is the most common form of primary lymphedema. Seventy percent of cases are unilateral, with lower extremity swelling being more common. This type of primary edema is most often due to hypoplastic lymphatic channels. This condition most often manifests clinically around menarche, suggesting that estrogen may play a role in its pathogenesis. Lymphedema tarda manifests later in life, usually in persons older than 35. It is thought to be due to a defect in the lymphatic valves, resulting in incompetent valve function.

The secondary causes of lymphedema are due to obstruction or infiltration of the lymphatic system, including malignancy, infection, obesity, trauma, congestive heart failure, portal hypertension, and post-therapeutic and postsurgical complications.

The most common cause from infection of lymphedema is filariasis. Medically, the most common cause is obesity. The most common postsurgical cause is from a mastectomy and therapeutically, radiation therapy is the most common cause reported.

Angiosarcoma arising in an area of long-standing lymphedema is termed Stewart-Treves syndrome. Most cases of Stewart-Treves syndrome occur in the arm after surgery for breast cancer. However, sometimes angiosarcomas can arise in a chronically lymphedematous leg. Lymphangiosarcomas are extremely aggressive tumors with a high local recurrence rate and a tendency to metastasize early to many areas.

DATA COLLECTING
History

Primary lymphedema can also be associated with various cutaneous syndromes. Patients often report that chronic swelling of an extremity preceded lymphedema. Eighty percent of patients present with lower extremity involvement, although the upper extremities, face, genitalia, and trunk can also be involved. The history confirms involvement of a distal extremity initially, with proximal involvement following. Patients with lymphedema often report painless swelling and leg heaviness.

Fevers, chills, and generalized weakness may be reported. Patients may have a history of recurrent episodes of cellulitis, lymphangitis, fissuring, ulcerations, and/or verrucous changes. Patients have a higher prevalence of bacterial and fungal infections. In primary lymphedema, patients have a congenital defect in the lymphatic system; therefore, the history of onset is more typical of the specific type.

Association with Genetic Disorders

Primary lymphedema is often associated with other anomalies and genetic disorders, such as yellow nail syndrome, Turner syndrome, Noonan syndrome, xanthomatosis, hemangiomas, neurofibromatosis type 1, distichiasis lymphedema, Klinefelter syndrome, congenital absence of nails, trisomy 21, trisomy 13, and trisomy 18.

A rare inherited disorder, distichiasis-lymphedema syndrome is characterized by the presence of extra eyelashes (distichiasis) and swelling of the arms and legs (lymphedema). Swelling of the legs, especially below the knees, and eye irritation are common in people with this disorder. Spinal cysts (epidural) with or without other abnormalities of the spinal column can accompany distichiasis lymphedema. Distichiasis-lymphedema syndrome is inherited as an autosomal dominant genetic trait due to a mutation of the FOX2 gene.

In secondary lymphedema, the associated history should be more evident, based on the primary etiology. If the disease is due to filariasis, the history should include travel or habitation in an endemic area. Other patients should have a clear history of a neoplasm obstructing the lymphatic system, recurrent episodes of lymphangitis and/or cellulitis, obesity, trauma, or lymphedema resulting after surgery and/or radiation therapy.

Physical Examination

The earliest symptom of lymphedema is nontender pitting edema of the affected area, most commonly the distal extremities. The face, trunk, and genitalia also may be involved. Radial enlargement of the area occurs over time, which progresses to a nonpitting edema resulting from the development of fibrosis in the subcutaneous fat. The distal extremities are involved initially, followed by proximal advancement. Patients have erythema of the affected area and thickening of the skin, which appears as peau d'orange and woody edema. With long-term involvement, an area of cobble-stoned, hyperkeratotic, papillomatous plaques is most commonly seen on the shins. The plaques can be covered with a loosely adherent crust, can be weepy or oozing a clear or yellow fluid, and/or can have a foul-smelling odor. Fissuring, ulcerations, skin breakdown, and lymphorrhea can also be seen. Superinfection is common and can manifest as impetigo with yellow crusts. A positive Stemmer sign (inability to pinch the dorsal aspect of skin between the first and second toes) may be elicited upon examination. The inability to tent the skin over the interdigital webs (Stemmer sign) is characteristic of lymphedema. Other associated physical findings specific for the cause of secondary lymphedema and genetic disorders involving lymphedema may be noted upon examination.

DATA MINING

A CBC and differential are helpful to determine an infectious origin. Liver function, BUN/creatinine levels, and urinalysis results should be checked if a renal or hepatic etiology is suspected. Specific markers should be checked if a neoplasm is suspected. Imaging is not necessary to make the diagnosis, but it can be used to confirm it, to assess the extent of involvement, and to determine therapeutic intervention. Lymphangiography can be used to evaluate the lymphatic system and its patency. Although it was once thought to be the first-line imaging modality for lymphedema, it is now rarely used because of its invasive nature and potential adverse effects.

Lymphoscintigraphy

Lymphoscintigraphy is the new criterion used to assess the lymphatic system. It allows for detailed visualization of the lymphatic channels with minimal risk. The anatomy and the obstructed areas of lymphatic flow can be assessed.

Ultrasonography

Ultrasonography can be used to evaluate the lymphatic and venous systems. Volumetric and structural changes are identified within the lymphatic system. Venous abnormalities such as deep vein thrombosis can be excluded based on ultrasonography findings.

MRI and CT Scan

MRI and CT scanning can also be used to evaluate lymphedema. These radiologic tests can be helpful in confirming the diagnosis and monitoring the effects of treatment. They are also recommended when malignancy is suspected.

Biopsy

A biopsy can be performed if the diagnosis is not clinically apparent, if areas of chronic lymphedema look suspicious, or if areas of chronic ulceration exist.

PROGRAMMED MANAGEMENT

The goal of therapy is to restore function, to reduce physical and psychological suffering, and to prevent the development of infection. The first-line treatment is complex physical therapy aimed at improving lymphedema with manual lymphatic drainage, massage, and exercise. The use of compression stockings, multilayer bandaging, or pneumatic pumps is necessary. Leg elevation is essential. Appropriate skin care and debridement are also stressed to prevent recurrent cellulitis or lymphangitis.

In secondary lymphedema, the underlying etiology (neoplasm or infection) should also be properly treated to relieve the lymphatic obstruction and to improve lymphedema. Weight loss is a necessity for obesity, which impairs lymphatic return. Few pharmacologic therapies have been found to be effective in the treatment of lymphedema. Benzopyrones (including coumarin and flavonoids) are a group of drugs that have been found to be successful in treating lymphedema when combined with complex physical therapy. They aid in decreasing excess edematous fluid, softening the limb, decreasing skin temperature, and decreasing the number of secondary infections. The benzopyrones successfully increase the number of macrophages, leading to proteolysis and protein reabsorption. Topical emollients and keratolytics may improve secondary epidermal changes. Diuretics have no role in the treatment of lymphedema.

Surgery is reserved for cases of lymphedema resistant to medical therapies. Several debulking procedures have been used and may involve the drainage of lymph fluid from the subcutaneous tissue via a silicone tube connected to a one-way valve. The Charles procedure consists of radical excision of the affected subcutaneous tissue with primary or staged skin grafting. Total superficial lymphangiectomy is a variant of this procedure, in which debulking of the entire limb is performed. Venous-lymphatic anastomosis may be performed in severe cases of lymphedema with a functioning venous system, and this procedure may be effective only in cases of secondary lymphedema.

Prophylactic lymphovenous anastomoses have been performed in patients undergoing extensive pelvic lymph node dissection who have a high risk of developing lymphedema. Recalcitrant cases may ultimately require amputation.

RENAL VEIN THROMBOSIS
Definition

Renal vein thrombosis (RVT) is relatively uncommon but may actually be underdiagnosed. RVT can be caused by trauma to the back, scar formation, tumors, or stricture. Hypercoagulable states increase the risk and are often noted in patients with nephrotic syndrome. The incidences of both renal venous and arterial thrombosis are much higher in patients with nephrotic syndrome compared to the general population.

Risk Factors

The risk of thrombosis varies among the causes of nephrotic syndrome. The risk is highest with membranous nephropathy followed by membranoproliferative glomerulonephritis (MPGN) and minimal change disease. The risk of thrombosis may also be related to the severity and duration of the nephrotic state and appears to be particularly increased with serum albumin concentrations ≤ 2.0 g/dL (20 g/L).[11]

RVT may be unilateral or bilateral and may extend into the inferior vena cava. RVT is more often chronic, but acute RVT can occur and has a more dramatic presentation. Acute RVT is most often due to trauma, severe dehydration (especially in infants), or a generalized hypercoagulable state. It is an uncommon complication of the nephrotic syndrome.

DATA COLLECTING
Acute Renal Vein Thrombosis

RVT typically presents with symptoms of renal infarction, including flank pain, microscopic or gross hematuria, a marked elevation in serum lactate dehydrogenase (without change in transaminases), and an increase in renal size on radiographic study. Bilateral RVT may manifest with acute renal failure.

Significant proteinuria is a rare complication of acute RVT in patients without underlying nephrotic syndrome. In a case report, a previously healthy individual with bilateral RVT presented acutely with lower abdominal and flank pain and proteinuria (2.3 g over 24 hours); both the thrombus and proteinuria disappeared after two courses of urokinase followed by intravenous heparin. Subsequent examination of renal biopsy tissue via light microscopy, immunofluorescence, and electron microscopy was normal.

Chronic Renal Vein Thrombosis

CRVT most often has an insidious onset and produces no symptoms referable to the kidney. A pulmonary embolus is usually the only clinical clue to the presence of renal or other deep vein thrombosis. Chronic RVT in patients with nephrotic syndrome may lead to increased proteinuria or progressively worsening kidney function.

The gold-standard diagnostic test for RVT is selective renal venography. However, less invasive procedures, including spiral computed tomography (CT) with contrast, magnetic resonance imaging (MRI), and Doppler ultrasonography are increasingly being used.

PROGRAMMED MANAGEMENT

There are no randomized trials to guide optimal therapy of hypercoagulability in nephrotic syndrome. There are two aspects to therapy of the hypercoagulable state in nephrotic syndrome that must be considered: anticoagulation to prevent thromboembolic events (including RVT, DVT, and PE) and dissolution or removal of the thrombus with thrombolytic therapy or thrombectomy, which are primarily considered in patients with acute RVT.

For the prevention of thromboembolism in patients with nephrotic syndrome, prophylactic anticoagulation, anticoagulation for asymptomatic RVT, and anticoagulation after a symptomatic thromboembolic event are the cornerstones of treatment for RVT.

Systemic fibrinolysis has been used in patients with RVT but carries the risk of bleeding, including intracranial bleeding, and is not recommended. Successful outcomes have been reported using local thrombolytic therapy with or without extraction catheter thrombectomy in nephrotic patients with acute RVT.

Surgical thrombectomy should be considered only in the rare patient with acute bilateral RVT and acute renal failure who cannot be treated with percutaneous thrombectomy and/or thrombolysis.

RETINAL VEIN OCCLUSION
Definition

Retinal vein occlusion (RVO) is the obstruction of the retinal veins, often as it constricts through the lamina cribrosa. The causes may be due to abnormal blood flow, hypercoagulability, atherosclerosis, vessel anomalies, or a combination of these factors classified according to where the obstruction is located. Obstruction of the retinal vein at the optic nerve is referred to as central retinal vein occlusion (CRVO), and obstruction at a branch of the retinal vein is referred to as branch retinal vein occlusion (BRVO). The two forms have both differences and similarities in pathogenesis and clinical presentation. RVO is a common vascular disorder of the retina and is one of the most common causes of blindness after diabetic retinopathy.

RVO is commonly subdivided into nonischemic and ischemic types. Two-thirds of patients with the ischemic type develop macular edema, macular ischemia, and neovascularization that may lead to blindness. Ischemic vein occlusions are the only vein occlusions that will likely develop neovascular complications and account for only one-third of all occlusions.

DATA COLLECTING

History

A history of systemic diseases, such as diabetes and hypertension, is often noted. The patient may be asymptomatic, but most complain of sudden painless unilateral loss of vision or loss of a visual field and sudden onset of floating spots or flashing lights. Nonischemic CRVO often presents with a subtle, intermittent visual loss that is painless with mild-to-moderate visual loss. Ischemic CRVO produces a more acute visual loss with or without pain and marked visual loss. Acuity may range anywhere from 20/20 to finger counting. Ischemic vein occlusions typically present with acuity worse than 20/200. An initial acuity better than 20/200 shows very low risk for developing severe permanent vision loss, and most cases are likely to resolve. If the vision loss is severe, there may be a relative afferent pupillary defect. Ischemic occlusions are likely to manifest with a relative afferent pupillary defect. If not, then the occlusions are probably nonischemic.[12]

Physical Examination

Ophthalmoscopic findings include retinal edema, superficial hemorrhage, disk swelling, cotton wool spots, and tortuous and dilated retinal veins. If there is a central retinal vein occlusion, these findings will encompass all four retinal quadrants. A hemi-central retinal vein occlusion will involve only the superior or inferior half of the retina. A branch retinal vein occlusion will present with findings in only one quadrant, which is usually the superotemporal quadrant, with the apex of the hemorrhage at an arteriovenous crossing. Associated hemorrhages may obscure the above findings. Neovascularization may be noted later in the disease.

DATA MINING

As there is association of systemic disease with vein occlusions, tests should include blood pressure monitoring, fasting blood glucose, lipid and cholesterol studies, FTA-ABS, complete blood count with differential, sickle index, antinuclear antibodies, angiotensin-converting enzymes, and viscosity studies to screen for hypercoagulable states.

PROGRAMMED MANAGEMENT

Management through preventive pan-retinal photocoagulation (PRP) is no longer recommended. PRP is now recommended when neovascularization has taken place. Patients will benefit from focal laser photocoagulation anywhere between 3 and 18 months after the occlusion's onset.[13-14] Monitor the patient monthly with serial ophthalmoscopy, fundus photography, and gonioscopy until resolution is noted.

TROUBLE-SHOOTING AND DEBUGGING

How to Differentiate Edema from Cardiac Disease from Edema from Varicose Veins

Edema in cardiac disease is caused by pump failure resulting in pitting edema of the legs and feet. The signs and symptoms of HF include rales in the lungs, a gallop rhythm, and distended neck veins from right-sided heart failure. In venous and lymphatic obstruction, the blood and lymph collect in the tissues. The veins of the legs have valves that prevent the backward flow of blood. In venous insufficiency, the incompetence of the valves occurs because of dilation of the veins and subsequent dysfunction of the valves themselves. Venous insufficiency leads to a stagnation of the blood and increased pressure in the veins causing venous hypertension. Venous insufficiency is a problem that is localized to the legs, ankles, and feet. One leg may be more affected than the other. In contrast, systemic diseases that are associated with fluid retention generally cause the same amount of edema in both legs, as in other parts of the body.

Diuretic therapy in patients with venous insufficiency tends to be of minimal value because of the continuous pooling of fluid in the lower extremities. Elevation of the legs during the day and the use of compression stockings may alleviate edema. Surgical treatment may also be needed to relieve chronic edema caused by venous insufficiency.

VARICOSE VEINS

Definition

Varicose veins are dilated and tortuous veins are due to a weakening in the vein's wall or the loss of competency of the valves.

Causes

The primary cause of varicose veins is incompetent venous valves that result in venous hypertension. Secondary varicose veins result from deep venous thrombosis and its sequelae or congenital anatomic abnormalities. The etiology of these varicose veins can be classified into primary, secondary, and congenital. A primary etiology occurs due to valvular insufficiency of the superficial veins, most commonly at the saphenofemoral junction. Secondary causes are varied. One cause is by deep vein thrombosis (DVT) that leads to chronic deep venous obstruction or valvular insufficiency. Long-term clinical sequelae have been called postthrombotic syndrome and include catheter-associated DVTs. Pregnancy-induced and progesterone-induced venous wall and valve weakness worsened by expanded circulating blood volume and an enlarged uterus compresses the inferior vena cava and venous return from the lower extremities. Trauma can also cause venous obstruction directly or indirectly. Congenital causes include any venous malformations, including avalvulia and Klippel-Trenaunay variants.

DATA COLLECTING

History

Patients may have a host of symptoms, but symptoms are usually caused by venous hypertension rather than the varicose veins themselves. Often, symptoms are purely aesthetic, and patients desire treatment of the unsightly nature of the tortuous, dilated varicosities. Complaints of pain, soreness, burning, aching, throbbing, heavy legs, cramping, muscle fatigue, pruritus, night cramps, and "restless legs" are usually secondary to the venous hypertension. Pain and other symptoms may worsen with the menstrual cycle, with pregnancy, and in response to exogenous hormonal therapy (oral contraceptives).

Also, pain associated with venous hypertension is usually a dull ache that worsens after prolonged standing and improves by walking or by elevating the legs. This is in contrast to the pain of arterial insufficiency, which is worse with ambulation and elevation. Subjective symptoms are usually more severe early in the progression of disease, less severe in the middle phases, and more severe again with advancing age. Patients who have become acclimatized to their chronic disease may not volunteer information about symptoms. After treatment, patients are often surprised to realize how much chronic discomfort they had accepted as "normal."

The venous history usually includes a history of venous insufficiency, the presence or absence of predisposing factors (heredity, trauma to the legs, occupational prolonged standing, and sports participation), superficial or deep thrombophlebitis, vascular disease, and a family history of vascular disease of any type.

Physical Examination

Varicose veins represent a significant clinical problem and are not just a "cosmetic" issue because of their unsightly nature. The clinical nature of the problem arises from the fact that varicose veins actually represent underlying chronic venous insufficiency with ensuing venous hypertension. This venous hypertension leads to a broad spectrum of clinical manifestations, ranging from symptoms to cutaneous findings like varicose veins, reticular veins, telangiectasias, swelling, skin discoloration, and ulcerations.

The physical examination should look for surgical scars from prior intervention, pigmentations and skin changes, visible, palpable veins in the subcutaneous skin larger than 3 mm, reticular veins, telangiectasias, eczema, and ulcers. The entire surface of the skin should be palpated with the fingertips because dilated veins may be palpable even where they are not visible. Distal and proximal arterial pulses are also palpated. Leg pain or tenderness may reveal a firm, thickened, thrombosed vein. These palpable thrombosed vessels are superficial veins, but an associated DVT may exist in as many as 40% of patients with superficial phlebitis.

DATA FILTERING (DIFFERENTIAL DIAGNOSIS)

Varices of recent onset are easily distinguished from chronic varices by palpation. Newly dilated vessels sit on the surface of the muscle or bone; chronic varices erode into underlying muscle or bone, creating deep "boggy" or "spongy" pockets in the calf muscle and deep palpable bony notches, especially over the anterior tibia. It is helpful to determine whether two venous segments are directly interconnected. With the patient in a standing position, a vein segment is percussed at one position while an examining hand feels for a "pulse wave" at another position. With the availability of duplex ultrasound, the Perthes maneuver/Linton test is rarely done. This is a physical examination technique in which a tourniquet is placed over the proximal part of the leg to compress any superficial varicose veins while leaving deep veins unaffected. The patient walks or performs toe-stands to activate the calf-muscle pump, which normally causes varicose veins to be emptied. However, if obstruction of the deep system exists, then activation of the calf-muscle pump causes a paradoxical congestion of the superficial venous system and engorgement of varicose veins, resulting in a positive test. To verify, the patient is then placed supine, and the leg is elevated (Linton test). If varices distal to the tourniquet fail to drain after a few seconds, again deep venous obstruction must be considered. This test is rarely performed in practice today with the advent of duplex imaging and assessment of the superficial and deep venous systems.

 JOB DESCRIPTION:

How to Do the Perthes Percussive Test

The Perthes percussive test is a classic maneuver that is useful to test whether venous segments are interconnected. With the patient in a standing position, a vein segment is tapped at one location while an examining hand feels for a pulse wave at another location. Propagation of a palpable pulse wave suggests that a fluid-filled vessel with open or incompetent valves connects the two locations. A pulse wave may be propagated after prolonged standing in the absence of true pathology because prolonged standing causes even normal veins to become distended and normal valves to float open. The Perthes test is most valuable when a bulging varicosity in the lower leg has no obvious connection with a varicosity in the upper thigh. A palpable pulse wave propagation between the two vessels is positive proof of the existence of an unseen connection.

 JOB DESCRIPTION:

How to Do the Trendelenburg Test

The Trendelenburg test is a classic physical examination maneuver that helps to distinguish superficial venous reflux from incompetence of the deep vein valves. The leg is elevated until all superficial veins have collapsed, and the point of suspected reflux from the deep system is occluded by manual compression or by a tourniquet. The patient is then asked to stand, and the distal varicosity is observed for refilling. If the distal varicosity remains mostly empty, the reflux pathway is principally through the peripheral varicosity that has been occluded. Inability to prevent rapid filling of the varicosity despite manual occlusion of the suspected high point of reflux suggests that another reflux pathway is involved. Rapid refilling of calf varices despite occlusion of the proximal trunk suggests deep system reflux or failure of the valves of multiple perforating veins.

DATA MINING

Ankle-Brachial Index

An ankle-brachial index is useful if arterial insufficiency is suggested. The duplex ultrasound has become the most useful tool for work-up and has replaced many of the physical examination maneuvers and physiologic tests once used for diagnosis. Duplex ultrasound with color-flow imaging is a special type of two-dimensional ultrasound that uses Doppler-flow information to add color for blood flow in the image. Vessels in the blood are colored red for flow in one direction and blue for flow in the other, with a graduated color scale to reflect the speed of the flow. Venous valvular reflux is defined as regurgitant flow with Valsalva that lasts longer than two seconds. Doppler auscultation can also be used. These compression-decompression maneuvers are repeated while gradually ascending the limb to a level at which the reflux can no longer be appreciated.

Magnetic Resonance Venography

Magnetic resonance venography (MRV) is the most sensitive and most specific test to find causes of anatomic obstruction. MRV is particularly useful because unsuspected nonvascular causes for leg pain and edema may often be seen on the scan image when the clinical presentation erroneously suggests venous insufficiency or venous obstruction. This is an expensive test used only as an adjuvant when diagnostic doubt still exists.

Venous Refilling Time

The maximum venous outflow (MVO) is a functional test to help detect obstruction to venous outflow. It can help detect more proximal occlusion of the iliac veins and IVC as well as extrinsic causes of obstruction in addition to DVTs. The venous refilling time (VRT) is a physiologic test also using plethysmography. The VRT is the time necessary for the lower leg to become infused with blood after the calf-muscle pump has emptied the lower leg as thoroughly as possible. In healthy subjects, venous refilling is longer than 120 seconds. In patients with mild and asymptomatic venous insufficiency, VRT is between 40 and 120 seconds. In patients with significant venous insufficiency, VRT is abnormally fast at 20 to 40 seconds. Such patients often complain of nocturnal leg cramps, restless legs, leg soreness, burning leg pain, and premature leg fatigue. A VRT of less than 20 seconds is markedly abnormal and is nearly always symptomatic. If the VRT is less than 10 seconds, venous ulcerations are likely.[15-17]

Muscle Pump Ejection Fraction

Muscle pump ejection fraction (MPEF) is used to detect failure of the calf muscle pump to expel blood from the lower leg. MPEF results are highly repeatable but require a skilled operator. The Trendelenburg test distinguishes patients with reflux at the sapheno-femoral junction (SFJ) from those with incompetent deep venous valves.

Contrast Venogram

A direct contrast venogram is an invasive venous imaging technique with a 15% chance of developing new venous thrombosis from the procedure itself. It is rarely used and has been replaced by duplex ultrasound. Its use is reserved for difficult or confusing cases.

ADVANCED MANAGEMENT

Surgical removal or obliteration of varicose veins is often for cosmetic reasons alone. Noncosmetic indications have developed that include symptomatic varicosities (pain, fatigability, heaviness, recurrent superficial thrombophlebitis, bleeding) or the treatment of venous hypertension after skin or subcutaneous tissue changes, such as lipodermatosclerosis, atrophie blanche, ulceration, or hyperpigmentation. Conservative treatment with stockings and external compression is an acceptable alternative to surgery, but worsening cutaneous findings or symptoms despite these measures usually warrant intervention.

Surgical Therapy

Current therapies are becoming less invasive with improved recovery, but long-term outcomes are uncertain. Therapies aim to remove the superficial venous system either through surgery, endovenous ablation, or sclerotherapy ablation. In 90% of cases in which venous hypertension is from superficial and perforator vein reflux, removal or obliteration of the greater saphenous vein (GSV) alone can resolve the venous hypertension. However, in the remaining 10%, additional treatment of the incompetent perforator veins may be needed. Additionally, if severe deep venous incompetence exists, treatment of the GSV alone usually does not resolve the venous hypertension. In both these cases, additional interventions with subfascial endoscopic perforating vein surgery (SEPS), perforator vein ablation, and/or venous reconstruction may be indicated.

Endovascular Therapy

Endovascular Techniques Involve Endovenous (EV) Laser and Radiofrequency (RF) Ablation

Minimally Invasive Techniques

Cutaneous electrodesiccation and sclerotherapy are less invasive alternatives. Chemical sclerosis with polidocanol and sodium tetradecyl sulfate is used to treat the GSV and its main tributaries.

Postoperative Therapy

After treatment of large varicose veins by any method, a 30- to 40-mm Hg gradient compression stocking is applied, and patients are instructed to maintain or increase their normal activity levels. Most practitioners also recommend the use of gradient compression stockings even after treatment of spider veins and smaller tributary veins.

Ace wraps and other long-stretch bandages should not be used. These elastic bandages fail to maintain adequate compression for more than a few hours. They often slip or are misapplied by patients, with a resulting tourniquet effect that causes distal swelling and increases the risk of DVT.

Activity is particularly important after treatment by any technique because all modalities of treatment for varicose disease have the potential to increase the risk of DVT. Activity is a strong protective factor against venous stasis. Activity is so important that most venous specialists will not treat a patient who is unable to remain active following treatment.

Complications

A correct diagnosis of superficial venous insufficiency is essential. Veins should be treated only if they are incompetent and if a normal collateral pathway exits. Removal of a saphenous vein with a competent termination will not aid in the management of nontruncal tributary varices. In the setting of deep system obstruction, varicosities are hemodynamically helpful because they provide a bypass pathway for venous return. Hemodynamically helpful varices must not be removed or sclerosed. Ablation of these varicosities will cause rapid onset of pain and swelling of the extremity, eventually followed by the development of new varicose bypass pathways. The most annoying minor complications of any venous surgery are dysesthesias from injury to the sural nerve or the saphenous nerve. Subcutaneous hematoma is a common complication, regardless of treatment technique used. It is easily managed with warm compresses, NSAIDs, or aspiration if necessary.

At the saphenofemoral junction, accidental treatment of the femoral vein by inappropriate radiofrequency or laser catheter placement, spread of the sclerosant (not visualizing the progression with ultrasound), or inappropriate surgical ligation can all lead to endothelial damage at the deep vein, causing deep vein thrombosis (DVT) formation with the potential for pulmonary embolism (PE) and even death.

Other complications, such as postoperative infection and arterial injury, are less common and may be kept to a minimum through strict precautions and good technique. Endovenous treatment techniques (with RF and laser therapy) have the potential for excessive tissue heating, which can lead to skin burns. This problem can be avoided if sufficient volumes of tumescent anesthetic are injected to elevate the skin away from the vein.

References

1. Perloff, J. K. Physical examination of the heart and circulation. Shelton, CT.: People's Medical Publishing House, 2009.
2. Eklöf, B., Rutherford, R. B., Bergan, J. J., et al.: Revision of the CEAP classification for chronic venous disorders: consensus statement. J Vasc Surg. 2004;40(6):1248–1252.
3. Chiesa, R., Marone, E. M., Limoni, C., et al.: Chronic venous disorders: correlation between visible signs, symptoms, and presence of functional disease. J Vasc Surg. 2007;46:322.
4. Callam, M. J., Harper, D. R., Dale, J. J., et al.: Chronic ulcer of the leg: Clinical history. Br Med J. 1987;294:1389.
5. In the clinic: Deep venous thrombosis. Ann Intern Med. 2008; 149: ITC3.
6. Qaseem, A., Snow, V., Barry, P., et al. Current diagnosis of venous thromboembolism in primary care: a clinical practice guideline from the American Academy of Family Physicians and the American College of Physicians. Ann Intern Med. 2007;146:454.
7. Alikhan, R., Cohen, A. T., Combe, S., et al.: Risk factors for venous thromboembolism in hospitalized patients with acute medical illness: analysis of the MEDENOX Study. Arch Intern Med. 2004;164:963.
8. Harvey, W. P.: Cardiac Pearls. Cedar Grove, NJ: Leannec Publishing, 1993, 43–112.
9. Brennan, M. J., Miller, L. T.: Overview of treatment options and review of the current role and use of compression garments, intermittent pumps, and exercise in the management of lymphedema. Cancer. 1998;83(12 Suppl American):2821–2827.
10. Child, A. H., Beninson, J., Sarfarazi, M.: Cause of primary congenital lymphedema. Angiology. 1999;50(4):325-326.
11. Wagoner, R. D., Stanson, A. W., Holley, K. E.: Renal vein thrombosis in idiopathic membranous glomerulopathy and nephrotic syndrome: incidence and significance. Kidney Int. 1983;23(2):368–374.
12. Keith, S., Humphries, R.: Current Diagnosis and Treatment of Emergency Medicine. 6th ed. New York: McGraw-Hill Co., 2008.
13. Mohamed, Q., McIntosh, R. L., Saw, S. M., et al.: Interventions for central retinal vein occlusion: an evidence-based systematic review. Ophthalmology. 2007;114(3):507-519, 524.
14. Madhusudhana, K. C., Newsom, R. S.: Central retinal vein occlusion: the therapeutic options. Can J Ophthalmol. 2007;42(2):193–195.
15. Naoum, J. J., Hunter, G. C.: Pathogenesis of varicose veins and implications for clinical management. Vascular. 2007;15(5):242–249.
16. Weiss, R. A., Feied, C. F., Weiss, M. A.: Vein Diagnosis and Treatment: A Comprehensive Approach, New York: McGraw-Hill, 2001, 119-150.
17. Pappas, P. J., Lal, B. K. L., Cerveira, J. J., et al.: The Management of Venous Disorders. In Rutherford, R. B., ed. Vascular Surgery. Philadelphia, PA: Elsevier, 2005, pp. 2220–2302.

Section IV

Disturbance of a Dead-End Vasculature

CHAPTER

13

Syncope

Thach Nguyen, Dayi Hu, Haiyun Wu,
Shi Wen Wang, and Brian Olshansky

Chapter Outline

DEFINITION

Syncope is an abrupt, transient loss of consciousness, with loss of postural tone, followed by complete, rapid recovery.

Strategic Programming

The initial and most critical part of the investigation of syncope requires a comprehensive history and physical examination (H and P) to prove the presence or absence of one or multiple episodes of hypotension causing general cerebrovascular ischemia. After the H and P, the physician can deduct a preliminary working diagnosis of syncope caused by transient hypotension and a short list of differential diagnoses (e.g., hypoglycemia, seizure). In order to rule in the working diagnosis and to rule out the differential diagnoses based on the H and P, tests (mainly about left ventricular function and structure.) are performed to establish the potential causes of syncope and the long-term and short-term risks of mortality. The dilemma is to avoid overtesting those who do not need excessive testing while not underdiagnosing those with life-threatening conditions. There is no "no gold standard" evaluation.

DATA COLLECTING

Investigation Master Plan

When a physician sees a patient suspected of having syncope, there are seven main areas of interest for data collecting (history and physical examination) based on a computational cardiac model (Table 13-1).

The main area of interest: The left ventricle (zone A). Syncope is a symptom resulting from a global decrease of cerebrovascular perfusion. The causes of hypotension can be structural abnormalities in the left ventricle (including aortic stenosis, severe left ventricular dysfunction, hypertrophic cardiomyopathy, or acute myocardial infarction), disruptive heart rate (such as is seen in severe brady- or tachyarrythmia), or of neurocardiogenic origin without any structural cardiac abnormality. The structural abnormality of the LV is a hardware problem, while cardioneurogenic syncope is due to a software problem. Rhythm disturbances can be due to a software problem if they are from sympathetic overstimulation (sinus tachycardia) or they can be due to a configuration set-up abnormality if the arrhythmia is secondary to re-entry circuit.

The upstream area: The pulmonary venous (capacitance) system, which does not contribute much to the syncopal process (zone B).

The downstream areas are the aorta and the distal peripheral arteries. The vascular tone (constriction or vasodilation) is important in the generation of hypotension-causing syncope (zone C).

The system configuration: If there is structural heart disease, there is disruption of the blood circulation. There is nothing wrong with the configuration of the system in the case of syncope of cardioneurogenic origin. If there is syncope due to re-entry tachycardia, this is a configuration problem (zone E).

The work-around configuration: None identified here (zone D).

The cardiovascular system: This is an index problem.

The network (the whole body): Syncope occurs due to low blood pressure causing decreased perfusion to the central nervous system. The

TABLE 13-1: Investigation Master Plan

	Index Problem	LV	Distal Peripheral Arteries	Symptom or Sign	Mechanism of Disease
Aortic Stenosis	Obstruction at the aortic valve level	High LVSP	Maximal dilation, inadequate con- striction	Systolic murmur of AS	Severity of index problem
Ventricular Tachycardia	Fast heart rate	Low LVSP	Overwhelmed constriction	Palpitations	Overwhelmed compensatory mechanisms
Neuro- Cardiogenic Syncope	Slow heart rate with inappropriate vasodilation	Low LVSP	Inappropriate vasodilation	None	Inappropriate compensatory mechanism

AS, aortic stenosis; LV, left ventricle; LVSP, left ventricular systolic pressure.

pulmonary venous (capacitance) system is not directly responsible for syncope because of its programmed delayed response to hypotension (zone F).

> ## DATA DECODING TIPS (CLINICAL PEARLS)
> ### One Main Question When Investigating Syncope
>
> Syncope is a common manifestation of many disease processes. The main question is whether the patient suffers an episode of hypotension causing significant decrease of global cerebral perfusion and syncope. Among all patients with syncope, patients with heart disease, particularly when there is impaired LV function, BBB, evidence of congestive heart failure, or a positive family history, are at particularly high risk for death. These patients require an aggressive initial approach and may need hospitalization and aggressive therapeutic interventions (including defibrillator implantation). The diagnosis of neurocardiogenic syncope is made by a taking a detailed history and obtaining a negative physical examination.

History

The key to the proper initial evaluation and ultimate management of the patient with syncope is a complete and carefully obtained history. While it is perhaps self-evident, the key problem in the evaluation and management of syncope relates to deficiencies in the history as narrated by the patient, reported by a witness, or not confirmed because of the absence of witnesses.

> ## DATA DECODING TIPS (CLINICAL PEARLS)
> ### Seven Questions to Guide the Investigative Process
>
> When evaluating syncope, the following questions need to be addressed: (1) Is it really syncope? (2) Is there hypotension that precipitates the syncopal episode? (3) What are the surrounding activities, events, or symptoms that could have caused hypotension? (4) Does the patient have a terrain susceptible for syncope (vulnerable to hypotension without adequate reflex compensatory mechanism) to raise blood pressure? (5) Is there a new compromising situation that makes the patient succumb to hypotension? (6) Is there a factor triggering the hypotension cascade? (7) Which tests are needed to prove these clinical suspicions (Table 13-2)?

Reconstruction of a Detailed History

In a common scenario of hypotension-induced syncope, at first the patient experiences lightheadedness or dizziness. As these symptoms become more severe, the patient may note that everything begins to fade and a black curtain falls down; slowly, the patient loses awareness and consciousness. The progression of these symptoms can vary from slow

TABLE 13-2: Details of a Complete History

Situations in which the event occurred, including body position, length of episode, number of episodes, physical activity, physical and mental stresses

Prodromal and post-syncopal symptoms: quantifying the type and duration or prodromal and recovery symptoms

Concomitant symptoms, including pain

Witnessed accounts

Past similar events: number and chronicity of prior syncopal and pre-syncopal episodes, length of time of problem (i.e., years, months, or days)

Medications taken by patient that may have played a role in syncope

Concomitant medical conditions

Family history of cardiac disease, syncope, or sudden death

to abrupt, according to how fast the decrease of cerebral blood flow is. If hypotension is gradual, the patient may be aware of the development of light-headedness and dizziness (a "prodrome") and be able to take measures to offset complete loss of consciousness in order to prevent significant injury. This is why it is of utmost importance to reconstruct the history and the sequence of these situational events (Table 13-2).

DATA DECODING TIPS (CLINICAL PEARLS)
Verification of the Syncopal Episode

Was it really syncope? Because there are various degrees of cerebral hypoperfusion, it is important to clarify the prodrome and the development from a mild first symptom of light-headedness to more severe dizziness culminating in the syncopal event. Is it cloudiness? Sleepiness? Confusion? Are there many prior episodes of dizziness on standing from a sitting or lying position? Does the patient experience imbalance when walking (at first)? Is there an abrupt or gradual loss of consciousness? Once supine, does the patient recover right away, become confused, develop fatigue, have transient neurologic abnormalities, stay unconscious for a period of time, or can he or she get up and call for help? Did the patient get hurt during the fall? Any injury related to the fall is strong objective evidence of syncope.[1]

Activities Surrounding the Syncopal Episode

All recent events that preceded syncope can be of importance. Did the patient engage in heavy physical activity prior to collapse? Had the patient just arisen from a lying position? Had the patient just taken medications that could cause hypotension? Had the patient just had a heavy coughing spell? These events may elucidate triggers for syncope.

Similarly, if there were prior episodes of syncope, the relationship between events that preceded syncope on prior occasions should be compared to any events that occurred before syncope on the most recent presentation.[1]

Family History
A family history of Wolff-Parkinson-White syndrome, familial cardiomyopathy, long QT syndrome, arrhythmogenic right ventricular dysplasia, hypertrophic cardiomyopathy, Brugada syndrome, or sudden cardiac death at a young age should be viewed with extreme concern.[1]

Drug History
Did the patient take vasoactive medications that can cause hypotension and orthostatic hypotension? Antiarrhythmic, or psychotropic drugs, diuretics, antihistamines, and antifungals can lead to serious ventricular (generally polymorphic) arrhythmias related to QT prolongation. Common medications in the elderly that can cause syncope are vasodilators and drugs that slow AV node conduction and sinus node function. These include calcium channel blockers, beta blockers, and antihypertensive medications.[1]

Comorbidities
It is important to recognize comorbidities. For example, does the patient have diabetes? Did he or she just take a large dose of insulin without eating?

Past Medical History
Failures of prior therapies are important. For example, if the patient receives a pacemaker and it is working but the patient is still passing out, presumably bradycardia is not the cause of syncope.[1]

Young Age
In younger patients, the cause of isolated syncope is generally neurocardiogenic, psychiatric, or situational (e.g., stress, prolonged standing, and dehydration). Young patients with frequent, recurrent episodes may need treatment to prevent debilitating consequences.[1]

Middle Age
Middle-aged patients (40–65 years), similar to younger patients, can have neurocardiogenic syncope, but a potentially serious cardiovascular cause must be considered as well.[1]

Old Age
Syncope in the elderly can be a tremendous diagnostic challenge. Fifty percent of elderly patients are amnesic of the episodes, and half of the episodes are unwitnessed. Elderly patients often take many medications, which further compromise autonomic reflexes and exacerbate hypotensive responses. Many patients have multifactorial causes for syncope.[1]

⊙ DATA DECODING TIPS (CLINICAL PEARLS)
Most Common Cause of Syncope in Elderly Patients

Always consider and rule out medications as a primary cause of syncope in elderly patients, even when cardiovascular disease is present, before undertaking an aggressive and perhaps risky evaluation.[1]

Physical Examination

The physical examination is less likely to provide guidance in the evaluation, but it can contain important diagnostic and prognostic information.

Vital Signs

A resting bradycardia or an irregular pulse can indicate sick sinus syndrome, various arrhythmias, atrioventricular (AV) block, or premature ventricular contractions.

Blood Pressure

Blood pressure should be checked with the patient lying down and after standing up for two minutes. Orthostatic hypotension is defined as a 20 mm Hg drop in systolic blood pressure or a 10 mm Hg drop in diastolic blood pressure within 3 minutes of standing. A decline in systolic blood pressure of about 20 mm Hg approximately one hour after eating has been reported in up to one third of elderly nursing home residents.[1]

Skin Turgor and Complexion

The patient can look normal or pale. Skin turgor can be normal or decreased.

Cardiovascular Exam

This exam is meant to detect aortic stenosis (AS), hypertrophic cardiomyopathy (HOCM), mitral stenosis, and pulmonic stenosis. This will rule in or out most "obstructive" lesions associated with syncope. It may also indicate the presence of left ventricular (LV) dysfunction. In a patient with known hypertension, a funduscopic examination should be performed to detect papilledema and/or retinal hemorrhages. These may be tell-tale signs of a transient hypertensive crisis causing syncope.[1]

Carotid Artery Exam

The patient should **be checked for** carotid bruit. Carotid sinus massage should be performed as an integral part of the examination in patients with a history suspicious of syncope related to maneuvers that exert spontaneous pressure on the carotid sinuses (e.g., tight collars, shaving).

JOB DESCRIPTION:

How to Perform Carotid Massage

The head of the patient is turned to the left, and the carotid artery is palpated at the angle of the right jaw. This is where the carotid sinus is located. Press this area with your index and middle fingers (some physicians prefer to use their thumb) and feel for carotid pulsation. An electrocardiogram records the rhythm strip. Press over the carotid sinus for 3 to 5 seconds, then let up for 5 to 10 seconds. Repeat this several times. Stop the pressure immediately if a response is obtained. Remember not to use prolonged carotid sinus stimulation because serious consequences can occur, such as prolonged cardiac asystole and even death. When carotid sinus pressure is not effective, it usually means that the exact spot of the carotid arterial pulsation at the angle of the jaw has not been located.[2]

A normal response to carotid sinus massage is a transient decrease in the sinus rate, a slowing of AV conduction, or both. Carotid sinus hypersensitivity is defined as a sinus pause longer than three seconds in duration and a fall in systolic blood pressure of 50 mm Hg or more. The response to carotid sinus massage can be classified as cardioinhibitory (asystole), vasodepressor (fall in systolic blood pressure), or mixed. Carotid sinus hypersensitivity is detected in approximately one-third of elderly patients who present with syncope or after falls. It is important to recognize, however, that carotid sinus hypersensitivity is also commonly observed in asymptomatic elderly patients.[1]

DATA COLLECTING TIPS (CLINICAL PEARLS)

Precautions When Doing Carotid Massage

Do not use carotid sinus pressure on a patient who has known cerebral vascular (or carotid) disease. Do not use simultaneous carotid sinus pressure over both right and left sides of the neck. Even though pressure over the eyeballs has been used and advocated as vagus nerve stimulation in the past, do not use it. Serious injury to the eye can and has ensued. Carotid sinus hypersensitivity has been noted in some patients with advanced aortic stenosis.[2]

DATA DECODING (PRELIMINARY DATA ANALYSIS)

Once the physician has obtained data about the patient through a comprehensive history and physical examination, a preliminary data analysis can be performed. The results culminate in a preliminary diagnosis and its causes.

History

History alone can positively identify characteristic "situational" syncope syndromes, such as deglutition syncope, emotional syncope, cough syncope, micturition syncope, trumpet player syncope, and carotid sinus syncope.[3]

Past History

While the patient's recall is invariably incomplete, preceding activities, sensations, and symptoms are of utmost importance. The relationship between prior events and syncope may be self-evident, but it is always possible that there is no relationship between the two.[1]

Orthostatic Hypotension

When orthostatic hypotension is abrupt and associated with reflex tachycardia, volume depletion should be suspected; when it is gradual and unaccompanied by increasing heart rate, autonomic dysfunction is most likely.

Skin Turgor and Complexion

Pallor can indicate anemia; when it is associated with decreased skin elasticity, it may indicate hypovolemia due to blood loss.

Position While Having Syncope

Syncope while sitting down suggests arrhythmias or seizure disorders. Syncope while standing for a long time suggests vasovagal syncope without underlying cardiac disease. If the episode occurred in a supine position, this would be unlikely to be related to, for example, orthostatic hypotension or neurocardiogenic syncope. Still, it could be neurally mediated or may be due to some other vagal reflex, such as coughing or vomiting. In addition, it could occur in a sitting position, such as during defecation or urination, and still be a neurally mediated type of syncope.[1]

Time and Duration of Syncope

Hypoglycemia is a rare cause of syncope occurring in the morning. Syncopal duration of less than one minute suggests vasovagal syncope, hyperventilation, or syncope related to another orthostatic mechanism. A longer duration of syncope suggests convulsive disorders, migraine, or arrhythmias.[4]

Arrhythmia

A patient with abrupt loss of consciousness (no prodrome), who recovers quickly ("classic" Stokes-Adams attack), may suffer from an arrhythmia. The classic form of Stokes-Adams attacks is due to transient asystole. Rapid ventricular tachyarrhythmias can also trigger abrupt loss of consciousness. In patients with syncope due to arrhythmias, the syncopal episode typically occurs with less than five seconds of warning and few if any prodromal or recovery symptoms (this is true if it is due to transient asystole; supraventricular tachyarrhythmias can cause syncope but usually have a longer prodrome). Demographic features suggesting that syncope results from an arrhythmia, such as ventricular tachycardia (VT) or AV block, include male gender, less than three prior episodes of syncope, and increased age.[1]

Neurocardiogenic Syncope

Features of the clinical history that indicate a diagnosis of neurally mediated syncope include palpitations, blurred vision, nausea, warmth, sweating, light-headedness, shivering, and the urge to defecate or urinate before syncope. Once they fall to the ground, patients tend to wake up and may be fatigued but fully alert. After syncope, patients can experience nausea, warmth, diaphoresis, or fatigue.[1]

Ischemia

Syncope provoked by exercise that is accompanied by chest pain or a history of unoperated or operated heart disease suggests a potential cardiac cause.

Seizure

Specific sensory and/or motor auras suggest a seizure. During a seizure, tongue biting, urinary incontinence, or fecal incontinence are common. After the episode, the patient does not regain complete consciousness immediately but may be confused. Features of the clinical history useful in distinguishing seizures from syncope include disorientation following an event, frothing at the mouth, aching muscles, feeling sleepy after the event, and unconsciousness lasting more than five minutes.[4]

Neurologic Disorders

A problem thought to be syncope may turn out to be epilepsy, hysteria, falls, coma, or stroke. If there are persistent neurologic deficits, this may indicate a transient ischemic event or a stroke. If loss of consciousness is prolonged, this may be due to drug or alcohol intoxication, head trauma, or an intracerebral bleed and not necessarily indicate syncope. It may instead be a coma or an altered state of consciousness.[3]

Frequent Falls in Elderly Patients

When viewed in their most broad definition of global hypoperfusion, symptoms related to syncope can manifest (especially in the elderly) with isolated transient loss of motor tone and hardly any impairment of consciousness. Therefore, a fall may be due to transient cerebral hypoperfusion. This can be difficult to discern, however, because patients often try to explain that they fell due to tripping or something similar rather than admitting to a transient change in level of consciousness. The elderly patient may fall or be found on the floor confused.[3]

DATA DECODING TIPS (CLINICAL PEARLS)

It is important to realize that information obtained from the history or physical examination may or may not be responsible for the cause for syncope. Drawing inferences as to the cause for syncope based on specific findings is also potentially fraught with error. For example, a systolic ejection murmur may indicate the presence of critical aortic stenosis, and while the mechanism of how aortic stenosis necessarily causes syncope is only partially understood (neurocardiogenic response with peripheral vasodilatation, decreased inotropic contraction, slowing of the heart rate, and decreased cerebral blood flow), the murmur may have nothing to do with syncope at all.[1]

DATA MINING (WORK-UP)

With the data gathered so far, the physician can formulate a main preliminary working diagnosis with a short list of differential diagnoses. Only the history can suggest the diagnosis for neurocardiogenic syncope (and the physical examination is negative). In other situations, even if the history and physical examination are suggestive of a particular diagnosis, there is a need to confirm the working diagnosis and rule out important or life-threatening conditions in the differential diagnoses (Table 13-3).

TABLE 13-3: Important Diagnoses to Be Ruled In and Differential Diagnoses to Be Ruled Out

Cardiac
Obstructive: hypertrophic cardiomyopathy, aortic stenosis, myxoma
Arrhythmic: complete AV block, sinus node disease, asystole, ventricular tachycardia, supraventricular tachycardia (SVT) (nonsustained and sustained)
Ischemic: transient hypotension and relative bradycardia
Noncardiac
Neurocardiogenic, orthostatic hypotension

Testing should be reserved for those individuals in whom there is concern for risk of sudden cardiac death (SCD) or total mortality, risk of recurrent syncope, and for those in whom the mechanism for syncope may have an impact on their overall clinical management.

Strategic Programming

All testing must be tailored to the patient based on the findings of the history and physical examinations and with knowledge of the sensitivity and specificity of each test. An abnormal test result does not necessarily indicate the cause for syncope and does not necessarily sanction a "wild goose chase." One goal in syncope evaluation is to convert a presumption into a definitive diagnosis. Some tests may provide clues to the diagnosis. These include carotid massage, electrocardiogram, tilt-table test, echocardiogram, EP test, treadmill test, and monitoring (i.e., Holter, transtelephonic, implantable loop recorder). A CT scan of the head, carotid Dopplers, an EEG, cardiac enzymes, and a neurology consult rarely play a role in the evaluation of true syncope.[1]

Unfortunately, most patients with syncope do not pass out in an environment at a time when physiological measurements can be made. The most accurate way to assess the cause for syncope, however, would be to monitor the patient with regard to pulse, electrocardiogram, electroencephalogram, blood pressure, and perhaps even cerebral blood flow measurements to determine the hemodynamics that may be responsible for syncope. Even in this case, the trigger for syncope can remain inscrutable. Therefore reliance on tests that attempt to reproduce the episodes of syncope is also fraught with error. For example, a tilt-table test can initiate an episode of syncope, but the predictive accuracy is a serious issue. Monitoring techniques may also be helpful, but they do not indicate the triggering mechanisms or the hemodynamics that may be responsible for and contribute to the episode.

For the evaluation of syncope, an attempt is made to evaluate (transient) orthostatic syncope or (functional) neurocardiogenic syncope and assess for structural heart disease. If the above evaluation is negative, then in the case of single episode of syncope, the evaluation is complete. In the case of recurrent problems, long-term follow-up for bradycardias and tachycardias is necessary. A diagnostic algorithm is suggested in Figure 13-1.

Observational Studies

Electrocardiogram

Every patient with syncope should receive an electrocardiogram (ECG). Although this may reveal diagnostic abnormalities in only 5 to 10% of patients (such as complete heart block), and abnormalities may be

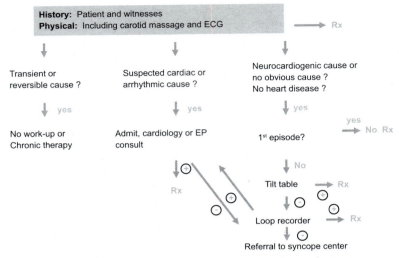

Figure 13-1 Evaluation and management strategies for patients with syncope. (Adapted from Olshansky B. Syncope: Mechanisms and Management. 2nd edition, Blackwell, 2005.)

nonspecific, it can provide helpful clues in another 20 to 30% of cases, such as old Q waves, various degrees and combinations of AV block and bundle branch block (BBB), preexcitation syndrome, LV hypertrophy, nonsustained ventricular tachycardia, long QT interval, evidence for Brugada syndrome, and evidence for arrhythmogenic right ventricular cardiomyopathy.

Echocardiogram

An echocardiogram alone is almost never diagnostic of the cause for syncope. It is of little help when there is no cardiac history and the physical examination and electrocardiogram are normal. Its chief usefulness is in providing an evaluation of ventricular function in patients with suspected heart disease and assessing obstructive valvular disease. It may pick up right ventricular dysfunction and atrial myxoma, but its main job is to determine if "structural heart disease." is present[1]

Holter Monitoring

This is rarely diagnostic and therefore minimally helpful, as the incidence of recurrent syncope while being monitored is rare (1–5%). Further, many asymptomatic and nonspecific abnormalities (such as PVCs, nonsustained ventricular tachycardia, sinus bradycardia, and sleep-related heart block and/or sinus pauses) may confuse the issue and lead to further unnecessary testing and therapy.[1]

Transtelephonic Monitoring

Transtelephonic monitoring enables the recording of an episode when the patient passes out. The patient must wear the monitor continuously (one such device is the size of a beeper). If the patient passes out, a button is pushed on his or her awakening. The device will store information from two to three minutes before the event.[1]

Implantable Loop Recorder

An implantable monitor is inserted surgically into a subcutaneous prepectoral pocket. It is capable of recording the heart rhythm for more than one year in patients with intermittent or rare episodes. The device is potentially highly cost-effective. It can eliminate the need for frequent and potentially unnecessary hospitalizations. The main shortcomings of this device are obviously the relative invasiveness of its implantation and its up-front cost. A more indirect pitfall is that monitor-obtained bradycardic manifestations of vasovagal syncope cannot be analyzed in the context of antecedent BP changes and may therefore lead to unnecessary pacemaker implants.[1]

 DATA MINING TIPS (CLINICAL PEARLS)
What Type of Monitor to Order

In general, if the symptom happens once a day, then the 24–48 hour Holter monitor is best. If the problem happens once a month, then the event monitor used as an endless loop recorder would be helpful. If the symptoms are rare and erratic but recurrent and otherwise unexplained, then an implantable loop monitor would help to reveal the problem.[1]

Signal-Averaged ECG

The signal-averaged electrocardiogram (SAECG) is only useful in the following situation—in a patient with syncope, known coronary artery disease (CAD), and normal (or only mildly abnormal) LV function. An abnormal SAECG would mandate electrophysiologic testing to assess the induction of VT in this small subgroup.[5] SAECG is generally not helpful to make a diagnosis and is not recommended. Similarly, T-wave alternans is rarely useful in making a diagnosis about the cause of syncope.

Provocative Testing

Exercise Stress Test

If the syncopal episode happens during or after exercise, then a stress test should be done to rule out ischemia as a cause of arrhythmia, angina, or exercise-induced syncope. Exercise stress testing is also useful for screening of rare cases of catecholaminergic polymorphic ventricular tachycardia.

Tilt-Table Testing

Head up tilt-table (HUTT) testing can be highly effective in uncovering and/or confirming neurocardiogenic syncope. Day-to-day variability in response and induction of neurocardiogenic syncope are common, unavoidable, and simply reflect the expected variability of the autonomic nervous system physiology. The sensitivity of the HUTT is always in question, but it can be increased with isoproterenol or nitroglycerin (possibly by different mechanisms).[6] These interventions, however, will decrease the specificity, which is a common problem with the tilt-table test.

The tilt-table test can cause various types of responses that may be responsible for syncope. The classic neurocardiogenic response is relative bradycardia and hypotension associated with syncope that resolves in the supine position. For some individuals, a more gradual hypotension without change in heart rate may indicate an autonomic syndrome. For other individuals there is an increase in heart rate associated with hypotension that might be an indication for postural orthostatic tachycardia syndrome ("POTS"), which tends to cause symptoms similar to those of syncope but does not cause true syncope in most cases.[1]

Tilt-table testing is useful when neurocardiogenic syncope is suspected but the diagnosis is uncertain. It should be one of the first tests considered when there is undiagnosed syncope and no structural heart disease present.[1] There is no reason to do a tilt-table test when the etiology is clear from the history.

DATA MINING TIPS (CLINICAL PEARLS)
When To Do a Tilt-Table Test

When episodes suggest but do not indicate neurocardiogenic cause
If there is recurrent syncope with no apparent cause at any age
When other evaluation is unrevealing
When therapies directed at other potential causes are ineffective
When the patient has a job that depends on the potential cause for syncope
If the family or the patient is very concerned about what the etiology might be, even if neurocardiogenic syncope is the most likely cause

Electrophysiology Testing

The main use for EP testing in syncope patients is to evaluate the inducibility and hemodynamic effects of monomorphic VT. It can be of some help to diagnose AV block and sinus node abnormalities, but the sensitivity and specificity are low. If the ejection fraction is < 0.40, VT can be induced in about 35% of patients, whereas for those with an ejection fraction >0.40, only 3% will have ventricular tachycardia induced, even if structural heart disease is present.[7] Patients with cardiomyopathy but no CAD are less likely to have VT induced (even if it is present clinically). The EP test is of no use for patients with long QT interval syndrome or hypertrophic cardiomyopathy.

Appropriateness of EP Studies

In the case of patients with CAD, syncope, and mild-to-moderate LV dysfunction (a LV ejection fraction > 35%), the yield to induce VT by EP testing is low. However, EP testing may still be appropriate in select patients with relatively preserved ventricular function but who have structural heart disease. If there is VT induced, then an ICD is needed.[8] In the case of patients with CAD, syncope, and low LV ejection fraction, in the interest of finding a diagnosis, an EP test may be helpful but it is probably not necessary. Even in the absence of syncope, patients with CAD and a LV ejection fraction <35% have a substantial survival benefit when treated with an ICD. The rationale for the implantation of an ICD is from the Multicenter Automatic Defibrillator Implantation Trial II (MADIT II), Sudden Cardiac Death in Heart Failure Trial (SCD-HeFT), and Defibrillators in Nonischemic Cardiomyopathy Evaluation (DEFINITE) trials.[9-11]

EP testing is most useful in patients with CAD (and no acute ischemia); patients with a LV ejection fraction less than 0.40; patients with left BBB; patients with an abnormal signal averaged ECG; and patients with ventricular ectopy of right ventricular outflow tract origin (LBBB morphology with inferior axis).

Induction of a previously undiagnosed syncopal SVT is relatively rare (about 10% of cases), but if induced, it can be treated by radiofrequency ablation during the same session. The induction of poorly tolerated atrial flutter of fibrillation is a much more difficult finding to interpret.

EP testing is fair, at best, in evaluating bradycardias.[12] Although an abnormal sinus node recovery time can indicate sinus node disease, its presence does not necessarily mean that the syncope is caused by sinus pauses. Furthermore, sinus node recovery time is an insensitive measure of sinus node dysfunction. No test provides a direct causal link to the clinical syncopal event—the link is only a putative one. Intra- or infra-Hisian block indicates a more likely causal link to syncope. Unfortunately, the sensitivity of EP testing to diagnose serious infranodal disease is only fair. Finally, EP testing is also not very well suited to evaluate abnormalities in AV nodal conduction.

A negative EP test does not rule out ventricular tachycardias as a cause of syncope, especially in patients with idiopathic dilated or nonischemic cardiomyopathies.[13] Further, EP testing is not well suited for the evaluation of polymorphic ventricular tachycardia.

A thorough but negative EP test, although not diagnostic, does indicate a generally good prognosis for predicting a relatively low two-year incidence of sudden cardiac death.

DATA CONVERTING (FORMULATING THE DIAGNOSIS OF SYNCOPE)

At this stage, the task of the physician is to convert useful information into active knowledge. The clinical process includes (A) confirming the diagnosis of syncope if it exists or denying it, and (B) assigning a cause to the syncopal episode.

The causes of syncope due to hypotension and resulting in cerebral hypoperfusion are clustered into four groups: (1) obstructive valvular disease (e.g., aortic stenosis), (2) contracted intravascular volume (e.g., prolonged diarrhea, excessive diuretics, bleeding), (3) excessive vasodilation (e.g., antihypertensive drugs, neurocardiogenic syncope), and (4) uncontrolled arrhythmia (e.g., atrial fibrillation [AF], SVT, nonsustained VT , VT, and ventricular fibrillation [VF]). Without any cardiovascular evidence of hypotension, other causes of syncope (such as neurological or psychological) are suggested. Common causes of syncope are listed in Tables 13-4 and 13-5.[1]

TABLE 13-4: Common Causes of Syncope

Noncardiovascular Disease
Reflex mechanisms
Neurocardiogenic
Micturition
Deglutition
Post-tussive
Defecation
Glossopharyngeal
Postprandial
Carotid sinus hypersensitivity
Hyperventilation
Dysautonomic storms (ganglionitis)
Valsalva maneuver
Orthostatic Hypotension
Dysautonomia
Fluid depletion
Illness, bed rest
Drugs
Psychogenic
Hysterical behavior
Panic disorder
Anxiety disorder

(continued)

TABLE 13-4: Common Causes of Syncope *(continued)*

Metabolic

Hypoglycemia
Hypoxia
Dehydration (intentional?)
Hyperventilation

Neurologic

Undiagnosed seizures
Improperly diagnosed confusional states, hypoglycemia, stroke, etc.
Drug-induced loss of consciousness (consider alcohol)

Cardiovascular Disease

Arrhythmic Etiology

AV block with bradycardia (due to structural changes or drugs)
Sinus pauses, bradycardia (vagal, sick sinus syndrome, drugs)
VT due to structural heart disease

Nonarrhythmic Etiology/Obstructive/Reflex Etiologies

Hypertrophic cardiomyopathy
Aortic stenosis

Syncope of Unknown Origin—About 50% of Patients

TABLE 13-5: Uncommon Causes of Syncope

Cardiovascular Disease

Arrhythmic Etiology

Supraventricular tachycardia (AVNRT, accessory pathway [WPW])
Long QT interval syndrome(s)
Idiopathic VT (Bellhassen, RVOT tachycardia)
Myocardial infarction causing bradycardias and tachycardias
Right ventricular dysplasia
Brugada syndrome
Hypertrophic cardiomyopathy

Nonarrhythmic Etiology

Pulmonary embolus
Pulmonary hypertension
Dissecting aortic aneurysm (Marfan syndrome)
Subclavian steal
Cardiac tumors—atrial myxoma
Cardiac tamponade

(continued)

TABLE 13-5: Uncommon Causes of Syncope *(continued)*

Cardiomyopathies (idiopathic, sarcoidosis, amyloidosis)
Myocarditis
Coronary anomalies: hypoplasia, spasm, bridging, aberrant ostia,
   anomalous origin
Congenital heart diseases

Noncardiovascular Disease

Circulating Mediators

Carcinoid syndrome
Systemic mastocytosis
Drugs/supplements—hormones (steroid), drugs (cocaine), ma huang,
   diuretics

Environmental—Heat Stroke, Cold Exposure

Blunt trauma—contusion and coronary thrombosis

AVNRT: atrioventricular nodal re-entry tachycardia, RVOT: right ventricular
   outflow tract, WPW: Wolff-Parkinson-White syndrome

Formulating the Diagnosis of Neurocardiogenic Syncope

Neurocardiogenic syncope is used to describe the autonomic responses that may ultimately lead to inappropriate vasodilatation, relative bradycardia, hypotension, and collapse. This reflex is a final common pathway of many potential autonomic inputs.[14] It may present as bradycardia and hypotension (classic vasovagal), hypotension alone, postural orthostatic tachycardia syndrome (POTS),[15] or a psychogenic or a "central" response (cerebral vasoconstriction).[16] It may be an isolated explainable event, a recurrent poorly understood reflex ("malignant neurocardiogenic syndrome"), or it may present in storms that ultimately abate. The neurocardiogenic reflex can be triggered by a severe viral syndrome or it may be caused by an inherited "dysautonomic" problem. There can be a genetic predisposition, and some patients are subject to multiple triggers.

DATA CONVERTING TIPS (CLINICAL PEARLS)

Need for Triggers on Susceptible Terrain to Ignite a Neurocardiogenic Syncopal Event

In real-world practice, the neurocardiogenic mechanism, generally benign, is the most common cause for syncope. Neurocardiogenic etiologies probably explain the majority of syncopal episodes, but many neurocardiogenic mechanisms for syncope exist.[17] The neurocardiogenic reflex may be transient, self-limited, persistent, or recurrent. It is there, hidden and ready to be used if there is a chance. The susceptible terrain can be related to a chronic condition (e.g., aortic stenosis) or a new acute illness or condition that makes the patient vulnerable or compromised (e.g., gastrointestinal bleed, dehydration from diarrhea, vasodilatation from alcohol intake). Then a trigger may arrive by chance, causing acute change in the vascular volume due to loss of vascular volume or inappropriate vasodilatation, such as new gastrointestinal bleeding, intense emotional stimuli,[18] intense physical activity, pain, the effects of alcohol or an inotropic stimulant, or an abrupt change of position from a lying or sitting position to a standing position. A sudden trigger ignites the inappropriate bradycardia and vasodilatation cascade, culminating in sudden loss of BP and presented as a syncopal episode. The reflex is there from birth. The susceptible terrain comes and goes. Without the susceptible terrain, even with the arrival of a trigger, there is no syncope. The unfortunate trigger needs to happen at the right time and in the right susceptible terrain in order to induce neurocardiogenic syncope (Table 13-6).

In a patient with neurocardiogenic syncope, there is a need to identify the chronic vulnerable terrain, a new compromising situation, and a triggering factor. Then the physician needs to add these three factors; if the result does not add up to three, there is no neurocardiogenic syncope.

FORMULA for the Diagnosis of Syncope (need three +)
Positive Vulnerable terrain (a)   (+)
Positive Compromising situation (b)   (+)
Positive Triggering factor (c)   (+)
Neurocardiogenic syncope happens if the total = 3   (+)

DATA FILTERING (DIFFERENTIAL DIAGNOSES)
Autonomic Failure

Pure autonomic failure (Bradbury-Eggleston syndrome) is an idiopathic, sporadic disorder characterized by orthostatic hypotension, usually in conjunction with evidence of more widespread autonomic failure, such as disturbances in bowel, bladder, thermoregulatory, and sexual function. Patients with pure autonomic failure have reduced supine plasma or epinephrine levels.[4]

Multiple system atrophy (Shy-Drager syndrome) is a sporadic, progressive adult-onset disorder characterized by autonomic dysfunction, parkinsonism, and ataxia in any combination.[4]

The third type of primary autonomic failure is Parkinson disease with autonomic failure. A small subset of patients with Parkinson disease may also experience autonomic failure, including orthostatic hypotension. In addition to these forms of chronic autonomic failure is a rare

TABLE 13-6: Identification of a Chronic Vulnerable Terrain, a New Compromising Situation, and a Triggering Factor

Event	Vulnerable Terrain Situation	New Compromising Triggering Factor (highlighted)
Urination Syncope		
Old age (+)	No long standing (−)	No straining (−) = no syncope
Old age (+)	Prolonged standing (+)	No straining (−) = no syncope
Old age (+)	Prolonged standing (+)	Straining (+) = syncope
Young age (−)	Prolonged stanging (+)	Straining (−) = no syncope
Defecation Syncope		
Old age (+)	Prolonged sitting (+)	No straining (−) = no syncope
Old age (+)	Prolonged sitting (+)	Straining (+) = syncope
Young age (−)	Prolonged sitting (+)	No straining (−) = no syncope
Old age (+)	No prolonged sitting (−)	Straining (+) = no syncope
Aortic Stenosis (AS)		
Mild AS (+)	Diarrhea (+)	No quick standing (−) = no syncope
Mild AS (+)	Diarrhea(+)	Quick standing (+) = syncope
Severe AS	No diarrhea	Syncope (due to severe AS)
Severe AS	No diarrhea	No quick standing (−) = no syncope
Syncope When Seeing Blood		
Psychiatric debility(+)	Chronic illness (+)	Seeing blood (+) = syncope
Psychiatric debility (−)	Chronic illness (+)	Not seeing blood = no syncope

acute panautonomic neuropathy. This neuropathy generally occurs in young people and results in widespread, severe sympathetic and parasympathetic failure with orthostatic hypotension, loss of sweating, disruption of bladder and bowel functions, fixed heart rate, and fixed dilated pupils.[4]

Postural Orthostatic Tachycardia Syndrome

This a milder form of chronic autonomic failure and orthostatic intolerance characterized by an increase of 30 beats/min or more in heart rate on standing for 10 minutes and the absence of a significant change in blood pressure.

Seizure

Tongue biting strongly indicates a seizure rather than syncope as the cause of loss of consciousness. Other findings suggestive of a seizure as the cause of the syncopal episode include (1) an aura before the episode, (2) horizontal eye deviation during the episode, (3) an elevated blood pressure and pulse during the episode, and (4) a headache following the event. Urinary or fecal incontinence can be observed in association with seizure or a syncopal episode but occurs more commonly in association with a seizure. Grand mal seizures are usually associated with tonic-clonic movements. It is important to note that syncope caused by cerebral ischemia results in decorticate rigidity, with clonic movements of the arms.[4]

Akinetic or petit mal seizures can be recognized by the patient's lack of responsiveness in the absence of a loss of postural tone. Temporal lobe seizures can also be confused with syncope. These seizures last several minutes and are characterized by confusion, changes in the level of consciousness, and autonomic signs such as flushing.[4]

Vertebral basilar insufficiency should be considered as the cause of syncope if it occurs in association with other symptoms of brainstem ischemia (diplopia, tinnitus, weakness or sensory loss, vertigo, and dysarthria). Migraine-mediated syncope is often associated with a throbbing, unilateral headache, scintillating scotomata, and nausea. Patients with seizures are more likely to have had a cut tongue, bed-wetting, prodromal déjà vu, mood changes, and hallucinations or trembling before loss of consciousness as well as postical confusion, muscle pain, headaches, observed convulsive movements, head turning, unresponsiveness during loss of consciousness, and turning blue as observed by a bystander.[4]

PROGRAMMED MANAGEMENT

Programmed management is the standard treatment according to the guidelines. If there is a reason not to follow the guidelines, then the

TABLE 13-7: Management Master Plan

Data Management	Keep BP in the high-normal range 140/90 mm Hg
	High–sodium diet (if having orthostatic hypotension)
	Preventive measures
	Pharmacologic therapy: distal vasoconstriction (midodrine)
System Configuration Correction	Aortic valve replacement in AS
	Pacing, if advanced AV block
Work-Around Management	Not applicable
System Recovery	Implanted cardiac defibrillator in sustained VT

physician needs to clarify why they being are not being followed. This strategy allows the greatest number of patients to receive comprehensive evidence-based management while also providing the physician with the freedom to have a tailored, personalized treatment plan for the patients who request it (Table 13-7).

Risk Stratification

Once the diagnosis of syncope is comfirmed, the patient is evaluated to determine whether there is increased risk of death. Patients with syncope of cardiovascular origin have a high mortality rate of 30% at two years and more than 80% at five years. The mortality is low (1-6% at two years) if the syncope is of noncardiovascular cause[1] (Table 13-8).

Management

In general, treatment depends on the causes of the syncope, as revealed by the evaluation process.

TABLE 13-8: Signs of High-Risk of Death Due to Syncope

Structural heart disease—prior myocardial infarction, LV dysfunction, right ventricular dysfunction, valvular heart disease, and BBB
Myocardial ischemia
Genetic heart disease (Wolff-Parkinson-White syndrome, long QT interval syndrome, Brugada syndrome, catecholaminergic polymorphic ventricular tachycardia, hypertrophic cardiomyopathy)

Structural Heart Disease

If there is structural heart disease, such as aortic stenosis or hypertrophic cardiomyopathy, then the treatment is to address these obstructive lesions and assess the long-term risk for arrhythmic death. If there is a transient destabilizing factor (e.g., dehydration due to heat, excessive diuretic use, or diarrhea), the patient is more susceptible to hypotension and syncope; however, once the transient cause is corrected, the long-term prognosis depends on the underlying disease regardless of the syncopal episode.

Ischemia

If the syncope is due to ischemia (a highly uncommon cause), then coronary revascularization is indicated. Even then, however, long-term risk assessment for SCD needs to be considered.

Transient Hypotensive Factors

If the syncope is a result of transient hypotension–caused dehydration, bleeding, diarrhea, or excessive sweating in a patient with or without heart disease, then the management is to treat the underlying reason for the episode.

ADVANCED MANAGEMENT

Significant Bradycardia and AV Block

If the patient has syncope due to significant bradycardia and AV block, then he or she needs a pacemaker. The indications for pacing related to syncope are listed in Table 13-9.[19]

DATA MANAGEMENT TIPS (CLINICAL PEARLS)

Limitation of Pacing

Even if the mechanism and the diagnosis are clear, the therapy administered may be ineffective. A pacemaker, for example, will prevent syncope recurrence in a patient with acquired, complete heart block but it may not be effective in a patient with bradycardia due to neurocardiogenic syncope. Even if a therapy is effective to prevent syncope, it may not prevent death. Beta blockers may prevent recurrent syncope in patients with long QT interval syndrome, but a beta blocker may not prevent death. Alternatively, a patient with syncope due to ventricular tachycardia could benefit from an ICD; it may prevent death, but it likely will not prevent recurrent syncope. A patient could collapse from ventricular tachycardia before an administered shock; some patients may require combination therapy, including ICD with drug therapy to decrease the incidence and the length of these episodes of VT.[19]

TABLE 13-9: ACC/AHA/HRS Guidelines Related to Syncope: PACEMAKER INDICATIONS

Sinus Node Dysfunction

CLASS I: Symptomatic bradycardia. (Level of Evidence: C)
CLASS IIa: Syncope of unexplained origin when clinically significant abnormalities of sinus node function are discovered or provoked in EP studies. (Level of Evidence: C)

Acquired Atrioventricular Block in Adults

CLASS I: Third-degree and advanced second-degree AV block, bradycardia with symptoms presumed to be due to AV block. (Level of Evidence: C)
Third-degree and advanced second-degree AV block at any anatomic level associated with arrhythmias and other medical conditions that require drug therapy that results in symptomatic bradycardia. (Level of Evidence: C)

Permanent Pacing in Chronic Bifascicular Block

CLASS IIa: Syncope not demonstrated to be due to AV block when other likely causes have been excluded, specifically ventricular tachycardia. (Level of Evidence: B)

Permanent Pacing Hypersensitive Carotid Sinus and Neurocardiogenic Syncope

CLASS I: Recurrent syncope caused by spontaneously occurring carotid sinus stimulation and carotid sinus pressure (induces asystole >3 seconds). (Level of Evidence: C)
CLASS IIa: Syncope without clear, provocative events and with a hypersensitive cardioinhibitory response of 3 seconds or longer. (Level of Evidence: C)
CLASS IIb: Significantly symptomatic neurocardiogenic syncope with bradycardia documented spontaneously or at the time of tilt-table testing. (Level of Evidence: B)
CLASS III: Not indicated for situational vasovagal syncope in which avoidance behavior is effective and preferred. (Level of Evidence: C)

Symptomatic Ventricular Tachycardia

If there is inducible monomorphic VT in a patient with structural heart disease (NOT in a patient with idiopathic VT and normal ventricular function), an ICD should be implanted. ICD therapy may need to be considered in patients at high risk for SCD and total mortality if there is HF present or impaired ventricular function regardless of the EP testing results (Table 13-10).

TABLE 13-10: Indications for Implantable Cardioverter Defibrillator

CLASS I: Syncope of undetermined origin with clinically relevant, hemodynamically significant sustained VT or VF induced at electrophysiologic study. (Level of Evidence: B)

Patients with LV ejection fraction < 35% due to prior MI who are at least 40 days post-MI and are in NYHA Functional Class II or III. (Level of Evidence: A) (WITH/WITHOUT SYNCOPE)

Patients with nonischemic dilated cardiomyopathy who have an LV ejection fraction ≤ 35% and who are in NYHA functional Class II or III. (Level of Evidence: B) (WITH/WITHOUT SYNCOPE)

Patients with LV dysfunction due to prior MI who are at least 40 days post-MI, have an LV ejection fraction < 30%, and are NYHA Functional Class I. (Level of Evidence: A) (WITH OR WITHOUT SYNCOPE)

Patients with nonsustained VT, MI, LV ejection fraction < 40%, and inducible VF or sustained VT at electrophysiologic study. (Level of Evidence: B) (WITH/WITHOUT SYNCOPE)

CLASS IIa: Unexplained syncope, significant LV dysfunction, and nonischemic DCM. (Level of Evidence: C)

To reduce SCD in patients with long QT syndrome who are experiencing syncope and/or VT while receiving beta blockers. (Level of Evidence: B)

Patients with Brugada syndrome who have had syncope. (Level of Evidence: C)

Patients with catecholaminergic polymorphic VT who have syncope and/or documented sustained VT while receiving beta blockers. (Level of Evidence: C)

CLASS IIb: Patients with syncope and advanced structural heart disease in whom thorough invasive and noninvasive investigations fail to define a cause. (Level of Evidence: C)

Neurocardiogenic Syncope

Treatments include lifestyle changes; avoiding things that cause syncope; and maintaining adequate hydration, salt load, and wearing support hose. There can be a lack of response to hydration and salt loading, however, but prior to an event that may cause neurocardiogenic syncope, hydration, especially with ice-cold water and salt loading, may be helpful. Tilt training may be effective. Dual chamber (DDDR-rate drop response) pacing has an insignificant role in the average patient with neurocardiogenic syncope.

The assessment of any medical therapy for neurocardiogenic syncope has been performed in relatively select populations. The POST trial, for example, was a group of patients that had very frequent recurrent episodes of neurocardiogenic syncope.[20] This study does not demonstrate a substantial benefit of beta blocker therapy for patients with neurocardiogenic syncope, and yet some patients seem to have responded. In patients with frequent, recurrent neurocardiogenic syncope who do not respond to other therapies, a beta blocker may be considered as an option but possibly may make the problem worse.

A first-line therapy for neurocardiogenic syncope after adequate hydration and avoidance approaches is fludrocortisone. Midodrine is an option, but it is a complex medication to take and does not necessarily benefit all patients. Although a selective serotonin reuptake inhibitors (SSRIs) may be beneficial, they do not universally work and have many adverse effects. There are some recent data on the use of pyridostigmine for neurocardiogenic syncope and orthostatic hypotension. Midodrine and and fludrocortisone may be very useful for patients with POTS.

 SMART THINKING:

Efficacy of Midodrine

Methodology: This is a double-blind, randomized, crossover trial. Twelve patients with a history of recurrent neurally mediated syncope, which was reproduced during head-up tilt, were randomized to receive a nonpressor dose of midodrine (5 mg) or placebo on day 1 and the opposite on day 3. One hour after drug or placebo administration, patients underwent 60-degree HUTT lasting 40 minutes (or until hypotension or bradycardia developed). *Results:* In patients in the supine position, midodrine produced no significant change in BP or heart rate. The responses to head-up tilt were significantly different on the midodrine and the placebo day: on the placebo day, 67% (8/12) of the subjects suffered neurally mediated syncope, whereas only 17% (2/12) of the subjects developed neurally mediated syncope on the midodrine day ($P < 0.02$). *Practical Applications:* These results indicate that midodrine significantly improves orthostatic tolerance during HUTT in patients with recurrent neurally mediated syncope.[21]

Training Exercises

These exercises are actually "mini-tilt table tests" that encourage the reflex and perhaps, in so doing, strengthen the individual's tolerance of it.[22] The use of tilt training is more than 90% effective and while much of this response may be placebo, the safety of this approach is such that it really does not matter what the beneficial mechanism might be. Patients are instructed to tilt against a wall for 15-30 minutes a day, as tolerated. This exercise may be primary therapy for some forms of neurocardiogenic syncope, and it appears highly effective in patients having vasovagal syncope with prodromal symptoms.[23]

Pacing

Recently, some studies revealed the efficacy of pacemaker implantation in decreasing recurrences in patients with vasovagal syncope. Because these studies were not blinded or placebo-controlled, the benefits observed might have been due to a bias in the assessment of outcomes or to a placebo effect of the pacemaker.

 SMART THINKING:

Does Pacing Therapy Reduce the Risk of Syncope Relapse?

Methodology: This is a randomized, double-blind, placebo-controlled study in which 29 patients (53 +/- 16 years; 19 women) with severe recurrent tilt-induced vasovagal syncope (median 12 syncopes in the lifetime) and one syncopal relapse after head-up tilt testing underwent implantation of a pacemaker and were randomized to pacemaker ON or to pacemaker OFF. *Results:* During a median of 715 days of follow-up, 8 (50%) patients randomized to pacemaker ON had a recurrence of syncope compared with 5 (38%) patients randomized to pacemaker OFF (P = NS); the median time to first syncope was longer in the pacemaker ON than in the pacemaker OFF group, although not significantly (97 [38-144] vs. 20 [4-302] days; P = 0.38). There was also no significant difference in the subgroups of patients who had a mixed response and in those who had an asystolic response during head-up tilt testing. *Practical Applications:* Active pacing does not prevent syncopal recurrence in patients with severe recurrent tilt-induced vasovagal syncope.[24]

TROUBLE-SHOOTING AND DEBUGGING

What Is the Most Effective Work-up Program for Syncope of Unknown Origin?

Establishing a diagnosis in patients with unexplained syncope is complicated by infrequent and unpredictable events. The cost-effectiveness of immediate, prolonged monitoring as an alternative to conventional diagnostic strategies has not been studied. *Methodology:* Prolonged monitoring with an implantable loop recorder with one-year monitoring. If patients remained undiagnosed after their assigned strategy, they were offered a crossover to the alternate strategy. Cost analysis of the two testing strategies was performed.

Results: 20 versus 47%, P = 0.029, at a cost of 1683 Canadian dollars per patient (P < 0.0001) and 8414 Canadian dollars per diagnosis (P < 0.0001). After crossover, a diagnosis was obtained in 1 of 5 patients undergoing conventional testing compared with 8 of 21 patients who completed monitoring (20 vs. 38%, P = 0.44). Overall, a strategy of monitoring followed by tilt and EP testing was associated with a diagnostic yield of 50% at a cost of 2937 Canadian dollars per patient and 5875 Canadian dollars per diagnosis. Conventional testing followed by monitoring was associated with a diagnostic yield of 47%, at a greater cost of 3683 Canadian dollars per patient (P = 0.013) and a greater cost per diagnosis (7891 Canadian dollars, P = 0.002). *Practical Applications:* A strategy of primary monitoring with implanted loop recorder monitoring is more cost-effective than conventional testing in establishing a diagnosis in recurrent unexplained syncope.[25]

What Is the Prognosis of Syncope after ICD in Patients with Severe HF?

Data from patients enrolled in the Sudden Cardiac Death and Heart Failure Trial (SCD-HeFT) were analyzed to determine whether syncope predicted outcomes in patients with CHF. *Methodology:* The outcomes (and associated clinical characteristics) in patients with and without syncope enrolled in SCD-HeFT were compared. *Results:* In the SCD-HeFT, 162 (6%) of patients had syncope before randomization, 356 (14%) had syncope after randomization (similar incidence in each randomized arm), and 46 (2%) had syncope before and after randomization. A QRS duration of 120 ms and the absence of beta blocker use predicted syncope during follow-up (hazard ratio [HR] 1.30 and 95% confidence interval [CI] 1.06 to 1.61, P = 0.014 and HR 1.25, 95% CI 1.01 to 1.56, P = 0.048, respectively). Syncope recurrence did not differ by randomization arm. However, in the ICD arm, syncope before and after randomization was associated with appropriate ICD discharges (HR 1.75, 95% CI 1.10 to 2.80, P = 0.019 and HR 2.91, 95% CI 1.89 to 4.47, P = 0.001, respectively). Post-randomization syncope predicted total and cardiovascular death (HR 1.41, 95% CI 1.13 to 1.76, P = 0.002 and HR 1.55, 95% CI 1.19 to 2.02, P = 0.001, respectively). The elevated relative risk of mortality for syncope versus nonsyncope patients did not vary significantly across treatment arms (ICD, HR 1.54, 95% CI 1.04 to 2.27; amiodarone, HR 1.33, 95% CI 0.91 to 1.93; and placebo, HR 1.39, 95% CI 0.96 to 2.02, test for difference P = 0.86). *Practical Applications:* For HF patients with ICDs, syncope was associated with appropriate ICD activations. ICD did not protect patients with HF having syncope.[26]

What Are the Causes for Athletes of Exercise-Induced Syncope? What Is the Management?

Syncope, dizziness, collapse, and loss of consciousness are among the most worrisome symptoms that occur in relation to exercise-induced syncope.[27-28] These dramatic symptoms can portend sudden and "unexpected" death. The cause is often uncertain and difficult to diagnose but is often related to an arrhythmia.

The trained athlete is unique. Exercise training increases vagal tone chronically but baroreceptor adjustments reduce the possibility of a neurocardiogenic reflex. Exercise-induced enhancement of sympathetic activity is blunted. Bikers or runners (dynamic activity) rarely pass out due to hemodynamic or autonomic effects. The muscle pump increases venous return and prevents this. Marathon runners can collapse from dehydration or hypotension during prolonged exertion or at the end of exercise. Such an event is not unusual or necessarily worrisome and may not require further evaluation. When an athlete stops exercising and there is maximal peripheral vasodilatation, the muscle pump may fail and the BP may drop to the point of causing syncope.[1]

It is highly unusual for an athlete to collapse from a benign cause at the onset of intense physical stress or even with prolonged, continued activity. Syncope during exercise tends to be worrisome and possibly related due to a malignant, arrhythmic, cause.[1]

Noncardiac causes for syncope include neurocardiogenic responses to exercise, dehydration (sometimes intentional, e.g., wrestlers), hyperventilation, Valsalva maneuver (e.g. weight lifters), and circulating mediators (e.g., histamine, serotonin). A variant of neurocardiogenic syncope is exercise-induced neurally mediated hypotension and bradycardia. Autonomic failure and loss of peripheral muscle pump function may participate in abrupt cardiovascular collapse with syncope.[1]

Supplements and drugs athletes take may cause tachy- and/or brady-arrhythmias or hemodynamic collapse. Ma huang (from the Chinese ephedra plant), androgens and creatine, easy to obtain over the counter, are potentially dangerous. Illicit drugs, such as cocaine taken to enhance performance, can have serious consequences causing syncope. It is important to rule out a possibility of seizure disorder.[1]

The cardiac causes for syncope are listed in Table 13-3. A young athlete with syncope who has significant coronary artery abnormalities will likely have other concomitant symptoms, including chest discomfort, and he or she often has ECG myocardial abnormalities present. Ischemia should always be considered a likely trigger in those older than 35. Polymorphic and monomorphic VT associated with structural heart disease can cause syncope and carry a poor prognosis in athletes. Exercise-induced "idiopathic" (no known structural heart disease) right and left VT can cause syncope and can be ablated with good long-term results and a good prognosis. High-grade or complete AV block or chronotropic incompetence causing syncope during exercise is rare in young athletes but may occur in elderly patients treated for heart disease.[29]

DATA COLLECTING

Evaluation of Syncope in the Athlete

The evaluation of syncope in an athlete is more complicated than for the nonathlete. Before allowing the patients return to exercise, the cause of syncope should be determined and treated properly. Any syncopal episode should be considered seriously and should be carefully evaluated, ruling out as needed hypertrophic cardiomyopathy, arrhythmogenic right ventricular dysplasia, coronary anomalies, and congenital long QT interval syndrome. Specific historical features to be collected are included in Table 13-11.[1]

🔴 DATA DECODING TIPS (CLINICAL PEARLS)
Important Questions from the History

An adequate history can require information available from team members, the family, friends, and witnesses. Symptoms must be scrutinized: Is syncope a single or a recurrent episode? Did exercise initiate the episode? Was exercise isometric (static) or isotonic (dynamic)? In what position did syncope occur? Did syncope occur with the start of exercise, with prolonged exercise, or at the end of exercise? Were there premonitory symptoms (e.g., palpitations, feelings of impending doom, diaphoresis, or chest pain), concomitant acute illnesses, "triggers," changes in dietary habits and/or medications, or the presence of emotional stress? Was there pallor, absence of a pulse, or concomitant acute illness? Was recovery immediate or prolonged? If syncope is prolonged, consider a hemodynamic-obstructive cause, such as aortic stenosis or hypertrophic cardiomyopathy. Syncope can be mimicked by seizures and hypoglycemia. To distinguish and exclude these potential causes, the episode and the circumstances surrounding the episode must be scrutinized carefully. The quality, severity, and length of the episode and the time required for recovery can help determine potential etiologies. The physical examination should concentrate on orthostatic vital signs (squatting and standing) and a complete cardiac and neurologic examination.[1]

TABLE 13-11: Details of History in Syncope of the Athlete

The circumstances and the timing of the episode related to exercise
The exercise type, the sport, and the length and intensity of exercise
Hydration status
Medication, illicit drug, and supplement use
Age
Degree of conditioning and exercise frequency
Presence of heart disease
Severity and length of the episode
Genetic screening and family history
Previous surgery and implanted devices
The temporal relationship to exercise
The type of athlete ("weekend-warrior" or full-time athlete).

DATA MINING

Diagnostic Testing for the Athlete

Any evaluation should be comprehensive, yet practical. All syncopal athletes should have at least an electrocardiogram and an echocardiogram.[1]

Arrhythmias can be difficult to reproduce during exercise, but the mechanisms for this are poorly understood. Arrhythmias and their hemodynamic influence can be difficult to induce. Exercise testing is a standard first-line approach and may yield a diagnosis. Even so, routine exercise testing may not be an adequate method to predict a cause for syncope. Sometimes a it is necessary for the individual to perform the same exercise that caused the event. An exercise test may be diagnostic even if it may not be possible to mimic the exact exercise situation that triggered the syncope. This is a useful and controlled approach to arrive at a diagnosis.[1]

An electrocardiographic monitor can provide crucial information and may be diagnostic. It is a first-line approach. Holter monitors, external endless loop recorders, and implanted monitors can help secure the diagnosis. The use of different techniques depends on the clinical situation. An exercise test may be useful; however, the specific activity associated with syncope such as soccer, basketball, or sprinting may be the only trigger for the arrhythmia. It may be necessary to monitor a patient during exercise, although there may be some danger in this approach.[1]

The Tilt-Table Test

In order for the tilt-table test to be diagnostic, must reproduce the symptoms exactly.[30] A tilt-table test may be useful to help diagnose a neurocardiogenic cause, but the results of such testing should always be considered nonspecific and be interpreted cautiously. Neurocardiogenic syncope is always the diagnosis of exclusion, especially if syncope occurs during intense exertion. Children have a different center of gravity and may need a more aggressive protocol. Likewise, an athlete may need a different protocol. Compensatory mechanisms such as the skeletal muscle pump can prevent neurocardiogenic syncope during exercise, although syncope may occur at exercise termination when the skeletal pump is less active. Dehydration or vasodilatation may also be contributing factors.

Electrophysiologic Testing

While this is a powerful tool, it can be misleading in the athlete. Unless the patient has underlying coronary artery disease and LV dysfunction, an EP test lacks sensitivity and is nonspecific. The test has limited, if any, use for patients with hypertrophic cardiomyopathy and right ventricular dysplasia. EP testing results may be useful to identify and ablate supraventricular and idiopathic ventricular tachycardias (with subsequent return of the athlete to full activity).

If all else fails, and there is a high suspicion of an ischemic etiology, a cardiac catheterization may be diagnostic. The decision to proceed with this or a myocardial biopsy requires a high degree of clinical suspicion and depends on concomitant symptoms. High-resolution echocardiography can image the proximal segments of the coronary arteries and rule out the anomalous origin of the coronary artery ostia.

TAKE-HOME MESSAGE

Data Collecting Collect all the data about the patient's history (of smoking, high-sodium, high-cholesterol diet, alcohol abuse, lack of exercise, HTN, DM, high cholesterol level), family history (of early sudden death due to heart disease, history of early CAD), social history (work and behaviors) and from a complete physical examination (signs of prior stroke, CAD, PAD, carotid murmur, weak peripheral pulses), all of which add weight to the clinical decision-making process. Syncope is a common manifestation of many disease processes. The main question is whether the patient has suffered an episode of hypotension causing significant decrease of global cerebral perfusion and syncope. Among all patients with syncope, patients with heart disease, particularly when there is impaired LV function, BBB, evidence for congestive heart failure, or a positive family history, are at particularly high risk for death. These patients require an aggressive initial approach and may necessitate hospitalization and aggressive therapeutic interventions (including defibrillator implantation).

Data Mining Recommend safe, appropriate, and efficacious investigation (including fasting lipid profile, fasting blood glucose, BUN and creatinine levels, weight, BMI, and waist circumference). When applied judiciously, tilt testing, long-term event monitoring, and EPS emerge as the most informative techniques available. Further diagnostic assessment should be directed based on the history and physical examination to understand the mechanisms for syncope better and to understand methods to treat that mechanism better. Make a diagnosis—the right diagnosis—but no routine battery of tests is helpful. Testing is based on the only gold standard evaluation—the history and physical exam.

Management Recommend safe, appropriate, and efficacious therapy to maintain the stable health status of the patient over time. Proper treatment first involves a careful understanding of the causes of syncope, based on a careful assessment of the patient initially and most importantly by the history and secondarily by the physical examination. Once there is a diagnosis, the treatment is easier. Treatment is aimed at reducing disability, recurrent syncope, and mortality.

Patient-Centered Care Get the patients involved in their own lifestyle modifications to increase compliance with diet, exercise, medication, office visits, and testing in order to provide continuity of care.

References

1. Olshansky, B., Hu, D., Pham, K., et al: Syncope. In Nguyen, T., Hu, D., et al., eds, Management of Complex Cardiovascular Problems: The Evidence-Based Medicine Approach. Philadelphia, PA.: Blackwell-Futura, 2007, pp 372–404.
2. Harvey, W. P.: Cardiac pearls. Cedar Grove, NJ: Leannec Publishing, 1993, 43–112.
3. Hypotension and syncope. In Libby, P. (ed): Braunwald's Heart Disease, A Textbook of Cardiovascular Medicine. Philadelphia, PA.: WB Saunders, 2008.
4. Park, M. K., ed: Pediatric Cardiology for Practitioners, 5th ed, Philadelphia, PA: Mosby Elsevier, 2008.
5. Winters, S. L., Stewart, D., Gomes, J. A.: Signal averaging of the surface QRS complex predicts inducibility of ventricular tachycardia in patients with syncope of unknown origin: A prospective study. J Am Coll Cardiol. 1987;10:775–781.
6. Bartoletti, A., et al.: 'The Italian Protocol': A simplified head-up tilt testing potentiated with oral nitroglycerin to assess patients with unexplained syncope. Europace. 2000;2(4):339–342.
7. Linzer, M., et al.: Predicting the outcomes of electrophysiologic studies of patients with unexplained syncope: preliminary validation of a derived model. J Gen Intern Med. 1991;6(2):113–120.
8. Strickberger, S. A., et al.: AHA/ACCF Scientific Statement on the Evaluation of Syncope. JACC. 2006;47:473–484.
9. Moss, A. J., Zareba, W., Hall, W. J., et al.: for the Multicenter Automatic Defibrillator Implantation Trial II Investigators Prophylactic Implantation of a Defibrillator in Patients with Myocardial Infarction and Reduced Ejection Fraction. N Engl J Med. 2002;346:877–883.

10. Bardy, G. H., Lee, K. L., Mark, D. B., for the Sudden Cardiac Death in Heart Failure Trial (SCD–HeFT) Investigators: Amiodarone or an Implantable Cardioverter-Defibrillator for Congestive Heart Failure. N Engl J Med. 2005;352(3):225–237.

11. Kadish, A., Dyer, A., Daubert, D. P., for the Defibrillators in Nonischemic Cardiomyopathy Evaluation (DEFINITE) Investigators: Prophylactic defibrillator implantation in patients with nonischemic dilated cardiomyopathy. N Engl J Med. 2004;350:2151–2158.

12. Fujimura, O., et al.: The diagnostic sensitivity of electrophysiologic testing in patients with syncope caused by transient bradycardia. N Engl J Med. 1989;321(25):1703–1707.

13. Middlekauff, H. R., Stevenson, W. G., Saxon, L. A.: Prognosis after syncope: impact of left ventricular function. Am Heart J. 1993;125(1):121–127.

14. Abboud, F. M.: Neurocardiogenic syncope. N Engl J Med. 1993;328(15):1117–1120.

15. Karas, B., et al.: The postural orthostatic tachycardia syndrome: A potentially treatable cause of chronic fatigue exercise intolerance and cognitive impairment in adolescents. Pacing Clin Electrophysiol. 2000;23(3):344–351.

16. Grubb, B. P., et al.: Cerebral syncope: loss of consciousness associated with cerebral vasoconstriction in the absence of systemic hypotension. Pacing Clin Electrophysiol. 1998;21 (4 Pt 1):652–658.

17. Grubb, B. P., Karas, B.: Diagnosis and management of neurocardiogenic syncope. Curr Opin Cardiol. 1998;13(1):29–35.

18. Engel, G. L.: Psychologic stress vasodepressor (vasovagal) syncope and sudden death. Ann Intern Med. 1978;89(3):403–412.

19. ACC/AHA/HRS 2008 Guidelines for Device-Based Therapy of Cardiac Rhythm Abnormalities. A Report of the American College of Cardiology/American Heart Association Task Force on Practice Guidelines (Writing Committee to Revise the ACC/AHA/NASPE 2002 Guideline Update for Implantation of Cardiac Pacemakers and Antiarrhythmia Devices) *Developed in Collaboration With the American Association for Thoracic Surgery and Society of Thoracic Surgeons* J Am Coll Cardiol. 2008; 51:1-62.

20. Sheldon, R., Rose, S., Connolly, S.: Prevention of Syncope Trial (POST): A randomized clinical trial of beta blockers in the prevention of vasovagal syncope; rationale and study design. Europace. 2003;5:71–75.

21. Kaufmann, H., Saadia, D., Voustianiouk, A.: Midodrine in neurally mediated syncope: A double-blind randomized crossover study. Ann Neurol. 2002;52(3):342–345.

22. Reybrouck, T., et al.: Tilt training: A treatment for malignant and recurrent neurocardiogenic syncope. Pacing Clin Electrophysiol. 2000;23(4 Pt 1):493–498.

23. van Dijk, N., Quartieri, F., Blanc, J. J., et al.: PC-Trial Investigators. Effectiveness of physical counterpressure maneuvers in preventing vasovagal syncope: the Physical Counterpressure Manoeuvres Trial (PC-Trial). J Am Coll Cardiol. 2006 Oct 17;48(8): 1652–1657.

24. Raviele, A., Giada, F., Menozzi, C., et al.: Vasovagal Syncope and Pacing Trial Investigators. A randomized, double-blind, placebo-controlled study of permanent cardiac pacing for the treatment of recurrent tilt-induced vasovagal syncope. The vasovagal syncope and pacing trial (SYNPACE). Eur Heart J. 2004;25: 1741–1748.
25. Krahn, A. D., Klein, G. J., Yee, R., et al: Cost implications of testing strategy in patients with syncope: randomized assessment of syncope trial. J Am Coll Cardiol. 2003;42:495–501.
26. Olshansky, B., Poole, J. E., Johnson, G., et al.: Syncope Predicts the Outcome of Cardiomyopathy Patients. Analysis of the SCD-HeFT Study. J Am Coll Cardiol. 2008; 51:1277–1282.
27. Maron, B. J., Fananapazir, L.: Sudden cardiac death in hypertrophic cardiomyopathy. Circulation. 1992;85(1 Suppl):I57–I63.
28. Maron, B. J., Gohman, T. E., Aeppli, D.: Prevalence of sudden cardiac death during competitive sports activities in Minnesota high school athletes. J Am Coll Cardiol. 1998;32(7):1881–1884.
29. Rosso, A., Alboni, P., Brignole, M.: Relation of clinical presentation of syncope to the age of patients. Am J Cardiol. 2005;96(10):1431–1435.
30. Lampert, R., Cannom, D., Olshansky, B.: Safety of sports participation in patients with implantable cardioverter defibrillators: a survey of heart rhythm society members. J Cardiovasc Electrophysiol. 2006; 17(1): 11–15.

Stable Coronary Artery Disease

Xiankai Li, Tuan D. Nguyen,
Sim Kui Hian, and Thach Nguyen

Chapter Outline

DEFINITION

Coronary artery disease (CAD) is a condition caused by obstruction of the blood flow in a coronary artery lumen, mostly due to atherosclerosis.

Patient Population in Focus

Patients with stable CAD present with their angina symptom at a fixed, predicted level of activity. These patients are (1) middle-aged with a high risk of CAD, having had stable angina pectoris by history, (2) asymptomatic or symptomatic with confirmed nonsignificant lesions in the coronary arteries, and (3) have a history of being stabilized from acute coronary syndrome (ACS) including non-Q myocardial infarction (non-Q MI) or ST segment elevation MI (STEMI).

Strategic Programming

The process of managing a patient with diverse presentations of chest pain is first to collect the data by a comprehensive interview and physical examination. The next step is to perform data processing in order to estimate the possibility of CAD and many other life-threatening conditions mimicking CAD. Using the method of data mining, many other noncardiac or cardiac conditions that trigger or aggravate angina, such as anemia, uncontrolled hypertension, thyroid disorders (thyrotoxicosis), heart rhythm abnormalities (tachyarrhythmias), and concomitant valvular heart disease can be ruled out. The reason for early recognition of CAD is to start aggressive preventive measures in order to avoid any major adverse cardiovascular (CV) events (MACE), such as myocardial infarction (MI), stroke, heart failure (HF) or death. Primary prevention is to prevent MACE in patients without diagnosed CAD. Secondary prevention is to prevent MACE in patients or populations with confirmed CAD.

DATA COLLECTING

Data collection by a physician occurs by interviewing and examining a patient in a structured, systematic, and scientific way. A formal data collection process is necessary because it ensures that data gathered are both defined and accurate and that subsequent decisions based on arguments embodied in the findings are valid.

Investigation Master Plan

When a physician sees a patient suspected of having stable CAD, there are seven main areas of interest for data collecting (history and physical examination) (see Table 14-1).

TABLE 14-1: Investigation Master Plan: Significant Lesion on a Major Coronary Artery

Index Problem	Mechanism	Symptoms	Signs	Tests
Significant coronary artery lesion	Significant obstruction of index artery	None	None	Angiogram: significant lesion
Upstream of index lesion	Compensatory prestenotic dilation	None	None	Angiogram: Prestenotic dilation
Downstream of index lesion	Compensatory poststenotic dilation or constriction from low flow	None	None	Angiogram: Poststenotic dilation or constriction
Downstream myocardium	Insufficient blood supplied to downstream myocardium	Chest pain	None	Ischemia on myocardial perfusion imaging
Work-Around of index lesion	Collaterals proliferation	No pain if a lot of collaterals	None	Collaterals on angiogram
Cardiovascular system	Wall motion abnormalities	Symptoms of LV dysfunction	S3 sound	Wall motion abnormalities on echocardiography
Network (Other systems) if there is severe LV dysfunction caused by CAD	Congestion in the pulmonary vascular system, poor renal perfusion	Symptoms of pulmonary congestion, RHF, renal insufficiency	Signs of pulmonary congestion, RHF, renal insufficiency	Pulmonary congestion on x-ray, high BUN and creatinine levels

BUN: blood urea nitrogen, CAD: coronary artery disease, LV: left ventricle, RHF: right heart failure.

The main area of interest: Index coronary lesion. The index lesion does not directly generate any symptoms or signs (zone A).

The upstream area of the index lesion is the proximal segment of the coronary artery, which dilates due to ischemia downstream. There are no signs or symptoms generated from this coronary segment (zone B).

The myocardium downstream to the index lesion. If the lesion is insignificant, the myocardium supplied by the index artery does not generate any symptoms or signs. If the lesion is severe enough, there are symptoms of angina (zone C).

The system configuration: There is nothing wrong with the configuration of the cardiovascular system (zone E).

The work-around configuration: The patient has collaterals to the distal segment of the index lesion. The more collateral the lesion has, the less pain the patient experiences (zone D).

The cardiovascular system: If there is longstanding stable CAD, the cardiovascular system is an end-organ, which bears the effect of obstruction of the coronary lesion, causing hypokinesis or akinesis of the myocardial segment supplied by the index artery. The symptoms of chest pain come from the area of the myocardium. If there is significant hypokinesis or akinesis, there will be symptoms and signs of left ventricular dysfunction.

The network (the whole body): Long-standing uncontrolled HF can cause right heart and kidney failure in the pulmonary and renal systems (zone F).

History
Typical Symptoms

Typical angina is usually described as a heavy chest pressure, discomfort, or squeezing feeling associated with shortness of breath or dizziness. The discomfort often radiates to the left shoulder, neck, or arm. It typically builds slowly in intensity over a few minutes. However, the main feature of typical angina is not the type, location, or associated characteristic of the pain but the fact that the discomfort is triggered by activities and relieved by rest.[1] While describing substernal chest pain or discomfort, the patient often clenches a fist and presses it over the midsubsternal area. This is known as the Levines sign, which is more specific to the diagnosis of angina than other signs.[2] During the interview with a patient with possible angina, to elicit an unbiased description of symptoms the patient should be asked: "What happens if you walk briskly up a hill, against the wind, in cold weather?" Be careful not to suggest to the patient that pain or discomfort might occur with this situation.[2]

◎ DATA DECODING TIPS (CLINICAL PEARLS)

Anatomic Identification of Coronary Lesions by a Detailed History

A patient who has typical angina at rest after a heavy meal may have significant left main artery disease. A patient with prior evidence of CAD has angina in the morning with regular activities (e.g., walking inside the house). The chest pain slowly disappears as the patient continues these regular activities. As the day goes on, even with higher levels of activity, the pain never comes back. This phenomenon is suggestive of chronic total occlusion (CTO). The mechanism is such that the collaterals collapse during the night. In the morning, the patient develops angina because of regular activities due to the mismatch between supply and demand. With chest pain as a trigger, the collaterals open up so that even at a higher level of activity as the day goes by, the pain never comes back. The same phenomenon repeats itself every day. These details in a patient's history help the physician to guess the patency of a recently stented artery without the need for coronary angiography.

Atypical Symptoms

Atypical symptoms can present as a sensation of burning, indigestion, stomach pain, jaw pain, burping, or breathlessness. These symptoms may be accompanied by less-specific symptoms, such as fatigue, nausea, or a sense of impending doom, especially in women. Symptoms can occur in atypical locations, such as between the shoulder blades, the jaw, the neck, or the arms.

A patient with asymptomatic CAD may develop any kind of noncardiac chest pain unrelated to the obstructive coronary lesion. If this patient undergoes a coronary angiogram, the incidental discovery of a coronary lesion does not prove the causal relationship between the lesion and the atypical or typical symptoms experienced by the patient. The most important feature suggestive of coronary origin is that the symptom is caused by exertion and relieved by rest.

The distress of angina is rarely sharp, localized, or spasmodic. It is also unlikely to be a darting, knife-like pain or in a localized area that can be pointed to. Angina attacks lasting more than thirty minutes are unusual, unless what is actually occurring is acute myocardial infarction (AMI). Administration of sublingual nitroglycerin (NTG) could relieve angina; however, NTG could also relieve discomfort from esophageal spasm.[2]

DATA DECODING TIPS (CLINICAL PEARLS)
Shortness of Breath as Angina Equivalent

In general, with activities, if a patient has SOB first, then most likely the patient has emphysema or heart failure. If the patient has chest pain first, then most likely the patient has CAD. However, some patients with CAD could experience SOB first with activities if they have lesions in the distal dominant right coronary artery (RCA), large obtuse marginal (OM) artery, or large diagonal artery. This is because the above branches supply one of the papillary muscles. When there is ischemia, transient mitral regurgitation could occur; pulmonary congestion, early edema, or SOB follow. Revascularization of the above branches could improve the symptom of SOB caused by ischemia.

Physical Examination

There are no typical findings in physical examination, but there are several nonspecific signs seen in patients with CAD. In some patients, an elevated blood pressure or tachycardia may be found, either as a precipitating factor or as a result of angina. Occasionally, a gallop rhythm (the third or fourth heart sound) may be heard due to transient ventricular dysfunction and an apical systolic murmur may be heard due to transient ischemic mitral regurgitation.

 JOB DESCRIPTION:

How to Search for an S3 or S4 Sound

The diastolic filling sound S3 at times may be heard only when the patient is turned to the left lateral position and one listens over the point of maximal impulse with the bell of the stethoscope barely making a seal with the skin of the chest wall.

An atrial gallop (S4) is frequently found in patients having CAD. As a rule, a ventricular (S3) diastolic gallop is not a loud sound. In fact, most gallops are faint and one needs to listen very carefully and specifically for them. They are very common; however, most ventricular (S3) gallops are usually heard every third or fourth rather than with every beat. On the other hand, an atrial (S4) gallop is more likely to be heard with almost every beat.[2]

DATA PROCESSING (FORMULATING A PRELIMINARY DIAGNOSIS)
Making the Diagnosis of Stable Angina

On many occasions, the only way to differentiate the diagnosis of angina or unstable angina in a patient with suspected CAD or with unstable

CAD is a detailed history. A patient who has stenting (PCI) less than one month before now develops chest discomfort. If you were to do a stress test, the stress test would be inconclusive because the pre-PCI nuclear scan would not reverse to normal until three months after PCI. Only a detailed history would help the physician to differentiate between significant angina, anxiety, pleuritic chest pain, or peptic ulcer disease. The same problem occurs with patients who have recently undergone open-heart bypass surgery (CABG) or with a recent (less than three years) normal coronary angiogram. If the symptoms are too confusing and not helpful, a repeat angiogram with or without IVUS is needed to confirm the patency of the coronary arteries.

DATA FILTERING (DIFFERENTIAL DIAGNOSES)

Gastrointestinal Disorders

Chest pain caused by peptic ulcer disease occurs usually 60 to 90 minutes after meals (gastric ulcer) or 3 to 4 hours after meals (duodenal ulcer) and is relieved by an antacid. This pain is usually epigastric in location but can radiate to the chest, shoulders, or back (if it is a duodenal ulcer). Symptoms are often worsened by a supine position (allowing acid reflux into the esophagus) and usually relieved by sitting upright or by acid-reducing drugs (if it is caused by gastroesophageal reflux, or GERD). Esophageal spasm can mimic angina. Mallory-Weiss tears of the esophagus can occur in patients who have had prolonged retching or vomiting. Aching or colicky pain from cholecystitis is usually localized in the right upper quadrant. Discomfort from pancreatitis is typically an intense aching epigastric pain that may radiate to the back.[1]

DATA DECODING TIPS (CLINICAL PEARLS)

Difference Between Pains Due to Gallstones and Pain from CAD

A patient with gallstones usually has pain in the right upper quadrant or in the epigastric area. The major feature is that the patient moves around while lying down and changes position of the body to find a comfortable position (to move the gallstone out of its obstructive location), whereas patients with angina try to stay still because they are afraid to start the anginal pain again. Biliary colic is triggered after a fatty meal, while angina is triggered by activity. If a patient with biliary colic receives morphine sulfate (MS) for pain, it could aggravate the pain by causing constriction of the neck of the gallbladder, while in a patient with chest pain from cardiac origin, MS would improve the pain and relieve the SOB by decreasing preload (venodilating effect).

Musculoskeletal Disorders

Chest pain can arise from musculoskeletal disorders, such as costo-chondritis, cervical disk disease, or herpes zoster. This pain can be elicited by direct pressure over the affected area or by movement of the patient's upper body or neck. The pain itself can be fleeting or last for hours.[1]

💿 DATA DECODING TIPS (CLINICAL PEARLS)
Chest Pain Due to Cervical Disk Disease

If there is suspicion of cervical disk involvement, the patient should be asked about the history of a motor vehicle accident that may have caused cervical whiplash. During the episode of chest pain, that patient might experience weakness or inability to move one of the arms (more often the left arm). As the pain is resolved, the patient can move the arm again. The presence of transient weakness of the upper extremity associated with chest pain strongly suggests cervical disk disease as the cause of chest pain. Magnetic resonance imaging (MRI) of the cervical spine would confirm this clinical suspicion. However, in a patient with chest or back pain associated with neurologic symptoms, there is a need to rule out thoracic aortic dissection.

Pericarditis

Pericarditis nearly always involves the surrounding pulmonary pleura. Patients would experience pleuritic pain on breathing, coughing, or change in position. Swallowing may also induce the pain because of the proximity of the esophagus to the posterior surface of the heart. The pain from infectious pericarditis is also frequently felt in the shoulder or neck[1] because the central diaphragm receives its sensory supply from the phrenic nerve, which arises from the third to fifth cervical segments of the spinal cord.

💿 DATA DECODING TIPS (CLINICAL PEARLS)
Pleuritic Chest Pain in Myocardial Infarction

A patient can present with typical pleuritic chest pain and be treated with nonsteroidal anti-inflammatory drugs (NSAIDs). On rare occasions, the pleuritic chest pain may be due to Löeffler syndrome, a post-MI peri-carditis. Subsequent enzyme measurements would confirm this clinical suspicion and post-MI work-up and management could be started (e.g., aspirin, beta blockers, stress test). Therefore be careful when seeing a patient with typical pleuritic pain, especially in the group with a high incidence of CAD. However, post-MI pericarditis was seen more frequently after thrombolytic therapy or without any reperfusion therapy. It is rare to see Löeffler syndrome after primary PCI.

Pulmonary Arterial Hypertension

Pulmonary arterial hypertension (PAH) can cause chest pain due to a reduction of coronary blood flow from a hypertrophied right ventricle.[3]

Angina without Atherosclerosis: Coronary Artery with Anomalies at the Origin

When a dominant RCA, a left main artery, or a left anterior descending artery (LAD) originates from the contralateral sinus (instead from the ipsilateral sinus), it courses to its (conventional) normal position through four pathways: interarterial, septal, retroaortic, or anterior. The last three courses are usually benign. The interarterial course is most serious because ischemia, syncope, and sudden death at a young age can happen due to compression of the coronary artery between the aorta and the pulmonary artery during systole.[1]

DATA DECODING TIPS (CLINICAL PEARLS)
No Angina and Sudden Death in Elderly Patients with Coronary Anomaly at the Origin

Elderly patients with abnormal coronary artery coming from the contralateral sinus through the interarterial pathway may not have sudden death or chest pain. The atherosclerosis on the wall of the aorta would limit its expansion during systole. However, patients can have angina from any atherosclerotic obstructive lesion in the anomalous coronary arteries due to usual risk factors.

Coronary Artery Fistula

Coronary artery fistula is an anomalous communication from the coronary artery to the cardiac chamber or vessel. It can cause heart failure if the shunt is large, pulmonary hypertension if the flow to the pulmonary artery is high, and arrhythmias or ischemia by the coronary steal phenomenon.[1]

Vasculitis

Patients with inflammation of the coronary arteries can have chest pain due to stenosis or small thrombi formation from aneurysmal changes, e.g., Takayasu disease or lupus erythematosus.

A summary of the characteristics of angina or pain from different causes is detailed in Table 14-2.[4]

DATA MINING

Data mining is an analysis technique that focuses on modeling and knowledge discovery for predictive rather than purely descriptive

TABLE 14-2: Differential Diagnoses of Angina

	Stable Angina	Unstable Angina	AMI	Aortic Dissection	Acute Abdomen (Peptic Ulcer, Acute Pancreatitis)
Pain Location	Left side of chest	Left side of chest	Retrosternal area	Changing localization, may radiate to arms or legs	Upper abdomen or other location
Characteristic	Tightness, heaviness, or squeezing	Tightness, heaviness, or squeezing	Tightness, heaviness, or squeezing, more severe, plus nausea, diaphoresis, dyspnea	Severe tearing pain	Burning or squeezing
Provoking Factors	Activity, meal, cold, or emotional stress	Activity, meal, cold, or emotional stress	Activity, meal, cold, or emotional stress	Hypertension	Heavy fatty meal
Duration	Short, 3-5 min	> 20 min	Much longer (>30 min)	Long	Long
Frequency	Frequent	More frequent	Infrequent	Infrequent	Frequent/Infrequent
Nitroglycerin	Relieves, the pain	Effective	Poorly effective	Not effective	Not effective

(continued)

TABLE 14-2: Differential Diagnoses of Angina (*continued*)

	Stable Angina	Unstable Angina	AMI	Aortic Dissection	Acute Abdomen (Peptic Ulcer, Acute Pancreatitis)
Pulmonary Edema	Rare	Occasional	Occasional	None	None
Blood Pressure	Normal or hypertension	Normal or hypertension or hypotension	Normal or hypotension or shock	Hypertension	Normal or hypertension
Fever	No	No	Rare	No	Often
WBC Court	Normal	Normal	Normal or elevated	Normal	Elevated
Cardiac Biomarkers	Normal	Normal or slightly elevated	Significantly elevated (troponin T/I, CK-MB)	Normal, or elevated when dissection to coronary arteries	Normal
ECG	Normal, or ST segment depression, or inverted T wave	Normal, or ST segment depression, or T wave inversion	ST segment elevation, evolving Q waves	Normal, or changing when dissection to coronary arteries	Normal

AMI: acute myocardial infarction, CK: creatine kinase, ECG: electrocardiogram, WBC: white blood cell.

purposes. In this chapter, as the patient has a preliminary clinical diagnosis of stable angina, there is a need to confirm (rule in) this clinical diagnosis and to rule out the most life-threatening differential diagnoses. The selection of a noninvasive modality for evaluating a specific patient depends on several factors, including availability of technology, local experience with a given modality, patient-specific factors, resting ECG abnormalities, and pretest probability of CAD.

Electrocardiogram (ECG)

A normal resting electrocardiogram (ECG) is usually seen in patients with angina. The abnormal ECG features include ST segment depression, old or new Q wave, or left ventricular hypertrophic changes. The ECG detects hypertrophy well and therefore detects conditions of pressure overload (such as uncontrolled HTN or aortic stenosis), but it is less reliable in detecting dilatation from volume overload, such as ischemic or diabetic dilated cardiomyopathy. Nonspecific arrhythmia (e.g., premature ventricular contractions [PVCs]) may be seen. The horizontal transient or downsloping ST segment depression may be reversed to baseline after chest pain is relieved.

2-D Echocardiography

A normal echocardiogram is frequently found in patients with stable CAD. Occasionally, it may reveal segmental wall motion abnormalities, which indirectly indicate ischemia, hibernating myocardium, or prior infarction. During an angina attack, transient systolic or diastolic LV dysfunction as well as transient mitral regurgitation may be detected. If the patient has pulmonary embolism (PE), the function of the right ventricle should be hyperdynamic, similar to the abnormality seen in dehydration or acute respiratory distress (e.g., exacerbation of COPD). The left ventricular (LV) function is an important factor in assessing the patient's level of activity, the cause of SOB, and especially the patient's prognosis.

Treadmill Exercise Testing (TET)

The reported sensitivity and specificity when patients with prior MI were removed from the analysis were 60% and 80%, respectively. The real value of exercise ECG lies in its availability and low cost. Further, the non-ST segment information (such as exercise metabolic equivalents [METS], time and heart rate and blood pressure recovery rates) is far more important than the ST changes. The major limitations of TET are its low sensitivity and inability to localize and quantify the ischemic burden and to assess LV function. Applicability of TET is also limited in patients with exercise limitations, women, obese patients, the elderly, and those with left bundle branch block (LBBB) and pacemakers.[5]

Myocardial Perfusion Imaging (MPI)

In order to increase the level of investigation by a noninvasive modality, gated single-photon emission computed tomography (SPECT) MPI provides information on the presence, extent, and severity of reversible defects (ischemia), fixed defects (scar), and global (ejection fraction) and regional (wall motion/thickening) LV function. The high sensitivity of stress MPI is due to the fact that perfusion abnormalities occur early in the ischemic cascade before wall motion abnormalities, ECG changes, and symptoms. As a result, SPECT allows earlier detection of CAD compared with imaging modalities that rely on the induction of wall motion abnormalities (stress echocardiography and MRI). Pharmacologic MPI is helpful in patients who cannot achieve an adequate exercise workload, such as ~85% of peak age-adjusted heart rate and > 5 METS and those with LBBB or pacemakers.[5]

DATA MINING TIPS (CLINICAL PEARLS)
False-Negative Myocardial Perfusion Imaging

In patients with left main or proximal three-vessel stenoses, the abnormality might be missed because of balanced ischemia. There is a need for 7% difference in the uptake of isotope between territories of the myocardium in order to see a difference. The sensitivity of SPECT is higher in three-vessel than one-vessel CAD; therefore one-vessel CAD disease may also be missed.[5]

Computed Tomographic Angiography

Computed tomographic angiography (CTA) can identify coronary artery lesions noninvasively. The sensitivity and specificity for CAD are high at 90–94% and 95–97%, respectively. The most valuable part is a negative predictive value of 93–99%. However, CTA cannot accurately identify lesions with heavy calcification, in-stent-restenosis, and cannot estimate the distal run-off for coronary artery bypass grafting (CABG).

TECHNOLOGY ASSESSMENT AND ECONOMIC ANALYSIS CT ANGIOGRAPHY FOR CORONARY ARTERIES:
Cost-Effectiveness Analysis

A 64-slice CTA is comparable to invasive coronary angiography for detecting true positive CAD. However, CTA is more costly because of its false-positive rates. After abnormal CTA results, invasive coronary angiography is performed to confirm the severity of the CAD lesions (which may require ad hoc PCI) or to provide the information about distal run-off flow for possible CABG if needed. These coronary angiograms add up the cost after CTA, especially if the rate of false-positive results is high or if the patient needs PCI or CABG. *Practical Applications: A* 64-slice CTA is best to rule out significant CAD by avoiding the costs and risks of unnecessary coronary angiography. But it is unlikely to replace coronary angiography in assessment for revascularization of patients, particularly if angiography and angioplasty are done in the same setting.[6]

Magnetic Resonance Imaging (MRI)

Magnetic resonance imaging (MRI) can detect CAD to evaluate regional LV function, by assessing myocardial perfusion, and by measuring global ventricular function and mass. Nonetheless, the clinical application of MRI for CAD is still limited because of the reimbursement problem in the U.S., high radiation exposure (more than CTA), and the logistics of getting the isotopes (in countries outside the U.S.).

Coronary Angiography

At this time, coronary angiography is still the method of choice to identify the lesions in the coronary arteries and to estimate their distal runoff if CABG is needed. The other advantage of coronary angiography is the ability to perform PCI in the same setting if needed.

 ## TECHNOLOGY ASSESSMENT AND ECONOMIC ANALYSIS:

Cost-Effectiveness of Different Diagnostic Pathways Prior to Coronary Angiography

In the care of patients with CAD, there is a need to evaluate the clinical and economic outcomes of different diagnostic strategies in low-risk chest pain patients in order to use the resources more cost effectively. In a study by Bedetti and coworkers, direct and indirect downstream costs were evaluated for the following strategies: coronary angiography (angio) after positive troponin I or T (cTn-I or cTnT), after positive exercise electrocardiography (ex-ECG), after positive exercise echocardiography (ex-Echo), after positive pharmacologic stress echocardiography (PhSE), after positive myocardial stress single-photon emission computed tomography with technetium Tc 99m sestamibi (ex-SPECT-Tc), and after direct angiography. The cost per patient regarding correctly identified results includes the estimated cost of the extra risk of cancer. The results are shown in Table 14-3.

Mechanism of Difference

Coronary angiography after abnormal enzyme level (troponin level) was not cost-effective because of frequent false positives of elevated troponin

TABLE 14-3: Comparative Cost Analysis of Various Diagnostic Pathways

	Positive Predictive Value (%)	Comparative Cost (as PhSE = 1)	Cost in $US
Ex-Troponin I	83.1	3.8	2.051.00
Ex-Troponin T	87.1	3.9	2.086.00
Ex-ECG	85.1	3.5	1.890.00
Ex-Echo	93.4	1.5	803.00
PhSE	98.5	1	533.00
Ex-Spect	89.4	3.1	1.634.00
Ex-Angio	18.7	56.3	29.999.00

level. Direct angiography after low-risk chest pain is also not cost-effective because of high-false negative results and the high cost for care of future breast cancer.

Practical Applications: Stress echocardiography–based strategies are cost-effective versus alternative imaging strategies because the risk and cost of radiation exposure are void. The calculated costs differ between countries and fluctuate at different periods according to the demand and supply balance of the market; therefore the selection of a pathway depends on the availability and cost-effectiveness of resources at the time the patient is seen and the tests are ordered.[7]

DATA CONVERTING

Once captured, the data need to be converted into *information* and *knowledge* in order to become clinically useful.

Confirming the Diagnosis of Stable Angina

For patients with new onset of typical angina, stable CAD is confirmed by abnormal stress test or myocardial perfusion scan. For patients with confirmed CAD after being stabilized by medical therapy or revascularization, a normal stress test or myocardial perfusion scan confirms the stability of CAD.

Risk Stratification

Once the diagnosis of stable CAD is confirmed, there is a need to stratify the annual mortality risk in order to start treatment. Aggressive treatment is for patients at high risk, while patients at low risk can have

TABLE 14-4: The Framingham Risk Stratification of Stable CAD

High Risk >3%

- Severe resting LV dysfunction (LVEF <35%)
- High-risk treadmill score (≤-11)
- Severe exercise LV dysfunction (LVEF <35%)
- Stress-induced large perfusion defect (especially anterior)
- Multiple, moderate-sized perfusion defects
- Large, fixed perfusion defect with LV dilation or increased lung uptake (thallium-201)
- Stress-induced moderate perfusion defect with LV dilation or increased lung uptake (thallium-201)
- Echocardiographic wall motion abnormality (>2 segments) at low dobutamine dose (≤10 mg/kg per min) or low HR (<102 bpm)
- Stress echocardiographic evidence of extensive ischemia

Intermediate Risk 1-3%

- Mild/moderate resting LV dysfunction (LVEF 35-49%)
- Intermediate-risk treadmill score (-11 < score < 5)
- Stress-induced moderate perfusion defect without LV dilation or increased lung intake (thallium-201)
- Limited stress echocardiographic ischemia with a wall motion abnormality only at higher doses of dobutamine involving ≤2 segments

Low Risk <1%

- Low-risk treadmill score (≥5)
- Normal or small myocardial perfusion defect at rest or with stress
- Normal stress echocardiographic wall motion or no change of limited resting wall motion abnormalities during stress

preventive measures. The list of factors affecting the annual mortality risks of patient with CAD is provided in Table 14-4.

PROGRAMMED MANAGEMENT

Strategic Programming

The management of patient with stable CAD consists of (1) control of angina symptoms, (2) prevention of new major CV events (MACE) such as MI, death, or stroke, and (3) optimal lifestyle, including return to work. The management of stable CAD includes the following general strategies (Table 14-5):

- Decreasing myocardial demand by medical therapy (e.g., beta blockers)

TABLE 14-5: Management Master Plan

Data Management	Medical treatment
System Configuration Correction	None
Root Cause Correction	Percutaneous coronary intervention
Work-Around Management	Coronary artery bypass graft surgery
System Replacement	None

- Increasing distal perfusion by mechanical revascularization (CABG or PCI)
- Administering antiplatelet drugs to prevent formation of thrombus at the lesion site
- Modifying plaque by administering cholesterol-lowering drugs

Prevention

As in any disease, the first measure is to prevent the disease before it appears (proactive approach) rather than to treat the disease (reactive approach). For patients with CAD, there is a need to stop smoking, to treat hypertension (HTN), to follow a low-sodium, low-cholesterol diet, and to exercise. The details of preventive measures for heart disease are discussed in detail in Chapter 4; controlling HTN in Chapter 7; lowering cholesterol in Chapter 5; and diet in Chapter 6.

In every country with limited health-care resources (including the U.S.), are the risk-lowering interventions (smoking cessation, antihypertensives, ASA, and statins) cost-effective in primary prevention? The rationale of such an approach is provided by the study that follows.

 BENEFITS, HARMS AND COST-EFFECTIVENESS ANALYSIS:

Is It Worth Preventing MI?

Methodology: Using data from the Framingham Heart Study and the Framingham Offspring study, life tables to model the benefits of the selected interventions were built. The effects of risk reduction are obtained as numbers of deaths averted and life-years saved within a 10-year period. Estimates of risk reduction by the interventions were obtained from meta-analyses and the estimates of cost savings were calculated from Dutch data. *Benefits:* The most cost-effective measure is smoking cessation therapy. ASA is the second most cost-effective therapy (2263 euros to 16,949 euros per year of life saved) followed by antihypertensives. Statins are the least cost-effective (73,971 euros to 190,276 euros per year of life saved). *Practical Applications:* A cost-effective strategy should offer a smoking cessation program for smokers as well as ASA for moderate and high-risk men older than 45 and for women aged 55 and older. Statin therapy is the most expensive option in primary prevention when the 10-year CAD risk is below 30%. However, if the price of generic statin decreases, its cost-effectiveness could improve.[8]

Diet and Exercise

The usual recommendations for a low-sodium, low-cholesterol diet and exercise apply for all patients with CVD. The details of a dietary approach and exercise are discussed in Chapters 6 and 4.

Aspirin

ASA is a weak platelet inhibitor indicated in all patients with stable CAD. However, what are the evidences of its benefits, harms, and cost-effectiveness?

BENEFITS, HARMS, AND COST-EFFECTIVENESS ANALYSIS: ASPIRIN

Methodology: In a meta-analysis of 195 RCTs, > 140,000 high-risk people with pre-existing CV disease, ASA was compared with no antiplatelet treatment. *Benefits:* Among almost 60,000 people (excluding those with acute ischemic stroke), ASA significantly reduced serious vascular events when compared with controls (OR 0.77, 95% CI 0.73 to 0.81). *Harms:* Low-dose ASA (< 100 mg/day) was associated with the lowest risk of bleeding (3.6%) and higher doses of ASA (100–325 mg/day, 325 mg/day) were associated with higher hemorrhagic event rates (9.1%, and 9.9%, respectively). The risk of intracranial hemorrhage with ASA was about 1/1000 (0.1%) treated for three years, which was not different from controls. However, an increased risk of intracranial hemorrhage (1.1%) with ASA doses > 325 mg/day was found. There was also a lower risk of GI hemorrhage with ASA doses of <100 mg/day (1.1%) than with ASA doses of 100–325 mg/day (2.4%) and ASA doses of > 325 mg/day (2.5%) *Practical Applications:* Among the patients at high risk of cardiac events, the large absolute reductions in serious vascular events associated with ASA far outweigh any absolute risks. Low-dose ASA, 75-150 mg/day, is best to lower the risk. Higher dose ASA (75 mg or more) is no more effective than lower-dose ASA at preventing CV events while causing more bleeding complications.[9]

Beta Blockers

In clinical practice, beta blockers (BBs) are used to reduce the myocardial oxygen demands in patients with angina by inhibiting sympathetic stimulation. BBs were proven to prevent reinfarction and to reduce CV death. BBs are also used for improving symptoms, preventing CV hospitalizations, and reducing cardiac events for patients with heart failure (HF). What is the effect of BBs on patient with stable CAD?

 BENEFITS, HARMS, AND COST-EFFECTIVENESS ANALYSIS:
Beta Blockers

There has been no RCT comparing BBs against placebo in patients with chronic stable CAD. ***Methodology:*** There was one RCT comparing metoprolol 200 mg once daily with verapamil 240 mg twice daily for a total of 809 patients with stable CAD. ***Results:*** There was no significant difference in either mortality or the combined outcome of mortality or a non-fatal CV event between those who took metoprolol verses those who took verapamil after a median follow up of 3.4 years (mortality: [5%] with metoprolol; [6%] with verapamil; OR 0.87, 95% CI 0.48 to 1.56). ***Practical Applications:*** In this RCT, metoprolol was shown to be effective at reducing mortality and improving quality-of-life scores in patients with stable angina.[10]

DATA MANAGEMENT TIPS (CLINICAL PEARLS)
How to Know the Patient is Well Betablockaded?

Beta blockers should be titrated to achieve a resting heart rate of 55-60 bpm and the heart rate should be below 90 beats per minute during moderate exercise, such as climbing stairs at a normal pace, or less than 85% of the maximum predicted heart rate during exercise stress testing.

How to Use BBs in Patients with COPD Not every patient with COPD has asthma. Many have only emphysema. So the anti-ischemic actions of beta blockers are mediated via beta-1 receptor inhibition. Inhibiting beta-2 stimulation with nonselective beta blockers can theoretically impair adrenergic-mediated coronary and bronchial vasodilation; therefore it is often recommended to use a beta-1 selective beta blocker such as metoprolol or atenolol for patients with emphysema. Carvedilol is not a selective BB. At the higher doses required to treat angina, there does not appear to be a significant difference between either selective or nonselective types of beta blockers causing bronchoconstriction.

Nitrates
No direct information about whether nitrates are better than no active treatment was found. The general clinical consensus is that nitrates are effective for treating the symptoms of stable angina.

> ### 🔴 DATA MANAGEMENT TIPS (CLINICAL PEARLS)
> #### Need for Treatment or Change of Strategy
>
> In the treatment of CAD, (1) when the symptoms are not responding to optimal medical treatment, (2) in patients who survive a cardiac arrest, (3) in patients who develop serious ventricular arrhythmias, or (4) in patients previously treated by PCI or CABG and now are developing recurrence of moderate or severe angina pectoris, there is a need to change strategy. Under each of those circumstances, physicians should change tactics or speed up the diagnostic process and start invasive testing or more aggressive treatment.

ADVANCED MANAGEMENT

Percutaneous Coronary Intervention

Although percutaneous coronary intervention (PCI) is invasive, it is optimal in treatment of patients who are refractory to medical treatments or at high risk for MACE in the near future. Recently, there have been many debates about the merits of PCI versus medical treatment in the treatment of stable CAD patients. The question is whether an initial management strategy of PCI with intensive pharmacologic therapy and lifestyle intervention (optimal medical therapy or (OMT) is superior to OMT alone in reducing the risk of CV events. The results were seen in the Clinical Outcomes Utilizing Revascularization and Aggressive Drug Evaluation (COURAGE) trial that follows

 ### EVIDENCE-BASED MEDICINE:

The COURAGE Trial

Methodology: Between 1999 and 2004, the COURAGE trial assigned 1149 patients to undergo PCI with OMT (PCI group) and 1138 to receive OMT alone (medical-therapy group). The primary outcome was death from any cause and nonfatal MI during a follow-up period of 2.5 to 7.0 years. *Results:* There were 211 primary events in the PCI group and 202 events in the medical-therapy group. The 4.6-year cumulative primary event rates were 19.0% in the PCI group and 18.5% in the medical-therapy group (P = 0.62). There were no significant differences between the PCI group and the medical-therapy group in the composite of death, MI, and stroke (20.0% vs. 19.5%; HR, 1.05; 95% CI, 0.87 to 1.27; P = 0.62), hospitalization for ACS (12.4% vs. 11.8%; HR, 1.07; 95% CI, 0.84 to 1.37; P = 0.56), or MI (13.2% vs. 12.3%; HR, 1.13; 95% CI, 0.89 to 1.43; P = 0.33). *Practical Applications:* As an initial management strategy in patients with stable CAD, PCI did not reduce the risk of death, MI, or other major CV events when added to optimal medical therapy.[11]

SMART THINKING:

What Should Not Be Done According to the COURAGE Trial?

In the discussions about the results of the Courage trial, we would like to highlight a few major features of the trial. First, roughly one-fourth of patients had Canadian Cardiac Society (CCS) functional Class 0 (never chest pain), one-fourth had CCS Class 1 (chest pain with very heavy activities), one-fourth had Class 2 (chest pain with very strenuous activities), and one-fourth had Class 3 (chest pain with regular activities). Second, all patients underwent angiography; two-thirds had a stress test and half had PCI. These data showed that the patients of the Courage trial are not the usual patients seen in daily practice. We never performed coronary angiography on patients CCS Class 0, 1, or 2 unless there was objective or functional evidence of high risk by stress test, stress echocardiography, or nuclear myocardial perfusion scan. The majority of patients (or at least a large minority) of the Courage trial underwent coronary angiography without appropriate indications. The second point is that the patients of the Courage trial underwent PCI by angiographic criteria, which are clearly by the steno-ocular reflex. According to conventional practice and guidelines, angiography has never been a criterion to risk-stratify patients (except for left main disease). In Table 14-4, which lists the risk stratification criteria for CAD, there is no mention of angiographic results. Because of the lack of clinical functional abnormalities in the patients who underwent PCI in the Courage trial, the results of PCI were skewed and not optimal.

The lesson, according to the Courage trial, is that the patient should undergo a comprehensive history and physical examination first because the diagnosis of angina is a clinical diagnosis. Then if there is a need to confirm or to rule out CAD, the patient should undergo a stress test with myocardial perfusion scan. Angiography is done if there is large area of ischemic change, and revascularization is performed if the angiographic lesions match the reversible ischemic change in the nuclear scan. In the past several years, if the lesion looked around 70% or more without concordant abnormality in the nuclear scan, we declined to perform PCI. These patients did well for many years afterward (personal experience). If the patient cannot go for revascularization for any reason, there is no indication for a coronary angiogram. Lesions on the coronary artery without objective or functional signs of ischemia should not be dilated. This has been the conventional practice for the last 25 years.

Coronary Artery Bypass Graft Surgery

The goals of coronary artery bypass graft surgery (CABG) are to reduce mortality, to reduce symptoms, to decrease the number of hospitalizations, and to decrease heart failure. If patients fail optimal medical therapy or PCI, CABG is best for provision of long-term treatment. In the U.S., if patients have (1) significant stenosis (>50%) of the left main stem, (2) significant proximal stenosis (≥70%) of the three major coronary arteries, and (3) significant stenosis of two major coronary arteries, including high-grade stenosis of the proximal LAD with LV dysfunction, CABG is indicated.

Caveats When Reviewing the Statistical Data on CABG

The results of a systematic review on CABG may not be easily generalized to current practice. The majority of patients in the RCTs were 65 years or younger; at present, more than 50% of CABG procedures are performed on patients over 65 years of age. In addition, in the RCTs almost all were high-risk male patients, but those with severe angina and left main artery disease were excluded. In the past RCTs, internal thoracic artery grafts were used in fewer than 5% of patients. Lipid-lowering agents (particularly statins) and ASA were used infrequently (ASA was used in 3% of patients at enrollment). Only about 50% of patients were taking beta blockers. Thus any systematic reviews, which include RCTs several decades ago, may underestimate the real benefits of CABG. By five years, 25% of patients receiving medical treatment had undergone CABG surgery and by 10 years, 41% had undergone CABG surgery. The underestimatation of effects would be greatest among patients at high risk. Moreover, patients with previous CABG have not been studied in the RCTs, although they now represent a growing proportion of those undergoing a second CABG.[12] In order to answer the question of difference, superiority, or noninferiority between PCI and CABG, the results of the SYNTAX trial (Synergy between PCI with Taxus and Cardiac Surgery), which was designed in the context of optimal therapy of modern medicine, follow.

 EVIDENCE-BASED MEDICINE:

The SYNTAX Trial After 2 Years

Methodology: This is an RCT that enrolled 1800 patients to either CABG (n = 897) or PCI (n = 903) with the Taxus DES. The primary endpoint was a 12-month MACE. Secondary outcome measures included overall MACE at different follow-up periods, rates of individual endpoints, quality-of-life, and cost-effectiveness measures. Patients who were deemed ineligible for CABG or ineligible for PCI were entered into one of the following two "nested" registries: 1077 into the CABG registry and 198 into the PCI registry. To be enrolled in the trial, patients needed to have left main artery disease, with or without additional coronary disease, or disease in all three vascular territories. ***Benefits:*** At two years, the MACCE rates for PCI were 23.4% while for CABG, they were 16.3%. ***Mechanism of Difference:*** The difference was driven primarily by increased repeat revascularization procedures in the DES group. The explanation for higher in-stent restenosis (ISR) is because the patients in the PCI arm of the SYNTAX trial typically received four or five stents. With the probability of ISR of 5% or 6% in any given stent, the total ISR rate is obtained by multiplying the single ISR rate by four or five in order to arrive at the 17.3% recurrence rate. ***Harms:*** Without repeat procedures, the combined rates of all-cause death/cerebrovascular events/MI were almost identical between the two groups, whereas the stroke rate, by contrast, was higher in the CABG-treated patients. However, after year 1, the stroke rate of 0.6% was similar between the 2 groups. Symptomatic graft-occlusion and stent-thrombosis rates were nearly identical in the two groups at 3.4% and 3.3%, respectively. ***Practical Applications:*** If the patient prefers PCI, then he or she would have a shorter hospital stay and fewer comorbidities caused by the surgery. However, the patient should be prepared for repeat PCI. If the patient selects CABG, the hospital stay is longer and it takes longer to recuperate after surgery. However, once the patient recovers, the prognosis is great and after year one, patients forget about the sternotomy (which they try to avoid by having PCI). The choice of modalities depends on the patient's preference, the expertise of the local physicians, and the availability of resources in the local area.[13]

Aspirin For Prevention of Cardiovascular Events in Asymptomatic Diabetics

Since daily low-dose ASA is shown to prevent CV events in patients with stable CAD, does ASA prevent CV events in asymptomatic diabetics? The answer lies in the results of the The Japanese Primary Prevention of Atherosclerosis with Aspirin for Diabetes (JPAD) study.

 EVIDENCE-BASED MEDICINE:

The JPAD

Methodology: The JPAD study randomized 2539 patients aged 85 or younger with type 2 diabetes without a history of atherosclerotic disease, structural heart disease, arrhythmic CV disease, stroke, cerebrovascular disease, or peripheral vascular disease to open-label ASA (81 mg/day or 100 mg/day) or no ASA. ***Results:*** Over a median follow-up of 4.4 years, 1262 patients on ASA experienced 68 atherosclerotic events as compared with 86 events among 1277 patients in the non-ASA group (5.4% vs. 6.7%, P = NS). The risk of fatal coronary or cerebrovascular events was significantly decreased in the ASA group. No other secondary endpoint, including death from any cause, showed a benefit from ASA. In a subgroup analysis, 1363 patients aged ≥65 years showed a significant ASA-related decrease in atherosclerotic events; younger patients showed no such difference. *Harms:* No increased risk in hemorrhagic stroke was demonstrated. There were 12 GI hemorrhagic events in the ASA group (including 4 patients who required transfusion) and 4 events in the non-ASA group. *Caveats:* The JPAD study was statistically underpowered for its primary endpoint of atherosclerotic events due to an unexpectedly low rate of clinical events. *Practical Applications:* In general, with negative results of other studies for primary prevention even for patients at high risk, there is no indication for ASA in asymptomatic patients with high-risk factors.[14]

Clopidogrel in Stable CAD

Clopidogrel is a thienopyridine derivative that inhibits the binding of adenosine diphosphate to its platelet receptors. In general, clopidogrel is not indicated for patients with de novo stable angina. It is indicated in patients with acute coronary syndrome (ACS) and patients undergoing PCI with stents. Also, it is an alternative for patients who cannot tolerate ASA. Is clopidogrel more clinically and cost-effective than ASA? The best data for using clopidogrel alone come from the Clopidogrel versus Aspirin in Patients at Risk of Ischemic Events (CAPRIE) trial, which follows.

 BENEFITS, HARMS, AND COST-EFFECTIVENESS ANALYSIS CLOPIDOGREL VERSUS ASA FOR STABLE CAD:

The CAPRIE Trial

Methodology: This is a RCT designed to assess the relative efficacy of clopidogrel (75 mg once daily) and ASA (325 mg once daily) in reducing the risk of a composite outcome of ischemic stroke, MI, or vascular death. The patients were stable after recent ischemic stroke, recent MI, or symptomatic peripheral arterial disease. Patients were followed for 1 to 3 years. *Benefits:* An intention-to-treat analysis showed that the patients treated with clopidogrel had an annual 5.32% risk of composite endpoints as compared with 5.83% with ASA (P = 0.043) with a relative-risk reduction of 8.7% in favor of clopidogrel (95% Cl 0.3-16.5). Corresponding on-treatment analysis yielded a relative-risk reduction of 9.4%. *Harms:* Equal numbers of adverse experiences in the clopidogrel and the ASA groups were reported: rash (0.26% vs. 0.10%), diarrhea (0.23% vs. 0.11%), upper GI discomfort (0.97% vs. 1.22%), intracranial hemorrhage (0.33% vs. 0.47%), and GI hemorrhage (0.52% vs. 0.72%), respectively. *Cost-Effectiveness Analysis:* For patients taking clopidogrel, the monthly cost will be $120.00 versus $3.00 (U.S.) per prescription, per month, for patients taking ASA. *Evidence-Based Applications:* Long-term administration of clopidogrel to patients with atherosclerotic vascular disease is only minimally more effective than ASA in reducing the combined risk of ischemic stroke, MI, or vascular death. Therefore clopidogrel is not clinically beneficial because the benefits did not outweigh the risks and is not financially effective because of its higher cost.[15]

Combination of ASA and Clopidogrel for Stable CAD

ASA is the prophylactic antiplatelet drug of choice for patients with CAD. Does the addition of clopidogrel to ASA provide additional benefit, especially for those at high risk of and those with established CAD? The answers depend on the results of the Clopidogrel and Aspirin versus Aspirin Alone for the Prevention of Atherothrombotic Events (CHARISMA) trial that follows.

 BENEFITS, HARMS, AND COST-EFFECTIVENESS ANALYSIS:

The CHARISMA Trial

Methodology: This is an RCT in which 15,603 stable patients with either clinically evident CV disease or multiple risk factors were randomized to receive clopidogrel (75 mg per day) plus low-dose ASA (75 to 162 mg per day) or placebo plus low-dose aspirin and followed for a median of 28 months. The primary efficacy endpoint was a composite of MI, stroke, or death from CV causes. *Results:* The rate of the primary efficacy endpoint was 6.8% with clopidogrel plus ASA and 7.3% with placebo plus ASA (relative risk, 0.93, 95% CI 0.83 to 1.05, P = 0.22). The rate of the primary endpoint among patients with multiple risk factors was 6.6% and 5.5%, respectively (relative risk, 1.2, 95% CI 0.91 to 1.59, P = 0.20), and the rate of death from cardiovascular causes also was higher with clopidogrel (3.9% vs. 2.2%, P = 0.01). *Harms:* The rate of severe bleeding was 1.7% and 1.3%, respectively (relative risk, 1.25, 95% CI 0.97 to 1.61%, P = 0.09). *Cost-Effectiveness Analysis:* There was a suggestion of benefit with clopidogrel treatment in patients with symptomatic atherothrombosis and a suggestion of harm in patients with multiple risk factors. For every 1000 people treated for an average of 28 months, five CV events were avoided and three major bleeds were caused. Overall, clopidogrel plus ASA was not significantly more effective than ASA alone in reducing the rate of MI, stroke, or death from CV causes. ***Evidence-Based Applications:*** According to the CHARISMA Trial, dual antiplatelet therapy is not better than single antiplatelet therapy and should not be used in stable CAD patients, even those with multiple high risk factors.[16]

Benefits and Risks of Warfarin on Top of ASA

In CAD patients with atrial fibrillation (AF), deep vein thrombosis (DVT), pulmonary embolism (PE), or prosthetic valve, is it beneficial to add moderate- to high-intensity oral anticoagulants to ASA in order to reduce CV events?

 BENEFITS, HARMS, AND COST-EFFECTIVENESS ANALYSIS:

ASA and Warfarin Versus ASA or ASA and Clopidogrel

Methodology: A systemic review (search date 2002, 22 RCTs) examined the effects of adding oral anticoagulants to ASA in people with CAD. It identified seven RCTs (12,333 people) of moderate or high intensity (international normalized ratio [INR] > 2) anticoagulation plus ASA compared with ASA alone, and three RCTs (8435 people) of low intensity (INR < 2) anticoagulation plus ASA compared with ASA alone. ***Benefits:*** Moderate- or high-intensity anticoagulation plus ASA reduced the composite outcome of mortality, MI, or stroke (composite measure: OR 0.88, 95% CI 0.80 to 0.97). Adding low-intensity anticoagulation to ASA, however, did not significantly reduce risk (composite measure: OR 0.91, 95% CI 0.79 to 1.06).[17] ***Harms:*** This review found a significant increase in major hemorrhage with moderate- or high-intensity anticoagulation plus ASA when compared with ASA alone (OR 1.74, 95% CI 1.39 to 2.17). Low-intensity anticoagulation plus ASA did not increase major hemorrhage when compared with ASA alone (OR 1.25, 95% CI 0.93 to 1.70)[18] ***Cost-Effectiveness Analysis:*** ASA and warfarin versus ASA and clopidogrel was not only associated with a significantly lower risk for all types of stroke, including thromboembolic stroke (NNT = 60) but also with an increased risk of major bleeds (number needed to harm, NNH = 300). Allocating 100 patients to ASA and warfarin (at INR ratio 2 to 3) with respect to ASA and clopidogrel could prevent 17 thromboembolic strokes while causing three major bleeds. ***Practical Applications:*** Moderate to high-intensity oral anticoagulants provide substantial protection against CV events, but the risks of serious hemorrhage are higher than for ASA alone (if INR> 2.6), and regular monitoring is required. Lower intensity anticoagulation is no more effective than ASA alone.[18]

TROUBLE-SHOOTING AND DEBUGGING

The guidelines for the treatment of CAD are published and available free on the websites of all major cardiology societies for any physician caring for a patient with stable CAD. When the signs and symptoms of CAD are not controlled satisfactorily as expected, then management requires the expertise and experience of a consultant cardiologist. The common questions from the referring physicians to the consultant cardiologist in the management of stable CAD follow.

Are Calcium Channel Blockers Beneficial for CAD?

Calcium antagonists include the following two general subclasses of agents: the dihydropyridines and nonselective calcium antagonists. The dihydropyridines—nifedipine, amlodipine, and felodipine—are primarily vasodilators that relax arterial smooth muscle contraction via inhibition of the L-type calcium channel. The primary anti-ischemic action is likely by the reduction in arterial pressure and, to a lesser extent, coronary vasodilation. The nonselective calcium antagonists, such as verapamil and diltiazem, also exert significant effect on nodal activity, AV conduction, and cardiac contraction. Many studies have shown that calcium antagonists improve anginal symptoms and exercise performance compared to placebo and are similar to beta blockers in terms of safety and antianginal efficacy.[19-20] In the International Verapamil-Trandolapril (INVEST) trial of over 22,000 patients with hypertension and coronary artery disease, compared to an atenolol-based regimen, treatment with a verapamil-based strategy resulted in a similar and significant reduction in the number of patients with angina from two-thirds at randomization to less than 25% after two years with no differences in the rates of death, MI, stroke, or cardiac-related hospitalization.[21] In general, dihydropyridines should be used in conjunction with a beta blocker to prevent potential reflex tachycardia from the calcium antagonist, unless additional heart rate suppression or nodal blocking is required, in which case a nonselective calcium antagonist could be used. Dihydropyridines are particularly effective in patients with a greater vasospastic component to their angina, such as Prinzmetal's angina. Neither verapamil nor diltiazem should be used in patients with depressed ventricular function because of their negative inotropic action, although amlodipine appears safe in patients with compensated heart failure.[22] The most common side effects of calcium antagonists are headaches, flushing, pedal edema (more common with dihydropyridines), and constipation (more common with verapamil).

How To Do Elective Surgery In Patients On Long Term Clopidogrel?

For patients on long term clopidogrel after drug-eluting stent, when the patients need elective surgery, these patients should be evaluated very carefully. The risks of stent thrombosis causing acute MI and other alternative non-surgical options should be discussed extensively with patients and family. Many surgeons agree to do surgery with clopidogrel on board. So the surgeons have to be sure that during surgery, all the sources of bleeding are well cauterized. If the patients really need surgery and if the benefits of the surgery outweigh the risks, then the patients should be prepared for surgery. If the patient is clinically stable, ideally they should undergo myocardial perfusion imaging or coronary angiogram to assure well patent coronary arteries. Seven days before surgery, clopidogrel is stopped. Three days before surgery, the patients are admitted to the hospital, receiving glycoprotein 2B3A inhibitors intravenously (mainly eptifibatide, because of its short half-life) . Aspirin is then stopped. Twelve hours before surgery, GP2B3AInhibitor is stopped. Twelve hours later, the patient can undergo surgery as usual. After surgery, clopidogrelcan be resumed as early as possible according to the clinical judgement of the surgeon.[23]

How to Suggest PCI and CABG in the Real World?

In any RCT comparing PCI versus CABG, patients are randomized for CABG or PCI if the patient is eligible for both. In the SYNTAX trial, the CABG registry was made up primarily of patients whose anatomy was deemed too complex for PCI, whereas the much smaller PCI registry was made up of patients ineligible for CABG because of too many comorbidities.

In the CABG registry of the SYNTAX trial, patients did extremely well, with lower rates of death, MI, revascularization, and MACE, than those CABG-treated patients in the randomized trial. In contrast, patients in the SYNTAX PCI registry did considerably worse than their PCI counterparts in the randomized study because of the many comorbidities. Therefore, for patients who are not eligible for PCI become of technical problems without any severe medical comorbidities, CABG is an excellent option. By contrast, for patients not eligible for CABG because of severe medical comorbidities (i.e., severe COPD, liver disease), PCI is only a viable option not because of the PCI technique but because of the poor prognosis caused by the comorbidities.[13]

How to Prescribe of Celecoxib (Celebrex)?

In practice, most cardiologists avoid using celecoxib for patients with CAD. However, what should be given to a patient with terrible joint pain despite trying all other recommended medications? Where are the data based on which the patient and physician can have a frank and honest discussion of the benefits and risks of the celecoxib? *Methodology:* This is a pooled meta-analysis of six RCTs involving celecoxib versus placebo in 7950 patients, comparing the dose regimens of 400 mg daily, 200 mg twice daily, and 400 mg twice daily, used for indications other than arthritis. The six RCTs are as follows: (1) The Adenoma Prevention with Celecoxib (APC) study, (2) the Prevention of Sporadic Adenomatous Polyps (PreSAP), (3) the ADAPT trial in Alzheimer's disease, (4) the MA-27 breast-cancer recurrence study, (5) a diabetic retinopathy study, CDME, and (6) the celecoxib/selenium trial. *Results:* The hazard ratio for the composite endpoint combining all the tested doses was 1.6. The HR was lowest for the 400-mg once-daily regimen (median follow-up, 35 months) (HR = 1.1, 95% CI, 0.6-2.0), intermediate for the 200-mg twice-daily regimen (median follow-up, 36 months) (HR = 1.8, 95% CI 1.1-3.1), and highest with an approximately threefold risk of adverse CV events for the 400-mg twice-daily dose regimen (median follow-up, 11 months) (HR = 3.1, 95% CI, 1.5-6.1). *Caveats:* The doses tested were higher than the 200-mg once-daily dose generally used in osteoarthritis. The new data do directly relate to doses recommended in the celecoxib label for rheumatoid arthritis, acute pain, dysmenorrhea, and familial adenomatous polyps. Another limitation was that none of the trials were specifically designed and prespecified to have a primary endpoint of adverse CV events. *Practical Applications:* In patients who need to take celecoxib V, the once-daily oral dosing had a lower risk than twice-a day dosing for the same total daily dose of 400 mg. There was a doubling of CV risk between low- and moderate-dose groups and a further doubling of risk between moderate- and high-dose groups. No conclusions can be drawn about the CV risk associated with the 200-mg once-daily dose.[24]

TAKE-HOME MESSAGE

Data Collecting Collect all the data about the patient's history (of smoking, high-sodium, high-cholesterol diet, alcohol abuse, lack of exercise, HTN, DM, high cholesterol level), family history (of early sudden death due to heart disease, history of early CAD), social history (work and behaviors) and from a complete physical examination (signs of prior stroke, CAD, PAD, carotid murmur, weak peripheral pulses), all of which add weight to the clinical decision-making process.

Data Mining Recommend safe, appropriate, and efficacious investigations (including fasting lipid profile, fasting blood glucose, BUN and creatinine levels, weight, BMI, waist circumference). Stress test, myocardial perfusion imaging, and coronary angiography are recommended if the MPI is positive.

Management Recommend safe, appropriate, and efficacious therapy to maintain the stable health status of the patient over time (low-sodium, low-cholesterol diet, stopping smoking, losing weight, not drinking alcohol, exercising). Standard medical treatment includes ASA, BBs, and statins. Other options include clopidogrel and calcium chanel blockers if BBs are contraindicated. Once the patient is refractory to medical treatment, then he or she may need PCI or CABG. On a long-term basis, for 3VD or diabetic patients and for those with, LM disease or proximal LAD lesion with LV dysfunction, CABG seems to be best. For other patients with well-controlled risk factors, PCI with DES is best.

Patient-Centered Care Get the patients involved in their own lifestyle modifications to increase compliance with diet, exercise, medication, office visits, and testing in order to provide continuity of care.

References

1. Morrow, D. A., Gersh, B.: Chronic coronary artery disease, in Libby, P. (ed.): Braunwald's Heart Disease, A Textbook of Cardiovascular Medicine. Philadelphia, PA: Saunders, 2008, pp. 1353–1417.
2. Harvey, W. P.: Cardiac Pearls. Cedar Grove, NJ: Leannec Publishing, 1993, pp. 43-112.
3. Rich, S., McLaughlin, V.: Pulmonry hypertension, in Libby, P. (ed.): Braunwald's Heart Disease, A Textbook of Cardiovascular Medicine. Philadelphia, PA: Saunders, 2008, pp. 1883–1914.
4. http://www.guideline.gov/summary/summary.aspx?doc_id=12790 (accessed 7/1/2008).
5. Iskandrian, A.: Evaluating the standard of care in CAD diagnosis in http://www.medscape.com/infosite/cardiodx/article-4 (accessed 5/9/2009).
6. Mowatt, G., Cummins, E., Waugh, N.: Systematic review of the clinical effectiveness and cost-effectiveness of 64-slice or higher computed tomography angiography as an alternative to invasive coronary angiography in the investigation of coronary artery disease. Technol Assess. 2008;12(17):iii-iv, ix–143.
7. Bedetti, G., Pasanisi, E. M., Pizzi, C., et al.: Economic analysis including long-term risks and costs of alternative diagnostic strategies to evaluate patients with chest pain. Cardiovasc Ultrasound. 2008;6:21.
8. Franco, O. H., der Kinderen, A. J., De Laet, C., et al.: Primary prevention of cardiovascular disease: cost-effectiveness comparison. Int J Technol Assess Health Care. 2007; 23(1):71–79.
9. Antithrombotic Trialists' Collaboration. Collaborative meta-analysis of randomised trials of antiplatelet therapy for prevention of death, myocardial infarction, and stroke in high risk patients. BMJ. 2002;324: 71–86.
10. Rehnqvist, N., Hjemdahl, P., Billing, E., et al.: Effects of metoprolol vs verapamil in patients with stable angina pectoris: the Angina Prognosis

Study in Stockholm (APSIS). Eur Heart J. 1996;17:76–81. [Erratum in: Eur Heart J 1996;17:483.]

11. Boden, W. E., O'Rourke, R. A., Teo, K. K., et al. and the COURAGE Trial Research Group.: Optimal medical therapy with or without PCI for stable coronary disease. N Engl J Med. 2007;356:1503–1516.

12. Yusuf, S., Zucker, D., Peduzzi, P., et al.: Effect of coronary artery bypass graft surgery on survival: Overview of 10-year results from randomized trials by the Coronary Artery Bypass Graft Surgery Trialists Collaboration. Lancet 1994;344:563–570.

13. The SYNTAX trial Presented by Dr. A. Pieter Kappetein (Erasmus Medical Center, Rotterdam, the Netherlands) at the European Society of Cardiology Congress September 2009 in Barcelona Spain.

14. Ogawa, H., Nakayama, M., Morimoto, T., et al.: Low-dose aspirin for primary prevention of atherosclerotic events in patients with type 2 diabetes: a randomized controlled trial. JAMA. 2008; 300:2180–2181.

15. CAPRIE Steering Committee. A randomised, blinded, trial of clopidogrel versus aspirin in patients at risk of ischaemic events (CAPRIE). Lancet. 1996;348:1329–1339.

16. Bhatt, D. L., Fox, K. A., Hacke, W., et al.: Clopidogrel and aspirin versus aspirin alone for the prevention of atherothrombotic events. N Engl J Med. 2006;354:1706–1717.

17. www.clinicalevidence.com (accessed: 7/1/2008).

18. Anand, S. S., Yusuf, S.: Oral anticoagulants in patients with coronary artery disease. J Am Coll Cardiol. 2003;41:62S–69S.

19. The Beta Blocker Pooling Project Research Group. The Beta Blocker Pooling Project (BBPP): subgroup findings from randomized trials in post infarction patients. Eur Heart J. 1988;9:8–16.

20. Dargie, H. J., Ford, I., Fox, K. M.: Total Ischaemic Burden European Trial (TIBET). Effects of ischaemia and treatment with atenolol, nifedipine SR and their combination on outcome in patients with chronic stable angina. Eur Heart J. 1996;17:104–112.

21. Pepine, C.J., Handberg, E.M., Cooper-DeHoff, R.M., et al. A calcium antagonist vs a non-calcium antagonist hypertension treatment strategy for patients with coronary artery disease. The International Verapamil-Trandolapril Study (INVEST): a randomized controlled trial. JAMA. 2003; 290:2805-2816.

22. Heart Failure: Insights From Clinical Trials. Abstract 2374:Heart Failure With Preserved and Impaired Left Ventricular Systolic Function in the Antihypertensive and Lipid-Lowering Treatment to Prevent Heart Attack Trial (ALLHAT)." Circulation. 114(2006): 571. 5 Nov. 2008.

23. Personal Communication with Ted Feldman, MD.

24. Solomon, S. D., Wittes, J., Finn, P. V., et al.: Cardiovascular risk of celecoxib in six randomized placebo-controlled trials: the cross trial safety analysis. Circulation. 2008; 117: 2104–2113.

Acute Coronary Syndrome

Thach Nguyen, Shao Liang Chen, Alexander Doganov, Dongminh Hou, and Steven Bailey

Chapter Outline

DEFINITION

Acute coronary syndrome (ACS) includes unstable angina (UA), non-Q myocardial infarction (non-Q MI), and ST segment elevation myocardial infarction (STEMI). However, in general practice, ACS includes patients with UA and non-STEMI (UA with positive cardiac biomarkers).

Strategic Programming

The first step is to identify patients with ACS through data collecting with a comprehensive history and physical examination. There is a need to find the causes of primary ACS, which is disruption or fissuring of a vulnerable atherosclerotic plaque or secondary ACS, such as anemia, hyperthyroidism, infection, tachyarrhythmias, or valvular heart disease.[1] The next step is to perform data processing in order to formulate a preliminary diagnosis and a short list of differential diagnoses (e.g., aortic dissection or pulmonary embolism). Then, using the method of data mining, tests could be ordered (troponin level, stress testing, coronary angiography) in order to confirm (data converting) the main diagnosis of UA or non–Q-MI and to rule out (data filtering) the differential diagnoses.

DATA COLLECTING

Investigation Master Plan

When a physician sees a patient with chest pain suspected of having ACS, there are seven main areas of interest in the history taking and physical examination, based on a cardiac computational model (Table 15-1).

The main area of interest: The lesion in the coronary artery. If there is significant stenosis, the patient would complain of different levels of chest pain. There are no physical findings directly related to the coronary stenosis. The source of the problem in ACS is the obstruction in the index coronary artery. This is a hardware problem causing disruption in the coronary flow and weakening the contractile function of the myocardial area supplied by the index coronary artery (zone A).

The area upstream to the lesion with hyperdynamic producing activities (compensatory state): In patients with ACS, there are no direct signs or symptoms related to the compensatory dilation of the coronary artery proximal to the coronary lesion. Since the patient does not have enough blood distributed to the distal segment, the reaction is to increase the cardiac output by increasing sympathetic output, causing an increased heart rate. The patient may feel palpitations and have diaphoresis (sweating) (zone B).

The area downstream to the lesion with hyperdynamic receiving capacity (compensatory state) or with down-regulatory program (disease state): In patients with ACS, the symptom of acceptable flow distal to the lesion is disappearance of chest pain. There are no direct signs of poststenotic dilation or chronic distal vasoconstriction due to low flow (zone C).

The system configuration: There is no abnormality in the setting up of the hardware devices of the cardiovascular system. The problem is the obstruction of a coronary artery, which supplies the blood to the myocardium (main part of the cardiovascular system) (zone E).

The work-around configuration: Because of stenosis in the coronary artery, the body develops collaterals in order to bring blood to the

TABLE 15-1: Investigation Master Plan: Significant Lesion on a Major Coronary Artery

Index Problem	Mechanism	Symptoms	Signs	Findings
Significant coronary artery lesion	Significant obstruction of index artery	None	None	Angiogram: significant lesion
Upstream of index lesion	Compensatory prestenotic dilation	None	None	Angiogram: Prestenotic dilation
Downstream of index lesion	Compensatory poststenotic dilation or constriction from low flow	None	None	Angiogram: Poststenotic dilation or constriction
Downstream myocardium	Insufficient blood supplied to downstream myocardium	Chest pain	None	Ischemia on myocardial perfusion imaging
Work-around of index lesion	Collaterals proliferation	No pain if a lot of collaterals	None	Collaterals on angiogram
Cardiovascular system	Wall motion abnormalities	Symptoms of LV dysfunction	S3, Signs of LV dysfunction	Wall motion abnormalities on echocardiography
Network: The pulmonary vascular system, the kidneys, the central nervous system		Symptoms of pulmonary congestion, RHF, poor renal perfusion, dizziness, near syncope	Signs of pulmonary congestion, RHF, renal insufficiency, low BP	Pulmonary congestion on CXR, high BUN and creatinine levels

BUN: blood urea nitrogen, CXR: chest x-ray, LV: left ventricle, RHF: right heart failure.

distal segment. If there are enough collaterals, there is no chest pain at the level of required activities (zone D).

The cardiovascular system: Because of significant stenosis of the lesion, the myocardium supplied by the diseased artery could show local wall motion abnormality (hypokinesis to akinesis). The symptom is poor exercise tolerance because of inadequate cardiac output to the level of activities required. The sign is a new S4, which shows a stiff ventricle requiring a stronger boost from the atrium (in patients older than 45 years of age). If the lesion is in the diagonal or obtuse marginal or dominant distal artery (PDA), then the patient can have papillary muscle dysfunction causing intermittent murmur of mitral regurgitation.

The network (the whole body): If the patient has a nonsignificant lesion, there is no reverberation to the lungs. If there is significant lesion causing LV dysfunction, then an elevated LV end diastolic pressure would cause elevation of the pulmonary venous pressure and subsequently shortness of breath (SOB). If during the pain, the arterial blood pressure is low enough, the patient could feel dizzy or pass out (see Table 15-1) (zone F).

History
Typical Symptoms
The principal presentations of UA are angina at rest or with minimal exertion, new-onset of severe angina, angina of increasing severity (more prolonged and more frequent episodes of angina compared with prior period), and postinfarction angina.

Atypical Symptoms
Some patients may have no chest discomfort but present solely with jaw, neck, ear, arm, shoulder, back, or epigastric discomfort or with unexplained dyspnea.[2] If these symptoms have a clear relationship to exertion or stress and are relieved promptly with NTG, they should be considered equivalent to angina. Occasionally, such "anginal equivalents" that occur at rest are the mode of presentation of a patient with ACS but without the exertional history or known prior history of CAD, and it may be difficult to recognize their cardiac origin.[2] Features that are not characteristic of myocardial ischemia are listed in Table 15-2.

Physical Examination
Typical Signs
The physical examination of the patient with ACS could be normal. Other indirect signs suggestive of severity of myocardial ischemia or LV dysfunction include diaphoresis, pale and cool skin, sinus tachycardia, S3 or S4 gallops, or rales in the lungs. The examination should be aimed at identifying potential precipitating causes of myocardial ischemia (uncontrolled hypertension, important comorbid conditions such as

---

TABLE 15-2: Features Not Characteristic of Myocardial Ischemia[2]

- Pleuritic pain (sharp or knife-like pain brought on by respiratory movements or cough)
- Primary or sole location of discomfort in the middle or lower abdominal region
- Pain that may be localized at the tip of one finger, particularly over the left ventricular apex or a costochondral junction
- Pain reproduced with movement or palpation of the chest wall or arms
- Very brief episodes of pain that last a few seconds or less
- Pain that radiates into the lower extremities

---

chronic obstruction pulmonary disease), and evidence of hemodynamic complications (congestive heart failure, new mitral regurgitation, or hypotension). In addition to vital signs, examination of the peripheral vessels should include assessment of the presence of bruits or absent pulses that suggest extracardiac disease.[2]

For patients whose clinical presentations do not suggest myocardial ischemia, the search for a noncoronary cause of chest pain should focus first on potentially life-threatening issues (aortic dissection, pulmonary embolism), and then turn to the possibility of other cardiac (percarditis) and noncardiac (esophageal spasm) diagnoses. A dissection is suggested by blood pressure or pulse abnormality or a new murmur of aortic regurgitation accompanied by back pain. Differences in the lung sounds in the presence of acute dyspnea and pleuritic chest pain raise the possibility of pneumothorax.[2]

DATA PROCESSING (PRELIMINARY DIAGNOSIS)

The diagnosis of unstable angina is made by the history of angina at rest or with minimal exertion, new onset of severe angina, angina of increasing severity (more prolonged and more frequent episodes of angina compared with prior period), and postinfarction angina. The diagnosis of ACS is made when the patient has positive enzymes without ST segment elevation on the ECG.

DATA FILTERING (DIFFERENTIAL DIAGNOSES)

The differential diagnoses of ACS include patients with noncardiac pain (pulmonary embolism, musculoskeletal pain, or esophageal discomfort) or cardiac pain not caused by myocardial ischemia (acute pericarditis). Esophageal rupture usually occurs after endoscopy or less commonly is of sudden onset after forceful vomiting. Examination may reveal a pneumothorax or subcutaneous emphysema. The patient with spontaneous pneumothorax may experience a sharp, sudden pleuritic chest pain that is associated with dyspnea. Physical exam may be normal or reveal decreased breath sounds and hyperexpansion on the affected side. A CXR during expiration may highlight the contrast between the pleural space and the lung parenchyma.

Other cardiac disorders causing myocardial ischemia rather than CAD include aortic stenosis and hypertrophic cardiomyopathy. Many factors that increase myocardial oxygen demand or decrease oxygen delivery to the heart can provoke or exacerbate ischemia in the presence of nonsignificant underlying CAD. For example, unrecognized gastrointestinal bleeding that causes anemia is a common secondary cause of worsening angina or the development of ACS. Acute worsening of chronic obstructive pulmonary disease (with or without superimposed infection) can lower oxygen saturation levels sufficiently to intensify ischemic symptoms in patients with CAD. Evidence of increased cardiac oxygen demand can be suspected in the presence of fever, signs of hyperthyroidism, sustained tachyarrhythmias, or markedly elevated blood pressure. Another cause of increased myocardial oxygen demand is an arteriovenous fistula in patients receiving dialysis or who have multiple myeloma.[2]

Acute Aortic Dissection

Acute aortic dissection usually causes sudden onset of excruciating, ripping pain. The ascending aortic dissections tend to manifest with pain in the midline of the front of the chest, while descending aortic dissections manifest with pain in the back. Aortic dissections usually occur in the presence of risk factors, including uncontrolled hypertension, pregnancy, atherosclerosis, coarctation of the aorta with bicuspid valve, and other conditions that lead to degeneration of the aortic media, such as Marfan syndrome or Ehlers–Danlos syndrome.[1]

⚬⚬ DATA DECODING TIPS (CLINICAL PEARLS)
Clinical Clues for Aortic Dissection

When a patient has chest or back pain associated with neurologic symptoms and HTN, dissection of the aorta is strongly suspected. The pain is typically maximal at onset. Check for any difference in symmetrical timing and strength of the pulses in the carotid, radial, and femoral arteries. Listen carefully for a transient diastolic murmur of acute aortic regurgitation. The chest x-ray may show a widened mediastinum.

Pulmonary Embolism

Pulmonary embolism (PE) may be asymptomatic but often may cause sudden onset of dyspnea and pleuritic pain. Massive pulmonary emboli could cause severe, persistent substernal pain due to distention of the large proximal pulmonary artery, while smaller emboli cause pulmonary infarction due to occlusion of the small distal pulmonary arteries.[1]

DATA DECODING TIPS (CLINICAL PEARLS)
Clinical Clues for Pulmonary Embolism

A patient is suspected of having PE if he or she is complaining of SOB, low oxygen saturation even while on an oxygen supplement, and has clear lungs (no rales, no wheezing). The patient should have sinus tachycardia. Patients with PE without tachycardia could have a small PE, are taking beta blockers, or are in severe end-stage heart failure. If the patient has severe PE, he or she could pass out and have shock because of low blood pressure. If the patient has an embolism in the distal pulmonary vasculature (pulmonary infarction) the presentation could manifest with pleuritic chest pain and less SOB.

DATA MINING (WORK-UP)
Investigation Master Plan

When a physician sees a patient with chest pain suspected of having ACS, there are seven main areas of interest for testing, as the heart is designed on a computational model (Table 15-3).

The main area of interest: The lesion in the coronary artery. If there is strong suspicion of a significant lesion, then a coronary angiogram is needed to identify the lesion. A CT angiogram is another good option (zone A).

The area upstream to the lesion: A coronary angiogram would show the dilating artery proximal to the lesion. A CT angiogram can do the same, unless there are too many calcifications or tortuosities present (zone B).

The area downstream to the lesion: A **coronary angiogram** can show the patency of the distal segment, the distal run-off, and the microvasculature. A **CT angiogram** can show the distal artery without information about the run-off flow or the distal microvasculature if the patient needs bypass surgery. A **myocardial perfusion imaging** (MPI) can discriminate between adequate blood supply or ischemia to the myocardial area supplied by the index artery. MPI cannot differentiate between a critical severe lesion and a chronic total occlusion with good collaterals because MPI shows function and not anatomy. An e**chocardiogram** can show the wall motion abnormality of the area supplied by the index artery. However, the wall motion abnormality is a late event, while MPI could detect the ischemia in the lesion that is not yet causing wall motion abnormality. **Troponin and creatine protein kinase** (CPK) level elevations

TABLE 15-3: Investigation Master Plan for Acute Coronary Syndrome

Index Problem	Mechanism	Direct Tests	Indirect Tests
Significant coronary artery lesion	Obstruction of index artery	Coronary angiogram, CT angio	
Upstream of index lesion	Compensatory prestenotic dilation	Coronary angiogram, CT angio	
Downstream of index lesion	Compensatory poststenotic dilation or constriction from low flow	Coronary angiogram, CT angio	Fractional flow reserve, myocardial perfusion imaging
Downstream myocardium	Insufficient blood supplied to downstream myocardium	Echocardiography, stress echo, myocardial perfusion imaging	ECG, exercise stress test, cardiac enzyme for myocardial damage
Work-around of index lesion	Collaterals proliferation	Coronary angiogram, CT angio	
Cardiovascular system	Wall motion abnormalities	Echocardiography	
Network The pulmonary vascular system	Pulmonary congestion	Chest XR	

CT: computed tomography, ECG: electrocardiogram, XR: x-ray.

would confirm the presence of damage in the myocardium downstream to the lesion (zone C).

The work-around configuration: A coronary angiogram can show the collaterals, while a CT angiogram can show the collaterals and the distal segment even if there is chronic total occlusion (not seen in a conventional angiogram) (zone D).

The cardiovascular system: The best test for checking the whole heart is echocardiography. An elevated level of a brain-natriuretic peptide (BNP) is evidence of LV overload.

The network (the whole body): In patients with ACS, a chest x-ray will help to assess the lung congestion, an indirect sign of LV dysfunction. The elevated liver enzymes would point to right-sided heart failure, causing severe liver congestion. One of the many causes of an elevated creatinine level is a lower renal perfusion from low cardiac output (zone F).

Clinical Investigation

In patients with ACS, the purpose of data mining is to perform noninvasive or invasive testing in order to detect ischemia, its severity (diagnosis), and to identify candidates at high risk for adverse outcomes (prognostication) in order to direct them to the procedures of coronary angiography and revascularization.[2.]

Troponin

Cardiac-specific troponin T and I (cTnT, cTnI) levels rise similarly to creatinine phosphate kinase (CPK) and is more specific and more sensitive for myocardial damage. Troponin also remains elevated even two weeks after the index event; even CPK-MB has returned to normal after three days. A newer method to rely on changes in serum marker levels (delta values) over an abbreviated time interval (2 hours) as opposed to the traditional approach of performing serial measurements over 6 to 8 hours[2] can identify and exclude MI within 6 hours of symptoms. Because these assays are becoming more sensitive and precise, this method permits the identification of myocardial damage while they are still in the normal or indeterminate range. As a result, high-risk patients with positive delta values can be selected earlier for more aggressive anti-ischemic therapy, and low-risk patients with negative delta values can be considered for early stress testing.[2]

> ### 🔴 DATA DECODING TIPS (CLINICAL PEARLS)
> #### Discordant Results Between Troponin and CPK
>
> When the troponin level is elevated, regardless of the results of CPK-MB, the prognosis is poor. In ACS patients who have had both CPK-MB and cTn measured, the hospital mortality was 2.7% in patients with both negative CK-MB and cTn, 3.0% in patients with positive CPK-MB and negative cTn, 4.5% in patients with negative CK-MB and positive/cTn, and 5.9% in patients with both positive CK-MB and cTn.[3]

> ### 🔴 DATA DECODING TIPS (CLINICAL PEARLS)
> #### Role of CPK and Troponin in Identifying Reinfarction
>
> Although CPK is important in the diagnosis of ACS, it lacks sensitivity when compared to troponin level. Troponin rises earlier and decreases later than CPK. In many institutions, CPK was deleted from the laboratory test panel to rule out MI. However, because troponin stays elevated long after the index event (two weeks), troponin could not be used to detect reinfarction. CPK MB returns to normal level after three days; therefore a second elevation of CPK MB later than three days after the index event could be used as confirmation of reinfarction.

Electrocardiogram

The electrocardiogram (ECG) usually shows nonspecific ST-T changes. There might be ST depression and symmetrical T-wave inversion. An ECG recording made during an episode of the presenting symptoms is particularly valuable. Transient ST segment changes (greater than or equal to 0.05 mV [i.e., 0.5 mm]) that develop during symptoms and resolve afterward strongly suggest acute ischemia. Patients with ischemia on current ECGs can be assessed with greater diagnostic accuracy if a prior ECG is available for comparison.[2]

The other common causes of ST segment and T-wave changes should include patients with LV aneurysm, pericarditis, myocarditis, Prinzmetal's angina, early repolarization (e.g., in young black males), apical LV ballooning syndrome (Takotsubo cardiomyopathy), and Wolff-Parkinson-White syndrome. Central nervous system events, drug therapy (tricyclic antidepressants or phenothiazines), or abdominal pathology can also cause deep T-wave inversion.[2]

Echocardiography

An A 2-D echocardiogram may reveal segmental wall motion abnormalities, which indirectly indicate ischemia, hibernating myocardium, or prior infarction. The left ventricular function is an important factor in the patient's prognosis. Transient systolic or diastolic dysfunction or transient mitral regurgitation may also be present during ACS.

Treadmill Exercise Testing (TET)

Once the patient is confirmed not to have non-Q MI, he or she can undergo TET. The real value of exercise ECG lies in its availability and low cost. Furthermore, the non-ST segment information (such as exercise metabolic equivalents [METS], time and heart rate, and blood pressure recovery rates) is far more important than the ST changes. The major limitations of TET are the low sensitivity and inability to localize and quantify the ischemic burden and assess LV function. Applicability of TET is also limited in patients with exercise limitations, women, obese patients, the elderly, and those with left bundle branch block (LBBB) and pacemakers.[4]

Stress Echocardiography

Echocardiography at rest, during exercise, or with infusion of dobutamine can help to assess the resting LV systolic, diastolic dysfunction and the extent of infarction and stress-induced ischemia. Of the noninvasive imaging techniques, it is perhaps the most versatile and provides the most ancillary information at the lowest cost. The predictive value of stress echocardiography (exercise or dobutamine) in detecting angiographically proven CAD varies widely, however, with overall accuracy rates ranging from 64 to 94%, without correction for referral bias. Poor image quality with a suboptimal acoustic window in up to 25% of patients and operator dependency are the major disadvantages of stress echocardiography. The use of contrast agents has improved the precision of wall motion analysis.[4]

Myocardial Perfusion Imaging (MPI)

In order to increase the level of investigation by noninvasive modality, gated single-photon emission computed tomography (SPECT) MPI provides information on the presence, extent, and severity of reversible perfusion defects (ischemia), fixed perfusion defects (scar), and global (ejection fraction and volumes) and regional (wall motion/thickening) LV function. The high sensitivity of stress MPI is due to the fact that perfusion abnormalities occur early in the ischemic cascade before wall motion abnormalities, ECG changes, and symptoms. As a result, SPECT allows earlier detection of CAD compared with imaging modalities that rely on the induction of wall motion abnormalities (stress echocardiography and MRI). Pharmacologic MPI is helpful in patients who cannot achieve an adequate exercise workload, such as ~85% of peak age-adjusted heart rate and > 5 METS, and those with LBBB or pacemakers.[4]

DATA MINING TIPS (CLINICAL PEARLS)
False-Negative Myocardial Perfusion Imaging

In patients with left main or proximal three-vessel stenoses, the abnormality might be missed because of balanced ischemia. There is a need for a 7% difference in the uptake of isotope between territories of the myocardium in order to see a difference. The sensitivity of SPECT is higher in three-vessel than one-vessel CAD and therefore 1-CAD disease could be missed too.[4]

Computed Tomographic Angiography

Computed tomographic angiography (CTA) can identify coronary artery lesions noninvasively. The sensitivity and specificity for CAD are high at 90–94% and 95-97%, respectively. The most valuable part is a negative predictive value of 93–99%. However, CTA cannot accurately identify lesions with heavy calcification, in-stent restenosis, and cannot estimate the distal run-off for coronary artery bypass grafting (CABG).

Coronary Angiography

At the present time, coronary angiography is still the method of choice to identify lesions in the coronary arteries and to estimate their distal run-off if CABG is needed. The other advantage of coronary angiogra-

TABLE 15-4: Comparison of Noninvasive Tests to Diagnose CAD[5]

Modality	Sensitivity	Specificity	Positive Predictive Value	Negative Predictive Value
Exercise ECG	52%	71%		
Stress Echo	85%	77%	71-100%	40-91%
Nuclear Stress (SPECT)	87%	64%		81-100%
Stress Perfusion MRI	91%	81%	86%	84%
CT Angiography	85%	91%	91%	83%

CAD: coronary artery disease, CT: computed tomography, ECG: electrocardiogram, SPECT: single-photon emission computed tomography, MRI: Magnetic resonance imaging.

phy is the ability to perform PCI in the same setting if needed. A comparison of the sensitivity, specificity, and negative and positive predictive value of different tests for the diagnosis of CAD is shown in Table 15-4.

Other Tests

Patients could undergo other tests to rule out the life-threatening conditions if indicated, such as CT scan of the chest to rule out aortic dissection, or lung scan or CT angiogram to rule out pulmonary embolism.

DATA CONVERTING (CONFIRMING THE MAIN DIAGNOSIS)

Once captured, the data need to be verified to become information, and converted into relevant knowledge in order to become clinically useful. Data converting means translating the data into a clinical diagnosis. In the case of unstable angina, the diagnosis is made by the history of increasing frequency and severity of angina. The diagnosis of non-Q MI is confirmed by an increase in cardiac enzymes (CPK-MB, or troponin level) regardless of the symptoms or ECG change.

Risk Stratification

Patients with ACS could be classified into low or high risk by different scoring systems, such as the Framingham or the Thrombolysis In Myocardial Infarction (TIMI) risk scores.

> ## 🔴 DATA DECODING TIPS (CLINICAL PEARLS)
> ### The Values of Traditional Risk Factors in the Diagnosis of ACS
>
> The presence or absence of the traditional risk factors (hypertension [HTN], male sex, diabetes mellitus [DM], old age) should not be used to determine whether an individual should be admitted or treated for ACS. These factors are less predictive in a single-patient visit to the emergency room than when studied longitudinally in a specific population. However, the presence of these risk factors does appear to relate to poor outcomes in patients with established ACS.[2]

TIMI Risk Scores

The TIMI risk scores are listed in Table 15-5. If there are fewer than two risk factors, then the patient belongs in the low-risk group. If there are three or four risk factors, then the patient is in the intermediate group. If there are more than four risk factors, then the patient belongs in the high-risk group. Even without calculating the TIMI risk score, elevated troponin levels and ST segment depression help to distinguish individuals at increased cardiovascular (CV) risk.[6]

PROGRAMMED MANAGEMENT

Strategic Programming

The goal of management is to prevent the UA patients from developing non-STEMI. For patients with elevated cardiac enzymes, the goal is to abort progression to STEMI. The standard management of ACS includes medical treatment, invasive testing, and mechanical revascularization. Without adequate treatment, 25% of ACS patients will progress to Q wave MI.

- The first most important strategy in ACS is to pacify the platelets. Without successful inhibition of 80% of platelets, long-term improvement of mortality and morbidity of ACS patients is not possible. This is achieved by administration of ASA and clopidogrel.

TABLE 15-5: TIMI Risk Scores for Acute Coronary Syndrome[6]

Age >65 years
Prior coronary stenosis >50%
Three or more risk factors for coronary artery disease (CAD) (hypertension, hypercholesterolemia, family history of CAD, active smoking, diabetes)
Prior use of aspirin within last 7 days
ST segment depression
Elevated cardiac biomarkers
Two or more episodes of rest angina in the last 24 hours

- The second strategy is to reverse the inflammatory environment, which starts and sustains the disease process. A statin is the main anti-inflammatory drug of choice, while the conventional nonsteroidal anti-inflammatory drugs (NSAIDs) could cause more harm than benefit to patients.
- The third strategy is to decrease oxygen demand with blockade of the beta-receptors.
- The fourth strategy is mechanical revascularization. The goal is to assure a distal TIMI–3 flow at the index artery. This strategy stresses the importance of complete mechanical revascularization in reversing all the significant obstructions in the coronary vasculature. This strategy also reemphasizes the failure of any oral or intravenous anti-platelet drug or anticoagulant to alleviate the result of a suboptimal PCI due to a high level of residual stenosis.

A summary of the management master plan based on a computational cardiac model is shown in Table 15-6.

TABLE 15-6 Management Master Plan for Acute Coronary Syndrome

Index Problem	Mechanism	Direct Treatment	General Treatment
Significant coronary artery lesion	Significant obstruction of index artery	PCI, antiplatelet drugs: aspirin, clopidogrel, anticoagulant	Statin (working in all vasculatures)
Upstream of index lesion	Compensatory prestenotic dilation		None
Downstream of index lesion	Compensatory poststenotic dilation or constriction from low flow		Nitroglycerin (working in downstream area)
Downstream myocardium	Insufficient blood supplied to downstream myocardium		Beta blocker Beta blocker to decrease O_2 demand, TMR, angiogenesis
Work-around of index lesion	Collaterals	CABG	
Cardiovascular system	Wall motion abnormalities		ACEIs, BBs

ACEI: angiotensin converting enzyme inhibitor, BB: beta blocker, CABG: coronary artery bypass graft surgery interventions, TMR: transluminal laser revascularization.

Aspirin

Because the main mechanism of ACS is thrombotic formation started with platelet aggregation, all patients with ACS should receive ASA as soon as possible. An ASA dose of 81 mg should be continued daily, unless there is a definite contraindication.

 BENEFITS, HARMS, AND COST-EFFECTIVENESS ANALYSIS:
Aspirin

Methodology: This is a systematic review, which includes 12 randomized controlled trials (RCTs) for a total of 5031 patients with UA. *Benefits:* Antiplatelet treatment (mostly medium dose ASA, 75–325 mg/day) reduced the combined outcome of vascular death, MI, or stroke at up to 12 months compared with placebo (8% with ASA vs. 13% with placebo; odds ratio [OR] 0.54, 95% confidence interval [CI]; P < 0.0001). *Harms:* There was an increase in major extracranial bleeding with ASA when compared with placebo, but the absolute risk was low (1.1% with ASA vs. 0.7% with placebo; OR 1.6, 95% CI 1.4 to 1.8).[7] *Practical Applications:* Antiplatelet treatment, mostly medium dose ASA 75–325 mg/day, reduced the risk of death, MI, and stroke when compared with placebo. The evidence suggested that there was a possible harmful effect without additional cardiovascular benefit from doses of ASA over 325 mg daily.[7]

Clopidogrel

Unlike ASA, clopidogrel does not block cyclooxygenase but interferes with adenosine-diphosphate–mediated platelet activation. In order to have full therapeutic efficacy, more than 80% of platelets need to be inhibited. In practice, ASA is used with clopidogrel as a double antiplatelet strategy. The results of the Clopidogrel in Unstable angina to prevent Recurrent Events (CURE) trial assessing the efficacy of clopidogrel follow.

 EVIDENCE-BASED MEDICINE:
The CURE Trial

Methodology: This is an RCT, which included 12,562 patients with ACS who were given either clopidogrel (300 mg orally within 24 hours of onset of symptoms followed by 75 mg/day) versus placebo. All participants received ASA (75–325 mg daily). Revascularization was performed during the index admission in only 23% of patients. *Benefits:* The proportion of patients experiencing cardiovascular death, MI, or strokes (primary outcome) at 30 days was 5.4% in the placebo group and 4.3% in the active group (relative risk

0.79, 95% CI 0.67 to 0.92). Beyond 30 days, the corresponding rates were 6.3% versus 5.2% (relative risk 0.82, 95% CI 0.70 to 0.95). Post-hoc subgroup analysis found that the reduction in death, MI, and stroke with clopidogrel was seen across all risk groups (low, medium, and high, as classified by the TIMI risk score.[8] *Harms:* Adding clopidogrel to ASA increased major bleeding complications when compared with placebo but not hemorrhagic strokes (major bleeding 3.7% with clopidogrel vs. 2.7% with placebo; RR 1.4, 95% CI 1.1 to 1.7; hemorrhagic stroke 0.1% with clopidogrel vs. 0.1% with placebo)[8] *Cost-Effectiveness Analysis:* For every 1000 people treated for an average of 9 months, 23 events would be avoided and 10 major bleeds would be caused. *Practical Applications:* Dual therapy with ASA and clopidogrel reduced the odds ratio of the composite outcome of death, reinfarction, and stroke with acceptable safety, especially in the management of patients with ACS in whom a noninterventional approach is intended.[8]

Low Molecular Weight Heparin

Low molecular weight heparins (LMWHs) include many types; however, only enoxaparin is available in the U.S. It has a more predictable anticoagulant effect, and routine laboratory monitoring is not required to assess its efficacy. LMWHs also have a great specificity for factor Xa binding and are resistant to inhibition by activated platelets. In addition, LMWHs cause less drug-induced thrombocytopenia. However, to confirm an adequate, subtherapeutic effect or to ensure the safety level of LMWH, there is no test available, especially in the case of persistent thrombus, new thrombotic formation, or a bleeding event during PCI or treatment, for which an exact level of anticoagulation is needed. There are many differences between various LMWHs; a systemic review of data combined from individual RCTs may not accurately reflect the benefits, harms, or cost-effectiveness of each individual LMWH. The data on enoxaparin, which is commonly used in the U.S., from the Efficacy and Safety of Subcutaneous Enoxaparin in Unstable Angina and Non-Q-wave MI (ESSENCE) trial are presented next.

 EVIDENCE-BASED MEDICINE:

The ESSENCE Trial

Methodology: This is an RCT comparing enoxaparin versus heparin in ACS patients receiving 1 mg/kg subcutaneous enoxaparin bid for 2 to 8 days (mean 2.6 days) versus intravenous dose-adjusted unfractioned heparin (UFH). *Results:* At 14 days, the risk of death, MI, or recurrent angina was significantly lower in patients assigned to enoxaparin than in those assigned to UFH (16.6% vs. 19.8%,

P = 0.019). At 30 days, the composite endpoint remained significantly lower in the enoxaparin group (19.8% vs. 23.3%, P = 0.016). The need for revascularization procedures at 30 days was also significantly less frequent in patients assigned to enoxaparin (27.0% vs. 32.2%, P = 0.001). At one-year follow-up the risk of death, MI, or recurrent angina was significantly lower for the enoxaparin group (35.7% heparin vs. 32.0% enoxaparin). *Harms:* The 30-day incidence of major bleeding complications was 6.5% in the enoxaparin group and 7.0% in the UFH group. The incidence of bleeding overall was significantly higher in the enoxaparin group (18.4% vs. 14.2%, P = 0.001), primarily because of ecchymoses at injection sites. *Practical Applications:* Treatment with enoxaparin plus ASA should be considered for at least 48 hours in patients with ACS to reduce the short-term and long-term risk of recurrent angina, MI, or death. Enoxaparin can be simply administered without the need for anticoagulation monitoring, which leads to cost savings while maintaining superior short-term and sustained long-term efficacy.[9]

Unfractionated Heparin

In addition to antiplatelet drugs, anticoagulant therapy is the second main cornerstone in the treatment of ACS. If UFH is selected, intravenous UFH should be started as soon as possible, titrated to an aPTT of 1.5 to 2.5 times control. However, the absorption of UFH is erratic, thus requiring frequent monitoring and titrations; its anticoagulant level is easier to be outside the therapeutic and safety windows. This might explain why there were equivocal results in the systemic review of UFH in patients with ACS.

 BENEFITS, HARMS, AND COST-EFFECTIVENESS ANALYSIS:

Unfractionated Heparin for ACS

Methodology: There are two systematic reviews that examined the outcomes at different time points (7 days and 12 weeks). Both included the same six RCTs in 1353 patients with ACS who were treated with UFH plus ASA or ASA alone for 2 to 7 days. *Results:* The first review found that UFH plus ASA reduced the risk of death or MI after 7 days compared with ASA alone (7.9% with UFH plus ASA vs. 10.4% with ASA; OR 0.67, 95% CI 0.45 to 0.99).[10] The second review found that UFH plus ASA did not reduce death or MI after 12 weeks compared with ASA alone (12% with UFH plus ASA vs. 14% with ASA; RR 0.82, 95% CI 0.56 to 1.20).[11] *Harms:* The second systematic review found that adding UFH to ASA did not significantly increase major bleeding compared with ASA alone (1.5% with UFH plus ASA vs. 0.4% with ASA; RR 1.99, 95% CI 0.52 to 7.65).[11] Mild thrombocytopenia may occur in 10 to 20% of patients who are receiving UFH, whereas significant thrombocy-topenia (platelet count <100,000) occurs in 1 to 5% of patients and typically appears after 4 to 14 days of therapy.[2] The rare (less than 0.2% incidence) heparin-induced thrombocytopenia (HIT) syndrome can occur both shortly after initiation of UFH or, rarely, in a delayed period (i.e., after 5 to 19 days or more).[2] *Practical Applications:* Because of the inconsistency of the results of UFH on patients with ACS and with the availability of LMWH (which is much more user-friendly by subcutaneous injection), the role of UFH is relegated to the rare situation in which there is a need for quickly reversing the effect of UFH by protamine, such as in the case of urgent PCI for ACS patients with active or high risk of bleeding.

How to Give Unfractionated Heparin

The recommended weight-adjusted regimen is to give an initial bolus of 60 U per kg (maximum 4000 U) and an initial infusion of 12 U per kg per hour (maximum 1000 U per h) in order to achieve an aPTT between 60 and 80 seconds. Measurements of aPTT should be made 6 hours after any dosage change and used to adjust UFH infusion. When two consec-utive aPTT values are therapeutic, the measurements may be made every 24 hours. In addition, a significant change in the patient's clinical con-dition (e.g., recurrent ischemia, bleeding, or hypotension) should prompt an immediate aPTT determination, followed by dose adjustment if nec-essary. Serial hemoglobin/hematocrit and platelet measurements are rec-ommended at least daily during UFH therapy to detect HIT.[2]

Beta Blockers

Reducing myocardial oxygen demand by decreasing heart rate and car-diac contractility, beta blockers are competitive antagonists to cate-cholamines. Evidences for the beneficial effects in the use of beta blockers (BBs) in patients with UA is based on limited RCT data done in the 1980s along with pathophysiologic considerations and extrapolation from experience with stable CAD or compensated chronic HF patients.[2]

 BENEFITS, HARMS, AND COST-EFFECTIVENESS ANALYSIS:

Beta Blockade in ACS

Methodology: There were two RCTs. The first RCT (338 people with at rest angina who were not already receiving a BB) compared nifedipine, metoprolol, or both versus placebo.[12] The second RCT (81 people with UA on optimal doses of nitrates and nifedipine) com-pared propranolol (≥ 160 mg/day) versus placebo.[13] *Results:* The first RCT found that metoprolol significantly reduced the composite outcome of recurrent angina and MI within 48 hours compared with nifedipine (28% with metoprolol vs. 47% with nifedipine; RR 0.66,

95% CI 0.43 to 0.98). The second RCT found no significant difference in the combined outcome of death, myocardial infarction, and requirement for CABG or PCI at 30 days (38% with propranolol vs. 46% with placebo; RR 0.83, 95% CI 0.44 to 1.30). *Harms:* Early aggressive IV beta blockade poses a substantial net hazard in hemodynamically unstable patients and could cause cardiogenic shock.[2] *Practical Applications:* There was a moderate net benefit for the ACS patients who were relatively stable and at low risk of shock. BBs are recommended to be initiated orally in the absence of contraindications (HF), within the first 24 hours.[2] Beta blockers without intrinsic sympathomimetic activity are preferred. Agents studied in the acute setting include metoprolol, propranolol, and atenolol, while carvedilol was studied in post-MI patients.

Contraindications of BBs

Patients with marked first-degree AV block (PR interval greater than 0.24 s), any form of second- or third-degree AV block in the absence of a functioning implanted pacemaker, a history of asthma, severe LV dysfunction with HF (e.g., rales or S3 gallop) or at high risk for shock (older age, female sex, time delay, higher Killip class, lower blood pressure, higher heart rate, ECG abnormality, and previous hypertension) should not receive BBs on an acute basis.[14] Patients with evidence of a low-output state (oliguria), sinus tachycardia, (which often reflects low stroke volume), significant sinus bradycardia (heart rate less than 50 beats per min), or hypotension (systolic blood pressure less than 90 mm Hg) should not receive acute BB therapy until these conditions have resolved.

Nitroglycerin

Nitroglycerin (NTG) not only vasodilates coronary arteries but also promotes coronary collateral flow and decreases cardiac preload. Although these effects have not been shown to decrease death or MI, NTG can clearly relieve the angina symptom. NTG tolerance can, however, occur in as little as 24 hours, such that patients might require a NTG-free interval or increased doses of intravenous NTG. The rationale for NTG use in ACS is extrapolated from pathophysiologic principles and extensive, although uncontrolled, clinical observations.[2]

Lipid-Lowering Drugs

As plaque rupture is the initial phase of thrombotic formation in ACS, plaque stabilization is the main treatment that turns off the disease process. Besides their role in lowering cholesterol levels, statin drugs seem able to stabilize the coronary plaques as the reduction in coronary events appears out of proportion to the degree of CAD regression. The benefit of early initiation of statin therapy during ACS occurs as early as in the first 30 days.[14]

EVIDENCE-BASED MEDICINE:

THE PROVE IT TIMI 22 Trial

Methodology: A total of 4162 patients with ACS were recruited in the Pravastatin or Atorvastatin Evaluation and Infection therapy-Thrombolysis in Myocardial Infarction -22 (PROVE IT TIMI 22) trial. Patients were randomized to intensive statin therapy (atorvastatin, 80 mg) or standard therapy (pravastatin, 40 mg). The composite triple endpoint of death, MI, or rehospitalization for recurrent ACS was determined in each group at 30 days. The composite triple and primary endpoints were assessed in stable patients from six months to the end of the study, after censoring for clinical events before six months. *Results:* The composite endpoint at 30 days occurred in 3.0% of patients receiving atorvastatin 80 mg versus 4.2% of patients receiving pravastatin 40 mg (hazard ratio [HR] = 0.72; 95% CI, 0.52 to 0.99; P = 0.046). In stable patients, atorvastatin 80 mg was associated with a composite event rate of 9.6% versus 13.1% in the pravastatin 40 mg group (HR = 0.72; 95% CI, 0.58 to 0.89; P = 0.003). *Cost-Effectiveness Analysis:* The NNT (number of patients needed to treat) to prevent one death was 84 patients.[15] *Practical Applications:* Intensive statin therapy early after ACS leads to a reduction in clinical events at 30 days, consistent with its greater early pleiotropic effects. In stable patients, intensive statin therapy provides long-term reduction in clinical events when compared with standard therapy. Thus, intensive statin therapy should be started in-hospital and continued almost indefinitely for ACS patients.

ADVANCED MANAGEMENT

Detection

Identification of High Risk ACS Patients with Negative Troponin Levels

In patients with UA when the troponin level is negative, the mortality is low. What is the best way to stratify these patients into lower risk or higher risk? Measuring the BNP may help to solve this problem.

 ## SMART THINKING:

Risk Stratification of Negative Troponin Patients by NT-proBNP

Methodology: There are two registries of 2614 patients from two independent registries, one serving as a derivation cohort comprising patients with evident ACS (Bad Nauheim ACS registry, n=1131) and the other serving as a validation cohort, including chest pain patients (PACS [Prognosis in Acute Coronary Syndromes] registry, n = 1483). NT-proBNP and TnT were measured upon admission. *Results:* The mortality rate was significantly lower among TnT-negative patients: 3.8% versus 8.2% (P = 0.009) in the Bad Nauheim ACS registry, and 2.8% versus 8.6% (P = 0.009) in the PACS registry. Among TnT-negative patients, receiver-operating characteristics curve analysis yielded an optimal cutoff value of 474 pg/mL for NT-proBNP that was able to discriminate patients at higher risk in the Bad Nauheim ACS and PACS registries (mortality rate 12.3% vs. 1.3%, P < 0.001, and 8.5% vs. 1.5%, P < 0.001, respectively). *Practical Applications:* Among ACS patients considered at low risk because of normal troponin values, NT-proBNP above 474 pg/mL is able to discriminate higher risk individuals.[16]

In the Jupiter trial for asymptomatic patients, a low level of C-reactive protein (CRP) would confer a very low level of morbidity and mortality. In patients with chest pain suspected to have UA without positive cardiac enzymes, a low CRP level would confer a low morbidity and mortality. Therefore patients with high NTproBNP or BNP and CRP should be given invasive testing. The patients with equivocal chest pain, low BNP and CRP can have noninvasive testing instead.[17]

Early Invasive or Selective Invasive Strategy

Even with recent improvements in the pharmacologic management of patients with ACS, the rates of death and MI remain quite high. As a result, the role of early coronary angiography and revascularization has been studied. No one would argue the pivotal role of coronary angiography in ACS patients who are refractory to medical therapy or who develop ischemia during a provocative test. However, routine early angiography is more controversial. The high-risk patients who should be considered for early catheterization are listed in Table 15-7. In all other patients, a decision should be based on the patient's risk, the available facilities, and the patient's preference. For women at low risk, a less aggressive strategy yielded a better outcome.[18]

2B3A Glycoprotein Inhibition

Glycoprotein IIb/IIIa inhibitors (PCI) are indicated in patients with ACS who are undergoing an invasive procedure. When is it best to initiate the therapy? Upstream or ad hoc before PCI? *Methodology:* This is a double-blinded RCT in which 9492 patients were randomly assigned to receive either early eptifibatide (two boluses, each containing 180 μg per kilogram of body weight, administered 10 minutes apart, and a standard infusion 12 hours before angiography) or a matching placebo infusion with provisional use of eptifibatide after angiography (delayed eptifibatide). *Results:* The primary endpoint occurred in 9.3% of patients in

> **TABLE 15-7:** High-Risk Features Favoring an Early Invasive Strategy[2]
>
> Recurrent angina/ischemia at rest or with low-level activities despite intensive anti-ischemic therapy
> Elevated troponin level
> New or presumably new ST segment depression
> Recurrent angina/ischemia with symptoms of heart failure, an S3 gallop, pulmonary edema, worsening rales, or new or worsening mitral regurgitation
> High-risk findings on noninvasive stress testing (large defect, increased lung uptake, transient dilation of the ventricle, early STT change, blood pressure decrease during TST, chest pain triggered by exercise)
> Left ventricular systolic dysfunction (ejection fraction <40% on a non-invasive study)
> Hemodynamic instability
> Sustained ventricular tachycardia
> Percutaneous coronary intervention within 6 months
> Prior coronary artery bypass graft surgery

the early eptifibatide group and in 10.0% in the delayed eptifibatide group (odds ratio, 0.92; 95% confidence interval [CI], 0.80 to 1.06; P = 0.23). At 30 days, the rate of death or myocardial infarction was 11.2% in the early eptifibatide group as compared with 12.3% in the delayed eptifibatide group (odds ratio, 0.89; 95% CI, 0.79 to 1.01; P = 0.08). Patients in the early eptifibatide group had significantly higher rates of bleeding and red-cell transfusion. There was no significant difference between the two groups in rates of severe bleeding or nonhemorrhagic serious adverse events. *Practical Applications:* In patients who had ACS without ST segment elevation, the use of eptifibatide 12 hours or more before angiography was not superior to the provisional use of eptifibatide after angiography. The early use of eptifibatide was associated with an increased risk of non–life-threatening bleeding and the need for transfusion. *Subgroup Analysis:* The most rational and evidence-based use of these agents is in the high-risk troponin-positive ACS patient. However, the bleeding risk is also increased, especially when used in conjunction with other antithrombotic agents. GPI is best used for bailout in case of procedural complications (e.g., thrombus). The evidence-base is not robust for either upstream use or for "routine" downstream use during PCI.[19]

Selective use of different levels of platelet inhibition gives the best protection to ACS patients without causing further harm. Low-risk patients in elective PCI benefit the most from a high loading dose of clopidogrel without the need for GPI. Patients with chest pain from progression of stable plaque, without platelet activation, would not benefit from GPI and may even be harmed. Biomarkers such as troponin I (evidence of possible distal platelet embolization), high TIMI risk score, elevated B-type natriuretic peptide level, and ST segment depressions help in identifying the high-risk patients undergoing PCI who benefit the most from GPI.

GFR Calculation to Avoid Drug Overdosing

Many ACS patients who underwent PCI had more bleeding. There is a question of drug overdosing because of the overestimated value of glomerular filtration rate (GFR). *Methodology:* The glomerular filtration rates (eGFRs) were estimated with the Cockcroft-Gault (C-G) and Modification of Diet in Renal Disease (MDRD) formulae in 46,942 non-ST elevation ACS patients from 408 CRUSADE (Can Rapid risk stratification of Unstable angina patients Suppress ADverse outcomes with Early implementation of the American College of Cardiology/American Heart Association Guidelines) hospitals. Formula agreement was shown continuously and by chronic kidney disease (CKD) stages. The in-hospital outcomes and the association between antithrombotic dose adjustment and bleeding for moderate CKD as determined by each formula were calculated. *Results:* The median (interquartile range [IQR]) eGFR was 53.2 mL/min (34.7, 75.1 mL/min) by C-G and 65.8 mL/min (47.6, 83.5 mL/min) by MDRD. The mean eGFR was higher with MDRD (9.1 mL/min), but this difference was greater in age, weight, and gender subgroups. Chronic kidney disease classification differed in 20% of the population and altered when antithrombotic dose adjustment was required by C-G versus MDRD (eptifibatide: 45.7% vs. 27.3%; enoxaparin: 19.0% vs. 9.6%). *Practical Applications:* Important CKD disagreements occur in 20% of ACS patients, affecting dosing adjustments in those already susceptible to bleeding. Dosing based on the Cockcroft-Gault formula is preferable, particularly in the small, female, or elderly patient.[20]

Timing of Invasive Intervention

Is early invasive management—angiography within 24 hours followed by PCI or CABG as appropriate—safe in patients with ACS? Overall does it have the same impact on the risk of death, new MI, or stroke compared with a delayed invasive strategy?

 EVIDENCE-BASED MEDICINE:

The TIMACS Trial

Question: Should patients with ACS (stratified at risk by the Global Registry of Acute Coronary Events [GRACE] scores) get early invasive management or not? *Methodology:* This is an RCT of >3000 patients with ACS who were "suitable" for revascularization to early (angiography as soon as possible within 24 hours, followed by PCI

TABLE 15-8: Rates of Death, MI, or Stroke Within Six Months According to GRACE Risk Level and HR (95% CI), Early vs. Delayed

Risk Level by GRACE Score*	Early (%)	Delayed (%)	HR (95% CI)	P
Low/intermediate (n = 2070)	7.7	6.7	1.14 (0.82-1.58)	0.43
High (n = 961)	14.1	21.6	0.65 (0.48-0.88)	0.005

*Low/intermediate risk = GRACE score <140; high risk = GRACE score ≥140.

or CABG) or delayed (any time after 36 hours, followed by PCI or CABG) invasive management. The median times to angiography were 14 hours and 50 hours, respectively. *Results:* The rates of primary composite endpoint (death, new MI, or stroke within six months) in the two groups of early or late interventions were similar, at 9.7% and 11.7%, respectively. The rates of major bleeding during the index hospitalization were 3.1% and 3.5%, respectively. *Harms:* No significant difference between the early and late strategies in rate of major bleeding was observed. *Cost-Effectiveness Analysis:* If there is an available catheterization laboratory and other resources are in place, the patient can undergo early angiography. This strategy might reduce the patient's length of stay and lower the cost. *Practical Applications:* Patients with ACS can be managed safely with either an early or a delayed invasive strategy. In the subset of patients at highest risk, early intervention appears to be superior. In all other patients with ACS, the decision regarding the timing depends on other factors, such as the availability of catheterization laboratories, the health care system environment, convenience, and economic considerations[21] (Table 15-8).

Revascularization in ACS Patients with CHF

Patients with non–ST-elevation ACS complicated by congestive heart failure (CHF) have a poor prognosis. The aim of the GRACE registry was to describe the use of revascularization and its impact on survival in this population.

 SMART THINKING:

Revascularization in ACS patients with HF in the GRACE Registry

Methodology: This is a registry of 29,844 patients with non–ST-elevation ACS. A total of 4953 patients had CHF at presentation:

20% of the patients with CHF underwent revascularization versus 35% of those without CHF (P < 0.001). **Results:** Hospital rates were not affected by revascularization (adjusted hazard ratio 0.97, 95% confidence interval 0.72 to 1.33, P = 0.87). Death from discharge to six-month follow-up was lower in patients who underwent revascularization than in those who did not (odds ratio 0.51, 95% CI 0.35 to 0.74, P < 0.001). This difference persisted after adjustment for GRACE risk score variables, country, and propensity for revascularization (odds ratio 0.58, 95% CI 0.40 to 0.85, P = 0.005). When revascularization as a time-varying covariate was taken into account in an adjusted Cox model regression, the rate of death was again lower in patients undergoing revascularization (hazard ratio 0.64, 95% CI 0.45 to 0.93, P = 0.02). **Practical Applications:** This observational study suggests a low use of in-hospital revascularization in non–ST-elevation ACS patients with CHF. The consistent reduction in postdischarge deaths suggests that broader application of revascularization in this high-risk group may be beneficial.[22]

Prevention of a New Myocardial Infarction

Without adequate medical and mechanical intervention, 25% of patients with ACS would develop non-Q MI. In order to prevent new MI, ASA, BBs, and statin drugs are the main medications. Stopping smoking is a must because smoking causes fissuring of vulnerable plaque. Lowering LDL cholesterol below 75 mg/dL is another goal to be obtained. Counseling on a low-salt and low-cholesterol diet should be reinforced regularly as well as exercise. Avoiding all unaccustomed strenuous activities, which are sudden, strenuous, and prolonged and that patients are not used to doing on a daily basis—such as shoveling snow, moving furniture, long and strenuous yard work—is recommended. What about sexual activity? Is it an unaccustomed strenuous activity?[23] The data of the Swedish trial showed that there was an increased risk of MI after sexual activity, especially among the less physically fit. However, sexual activities do not trigger MI if couples do not abstain or practice on a regular basis >2 times a week[23] (Table 15-9).

TABLE 15-9: Measures to Prevent Acute Myocardial Infarction

ASA and/or clopidogrel	(Compliance with medications)
Beta blockers every day	(Compliance with medications)
Cholesterol-lowering drug	(Compliance with medications)
Exercise every day	
No unscheduled strenuous activities	
Stop smoking	
Control diabetes	

Comprehensive Care

In order to overcome the acute phase of ACS, patients need a comprehensive care plan, which includes medication, mechanical revascularization if needed, change in diet, changes in lifestyle, and increased exercise. Once the unstable condition of ACS is converted into a more controlled and stable coronary artery disease (CAD) condition, oral medication is the next line of long-term medical intervention. Usually, these patients have to take many other medications either for CAD, DM, hypercholesterolemia, arthritis, congestive heart failure, or chronic obstructive pulmonary disease. Therefore some patients feel that they are overmedicated and/or many cannot afford to pay for all these drugs. In these situations, many patients rebel by stopping some or all medications. We have to try to explain to patients the importance of each cardiovascular drug and the reason why that particular drug should be taken and not missed, which medications the patients can omit, and when, why, and whether they can be exchanged for something else. In order to emphasize the importance of each modality and its priority rank of a comprehensive care program, we give the patient a set of seven questions asking the reasons and the importance ranking of the medications or modalities of treatment. The desired importance and priority (necessity) ranking are shown in Table 15-10.[24]

The answer to question 1 is ASA, because it is the agent to block the first step of the coagulation cascade: platelet aggregation. It is also universally affordable. The indication for ASA is nearly absolute, except

TABLE 15-10: Priority Rank of Different Medications or Modalities of Treatment

Question	Answer
If you can afford to buy only one medication to take every day, which one should you buy?	ASA
If you can afford to buy a second medication to take every day, which one should you buy?	Thienopyridines
If you can afford to buy a third medication every day, which one should you buy?	Beta blocker
Which is the next most important modality of treatment?	Low-cholesterol diet
Which one is the next most important modality of treatment?	Exercise
Which one is the next most important medication?	Cholesterol-lowering drug
Which one is the next optional modality of treatment?	PCI or CABG

for rare contraindication or intolerance. The second most important medication for ACS is clopidogrel. It should be taken for nine months as suggested in the CURE trial, or one month after BMS stenting, or >1 year after DES stenting. Premature discontinuation of clopidogrel in a patient receiving DES could cause early thrombosis of the stent, resulting in AMI and mortality. The answer to question 3 is a BB because it decreases mortality and prevents MI and hospital readmission in patients with LV dysfunction.[24]

The answer to question 4 is a low-cholesterol diet. We don't think a patient with CAD should take cholesterol-lowering drugs without trying a low-cholesterol diet first. Then, after failure to achieve a low LDL level of 75 mg/dL (which happens most of the time), the patient should be given cholesterol-lowering medication. In the case of ACS, statins should be given to patients even without looking at the cholesterol level because of their anti-inflammatory effects (even before a fasting lipid profile is done). Adherence to a low-salt and a low-cholesterol diet would help to curb obesity, another strong and stubborn risk factor for ACS.[24]

TROUBLE-SHOOTING AND DEBUGGING

In caring for patients with ACS, every physician has to adhere to the evidence-based guidelines for treatment. However, the more complex problems and the more esoteric questions require the expertise of a consultant cardiologist.

What Causes False Elevation of Troponin Level?

Because cTnT and cTnI generally are not detected in the blood of healthy persons, the cutoff values for elevated cTnT and cTnI levels are set to slightly above the upper limit of the performance characteristics of the assay for a normal healthy population.[25]

Although troponin accurately identifies myocardial necrosis, it can be elevated by other noncoronary causes, such as tachyarrhythmia, cardiac trauma by interventions, chest trauma from motor vehicle accidents, HF, LV hypertrophy, myocarditis, and pericarditis as well as severe noncardiac conditions such as sepsis, burns, respiratory failure, acute neurologic diseases, pulmonary embolism, pulmonary hypertension, drug toxicity, cancer chemotherapy, and renal insufficiency.[26] Among patients with end-stage renal disease and no clinical evidence of acute myocardial necrosis, 15 to 53% show increased cTnT, but fewer than 10% have increased cTnI; dialysis generally increases cTnT but decreases cTnI.[27] If the patient with CKD has a prior level of troponin, this level could be considered as baseline and any later significantly higher level can label the patient with the diagnosis of ACS.

How to Deal with False-Positive Results Due to Technical Problems

Currently, there are two major commercial immunoassays that measure cTnI levels. The Access System (Beckman Coulter, Fullerton, Calif) uses monoclonal mouse antibodies as both the capture and the conjugate antibodies. The AxSYM system (Abbott Co., Abbott Park, IL) uses monoclonal mouse antibodies as the capture antibody and goat anti-cTnI as the conjugate antibody.[28]

Heterophilic antibodies can cause false-positive cTnI results. The antibodies bind to the capture and the conjugate antibodies, simulating cTnI. Using antibodies from two different species, as in the AxSYM system, might decrease the false positivity due to heterophilic antibodies.[29] Persons with more frequent exposure to animal proteins (such as veterinarians, farmers, and pet owners) can also develop heterophilic antibodies. In a similar fashion, rheumatoid factor can interfere with the immunoassay. Five percent of healthy patients might have circulating rheumatoid factor, and about 1% of patients who have elevated cTnI levels because of the rheumatoid factor.[24]

What Are the Problems and the Scope of ASA Resistance?

Aspirin is well recognized as an effective antiplatelet drug for secondary prevention in subjects at high risk of cardiovascular events. However, most patients receiving long-term aspirin therapy still remain at substantial risk for thrombotic events due to insufficient inhibition of platelets, specifically via the thromboxane A2 pathway. To date, only a limited number of clinical studies have convincingly investigated the importance of aspirin resistance. Of these, few are of a sufficient scale, well designed, and prospective, with aspirin used at standard doses. Also, most studies do not sufficiently address the issue of noncompliance as a frequent but easily preventable cause of resistance to this antiplatelet drug. If there is suspicion of ASA resistance, clopidogrel may be used instead.[30]

What to Use If the Patient Is Allergic to Clopidogrel

Ticlodipine is not widely used in the U.S., unless there are side effects with clopidogrel. An RCT for ticlodipine (652 patients) found that ticlopidine plus conventional treatment significantly reduced the combined outcome of vascular deaths and MI after six months compared with conventional treatment alone (RR 0.5, 95% CI 0.2 to 0.9).[31] Diarrhea, rash, and reversible neutropenia have been reported in 1–2% of people taking ticlopidine.[32] The number of patients who need to be treated (NNT) in order to prevent one major cardiovascular event is 16.

Does a Proton Pump Inhibitor Decrease the Effectiveness of Clopidogrel?

Combination of clopidogrel and omeprazole (or other drugs): Aspirin-clopidogrel antiplatelet dual therapy is widely prescribed worldwide in conjunction with a proton pump inhibitor (PPI) to prevent gastrointestinal bleeding. There are questions about the efficacy of clopidogrel in conjunction with a PPI because PPIs may attenuate clopidogrel's antiplatelet response by interfering with CYP2C19-mediated clopidogrel metabolism. In order to be objective in the assessment of this problem, the exact results of three studies are reported so that readers can judge the studies according to the methodologies used and the outcomes presented. These three studies are the latest in a series of reports with inconsistent results trying to assess the clinical impact of combining the two classes of drugs.

In the first study, clopidogrel activity on platelets was tested by vasodilator-stimulated phosphoprotein (VASP) phosphorylation. *Methodology:* This is a double-blind placebo-controlled trial in which 124 consecutive patients undergoing coronary artery stent implantation received aspirin (75 mg/day) and clopidogrel (loading dose, followed by 75 mg/day) and were randomized to receive either omeprazole (20 mg/day) or placebo for 7 days. Clopidogrel effect was tested on days 1 and 7 in both groups by measuring platelet phosphorylated-VASP expressed as a platelet reactivity index (PRI). The main endpoint compared PRI value at the 7-day treatment period in the two groups. *Results:* Data for 124 patients were analyzed. On day 1, mean PRI was 83.2% (standard deviation [SD] 5.6) and 83.9% (SD 4.6), respectively, in the placebo and omeprazole groups (P = NS), and on day 7, 39.8% (SD 15.4) and 51.4% (SD 16.4), respectively (P < 0.0001). Omeprazole significantly decreased clopidogrel inhibitory effect on platelet P2Y12 as assessed by the VASP phosphorylation test.[33]

The second study is a population-based nested case-control study among patients aged 66 or older who commenced clopidogrel between April 1, 2002 and December 31, 2007 following hospital discharge after treatment of AMI. The cases in our study were those readmitted with AMI within 90 days after discharge. A secondary analysis considering events within one year was performed. Event-free controls (at a ratio of 3:1) were matched to cases on age, PCI, and a validated risk score. *Results:* Among 13,636 patients prescribed clopidogrel following AMI, 734 cases readmitted with MI infarction and 2057 controls were identified. After extensive multivariable adjustment, current use of PPI was associated with an increased risk of reinfarction (OR 1.27, 95% CI 1.03-1.57). There was no association with more distant exposure to PPI or in multiple sensitivity analyses. In a stratified analysis, pantoprazole, which does not inhibit cytochrome P450 2C19, had no association with readmission for MI (adjusted OR 1.02, 95% CI 0.70-1.47). *Interpretation:* Among patients receiving clopidogrel following AMI, concomitant therapy with PPI other than pantoprazole was associated with a loss of the beneficial effects of clopidogrel and an increased risk of reinfarction.[34]

In the third study, recently presented at the Annual Scientific Meeting of the SCAI, the one-year risk of cardiovascular events increased more than 50% in patients taking a PPI on top of clopidogrel as compared with patients not taking a PPI, and the risk seems to be a class effect according to a retrospective cohort study of more than 16,700 patients who received clopidogrel poststenting.

The study compared major adverse CV events among members of the Medco Health Solutions pharmacy and medical claims database. In all, 9862 patients never made a prescription claim for a PPI over the 12 months post-PCI and were classified as having no PPI therapy for the purposes of the study, while 6828 filed prescription claims for a PPI: esomeprazole (Nexium, AstraZeneca), omeprazole, pantoprazole (Protonix, Wyeth), lansoprazole, or rabeprazole (Aciphex, Eisai/Ortho-McNeil-Janssen Pharmaceuticals). Prescription status was then correlated with hospitalization for stroke/TIA, ACS, cardiovascular death, or coronary revascularization based on ICD-9 or CPT-4 codes. The one-year risk of MACE was significantly higher in PPI-treated subjects, at 25.1%, as compared with patients who did not take a PPI, at 17.9% (hazard ratio 1.51; 95% CI 1.39-1.64; P<0.0001). According to investigators, PPI effect was "consistent across subgroups," with no single patient subset being significantly more likely to develop an adverse cardiovascular event.

The hospitalization rates for upper GI bleeding were low across all groups of PPI use, in the range of 1.1%. In patients who were not treated with clopidogrel, there was no increased risk of CV events compared with patients taking neither a PPI nor clopidogrel. The data on concomitant H2-receptor–antagonist therapy showed no effects on CV events. In an analysis of 472 patients taking clopidogrel and an H2 blocker, the incidence of CV events was 20.3% for patients taking H2 blockers and 17.8% in patients not taking these agents, a statistically nonsignificant difference.[35]

How to Explain the Problem of Drug Interaction Between Clopidogrel and Other Drugs

Clopidogrel is a pro-drug and is converted in the liver by the members of the cytochrome P450 (CYP) family (predominantly the 3A and 2C groups) to a series of metabolites, the last of which, the thiol metabolite, is an antagonist of the platelet purinergic receptor known as P2Y12.[36] Although the finding that atorvastatin can interfere with the effect of clopidogrel (probably through competition for CYP3A4)[37] has been replicated in ex vivo studies, other studies dispute the presence of the interaction,[38] and clinical observations from several databases have failed to support the hypothesis that rates of MI or stent thrombosis are elevated among patients treated with atorvastatin and clopidogrel compared to clopidogrel alone.[39] It is theoretically possible that the databases reflect a balance between the effects of atorvastatin in preventing myocardial infarction on the one hand, and its diminishing of the in vivo effect of clopidogrel on the other. However, it is also possible that the degree to which the decreased biologic effect of clopidogrel is not clinically significant and/or that the wrong measure of platelet activity was tested in the ex vivo studies. Another issue, statistical confounding, is also important in interpreting the findings of any study. It is likely that patients with more severe disease (and therefore at high risk) were more likely to receive more drugs (e.g., calcium-channel blockers). It is possible that unmeasured confounders played an important role by increasing platelet activation or decreasing clopidogrel metabolism.[40] *Solutions:* A statement released at the time of the Clopidogrel Medco Outcomes study, the Society of Cardiac Angiography and Interventions (SCAI), notes that, while this particular study is the largest to date to address the question of a PPI-clopidogrel interaction, two other, smaller studies have found disparate results. SCAI believes more research is needed. Recently, the results of the COGENT trial presented at the Transcatheter Therapeutic 2009 in San Francisco showed no differences in CV death and MI between the two groups of ACS patients receiving omeprazole or placebo with dual antiplatelet therapy (clopidogrel and aspirin). However, given the thousands of patients who receive stents each year, SCAI recommends the use of alternative medications for GI symptoms in patients with stents when appropriate. Other effective treatments for heartburn and ulcers include histaminergic (H_2) blockers (Zantac [ranitidine, Boehringer Ingelheim], Tagamet [cimetidine, GlaxoSmithKline]), or antacids.[41]

Is Prasugrel a Promising Drug?

Dual-antiplatelet therapy with ASA and a thienopyridine is the cornerstone in the prevention of MACE for ACS patients. Newer drugs are designed to have better efficacy and lower side effects. Prasugrel is a new antiplatelet drug and was assessed in the RCT that follows. *The TRITON- TIMI 38 Trial Question:* Is prasugrel as good as clopidogrel in patients with ACS undergoing PCI? *Methodology:* This is an RCT in which 13,608 patients with moderate-to-high-risk ACS and being scheduled for PCI were randomly assigned to receive prasugrel (a 60-mg loading dose and a 10-mg daily maintenance dose) or clopidogrel (a 300-mg loading dose and a 75-mg daily maintenance dose) for 6 to 15 months. *Results:* The primary efficacy endpoint occurred in 12.1% of patients receiving clopidogrel and 9.9% of patients receiving prasugrel (HR for prasugrel vs. clopidogrel, 0.81; 95% CI, 0.73 to 0.90; $P < 0.001$). Significant reductions were found in the prasugrel group in the rates of MI (9.7% for clopidogrel vs.

7.4% for prasugrel; P < 0.001), urgent target vessel revascularization (TVR) (3.7% vs. 2.5%; P < 0.001), and stent thrombosis (2.4% vs. 1.1%; P < 0.001). *Harms:* Major bleeding was observed in 2.4% of patients receiving prasugrel and in 1.8% of patients receiving clopidogrel (HR, 1.32; 95% CI, 1.03 to 1.68; P = 0.03). Also greater in the prasugrel group was the rate of life-threatening bleeding (1.4% vs. 0.9%; P = 0.01), including nonfatal bleeding (1.1% vs. 0.9%; HR, 1.25; P = 0.23) and fatal bleeding (0.4% vs. 0.1%; P = 0.002). *Practical Applications:* In patients with ACS being scheduled for PCI, prasugrel therapy was associated with significantly reduced rates of ischemic events, including stent thrombosis, but with an increased risk of major bleeding, including fatal bleeding. The overall mortality was similar between the treatment groups.[42]

What Is the Efficacy and Harm of the New Factor Xa Inhibitor Fondaparinux?

Fondaparinux, a synthetic pentasaccharide, is a factor Xa inhibitor that selectively binds antithrombin and rapidly inhibits factor Xa. The efficacy and risk profile of fondaparinux were assessed in the Organization for the Assessment of Strategies for Ischemic Syndromes (OASIS)-5 trial. The report follows.[43] *The OASIS-5 Trial Question:* When used among patients with ACS, does fondaparinux, a new anticoagulant, prevent more ischemic events and have fewer side effects compared with enoxaparin? *Methodology:* A group of 10,021 patients were randomized to fondaparinux (2.5 mg/day, n = 10,057) or enoxaparin (1.0 mg/kg twice daily). Patients who underwent PCI in the enoxaparin group were to receive UFH if the last dose of study medication was received > 6 hours prior to PCI. The primary analysis was a test for noninferiority between the treatment groups. *Results:* The primary endpoint of death, MI, or refractory ischemia at day 9, occurred in 5.7% of the enoxaparin group and in 5.8% of the fondaparinux group, meeting the prespecified criteria for noninferiority of fondaparinux compared with enoxaparin (hazard ratio [HR] 1.01, 95% CI 0.90-1.13, P = 0.007 for noninferiority). At 30 days, there was no difference in the composite of death, MI, or refractory ischemia (8.0% for fondaparinux vs. 8.6% for enoxaparin, P = NS), but mortality was significantly lower in the fondaparinux group (2.9% vs. 3.5%, P = 0.02), a reduction maintained at six months (5.8% vs. 6.5%, HR 0.89, P = 0.05). Stroke was also lower at six months in the fondaparinux group (1.3% vs. 1.7%, P = 0.04), but there was no difference in MI (6.3% vs. 6.6%, P = NS). The composite endpoint that combined efficacy and safety (death, MI, refractory ischemia, or major bleeding) at 180 days was lower in the fondaparinux group (HR 0.86, P<0.001). *Harms:* Major bleed by day 9 was lower in the fondaparinux group (2.1% vs. 4.1%, HR 0.52,

P < 0.001), as was minor bleed (1.1% vs. 3.2%, P < 0.001) and any bleed (3.3% vs. 7.3%, HR 0.41, p < 0.001). Occurrence of thrombus formation on the catheter during PCI occurred more frequently in the fondaparinux group (n = 29 vs. n = 8, HR 2.99, P=0.08).[43]

Subgroup Analysis: Results were similar across most subgroups. However, in patients age <65 years, no benefit of fondaparinux was observed (composite of death, MI, refractory ischemia, or major bleeding 7.4% for fondaparinux vs. 7.5% for enoxaparin, HR 0.99, P = NS), but benefit was observed in the age > 65 years subgroup (12.1% vs. 15.4%, HR 0.77, P < 0.001). In patients who underwent PCI, there was no difference in death or MI (6.2% for fondaparinux vs. 5.8% for enoxaparin, P = NS), but bleeding was lower in the fondaparinux group (2.3% vs. 5.1%, P<0.001), although it should be noted that 54% of patients in the enoxaparin group also received UFH per protocol.[43] *Practical Applications:* Among patients with non-ST elevation ACS, treatment with fondaparinux was noninferior for the primary composite endpoint of death, MI, or refractory ischemia at day nine compared with treatment with enoxaparin. Additionally, there were significant reductions in major bleeding at 9 days and the secondary endpoint of mortality at 6 months.[43]

PROVOCATIVE DATA Delipidated HDL: A New, Autologous Option for Plaque Regression?

Pre-beta HDL is the most effective form of HDL for lipid removal from arterial plaque via reverse cholesterol transport. Plasma delipidation, through apheresis, converts alpha HDL to pre-beta HDL and may lead to regression of atherosclerosis as demonstrated in a rabbit model. *Question:* Could reinfusion of a patient's own HDL, after it has essentially been stripped of its lipid content, safely increase the proportion of pre-beta HDL in the body? *Methodology:* A group of 28 patients with ACS scheduled for cardiac catheterization were randomized to either HDL delipidation and reinfusion or undelipidated plasma reinfusion. The HDL apheresis/reinfusion procedure was repeated seven times, once per week, and IVUS was performed two weeks after the final procedure. Weekly lipid apheresis/reinfusion schedule was performed according to the protocol from the ApoA-1 Milano (ETC-216, Pfizer) study, which showed improvements in atherosclerotic burden following an infusion regimen of a recombinant HDL mimetic.[44] *Results:* The apheresis procedure increased the proportion of pre-beta HDL (from about 5.6% in the sample to 92.8%) and reduced the proportion of alpha HDL (from about 92.8% of the sample to 20.9%). Associated with the increase in pre-beta HDL was a fivefold rise in cholesterol efflux seen in patients receiving the delipidated plasma versus the control group. All reinfusion sessions were well tolerated, and there was no signal of an adverse biochemical or hemodynamic reaction to therapy. In the exploratory IVUS analyses, reductions in total atheroma volume and in plaque burden were greater in the delipidation group as compared with the control group, although the differences from baseline were not statistically significant—probably due to the small study size. *Practical Applications:* This is a very promising drug.[44]

TAKE-HOME MESSAGE

Data Collecting Collect all the data about the patient's history (of smoking, high-sodium, high-cholesterol diet, alcohol abuse, lack of exercise, HTN, DM, high cholesterol level), family history (of early sudden death due to heart disease, history of early CAD), social history (work and behaviors) and from a complete physical examination (signs of prior stroke, CAD, PAD, carotid murmur, weak peripheral pulses), all of which add weight to the clinical decision-making process.

Data Mining Recommend safe, appropriate, and efficacious investigation (including cardiac enzymes, fasting lipid profile, fasting blood glucose, BUN and creatinine levels, weight, BMI, waist circumferences). An early invasive strategy seems warranted in high-risk patients.

Management Recommend safe, appropriate, and efficacious therapy to maintain the stable health status of the patient over time (low-sodium, low-cholesterol diet, stopping smoking, losing weight, not drinking alcohol, exercising). Patients with UA should be admitted and placed on bed rest with continuous ECG monitoring. All patients should receive regular ASA (160 to 324 mg), clopidogrel, a statin, and UFH or LMWH as soon as possible. If there are no contraindications, BBs should be administered. Patients who fail medical therapy with positive cardiac enzymes or have a positive stress test should have invasive therapy. In intermediate-risk patients, the choice of early conservative or early invasive strategies depends on the physician's experience and the patient's preference. Low-risk women should receive medical treatment first.

Patient-Centered Care Get the patients involved in their own lifestyle modifications to increase compliance with diet, exercise, medication, office visits, and testing in order to provide continuity of care. All patients should receive intensive counseling on risk factor modification (stopping smoking, losing weight, or exercising). Long-term treatment includes ASA, clopidogrel, beta blockers, and a statin drug.

References

1. Approach to the Patient with Chest Pain. In Libby, P., (ed.), Braunwald's Heart Disease, A Textbook of Cardiovascular Medicine. Philadelphia, PA.: Saunders, 2008, pp. 1195-1206.

444 Evidence-Based Cardiology Practice

2. ACC/AHA 2007 Guidelines for the Management of Patients With Unstable Angina/Non–ST-Elevation Myocardial Infarction—Executive Summary. J Am Coll Cardiol. 2007;50;652–726.
3. Dokainish, H., Pillai, M., Murphy, S.A., et al.: TACTICS-TIMI-18 Investigators. Prognostic implications of elevated troponin in patients with suspected acute coronary syndrome but no critical epicardial coronary diseasea TACTICS-TIMI-18 substudy. J Am Coll Cardiol. 2005;45:19–24.
4. Iskandrian A. Evaluating the Standard of Care in CAD Diagnosis at http://www.medscape.com/infosite/cardiodx/article-4 (accessed 5/9/2009).
5. Data from Sarawak General Hospital, personal communication. Sim kui Hian MD, 5/2009.
6. Antman, E. M., Cohen, M., Bernink, P. J., et al.: The TIMI risk score for unstable angina/non-ST elevation MI: A method for prognostication and therapeutic decision making. JAMA. 2000; 284:835–842.
7. Antithrombotic Trialists' Collaboration. Collaborative meta-analysis of randomised trials of antiplatelet therapy for prevention of death, myocardial infarction, and stroke in high risk patients. BMJ. 2002;324: 71–86.
8. Yusuf, S., Zhao, F., Mehta, S., et al.: The Clopidogrel in Unstable angina to prevent Recurrent Events (CURE) trial. N Engl J Med. 2001;345: 494–502.
9. Cohen, M., Demers, C., Gurfinkel, E. P., et al. and the ESSENCE study group: A Comparison of Low-Molecular-Weight Heparin with Unfractionated Heparin for Unstable Coronary Artery Disease. N Engl J Med. 1997;337:447–452.
10. Eikelboom, J. W., Anand, S. S., Malmberg, K., et al.: Unfractionated heparin and low molecular weight heparin in acute coronary syndrome without ST elevation: a meta-analysis. Lancet. 2000;355:1936–1942.
11. Oler, A., Whooley, M. A., Oler, J., et al.: Adding heparin to aspirin reduces the incidence of myocardial infarction and death in patients with unstable angina: a meta-analysis. JAMA. 1996;276:811–815.
12. Gottlieb, S. O., Weisfeldt, M. L., Ouyang, P., et al.: Effect of the addition of propranolol to therapy with nifedipine for unstable angina pectoris: a randomized, double-blind, placebo-controlled trial. Circulation. 1986;73:331–337.
13. HINT Research Group. Early treatment of unstable angina in the coronary care unit: a randomized, double blind, placebo controlled comparison of recurrent ischaemia in patients treated with nifedipine or metoprolol or both. Br Heart J. 1986;56:400–413.
14. Chen, Z. M., Pan, H. C., Chen, Y. P., for the COMMIT (Clopidogrel and Metoprolol in Myocardial Infarction Trial) collaborative group. Early intravenous then oral metoprolol in 45,852 patients with acute myocardial infarction: randomised placebo-controlled trial. Lancet. 2005;366(9497):1587–1589.
15. Kausik, K. R., Cannon C. P., McCabe, C. H., et al. for the PROVE IT TIMI 22 Investigators: Early and Late Benefits of High-Dose Atorvastatin in Patients With Acute Coronary Syndromes J Am Coll Cardiol. 2005; 46:1405–1410.

16. Weber, M., Bazzino, O., Navarro Estrada, J. L. et al.: N-terminal B-type natriuretic peptide assessment provides incremental prognostic information in patients with acute coronary syndromes and normal troponin T values upon admission. J Am Coll Cardiol. 2008; 51(12): 1188–1195.

17. Ridker, P. M., Danielson, E., Fonseca, F. A. H., et al., for the JUPITER Study Group: Rosuvastatin to prevent vascular events in men and women with elevated C-reactive protein. N Engl J Med. 2008;359: 2195–2207.

18. O'Donoghue, M., Boden, W. E., Braunwald, E., et al.: Early invasive vs conservative treatment strategies in women and men with unstable angina and non-ST segment elevation myocardial infarction: a meta-analysis. JAMA. 2008 2;300(1):71–80.

19. Giugliano, R. P., White, J. A., Bode, C., et al.: Early versus delayed provisional eptifibatide in acute coronary syndromes. N Eng J Med. 2009 360:2176–2190.

20. Melloni, C., Peterson, E. D., Chen, A. Y.: Cockcroft-Gault Versus Modification of Diet in Renal Disease: Importance of Glomerular Filtration Rate Formula for Classification of Chronic Kidney Disease in Patients with Non–ST Segment Elevation Acute Coronary Syndromes. J Am Coll Cardiol. 2008;51:991–996.

21. Mehta, S. R., et al.: Randomized comparison of early vs delayed invasive strategies in high risk patients with non-ST segment elevation acute coronary syndromes: Main results of the Timing of Intervention in Acute Coronary Syndromes (TIMACS) Trial. N Eng J Med. 2009;360: 2165–2175.

22. Philippe Gabriel Steg, P. G., Kerner, A., de Werf, F. V., for the Global Registry of Acute Coronary Events (GRACE) Investigators: Impact of In-Hospital Revascularization on Survival in Patients With Non–ST-Elevation Acute Coronary Syndrome and Congestive Heart Failure Circulation. 2008;118:1163–1171.

23. Möller, J., Ahlbom, A., Hulting, J.: Sexual activity as a trigger of myocardial infarction. A case-crossover analysis in the Stockholm Heart Epidemiology Programme (SHEEP). Heart. 2001;86(4):387–390.

24. Nguyen, T., Tan, H. C., Agarwal, B., et al.: Acute coronary syndrome. Boston: Blackwell Futura, 2007, pp. 1–49.

25. Coudrey, L.: The troponins. Arch Intern Med. 1998;158:1173–1180.

26. Bonnefoy, E., Godon, P., Kirkorian, G., et al.: Serum cardiac troponin I and ST segment elevation in patients with acute pericarditis. Eur Heart J. 2000;21:1832–1836.

27. Heeschen, C., Goldmann, B. U., Moeller, R. H., et al.: Analytical performance and clinical application of a new rapid bedside assay for the detection of serum cardiac troponin I. Clin Chem. 1998;44: 1925–1930.

28. Volk, A. L., Hardy, R., Robinson, C. A., et al.: False-positive cardiac troponin I results–Two case reports. Lab Med. 1999;30:610–612.

29. Fitzmaurice, T. F., Brown, C., Rifai, N., et al.: False increase of cardiac troponin I with heterophilic antibodies. Clin Chem. 1998;44:2212–2214.

30. Gasparyan, A. Y., Watson, T., Lip, G., et al.: The role of aspirin in cardiovascular prevention implications of aspirin resistance. J Am Coll Cardiol. 2008;51:1829–1843.

31. Balsano, F., Rizzon, P., Violi, F., et al., and the Studio della Ticlopidina nell'Angina Instabile Group: Antiplatelet treatment with ticlopidine in unstable angina: a controlled multicentre clinical trial. Circulation. 1990;82:17–26.

32. Gurbel, P. A., Bliden, K. P., Hayes, K. M., et al.: The relation of dosing to clopidogrel responsiveness and the incidence of high post-treatment platelet aggregation in patients undergoing coronary Stenting. JACC. 2005;49:1392–1396.

33. Gilard, M., Arnaud, B., Cornily, J. C., et al.: Influence of Omeprazole on the Antiplatelet Action of Clopidogrel Associated With Aspirin The Randomized, Double-Blind OCLA (Omeprazole CLopidogrel Aspirin) Study, Am Coll Cardiol, 2008;51:256–260.

34. Lau, W. C., Gurbel, P. A.: The drug–drug interaction between proton pump inhibitors and clopidogrel. Canadian Association Medical Journal. 2009;180:699–700.

35. Stanek, E. J.: Results of the Clopidogrel Medco Outcomes study at a late-breaking clinical trial during the first day of the Society for Cardiovascular Angiography and Interventions. (SCAI). 2009 Scientific Sessions.

36. Savi, P., Pereillo, J. M., Uzabiaga, M. F., et al.: Identification and biological activity of the active metabolite of clopidogrel. Thromb Haemost. 2000;84:891–896.

37. Lau, W. C., Waskell, L. A., Watkins, P. B., et al.: Atorvastatin reduces the ability of clopidogrel to inhibit platelet aggregation: a new drug-drug interaction. Circulation. 2003;107:32–37.

38. Saw, J., Steinhubl, S. R., Berger, P. B., et al.: Lack of adverse clopidogrel-atorvastatin clinical interaction from secondary analysis of a randomized, placebo-controlled clopidogrel trial. Circulation. 2003;108:921–924.

39. Lotfi, A., Schweiger, M. J., Giugliano, G. R., et al.: High-dose atorvastatin does not negatively influence clinical outcomes among clopidogrel treated acute coronary syndrome patients—a Pravastatin or Atorvastatin Evaluation and Infection Therapy-Thrombolysis in Myocardial Infarction 22 (PROVE IT TIMI 22) analysis. Am Heart J. 2008;155:954–958.

40. Kleiman, N. S.: Clopidogrel and calcium-channel antagonists another drug–drug interaction for the ever-wary clinician? J Am Coll Cardiol. 2008;52:1564–1566.

41. http://www.medscape.com/viewarticle/589083 (Accessed 6/7/2009).

42. Wiviott, S. D., Braunwald, E., McCabe, C. H., and the TRITON-TIMI 38 Investigators: Prasugrel versus clopidogrel in patients with acute coronary syndromes. N Engl J Med. 2007; 357:2001–2015.

43. OASIS-5 Investigators: Comparison of fondaparinux and enoxaparin in acute coronary syndromes. N Engl J Med. 2006;354.

44. http://www.medscape.com/viewarticle/574643 (Accessed 6/7/2009).

Prehospital Management of Acute ST Segment Elevation Myocardial Infarction

CHAPTER

16

*Marko Noc, Peter Radsel,
Nguyen Ngoc Quang, Tom Ploj,
Pham Gia Khai, and Nguyen Lan Viet*

Chapter Outline

INTRODUCTION

Prompt diagnosis of acute ST segment elevation myocardial infarction (STEMI) followed by immediate reperfusion is a crucial step in reducing hospital morbidity and mortality. The presence of typical chest discomfort and the STEMI pattern in the electrocardiogram (ECG) usually indicate transmural ischemia due to acute occlusion of a major coronary artery in the absence of adequate collateral flow to distal vessels.

Strategic Programming

The first step is to identify patients with STEMI through data collecting with a short and focused exam in order to find the clinical signs or symptoms requiring intermediate attention and correction of any abnormality, if needed. The next step is to perform an electrocardiogram (ECG) (data processing) in order to formulate a preliminary diagnosis and a short list of differential diagnoses (conditions mimicking STEMI, such as aortic dissection, myocarditis, pericarditis or impending stroke, acute abdomen, gallbladder or pancreas problem, or pulmonary embolism). Then, using the method of data mining, tests may be ordered (e.g., troponin level, coronary angiography) in order to confirm (data converting) the main diagnosis of STEMI and to rule out (data filtering) the differential diagnoses.

DATA COLLECTING

Physical Examination

The history interview and the physical examination in a patient with ST segment elevation are used to confirm the diagnosis of AMI so the patient can receive medical or mechanical reperfusion as quickly as possible. Factors requiring immediate attention are listed in Table 16-1.

Risk Stratification

Other factors suggesting a poor prognosis in general are as follows: advanced age, female gender, high white blood cell count, anemia, diabetes mellitus, high brain natriuretic peptid level, and chronic kidney disease (CKD).

TABLE 16-1: Factors Requiring Immediate Attention and Correction

Hypotension (blood pressure <100 mm Hg)
Sinus tachycardia (heart rate >100 BPM)
Persistent chest pain
Persistent ST segment elevation
Congestive heart failure

FORMULA TO MEMORIZE:

Which STEMI Patient Will Not Die in the Next 24 Hours?

In patients with STEMI, if the heart rate is below 100 beats per minute (BPM) and the blood pressure is above 100 mm Hg, the chance of the patient's dying in the near future is low.

Mortality is low if:
   Heart Rate < 100 BPM
   Blood Pressure > 100 mm Hg

These patients may develop ischemia or reinfarction but mortality is still minimal in the next 24 hours.[1] A very low heart rate (<50 BPM) might be detrimental because it can represent advanced atrioventricular blockage or agonal rhythm.[2]

DATA MINING (WORK-UP)
Electrocardiogram

Because 12-lead electrocardiography (ECG) is the cornerstone of the STEMI diagnosis, it should be recorded as soon as possible at the first medical contact.[3] It is important to emphasize that it is the initial ECG that dictates the treatment of patients with suspected acute coronary syndrome (ACS) and especially the need for acute reperfusion if ST segment elevation or new left bundle branch block (LBBB) is present. Cardiac enzymes, including cardiac-specific troponin, are often normal at the early stage of evolving STEMI and usually serve as early risk-stratification in patients with non–ST-elevation ACS.

Electrocardiographic Patterns in STEMI

The initial ECG is diagnostic of acute myocardial infarction (AMI) in approximately 50% of patients, abnormal but nondiagnostic in about 40% of patients, and normal in 10% of patients. Normal or atypical initial ECG in a patient with evolving STEMI may be due to the absence of ischemia at the time of recording, to spontaneous reperfusion, a delay in evolution in the typical pattern, an initially small infarct that becomes electrocardiographically visible only after extension, or involvement of ECG silent areas. However, it is important to emphasize that serial ECG tracings increase sensitivity of this examination to more than 90%. Such serial recordings are also very useful in patients with on-and-off chest discomfort.

Because the ECG lead reflects electrical activity of a particular part of the myocardium, location of ST elevation also pinpoints the affected coronary artery. It is important to realize that ST elevation in leads adjacent to the myocardium with transmural ischemia is usually also reflected as reciprocal ST depression in contralateral leads. However, precise anatomic location of occlusion based on ECG pattern is not always possible because of factors such as relationship and distance between the heart and electrode, individual differences in coronary anatomy, and site of coronary occlusion. It is the urgent coronary angiography that definitely determines the site and morphology of the suspected occlusion, the size and territory of the affected vessel, the degree of anterograde coronary the flow, and the presence of collateral flow distal to the occlusion.

⊙ DATA DECODING TIPS (CLINICAL PEARLS)
Earliest ECG Changes During AMI

The earliest change of the ECG during STEMI is the widening of the QRS complex due to the delay of the ascending branch of the R wave. This is a result of ischemia in the right side of the septum. The second subtle change in the ECG is the fusion of the ascending branch of the T wave into the QRS complex.

DATA CONVERTING (FORMULATING A DIAGNOSIS)

There is general agreement between leads with ST elevation and the affected coronary artery. ST elevation in precordial leads (V1-V4) usually reflects anteroseptal ischemia related to the occlusion of the left descending coronary artery (LAD) (Figure 16-1).

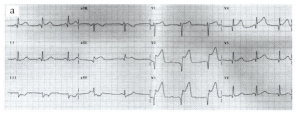

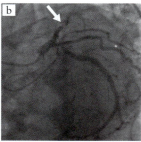

Figure 16-1 Anteroseptal STEMI (ST elevation in V1-V4) (A) due to acute thrombotic occlusion of the LAD (B, arrow).

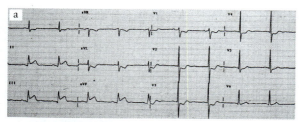

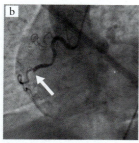

Figure 16-2 Inferior STEMI (ST elevation in II, III, aVF) (A) due to occlusion of the RCA (B, arrow). There is also evidence of some ST depression in precordial leads due to transmural ischemia of the posterior wall supplied by the posterolateral branch of the occluded dominant RCA.

ST elevation in inferior leads (ll, lll, aVF) argues for involvement of the inferior wall due to occlusion of a right coronary artery (RCA) or a dominant left circumflex artery (LCX) proximal to the origin of the posterior descending artery (Figure 16-2).

ST elevation in leads l, aVL, and V4-6 reflects the lateral wall supplied by either a proximal diagonal branch from the LAD, a marginal branch from the LCX, or the Ramus intermedius (Figure 16-3).

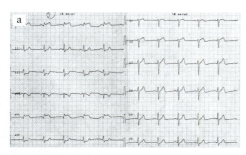

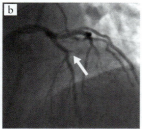

Figure 16-3 Lateral STEMI (ST elevation in l, aVL) (A) due to occlusion of the large first diagonal branch (B, arrow).

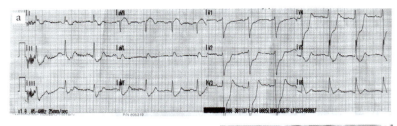

Figure 16-4 Posterior STEMI (ST depression in leads V1-V4) (A) due to occlusion of the midportion of the LCX (B, arrow).

Isolated transmural posterior ischemia is usually demonstrated only as ST depression rather than elevation in leads V1-V4 and is caused by occlusion of dominant RCA or dominant LCX proximal to the posterior left ventricular branch (Figure 16-4). This is a reciprocal phenomenon related to the posterior wall transmural ischemia. It is important to notice that a similar ECG may be obtained in a patient with subendocardial rather than transmural ischemia in the LAD territory. A recording with the ECG leads in the back could show ST segment elevation.

In the real world, different ECG patterns with ST elevation often combine. As previously discussed, this depends on individual variations in coronary anatomy and the site of occlusion, which may be located in the proximal, mid- or distal part of the vessel. For example, proximal occlusion of a large LAD prior to the origin of a large first diagonal branch will result in ST elevation in the anterior and lateral leads (Figure 16-5).

If the LAD goes around the apex of the left ventricle and ends as a posterior descending artery, ST elevation may be present not only in the precordial but also in the inferior leads. Occlusion of dominant RCA before the crux or of dominant LCX before the origin of the posterolateral branch will result in ST elevation in the inferior leads as well as ST depression in leads V2-V4 (Figure 16-6).

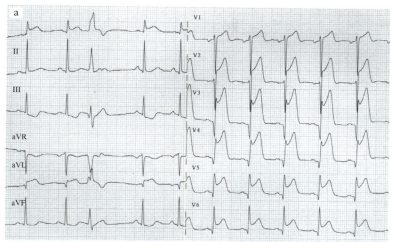

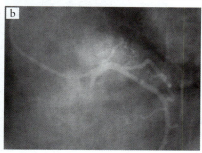

Figure 16-5 Large anteroseptal and lateral STEMI (ST elevation in all precordial leads as well as in I and aVL) (A) due to the ostial occlusion of LAD (B, arrow).

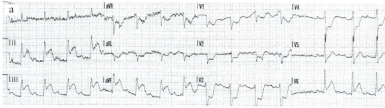

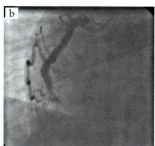

Figure 16-6 Large inferior, posterior, and lateral STEMI (ST elevation in II, III, aVF, V5-6; ST depression in V2-4) (A) due to acute occlusion of dominant RCA (B, arrow) supplying large descending posterior and posterolateral branches.

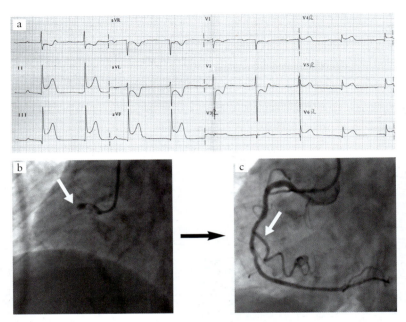

Figure 16-7 Right ventricular STEMI (ST elevation in V4R-V6R) in a patient with concomitant inferior and posterior left ventricular infarction (A) due to proximal RCA occlusion (B, arrow). After reestablishment of anterograde flow by PPCI, a large acute marginal branch responsible for right ventricular involvement was seen (C, arrow).

STEMI of the Right Ventricle

STEMI involving the free wall of the right ventricle (RV) may be caused by occlusion of the RCA proximal to the origin of a significant RV branch, unless there is adequate collateral flow, predominantly from the LAD territory. Right ventricular infarction is therefore usually associated with inferior left ventricular infarction. Isolated RV infarction is rare and may be caused by acute occlusion of the nondominant RCA supplying only the RV free wall. RV infarction is diagnosed by the presence of ST elevation in the right precordial leads and especially V4R (Figure 16-7). The sensitivity and specificity of ST elevation in this lead alone have been estimated as between 82% and 100% and between 68% and 77%, respectively. Since ST elevation in right precordial leads is the most reliable sign of concomitant RV involvement, it is reasonable to record these leads in every patient with evolving inferior STEMI.[4, 5]

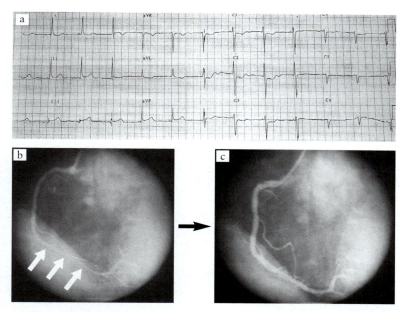

Figure 16-8 ST elevation in inferior leads (II,III, aVF) and ST depression in precordial leads (V1-V3) (A) associated with typical chest discomfort which minimally presents at the time of urgent coronary angiography. Coronary spasm with preserved anterograde flow was documented in the distal part of RCA (B, arrow). Following intracoronary injection of nitroglycerin, chest discomfort completely resolved and the ECG normalized. Repeat RCA injection revealed patent RCA without any evidence of spasm (C). A diagnosis of Prinzmetal angina was therefore established, and the patient was treated with a long-acting nitrate and a calcium channel blocker.

DATA FILTERING (DIFFERENTIAL DIAGNOSES)

ECG Changes Simulating STEMI

STEMI patterns with or without concomitant chest discomfort may also be documented in conditions other than acute coronary occlusion. Such conditions include vasospastic Prinzmetal angina (Figure 16-8), acute myopericarditis (Figure 16-9), stress cardiomyopathy (Figure 16-10), left ventricular aneurysm, hypertrophic cardiomyopathy, acute cor pulmonale, myocardial infiltrative diseases, hyperkalemia, cerebrovascular accidents, and cocaine abuse. In African-American young men, the most common cause of ST elevation is so-called early depolarization (or high J point elevation), which is a normal physiologic variant. In the presence

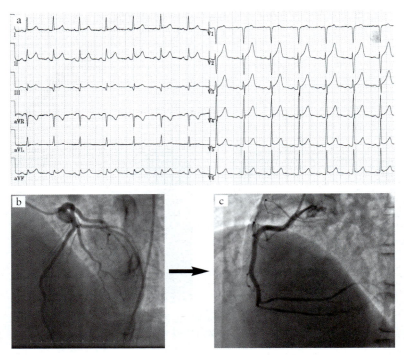

Figure 16-9 Because of typical ischemic chest discomfort associated with ST elevation in inferior leads (II,III, aVF) (A), STEMI was suspected. Urgent coronary angiography revealed widely patent left (B) and right (C) coronary arteries with normal anterograde flow. A diagnosis of acute viral myopericarditis was subsequently confirmed by serological tests.

of obvious ST elevation and ongoing chest discomfort, urgent coronary angiography should be performed to exclude acute coronary occlusion or significant stenosis and to define coronary anatomy as well as the status of the epicardial blood flow. Coronary spasm and its response to intracoronary nitroglycerin can be evaluated in patients with suspected Prinzmetal angina. Information on coronary anatomy should be complemented by LV assessment, either by contrast ventriculography or urgent echocardiography to correlate the coronary findings with the LV wall motion abnormality (Figure 16-11).

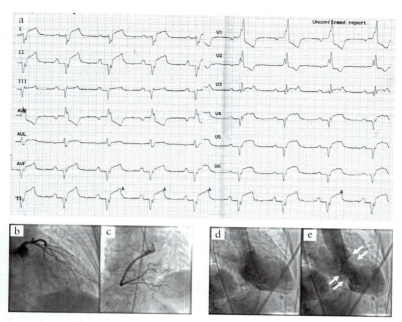

Figure 16-10 Because of typical chest pain and new onset of right bundle branch block with ST elevation in precordial leads (A), proximal occlusion of LAD was suspected. Urgent coronary angiography revealed no evidence of coronary artery disease and normal anterograde flow in the left (B) and right (C) coronary arteries. Subsequent left ventriculography revealed a typical apical ballooning pattern (D and E). A diagnosis of stress-induced cardiomyopaty was therefore established.

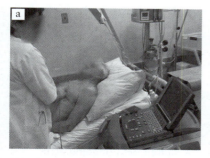
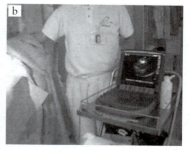

Figure 16-11 Urgent echocardiography using a portable device in the emergency room (A) and in the catheterization laboratory (B)

Conduction Delays and Diagnosis of Acute Coronary Occlusion

Conduction delays may not interfere with, may mask, or may falsely suggest the diagnosis of acute coronary occlusion. In right bundle branch block (RBBB), the pattern of infarction is usually not altered. It is important to notice, however, that sometimes the new development of RBBB will unmask acute anteroseptal STEMI (Figure 16-12).[6] In left bundle branch block (LBBB), the pattern of early activation is altered, and the initial septal vector is directed from right to left. Numerous

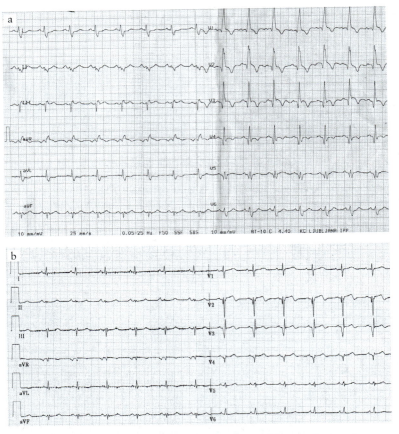

Figure 16-12 New onset of RBBB in a patient with ongoing acute chest discomfort (A). Urgent coronary angiography demonstrated acute occlusion of the proximal LAD. Following successful PPCI, RBBB immediately dissolved, and a typical ST-T evolution pattern of anteroseptal STEMI was seen in precordial leads (B).

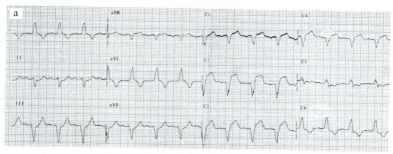

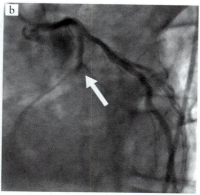

Figure 16-13 A patient presenting with acute ischemic discomfort and onset of new LBBB (A), which was established by examination of old ECG recordings. Urgent coronary angiography revealed acute occlusion of the mid-LAD (B).

attempts at defining diagnostic criteria for STEMI in the presence of LBBB were unsuccessful. However, the presence of Q waves in at least two leads (l, aVL, V5, or V6), R-regression from V1-V4, and striking ST deviation beyond what can be explained by a conduction defect argue for AMI.[7] Sometimes acute coronary occlusion or critical stenosis may also be manifested as the onset of new LBBB (Figure 16-13). It is very rare that we can obtain unequivocal diagnosis in these settings because previous ECG recordings are usually not available at the time of admission. In the presence of Wolff-Parkinson-White (WPW) syndrome, the initial vector may be directed toward the left ventricular cavity, precluding the appearance of a Q wave. Changes in ST-T segment masked by WPW are therefore recognizable in the presence of normal intraventricular conduction. Also in patients with pacemaker rhythm, acute coronary occlusion or critical stenosis may be electrocardiographically silent (Figure 16-14).

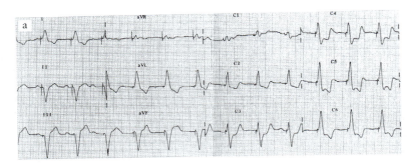

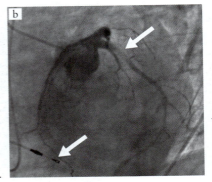

Figure 16-14 Pacemaker rhythm with "spikes" in a patient with severe chest discomfort and permanent pace (A). Urgent coronary angiography revealed a "hazy" thrombotic lesion of LCX with some degree of spontaneous reperfusion (B, arrow). Cineangiography also revealed the tip of the permanent pacemaker in the apex of the right ventricle.

DATA DECODING TIPS (CLINICAL PEARLS)

ECG Changes Due to AMI in Patients with BBB and Pacemakers

Patients with pacemakers should have a magnet put on top of the pacemaker site so there is fixed pacing. The few intrinsic beats between the paced beats can show ST segment elevation. Without using the magnet, if the patient does some exercise with the legs or arms to increase the heart rate (which is higher than the pacing threshold), an ECG could be recorded and the ST-T changes could be evaluated for AMI. However, after a paced beat, the T wave can become inverted. If there is ST elevation in the intrinsic beat, then the ST elevation is most helpful. In patients with RBBB, the ST changes of AMI can be seen normally (ST segment elevation). In patients with LBBB, there is delay of the ascending branch of the R wave suggestive of AMI. If there is a prior ECG documenting LBBB and the new ECG shows further ST elevation, a diagnosis of AMI can be made based on these new ECG changes.

In the absence of typical ECG changes and ongoing chest discomfort despite adequate initial medication, urgent echocardiography may demonstrate significant abnormal wall motion as well as acute extracardiac pathologies, including aortic dissection type A and "acute cor pulmonale" due to massive pulmonary embolism. Significant LV wall motion abnormalities may pinpoint the territory of acute coronary occlusion and facilitate the decision to perform urgent coronary angiography.

Hidden STEMI

In some patients without previously described conduction delays, acute coronary occlusion may not be associated with the typical STEMI pattern. Again, adequate initial therapy, including nitroglycerin, acetylsalicylic acid, oxygen, and morphine, does not result in cessation of chest discomfort. Urgent echocardiography and coronary angiography are very helpful in determining the cause of acute chest discomfort and may be followed by immediate percutaneous or surgical revascularization (Figures 16-15 and 16-16). Examples of this are "hidden" acute

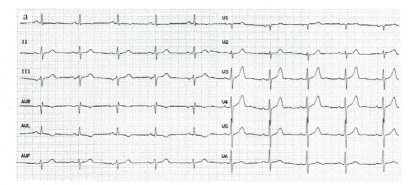

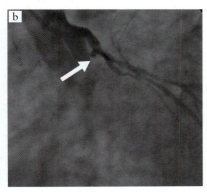

Figure 16-15 A patient with severe chest discomfort and an unremarkable ECG recording (A). Despite adequate initial medical therapy, severe chest pain persisted. Urgent coronary angiography revealed ostial occlusion of the LAD (B, arrow).

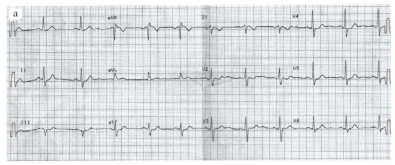

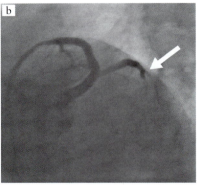

Figure 16-16 Absence of remarkable ST changes (A) in a patient with ongoing chest discomfort. Urgent coronary angiography revealed proximal occlusion of the left circumflex artery (B, arrow).

proximal LAD (Figure 16-15) and proximal LCX (Figure 16-16) occlusion. It is important to notice that isolated ST elevation in aVR with or without concomitant ST depression in precordial leads may pinpoint the *critical left main stenosis* (Figure 16-17).

PROGRAMMED MANAGEMENT

Because timely primary percutaneous coronary intervention (PPCI) is currently the gold standard of acute reperfusion therapy in STEMI, these patients should immediately be transferred directly from the field to the cardiac unit center with "24-7" access to interventional cardiology and cardiac intensive care.[8] Such a "STEMI fast track," including early symptom recognition, prehospital 12-lead ECG, "phone cath lab alert," and direct transportation to PPCI, is the most effective way to reduce time delays from symptom onset to mechanical reperfusion

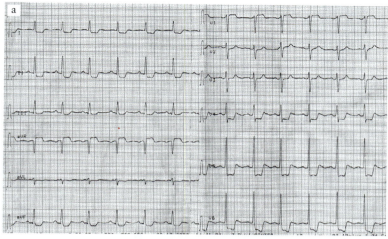

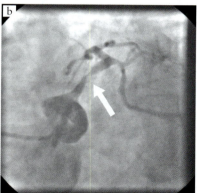

Figure 16-17 Elevation in aVR and ST depression in lateral and inferior leads (A) associated with critical left main stenosis (B).

(Figure 16-18). It is therefore necessary that each community designs an effective PPCI network that would timely capture the majority of patients with STEMI.[3] If there is a delay in PPCI, the patient should be treated for fibrinolytic therapy.

EMS-to-Balloon Times: A New Standard of Care

More evidence that a coordinated regional approach to the treatment of STEMI patients, with prehospital triage and cath-lab activation, leads to a consistent reduction in door-to-balloon times, has come from a new study.[9] This entails prehospital triage of STEMI patients in which

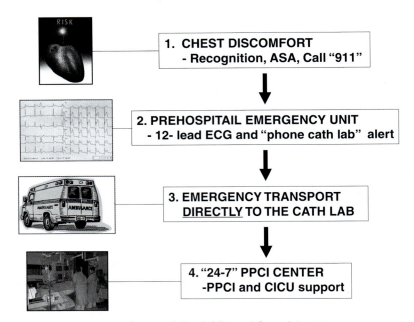

Figure 16-18 STEMI fast track in Ljubljana (Slovenia). ASA-acetylsalycilic acid; PPCI-primary percutaneous coronary intervention; CICU-cardiac intensive care unit; 24-7-hospital with permanent availability of interventional cardiology team.

paramedics perform ECGs in the ambulance and patients are brought to the nearest primary PCI-capable hospital with already activated catheterization laboratories. In a pooled analysis of 10 independent, prospective, observational registries involving 72 hospitals, data were collected on all consecutive patients with a prehospital ECG diagnosis of STEMI. In total, paramedics transported 2712 such patients directly to a PCI hospital. A primary PCI was performed on 2053 patients (76%), and 86% of these had a door-to-balloon time of less than 90 minutes, well above the ACC benchmark of 75%. In addition, door-to-balloon times were less than 60 minutes in 50% of patients, less than 45 minutes in 25% of patients, and less than 30 minutes in 8% of patients. Another measure—emergency medical services (EMS)-to-balloon time (E2B)—was less than 90 minutes in 68% of patients. In this study, 24% of patients for whom the catheterization laboratories were activated did not have primary PCI. The most important lesson of this study is that reperfusion with primary PCI can be provided more rapidly if EMS is placed in its rightful position as the front line for integrated STEMI care.[10]

Local Fibrinolytic Therapy or Transfer for Coronary Intervention

As more patients with STEMI prefer PCI, the problem is the availability of the cardiac catheterization laboratories with PCI capability. Only 20% of U. S. hospitals have cardiac catheterization laboratories, and even fewer have the capability of performing emergency PCI. Although transfer of the MI patient to a facility that can perform PCI is possible, 87% of transferred patients had more than a two-hour delay, which may theoretically outweigh any added benefit. An excellent mortality result is dependent on short door-to-balloon time, optimally less than 90 minutes, which is not easily attainable in every U. S. cardiac catheterization laboratory. Furthermore, in the large NIMR 2-3 registry of more than 300,000 patients, the result of PCI was excellent if performed by experienced operators in high-volume interventional laboratories. while there was no difference in mortality between FT or mechanical interventions in low-volume hospitals.[11] It is reasonable to transfer a patient for acute PCI if delay is not more than 90 minutes. If there is a delay or the time of transportation is too long because of the distance between the local hospital and the PCI center, then FT is the best choice. This strategy is reconfirmed by the positive results of the NORDISTEMI trial presented at the European Society of Cardiology Congress in September 2009, Barcelona, Spain.

 BENEFITS, HARMS, AND COST-EFFECTIVENESS ANALYSIS:

Simple Formula to Decide Local FT or Distal Transfer for PCI

Methodology: This is a systematic review and meta-analysis. *Results:* There were 22 studies included in the meta-analysis, with 3760 and 3758 patients randomized to primary angioplasty and FT, respectively. The mean (SE) angioplasty-related time delay (over and above time to FT) was 54.3 (2.2) minutes. For this delay, mean event probabilities were lower for primary angioplasty for all outcomes. Mortality within 1 month was 4.5% after angioplasty and 6.4% after FT (OR = 0.68, 95% CI 0.46 to 1.01) For nonfatal reinfarction, OR = 0.32 (95% CI 0.20 to 0.51); for non-fatal stroke OR = 0.24 (95% CI 0.11 to 0.50). For all outcomes, the benefit of angioplasty decreased with longer delay from initiation. *Practical Applications:* The benefit of primary angioplasty over FT depends on the additional time delay. For delays of 30 to 90 minutes, angioplasty is superior for one-month fatal and nonfatal outcomes. For delays of around 90 minutes, FT may be the preferred option as assessed by six-month mortality; there is considerable uncertainty for longer time delays.[11]

Who Benefits the Most and Who Does Not Benefit from an Expedited PCI?

The patients who need an expedited process for PCI are the ones with high risks and with short interval from symptom onset to presentation. Physicians can make a difference in mortality of these patients by focusing on and making a real effort to shorten the door-to-balloon time. While patients with low risk and a long interval between symptom onset to presentation also need to have a short door-to-balloon time, they do not benefit from an expedited PCI because the window of myocardial salvage has passed or the MI is too small to be helped by invasive interventions.[12] These standards are used to rationalize the fairness in triage and to give priority to patients who should go for PCI first or be transferred first when two patients arrive at the same time in the same emergency room or are transferred from different hospitals. An example of two patients is as follows: one young patient arrives at the ER 8 hours after onset of chest pain with ST elevation in leads 2,3, F, while a much older patient arrives 2 hours from the onset of chest pain and with ST elevation in leads V1-V6. The second patient should be given priority because his AMI is larger with higher risk and the chance for recovery is higher.

Intermittent Occlusion of the Brachial Artery to Induce Preconditioning

Occluding the brachial artery to induce ischemic preconditioning in coronary stenting was recently shown to reduce myocardial necrosis as a result of the procedure and was also shown to reduce ischemic chest pain and ECG abnormalities during PCI. In this study, 108 patients with STEMI underwent conventional PCI, while 105 patients underwent ischemic conditioning in the ambulance. In the ambulance patients, the paramedic obtained the electrocardiogram, transmitted the data to the hospital, and, when the attending physician confirmed STEMI, had a blood-pressure cuff placed around the patient's upper arm and inflated to 200 mm Hg for five minutes. The conditioning process was repeated four times.

For the primary endpoint, the myocardial salvage index at 30 days, an assessment of the myocardial area at risk showed significantly lower final infarct size among those who underwent conditioning. Interestingly, the benefit appeared driven by large infarcts caused by left anterior descending (LAD) lesions.[13]

TROUBLE-SHOOTING AND DEBUGGING

Whom to Rush for Rescue PCI?

Given the association between bleeding events and subsequent ischemic events, it might be reasonable to select moderate- and high-risk patients for PCI after fibrinolysis and to treat low-risk patients with medical therapy. As noted previously, patients with cardiogenic shock, severe heart failure, or hemodynamically compromising ventricular arrhythmias are excellent candidates. An ECG estimate of potential infarct size in patients with persistent ST segment elevation (less than 50% resolution at 90 minutes following initiation of FT in the lead, showing the worst initial evaluation) and ongoing ischemic pain is useful for selecting other patients for rescue PCI. Anterior MI or inferior MI with right ventricular involvement or precordial ST segment depression usually predicts increased risk. Conversely, patients with symptom resolution, improving ST segment elevation (less than 50% resolution), or inferior MI localized to three ECG leads probably should not be referred for angiography. Likewise, it is doubtful that PCI of a branch artery (diagonal or obtuse marginal (OM) branch) will change prognosis in the absence of high-risk criteria noted above. However, we don't have the angiographic diagnosis of a diagonal causing AMI unless we do an angiogram. It is agreed that PCI of a large diagonal or OM does not decrease mortality, however, if the IRA is a large diagonal, large OM in a LCX-dominant or large PDA in a RCA-dominant, then opening a diagonal or OM branch may decrease the probability of mitral regurgitation due to papillary muscle dysfunction.

When to Perform PCI After FT

Previous studies of PCIs performed in the early plain old balloon angioplasty (POBA) era have shown no advantage of immediate intervention compared with delayed intervention or with a conservative approach after full-dose FT for STEMI. Later, combined low-dose FT and immediate PCI were thought to increase the patency rate of infarct-related artery (IRA) and reduce the need for rescue PCI. With better interventional techniques, equipment, the availability of stents, safer anticoagulants, antiplatelet drugs, and effective bleeding prevention at the arterial access site, PCI after FT showed fewer bleeding complications. However, the best subsequent management of patients after FT remains unclear. The benefits and harms of FT and immediate PCI or FT and only rescue PCI were studied in the CARESS-AMI trial that follows. The CARESS-AMI *Trial Question:* What is the best management after FT: FT and immediate PCI or FT and delayed PCI unless patients need rescue PCI? *Methodology:* This is an RCT in which 600 patients aged 75 years or younger with one or more high-risk features (extensive ST segment elevation, new-onset left bundle branch block, previous MI, Killip class >2, or LV ejection fraction < or = 35%) with STEMI treated by FT and abciximab at a noninterventional hospital were randomized to immediate transfer for PCI, or to standard medical therapy with transfer for rescue angioplasty. *Results:* Of the 299 patients assigned to immediate PCI, 289 (97.0%) underwent angiography and 255 (85.6%) received PCI. Rescue PCI was done on 91 patients (30.3%) in the standard care/rescue PCI group. The primary outcome occurred in 13 patients (4.4%) in the immediate PCI group compared with 32 (10.7%) in the standard care/rescue PCI group (hazard ratio 0.40; 95% CI 0.21-0.76, log rank P = 0.004). *Harms:* Major bleeding was seen in ten patients in the immediate group and seven in the standard care/rescue group (3.4% vs. 2.3%, P = 0.47). Strokes occurred in two patients in the immediate group and four in the standard care/rescue group (0.7% vs. 1.3%, P = 0.50) *Evidence-Based Applications:* Immediate transfer for PCI improves outcome in high-risk patients with STEMI treated at noninterventional hospitals with half-dose reteplase and abciximab.[14.]

The previous data were confirmed again in the TRANSFER-AMI trial.[15] TRANSFER-AMI is a "pharmacoinvasive" study that tested the best combination of early pharmacotherapy and transfer to PCI—a field crowded with a mix of positive and negative studies. The 30-day results showed that a strategy of transferring STEMI patients for PCI within six hours of receiving thrombolysis at a non-PCI center is superior to the more standard wait-and-see strategy. Immediate transfer after fibrinolysis was associated with a significant 41% relative reduction in the primary endpoint composite of 30-day deaths, repeat MI, CHF, severe recurrent ischemia, or shock. Rates of reinfarction, recurrent ischemia, and death/MI/ischemia were also lower in the pharmacoinvasive group. At six months, there were continued trends toward fewer deaths, reinfarction, and death/reinfarction with the pharmacoinvasive strategy. Based on the shorter hospital length of stay with this approach and the fact that most patients undergoing standard therapy end up in the catheterization laboratory at some point, the pharmacoinvasive strategy is likely to be cost-effective.[15]

TAKE-HOME MESSAGE

Data Collecting Collect all the data about the patient's history (of smoking, high-sodium, high-cholesterol diet, alcohol abuse, HTN, DM, high cholesterol level), family history (of early sudden death due to heart disease, history of early CAD), and from a focused physical examination (signs of prior stroke, CAD, PAD, carotid murmur, weak peripheral pulses), all of which add weight to the clinical decision-making process.

Data Mining Recommend safe, appropriate, and efficacious investigation (including ECG, electrolyte, BUN, and creatinine levels, and weight). The ECG should therefore already be recorded in the prehospital setting at the first medical contact. In the absence of typical ECG changes and ongoing chest discomfort despite adequate initial medication, hidden acute coronary occlusion or extracardiac disease such as type A aortic dissection or acute pulmonary embolism should be suspected. Urgent echocardiography and coronary angiography are very helpful in establishing the exact diagnosis.

Urgent coronary angiography represents the easy and safe gold standard imaging technique to obtain accurate information about coronary anatomy and infarct-related artery, which is essential for further percutaneous or surgical revascularization. Coronary angiography will also confirm the absence of acute thrombotic coronary occlusion in patients with acute myopericarditis, coronary spasms, stress cardiomyopathy, and other noncoronary conditions that may resemble STEMI. This information is crucial to confirm the diagnosis and tailor further management.

Management Recommend safe, appropriate, and efficacious therapy to maintain the stable health status of the patient over time (fibrinolytic therapy, PCI, transfer to the closest hospital). Patients with signs of ongoing STEMI are best managed in tertiary cardiac centers with 24-7 availability of an interventional cardiology team and skilled cardiac intensive care.

References

1. Lee, K., Woodlief, L. H., Topol, E., et al. for the GUSTO-I investigator: Predictor of 30-day mortality in the era of reperfusion for AMI. Circulation. 1995;91:1659–1668.
2. Crimm, A., Severance, H. W., Coffey, K., et al.: Prognostic significance of isolated sinus tachycardia during the first three days of AMI. Am J Med. 1984;73:983–988.
3. Ting, H. W., Krumholz, H. M., Bradley, E. H., et al.: Implementation and integration of prehospital ECGs into systems of care for acute coronary syndrome. Circulation. 2008;118:1066–1079.
4. Andersen, H. R., Falk, E., Nielsen, D.: Right ventricular infarction: Diagnostic accuracy of electrocardiographic right chest leads V3R to V7R investigated prospectively in 43 consecutive fatal cases from a coronary care unit. Br Heart J. 1989;62:328.
5. Lopez-Sendon, J., Coma-Cannella, J., Alcasena, S., et al.: Electrocardiographic findings in acute right ventricular infarction: Sensitivity and specificity of electrocardiographic alterations in right precordial leads V4R, V3R, V1, V2 and V3. Am Coll Cardiol. 1985;8:1273.
6. Rosenbaum, M. B., Girotti, L. A., Lazzari, J. O., et al.: Abnormal Q waves in right sided chest leads provoked by onset of right bundle branch block in patients with anteroseptal infarction. Br Heart J. 1982;47:227.
7. Hands, M. E., Cook, E. F., Stone, P. H., et al.: Electrocardiographic diagnosis of myocardial infarction in the presence of complete bundle branch block. Am Heart J. 1988;116:23.
8. Rokos, I. C., French, W. F., Koenig, W. J., et al.: Integration of prehospital electrocardiograms and ST-elevation myocardial infarction receiving center (SRC) networks: Impact on door-to balloon times across

10 independent regions. J Am Coll Cardiol Cardiovasc Intervent. 2009; 2:339–346.

9. Granger, C. B.: Accelerating ST segment elevation myocardial infarction care. Emergency medical services take center stage. J Am Coll Cardiol Cardiovasc Intervent. 2009;2:347-349.

10. Tadel Kocjančič, S., Zorman, S., Jazbec, A., et al.: Effectiveness of primary percutaneous coronary intervention for acute ST-elevation myocardial infarction 10. from a 5-year single center experience. Am J Cardiol. 2008;101:162–168.

11. Magid, D. J., Calonge, B. N., Rumfeld, J. S., et al., for the National Registry of Myocardial Infarction 2 and 3 Investigators: Relations between hospital primary angioplasty volume and mortality for patients with AMI treated with primary angioplasty vs. thrombolytic therapy. JAMA. 2000;284:3131–3138.

12. Bruce, R., Brodie, B. R., Hansen, C., et al.: Door-to-balloon time with primary percutaneous coronary intervention for acute myocardial infarction impacts late cardiac mortality in high-risk patients and patients presenting early after the onset of symptoms. J Am Coll Cardiol. 2006;47:289–295.

13. Bøtker, H.E., et al.: Upper-Limb Ischemia During Ambulance Transfer Reduces Myocardial Perfusion Injury in STEMI Presented during a clinical-trials session of the i2 Summit at the American College of Cardiology 2009 Scientific Sessions, Orlando, FL, March 2009.

14. Di Mario, C., Dudek, D., Piscione, F., et al.: for the CARRESS-in-AMI Investigators. Immediate angioplasty versus standard therapy with rescue angioplasty after thrombolysis in the combined abciximab reteplase stent study in acute myocardial infarction (CARESS-in-AMI): an open, prospective, randomized, multicentral trial. Lancet. 2008;371:559-68.

15. Cantor, W.J., Fitchett, D., Borgundvaag, B., et al.: TRANSFER-AMI Trial Investigators. Routine early angioplasty after fibrinolysis for acute myocardial infarction. N Engl J Med. 2009;360:2705-18.

Management of ST Segment Elevation Myocardial Infarction

CHAPTER

17

Thach Nguyen, Dayi Hu, Dobrin Vasilev, Rong Lin Zhang, Nguyen Duc Cong, GimHoi Choo, and Do Quang Huan

Chapter Outline

DEFINITION

ST segment elevation myocardial infarction (STEMI) is acute myocardial infarction manifested in patients by ST segment elevation or new left bundle branch block (LBBB) in a 12-lead electrocardiogram (ECG).

Patient Population in Focus

Patients with chest pain or equivalent symptoms who present with ST segment elevation or new LBBB in a-12 lead ECG are the focus of this chapter.

Strategic Programming

The first step is to identify the patients with STEMI through data collecting (i.e., a short and focused history and physical examination: history of chest pain, high blood pressure, heart rate, rales in lungs) and data mining (an ECG) confirming the abnormal ST changes. The next step is to perform basic testing preparing the patient for emergency angiogram if indicated (CBC, electrolytes, blood glucose, BUN and creatinine levels, PT, PTT, troponin level) in order to confirm (data converting) the main diagnosis of STEMI and start treatment.

The goal of the treatment is to achieve successful reperfusion in the infarct-related artery (IRA), defined as early, complete restoration of the coronary blood flow with a Thrombolysis In acute Myocardial Infarction (TIMI) 3 flow and a TIMI grade 4 myocardial perfusion.[1] This brisk flow allows sufficient microvascular perfusion to reduce the infarct size, to preserve the LV function, and, most importantly, to reduce mortality.

PROGRAMMED MANAGEMENT

The strategies that guide cardiologists for the next 120 minutes from the first encounter with the patient in the emergency room are listed in Table 17-1.

Fibrinolytic Therapy

The indications for fibrinolytic therapy (FT) are for patients presenting with chest discomfort within 12 hours of onset and with ST segment elevation (1 mm in at least two limb leads and 2 mm in two or more contiguous precordial leads suggestive of STEMI) or new LBBB. The advantage of FT is by earliest restoration of flow due to its quick and simple intravenous administration (door-to-needle = 30 minutes). It does not restore full epicardial or microvascular flow to the majority of patients or sustain its patency thereafter. The contraindications of FT are listed in Table 17-2.[2]

Unfractionated heparin (UFH) is used after FT with tPA or retavase to prevent propagation of thrombus, formation of new mural

---

TABLE 17-1: Management Strategies for Patients with STEMI

1. **Data collecting:** Quickly screen patients for indications and risks of fibrinolytic therapy or primary coronary intervention (PCI).
2. **Data management:** Start fibrinolytic therapy at the local hospital or send the patient quickly to the cardiac catheterization laboratory for emergency PCI.
3. **Root-cause correction:** Start fibrinolytic therapy or PCI with the lowest (<90 minutes) door-to-balloon time.
4. **Work-around configuration correction:** CABG if indicated
5. Prevent left ventricular remodeling (to avoid left ventricular dilation)
6. Observe and treat reinfarction and mechanical complication of AMI: e.g., new ventricular septal defect (VSD), perforation, rupture of the papillary muscle.

TABLE 17-2: Contraindications of Fibrinolytic Therapy

Absolute Contraindications

Any prior intracranial bleeding
Known structural cerebrovascular lesion (e.g., arteriovenous malformations)
Known malignant intracranial neoplasm (primary or metastatic)
Ischemic stroke within three months, EXCEPT for ischemic stroke within three hours
Suspected aortic dissection
Active bleeding or bleeding diathesis (excluding menses)
Significant closed head trauma or facial trauma within three months

Relative Contraindications

History of chronic, severe, poorly controlled hypertension
Severe. uncontrolled hypertension on presentation (systolic blood pressure >180 mm Hg, diastolic blood pressure >110 mm Hg)
History of prior ischemic stroke within three months, dementia, or known intracranial pathology (not covered in absolute contraindications)
Traumatic (longer than 10 minutes) cardiopulmonary resuscitation or major surgery (<3 weeks)
Noncompressive vascular puncture
For streptokinase/anistreplase: prior exposure (more than five days ago) or prior allergic reaction to these agents
Pregnancy
Active peptic ulcer
Current use of anticoagulants: the higher the international normalized ratio (INR), the higher the risk of bleeding

---

thrombosis, systemic embolism, and coronary reocclusion. The aPTT is maintained at 1.5 to 2 times control (50-70 seconds). There is no need for UFH after administration of streptokinase.

BENEFITS, HARMS, AND COST-EFFECTIVENESS ANALYSIS:

Fibrinolytic Therapy Trialists' (FTT) Collaborative Group

Methodology: This is a meta-analysis to review all fibrinolytic therapy trials versus controls that randomized more than 1000 patients with suspected AMI (ST elevation or LBBB). *Results:* The nine trials included 58,600 patients with 6177 (10.5%) deaths, 564 (1.0%) strokes, and 436 (0.7%) major noncerebral bleeds. *Benefits:* There was highly significant mortality reduction of 10 per 1000 for those presenting within 0 to 6 hours, 20 per 1000 for those presenting within 7 to 12 hours, and a statically uncertain benefit of 10 per 1000 for those presenting at 13 to 18 hours. The benefit was observed irrespective of age, sex, blood pressure, heart rate, presence of diabetes, or previous history of MI. *Harms:* FT was associated with one excess death and four extra strokes per 1000 during days 0-1. *Practical Applications:* FT is beneficial for patients with AMI when indicated.[3]

Low Molecular Weight Heparin After Fibrinolytic Therapy

Low molecular weight heparin (LMWH) is very user friendly by subcutaneous injection instead of prolonged infusion as by UFH. Therefore LMWH was tried in patients with STEMI after receiving FT.

EVIDENCE-BASED MEDICINE:

The Extract TIMI-25 trial

Methodology: The EXTRACT-TIMI 25 trial was a double-blind, randomized clinical trial (RCT) comparing enoxaparin and UFH in 20,506 patients with STEMI who were scheduled to undergo FT and receive enoxaparin throughout the index hospitalization or weight-based UFH for at least 48 hours. The primary efficacy endpoint was death or nonfatal recurrent MI through 30 days. *Results:* The primary endpoint occurred in 12.0% of patients in the UFH group and 9.9% of those in the enoxaparin group ($P < 0.001$). Nonfatal reinfarction occurred in 4.5% of the patients receiving UFH and 3.0% of those receiving enoxaparin ($P < 0.001$); 7.5% of patients given UFH died, as did 6.9% of those given enoxaparin ($P = 0.11$). The composite of death, nonfatal reinfarction, or urgent revascularization occurred in 14.5% of patients given UFH and 11.7% of those given enoxaparin ($P < 0.001$). *Harms:* Major bleeding occurred in 1.4% and 2.1%, respectively ($P < 0.001$). *Mechanism of Difference:* Because prior trials reported that bleeding with enoxaparin was increased in elderly patients, a novel dosing regimen was devised for patients 75 or older, and strict attention was paid to dose reduction in patients with significantly impaired renal function to minimize the accumulation of anti-Xa activity. *Evidence-Based Applications:* In patients receiving FT for STEMI, treatment with enoxaparin throughout the index hospitalization is superior to treatment with UFH for 48 hours but is associated with an increase in major bleeding episodes. These findings should be interpreted in the context of net clinical benefit.[4]

TABLE 17-3: Angiographic Exclusions Precluding Performance of PCI in STEMI

Unprotected LM > 60%
IRA with TIMI 3 flow and lesion morphology at extremely high risk for abrupt closure (extremely long lesion or severe angulated lesion)
Multivessel disease with TIMI-3 flow in the IRA, now stable and pain-free
IRA supplies a small or secondary vessel supplying a small amount of myocardium in which the risk of PCI may outweigh the benefit
Inability to clearly identify the IRA

Primary Coronary Intervention (PCI)

Direct PCI includes patients who presented with AMI without prior FT undergoing plain balloon angioplasty (POBA), bare-metal stenting (BMS), or drug-eluting stenting (DES). The efficacy of POBA was limited because of recurrent ischemia in 10% to 15% and early reocclusion (4%) and late restenosis in 31% to 45%.[5] For patients not eligible for coronary stenting because of their vessel size or anticoagulation problems, POBA is the best way to achieve emergent TIMI 3 flow. Contraindications for PCI are listed in Table 17-3.

DES versus BMS

The problem of safety after DES and BMS in the setting of AMI is studied in several RCTs. The results of the HORIZON-AMI trial follow.

 EVIDENCE-BASED MEDICINE:

The HORIZON-AMI Trial

Question: Does DES cause more acute stent thrombosis and higher mortality and morbidity compared with BMS? ***Methodology:*** Following emergent angiography, 3006 patients were then randomized in a 3:1 fashion to DES or BMS and followed for one year. All patients were treated with ASA for the entire study duration, with an additional antiplatelet recommended for at least one year following PCI. Angiographic follow-up was performed at 13 months in order not to interfere with the 12-month clinical follow-up. ***Results:*** At 12 months, treatment with the DES reduced ischemic target lesion revascularization (TLR) by 41% compared with BMS. MACE, a composite of all-cause mortality, reinfarction, stroke, and stent thrombosis, was equivalent with the two stents. ***Cost-Effectiveness Analysis:*** The benefit of a 3% absolute difference means that there is a need to treat about 30 patients in order to benefit one TLR (Table 17-4).

Practical Applications: The real strength of the study was the reassurance of the safety of the DES; there was no difference in mortality or stent thrombosis when compared with BMS in the setting of AMI.[6]

Direct Thrombin Inhibition During PCI

Direct thrombin inhibitor (DTI) given to patients undergoing primary PCI is more convenient because of the small bolus dose and the short infusion time. It is also safer because it does not cause a higher rate of complications when compared to the conventional treatment.

 EVIDENCE-BASED MEDICINE:

The HORIZONS-AMI Trial

Methodology: A group of 3602 patients with STEMI were undergoing primary PCI within 12 hours of onset of symptoms and were randomized into UFH plus a glycoprotein 2B3A inhibitor (GPI) or bivalirudin alone. The two primary end points were major bleeding and combined adverse clinical events (combination of major bleeding and death, reinfarction, TVR for ischemia, and stroke) within 30 days. *Results:* Anticoagulation with bivalirudin alone, as compared with UFH plus GPI, resulted in a reduced 30-day rate of net adverse clinical events (9.2% vs. 12.1%; relative risk, 0.76; 95% CI 0.63 to 0.92; P = 0.005). Treatment with bivalirudin alone, as compared with UFH plus GPI, resulted in significantly lower 30-day rates of death from cardiac causes (1.8% vs. 2.9%; relative risk, 0.62; 95% CI, 0.40 to 0.95; P = 0.03) and death from all causes (2.1% vs. 3.1%; relative risk, 0.66; 95% CI, 0.44 to 1.00; P = 0.047). At one year, the benefits of bivalirudin monotherapy were maintained. There was a 16% reduction in the one-year rate of composite net adverse clinical events as well as a significant 39% reduction in major bleeding. There was also a significant 31% reduction in all-cause mortality and 43% reduction in cardiac mortality or an absolute reduction of 1.4% and 1.7%, respectively. The type of stent used—either DES or BMS—did not affect any of the endpoints. *Harms:* A lower rate of major bleeding (4.9% vs. 8.3%; relative risk, 0.60; 95% CI, 0.46 to 0.77; P < 0.001) was reported. There was an increased risk of acute stent thrombosis within 24 hours in the bivalirudin group but no significant increase was present by 30 days. *Evidence-Based Applications:* When bivalirudin is given alone during direct PCI, it has fewer bleeding complications and fewer adverse clinical events as compared with UFH plus GPI.[7]

Stent Thrombosis with Bivalirudin

The results of the HORIZONS AMI trial showed that bivalirudin monotherapy resulted in fewer incidents of major bleeding, comparable rates of ischemia, and improved survival rates compared with UFH plus

TABLE 17-4: HORIZONS-AMI: Primary Efficacy and Safety Endpoints

Endpoint	Taxus, n = 2257 (%)	Express BMS n = 749 (%)	Hazard Ratio (95% CI)
Ischemic target lesion revascularization	4.5	7.5	0.59 (0.43–0.83)
Safety MACE	8.1	8.0	1.02 (0.76–1.36)
All-cause mortality	3.5	3.5	0.99 (0.64–1.55)
MI	3.7	4.5	0.81 (0.54–3.22)
Stroke	1.0	0.7	1.52 (0.58–4.00)
Stent thrombosis	3.1	3.4	0.92 (0.58–1.45)
Binary restenosis per lesion at 13 mo	10.0	22.9	0.44 (0.33–0.57)
Binary restenosis per patient at 13 mo	10.9	24.9	0.4 (0.33–0.57)

BMS: bare metal stent, CI: confidence interval, MACE: major adverse cardiovascular events, MI: myocardial infarction.

a GPI at 30 days and one year. However, there were 107 cases of definite or probable stent thrombosis (3.3%) by one year. Of those, 0.9% happened in the first 24 hours (acute), 1.6% between one and 30 days (subacute), and 1% between one month and one year (late).

The most important factor influencing acute stent thrombosis appeared to be the use of early nonrandomized UFH before patients had been randomized to the study drug. Patients who received such treatment had significantly lower rates of stent thrombosis within the first 24 hours regardless of which treatment group they were assigned to.

A 600-mg loading dose of clopidogrel also appeared to be important in reducing stent thrombosis, particularly subacute stent thrombosis in the bivalirudin group. Other usual factors that affected acute and subacute stent thrombosis in HORIZONS AMI were vessel flow, lesion characteristics, and number and length of stents, while patient-related factors including cigarette smoking, were predictors of late stent thrombosis.

While stent thrombosis within one year occurred with similar frequency in both randomized treatment arms, it was more common with bivalirudin, especially within the first five hours, unless the patient received prior UFH. Stent thrombosis between 24 hours and one year was more common in the heparin-GPI arm. The type of stent implanted (drug eluting or bare metal) did not affect the risk of stent thrombosis during any time interval up to one year.[8]

Indicators of Excellence

The results of PCI in STEMI are operator- and institution-dependent. The indicators of excellence in interventional service are listed in Table 17-5.

TABLE 17-5: Indicators of Excellence in Providing Interventional Service for STEMI

Door-to-balloon time <90 minutes
TIMI 2 or 3 flow attained in >90% of patients
Emergency CABG <2%
Actual performance of PCI in >85% brought to the laboratory
Risk-adjusted in-hospital mortality rate 3% in patients without cardiogenic shock

CABG: coronary artery bypass graft surgery, PCI: percutaneous coronary interventions, STEMI: ST segment elevation myocardial infarction, TIMI: thrombolysis in myocardial infarction.

If these results are not met when compared to those at the national level, then the focus of treatment for STEMI patients in that particular hospital should be the use of FT with further referral to PCI when indicated.[9]

Adjunctive Medical Management

Acetylsalicylic Acid

The effect of aspirin (ASA) occurs within 15 to 30 minutes after ingestion of a nonenteric-coated aspirin. ASA (100 to 300 mg) should be given as early as possible, preferably in the emergency room. Also, intravenous, chewable, or high-dose (>500 mg) oral administration of ASA can induce therapeutic effects rapidly.

Thienopyridine

Clopidogrel is a thienopyridine derivative that inhibits the binding of adenosine diphosphate to its platelet receptors. It exerts its full effectiveness when >80% of platelets are inhibited, usually 24 hours after a loading dose of 300 to 600 mg.[10] The benefits and harms of clopidogrel in AMI were studied in the Clopidogrel as Adjunctive Reperfusion Therapy–Thrombolysis in Myocardial Infarction 28 (CLARITY-TIMI 28) Study that follows.

 EVIDENCE-BASED MEDICINE:

The CLARITY-TIMI 28 Study

Methodology: A group of 3491 patients (18 to 75 years of age) receiving FT within 12 hours of STEMI were randomized to clopidogrel (300 mg oral loading dose; 75 mg oral daily maintenance dose) or placebo.[11] *Results:* The primary composite efficacy endpoint of an occluded infarct artery on angiography or death or recurrent MI before angiography (between 48 and 192 hours after the start of study medication) occurred in 21.7% of the placebo group and 15.0% of the clopidogrel group (OR 0.64; 95% CI 0.53 to 0.76;

P<0.001). **Harms:** The rate of TIMI major bleeding through 30 days was 1.7% in the placebo group and 1.9% in the clopidogrel group (P = 0.80). **Mechanism of Difference:** The benefit of clopidogrel was driven largely by the reduction in rate of an occluded infarct artery, which appears to have been accomplished by preventing infarctrelated reocclusion rather than by facilitating early reperfusion. **Evidence-Based Applications:** Clopidogrel should be given to all patients with AMI undergoing FT or PCI.[11]

Beta Blockers

The majority of RCTs of BBs during STEMI were done in the FT era. The systemic review of RCTs of BBs in STEMI has found that BBs given within hours of infarction reduce both mortality and reinfarction. BBs may reduce the rates of cardiac rupture and ventricular fibrillation. In patients with moderate heart failure (NYHA class II or III), BBs were found to decrease readmission, mortality, and sudden death. The benefits of BBs were evidenced in patients with STEMI after FT or before PCI. The results of the Clopidogrel and Metoprolol in Myocardial Infarction Trial/Second Chinese Cardiac Study, COMMIT/CCS-2, which was conducted in the present era when patients received optimal therapy, follow.

 EVIDENCE-BASED MEDICINE:

The COMMIT/CCS-2 Study

Methodology A group of 45,852 patients were randomized within 24 hours of onset of suspected MI to receive metoprolol (up to three doses of 5 mg IV each in the first 15 minutes, followed by 200 mg orally daily) or matching placebo. Fifteen minutes after the IV doses, a 50-mg tablet of metoprolol or placebo was administered orally and repeated every 6 hours during days 0 to 1 of hospitalization. From day 2 onward, 200 mg of controlled-release metoprolol or placebo was administered orally daily until discharge from the hospital or up to a maximum of four weeks in hospital (in survivors, the mean was 15 days). The two prespecified coprimary outcomes were the composite of death, reinfarction, or cardiac arrest and death from any cause during the scheduled treatment period. **Results:** Neither of the co-primary study endpoints was significantly reduced by allocation to metoprolol. **Cost-Effectiveness Analysis:** For every 1000 patients treated, metoprolol was associated with five fewer episodes of reinfarction, five fewer episodes of ventricular defibrillation, but 11 more episodes of cardiogenic shock. **Mechanism of Difference:** The excess of cardiogenic shock was seen chiefly from days 0 to 1 after hospitalization, whereas the reductions in reinfarction and ventricular fibrillation appeared from day 2 onward. Metoprolol produced an average relative increase of 30% in cardiogenic shock, with higher rates for those over 70 years of age, systolic blood pressure <120 mm Hg, presenting heart rate >110 bpm, or with Killip class >1. Metoprolol allocation was associated with significantly more persistent hypotension and more cases of bradycardia. ***Evidence-Based Applications:*** It is reasonable to administer IV beta blocker therapy on days 0 to 1 of hospitalization for STEMI when hypertension is present and the patient is not at an increased risk of cardiogenic shock on the basis of the risk factors defined earlier. Patients with sinus tachycardia or atrial fibrillation should have left ventricular (LV) function rapidly evaluated before administration of IV beta blockers. From day 2 onward, when beneficial effects on reinfarction and ventricular fibrillation are seen, administration of 200 mg of controlled-release oral metoprolol daily appears to be safe in hemodynamically stable patients with STEMI who are free of contraindications.[12]

 CONCRETE INSTRUCTION

How to Give Beta Blockers

Intravenous metoprolol may be given in 5-mg increments by slow intravenous administration (5 mg over 1 to 2 minutes), repeated every 5 minutes for a total initial dose of 15 mg. In patients who tolerate the total 15-mg IV dose, oral therapy can be initiated 15 minutes after the last intravenous dose at 25 to 50 mg every 6 hours, for a total of 48 hours. Thereafter, patients should receive a maintenance dose of up to 100 mg twice daily. Monitoring during intravenous beta blocker therapy should include frequent checks of heart rate and blood pressure and continuous ECG monitoring as well as auscultation for rales and bronchospasm. It is prudent to initiate a dose of 50 mg of metoprolol orally every 6 hours, transitioning to a dose equivalent to 200 mg per day orally or the maximum tolerated dose.

Angiotensin-Converting Enzyme inhibitors (ACEIs)

Several large-scale randomized trials have demonstrated that ACEIs improved mortality when started during the course of AMI. The indications for ACEIs in the early treatment of AMI were studied in a systematic overview of individual data from 100,000 patients in randomized trials by the ACEI Myocardial Infarction Collaborative Group.

 SMART THINKING:

ACEIs in Myocardial Infarction

Methodology: This meta-analysis of data from all randomized trials involved more than 1000 patients in whom ACEI treatment started in the acute phase (0 to 36 hours) of MI and continued for a short time

(4 to 6 weeks). ***Results:*** Thirty-day mortality was 7.1% among patients allocated to ACEI and 7.6% among control subjects, corresponding to a 7% (SD, 2%) proportional reduction (95% CI, 2% to 11%; 2P < 0.004). ***Cost-Effectiveness Analysis:*** This represented avoidance of approximately 5 deaths per 1000 patients, with most of the benefit observed within the first week. The proportional benefit was similar in patients at different underlying risks. The absolute benefit was particularly large in some high-risk groups (i.e., Killip class 2 to 3, heart rate > or = 100 bpm at entry) and in anterior MI. ACE-inhibitor therapy also reduced the incidence of nonfatal cardiac failure (14.6% vs. 15.2%, 2P = 0.01). ***Harms:*** ACEI treatment was associated with an excess of persistent hypotension (17.6% versus 9.3%, 2P < 0.01) and renal dysfunction (1.3% versus 0.6%, 2P < 0.01). ***Practical Applications:*** ACE inhibitors save lives when started early. It is reasonable to give ACEIs to everyone with AMI. However, more benefits were seen in the sickest patients.[13]

Angiotensin II Receptor Blockers (ARBs)

Angiotensin receptor blockers act on the angiotensin receptor level. In the Valsartan in Acute Myocardial Infarction (VALIANT) trial, patients with STEMI complicated by left ventricular (LV) dysfunction, ARBs were compared with ACEIs.

 EVIDENCE-BASED MEDICINE:

The VALIANT Trial

Methodology: Patients with acute MI receiving conventional therapy were randomly assigned to additional therapy with valsartan (4909 patients), valsartan plus captopril (4885 patients), or captopril (4909 patients). The primary endpoint was death from any cause. ***Results:*** During a median follow-up of 24.7 months, 979 patients in the valsartan group died, as did 941 patients in the valsartan and captopril group, and 958 patients in the captopril group (HR in the valsartan group as compared with the captopril group, 1.00; 97.5% CI, 0.90 to 1.11; P = 0.98; HR in the valsartan and captopril group as compared with the captopril group, 0.98; 97.5% CI, 0.89 to 1.09; P = 0.73). The upper limit of the one-sided 97.5% confidence interval for the comparison of the valsartan group with the captopril group was within the prespecified margin for noninferiority with regard to mortality (P = 0.004). ***Harms:*** The valsartan and captopril group had the most drug-related adverse events. With monotherapy, hypotension and renal dysfunction were more common in the valsartan group, and cough, rash, and taste disturbance were more common in the captopril group. ***Practical Applications:*** Valsartan is as effective as captopril in acute MI patients. However, combining valsartan with captopril increased the rate of adverse events without improving survival. It is reasonable to give the ARB to AMI patients if they cannot tolerate the ACEI.[14]

Lipid-Lowering Drugs

There were no major RCTs for statin therapy in patients with STEMI. There were RCTs conducted in order to clarify the benefits of statins on patients with ACS. The results of a systemic review of RCTs for use of statins in ACS patients follow.

 SMART THINKING:

Statins in Acute Coronary Syndrome

Methodology: This is a systematic review with 9553 ACS patients who started statin therapy within 12 days of hospital presentation. *Results:* The incidence of all-cause mortality was 3.4% in the statin group versus 4.6% in the less-intensive lipid reduction group over a weighted mean follow-up of 22.9 months (relative risk [RR] 0.74; 95% CI 0.61, 0.90; P = 0.003). The incidence of cardiovascular mortality in the statin versus the less intensive lipid reduction group was 2.4% versus 3.3% (RR 0.74; 95% CI 0.58, 0.93; P = 0.010), unstable angina was 4.1% versus 5.0% (RR 0.81; 95% CI 0.68, 0.98; P = 0.027), revascularization was 11.2% versus 12.9% (RR 0.86; 95% CI 0.78, 0.96; P = 0.006), stroke was 1.1% versus 1.2% (RR 0.90; 95% CI 0.62, 1.30; P = 0.56), and MI was 6.6% versus 7.0% (RR 0.94; 95% CI 0.81, 1.09; P = 0.41). *Cost Effectiveness Analysis:* A total of 84 patients would need to be treated to prevent one death. *Practical Applications:* The benefit of early initiation of statin therapy during ACS is confirmed. Furthermore, this approach significantly reduces unstable angina and the need for revascularization. High doses of statins should be started early, regardless of the patient's lipid levels.[15]

Indicators of Excellence

For patients with STEMI, comprehensive management requires early administration of antiplatelet agents, early beta blockade, early medical or mechanical reperfusion, ACE inhibition, early cardiac rehabilitation, education to stop smoking, and AMI prevention methods for patients and family. In real life, in addition to the above measures, the comprehensive management of STEMI patients requires (1) prescribing the same doses of drug with proven benefit as used in the randomized clinical trials, and (2) instructing patients about the absolute or relative necessity of a particular drug or modality of treatment in order to increase compliance.

TABLE 17-6: Performance Indicators of Comprehensive Care for STEMI Patients

Indicator	Benchmark	St Mary Medical Center, Hobart IN (Second Quarter of 2009)
ASA administration within 24 hours after arrival	94%	96%
ASA prescribed at discharge (if no contraindications)	93%	100%
Beta blocker prescribed at discharge	93%	96%
ACEI or ARB prescribed at discharge in patients with EF<40%	90%	71%
Door to needle time (for FT) <30 minutes	41%	N/A
Door to balloon time < 90 minutes	77%	50%
Adult smokers receive smoking cessation advice and counseling	95%	100%
AMI mortality	7.34%	6.9%

AMI: acute myocardial infarction, ASA: aspirin, ACEI: angiotensin converting enzyme inhibitor, ARB: angiotensin receptor blocker, EF: ejection fraction, FT: fibrinolytic therapy.

In order to evaluate the completeness in the management of patients with STEMI, a checklist for excellent performance indicators is shown in Table 17-6. All the benchmarks are set by the Center of Medicare and Medicaid Services.[16]

ADVANCED MANAGEMENT

STEMI with Patent Coronary Arteries

On several occasions, many young patients (mostly women) present with STEMI; however, their angiograms are negative. These patients were treated with standard therapy: aspirin, clopidigrel, beta blockers, and ACEIs, as indicated. However, they did not all improve. The conditions causing AMI without having significant atherosclerosis are listed in Table 17-7.

Coronary Vasculitis

In the case of young female patients with AMI following a recent pregnancy, it is believed that the AMI is due to coronary vasculitis secondary to immunologic sensitization during pregnancy. Usually the coronary angiogram shows distal low flow without significant lesion. The left ventricular function could be depressed. There was no indication for PCI.

TABLE 17-7: Acute Myocardial Infarction without Significant Coronary Lesion

Coronary vasculitis
Spontaneous coronary artery dissection
Antiphospholipid syndrome
Systemic lupus erythematosus

The best treatment is by plasmapheresis, intravenous immunoglobulin, and steroids. During plasmapheresis, blood is taken out of the body. Plasma is then separated by a cell separator. After that, the blood cells are returned to the body while the plasma that contains the harmful antibodies is discarded. The preload-sensitive patient can receive albumin infusion for volume replacement to ward off hypotension during therapeutic plasmapheresis. The result is the nonselective removal of all proteins, including the culprit antibodies.[17]

STEMI in Pregnant Women

In young, pregnant women presenting with AMI, the most common cause is spontaneous coronary artery dissection (SCAD). The incidence of SCAD is underestimated because of the high rate of sudden death (up to 50%) in affected patients prior to any medical contact. Pregnancy and the early puerperium period are recognized as predisposing factors. The physiologic and hormonal changes that occur in pregnancy may cause medial dissection of the coronary artery through impairment of collagen synthesis, proliferation of myocytes, and alteration in the mucopolysaccharide and protein content in the media layer. The increased blood volume and cardiac output during pregnancy also facilitate intimal rupture and medial dissection. Other possible mechanisms of SCAD include rupture of an atherosclerotic plaque or vasa vasorum, an underlying connective tissue disorder, cystic medial necrosis, and increased shear stress.

The optimal treatment of SCAD depends on the patient's clinical presentation, hemodynamic condition, the location and magnitude of the coronary dissection, and the number of vessels affected. In general, the principle for management of coronary dissection after PCI is applied as follows: If there is dissection with distal TIMI 3 flow, then the patient is stable. There is no need for immediate stenting unless there is a question of future deterioration. Medical therapy, including beta-adrenergic blockade to control heart rate and blood pressure, aspirin to prevent thrombosis, and a vasodilator to prevent vasospasm, are appropriate for hemodynamically stable patients with limited coronary dissection.

🔵 DATA MANAGEMENT TIPS (CLINICAL PEARLS)
Invasive Treatment of AMI in Pregnant Patients

The role of anticoagulation is unknown, although complete angiographic resolution of SCAD has been reported. Fibrinolytic therapy, although beneficial in some patients, may cause propagation of the dissection and possible subsequent deterioration. Fibrinolytic therapy can also cause increased risk of maternal and fetal hemorrhage. Patients with chest pain from persistent impairment of coronary blood flow need emergent stent placement. The safety and effectiveness of paclitaxel-eluting stents have not been established in pregnant or lactating women. Patients with multivessel dissection, left main dissection, or failed stent placement should have coronary artery bypass grafting.[18-19]

STEMI Due to Antiphospholipid Syndrome

Antiphospholipid syndrome (APS) is the association of persisting antiphospholipid (aPL) antibodies with a thrombotic event. Unlike the congenital thrombophilias that mainly predispose to venous thrombosis, aPL antibodies can cause thrombosis in any vascular bed, including the coronary artery circulation, causing AMI in structurally normal coronary arteries. It is crucial not to miss this diagnosis as patients are more likely to have recurrent thrombotic episodes and the recommended treatment is high-dose oral anticoagulation; standard secondary prevention of atherosclerosis with antiplatelet agents and risk-factor modification is ineffective.

🔵 DATA MINING TIPS (CLINICAL PEARLS)
How to Do Work-Ups for Patients Suspected of APS

Current laboratory criteria for diagnosing APS require two positive tests of either lupus anticoagulant and/or anticardiolipin antibodies at least 12 weeks apart. Recently, anti-β-2 glycoprotein-1 antibodies have been added to the diagnostic criteria. It is difficult to test for and interpret the results of screens for aPL antibodies because there is heterogeneity of aPL antibodies between individuals and a lack of national and international standardization of the assays.

There are a number of assays to diagnose lupus anticoagulant, including the dilute Russell viper venom and activated partial thromboplastin time assays. The principle of the lupus anticoagulant assays is that phospholipid is required for coagulation to proceed; therefore in the presence of an aPL antibody, the phospholipid clotting time is prolonged because of the aPL antibody binding the phospholipid. The second stage is to add excess phospholipid (usually platelet extract), which removes the aPL antibodies and shortens the clotting time. Anticoagulation interferes with the lupus anticoagulant, making the results difficult to interpret. If a patient is taking oral anticoagulation, (warfarin), he or she should be switched to LMWH for 2 weeks and then have LMWH omitted for 24 hours prior to the test. Initially negative tests do not exclude aPL antibodies. The test should be repeated on two occasions before the diagnosis is formally excluded. It is important to perform two sets of tests separated by 12 weeks because aPL antibodies can become transiently positive.[20]

Patients with AMI due to thrombi caused by APS should undergo coronary angioplasty and thrombectomy should be performed if needed. The indications and contraindications for FT and PCI are the same as they are for any STEMI patients. For secondary thromboprophylaxis, patients should be treated with high-dose warfarin. Aspirin was ineffective in preventing recurrent thrombosis in APS.[20]

AMI from Cocaine

Cocaine has multiple cardiovascular and hematologic effects that likely contribute to the development of myocardial ischemia and/or MI. Cocaine blocks the reuptake of norepinephrine and dopamine at the presynaptic adrenergic terminals, causing an accumulation of catecholamines at the postsynaptic receptor and thus acting as a powerful sympathomimetic agent. Self-reported use of cocaine can be obtained easily and nonintrusively; however, a potentially significant drawback is denial or underreporting by patients. As the use of cocaine may influence treatment strategies, patients being evaluated for possible acute coronary syndrome (ACS) should be routinely queried about the use of cocaine.[21]

DATA DECODING TIPS (CLINICAL PEARLS)
Caveats in Management of Patients with Cocaine-Induced MI

Cocaine-associated chest pain may be caused not only by MI but also by aortic dissection; these must be considered in the differential diagnosis. Compared with nonusers, long-term cocaine users have a higher left ventricular mass index and thickness of the posterior wall. Patients with cocaine-associated chest pain, unstable angina, or MI should be treated similarly to those with traditional ACS or possible ACS, with some notable exceptions. Unlike patients with ACS unrelated to cocaine use, cocaine users should be provided with intravenous benzodiazepines as early management. Beta blockers should not be administered to patients with ST-elevation MI precipitated by cocaine use because of the risk of exacerbating coronary spasm; beta blockers are contraindicated in cocaine-induced ACS. Cessation of cocaine use should be the primary goal of secondary prevention for cocaine-induced ACS.[21]

STEMI Patients with Renal Dysfunction

Renal impairment is a strong independent indicator of increased mortality in patients who are admitted with STEMI. Patients with creatinine clearance <75 mL/min have high in-hospital mortality rates (5.1% vs. 0.8%) or 6 month-mortality of 7.4% vs 1.1%. However, the overall mortality in STEMI patients on long-term dialysis was worse: 59% in one year, 73% in two years, and 89% in five years.[22]

 DATA MANAGEMENT TIPS (CLINICAL PEARLS)
Diagnosis of Fluid Overload and Ischemia in ESRD Patients

Patients with end-stage renal disease (ESRD) may present with atypical symptoms. The nonspecific ST-T changes of LV hypertrophy can make the diagnosis of STEMI more difficult. The volume overload associated with elevation of LV diastolic pressure may produce anginal symptoms and shortness of breath, sometimes indistinguishable from the symptoms of acute ischemia.[23] In this immediate peri-infarction period, echocardiography can provide useful information about the LV, RV systolic function, and volume status.[24] Dialysis is better deferred in the first 24 hours of STEMI unless dictated by acute metabolic derangement or volume overload. Emergent PCI can be performed with low-osmolar contrast agents in order to decrease acute volume stress. Modification of dialysis runs may be required for low-output states.[23]

Management of Late AMI

Is there a place for the late opening of the IRA, beyond the 12-hour window for myocardial salvage? The rationale included the prevention of infarct expansion and ventricular remodeling leading to ventricular dilatation, the provision of electrophysiologic stability lessening the likelihood of malignant ventricular arrhythmias, and the ability of collaterals emanating from the recanalized artery to perfuse ischemic but still viable myocardium.[25] There were also reasons that late reperfusion might be harmful, including the risk of inducing myocardial stunning, microvascular damage, and intramyocardial hemorrhage leading to an increased likelihood of myocardial rupture. However, in reality, is the patency of the late opened IRA translated into better mortality and morbidity?

EVIDENCE-BASED MEDICINE:

PCI for Persistent Occlusion After AMI

Methodology: This is an RCT involving 2166 stable patients who had total occlusion of the IRA 3 to 28 days after MI and who met a high-risk criterion (an ejection fraction of <50% or proximal occlusion). *Results:* The four-year cumulative primary event rate was 17.2% in the PCI group and 15.6% in the medical therapy group (HR for death, reinfarction, or heart failure in the PCI group as compared with the medical therapy group, 1.16; 95%CI, 0.92 to 1.45; P = 0.20). Rates of myocardial reinfarction (fatal and nonfatal) were 7.0% and 5.3% in the two groups, respectively (HR 1.36; 95% CI, 0.92 to 2.00; P = 0.13). Rates of nonfatal reinfarction were 6.9% and 5.0%, respectively (HR 1.44; 95% CI, 0.96 to 2.16; P = 0.08). Rates of NYHA Class IV heart failure (4.4% vs. 4.5%) and death (9.1% versus 9.4%) were similar. There was no interaction between treatment effect and any subgroup variable (age, sex, race or ethnic group, infarct-related artery, ejection fraction, diabetes, Killip class, and the time from MI to randomization). *Practical Applications:* In stable patients, PCI after day 3 of MI did not reduce the occurrence of death, reinfarction, or heart failure, and there was a trend toward excess reinfarction during four years of follow-up.[25]

Glycoprotein 2b3a Inhibition in AMI

Glycoprotein 2b3a Inhibitor (GPI) is a strong and effective antiplatelet drug. In the setting of comprehensive care of STEMI patients in the 21st century, does GPI still have a role in the management of patients with AMI undergoing PCI?

EVIDENCE-BASED MEDICINE:

The BRAVE-3 trial

Question: Does GPI improve mortality and morbidity in patients with AMI undergoing PCI? *Methodology:* This is a randomized, multicenter, double-blind, placebo-controlled trial of 800 patients with acute MI presenting within 24 hours of symptoms and undergoing PCI. All participants received ASA 500 mg, UFH 5000 IU, and pretreatment with 600 mg of clopidogrel, and they were then assigned to either abciximab (usual bolus and perfusion regimen) or placebo. In both groups, 44% of patients received a DES, and 50% received a BMS in each arm. The primary endpoint was left ventricular (LV) infarct size as determined by single-photon-emission computed tomography (SPECT) performed 5 to 10 days after enrollment. Secondary endpoints included the 30-day combined incidence of death, MI, urgent revascularization, and stroke as well as the incidence of bleeding and profound thrombocytopenia. *Results:* There was no difference between the two treatment arms in the primary endpoint or in most of the secondary endpoints (the 30-day combined incidence of death, MI, urgent revascularization, and stroke was 5% in the abciximab group versus 3.8% in the placebo group). *Harms:* There was, however, a 1.5% incidence of profound thrombocytopenia in the abciximab group, and these patients also had a slightly higher rate of TIMI minor bleeding compared with the placebo group. ***Evidence-Based Applications:*** Routine use of the GPI abciximab in acute ST-elevation MI (STEMI) patients undergoing PCI after pretreatment with a loading dose of 600 mg of clopidogrel does not add any measurable benefit. If the patient has a heavy thrombotic burden after PCI, he or she could have short-term GPI or UFH to clear the thrombi.[26]

TROUBLE-SHOOTING AND DEBUGGING

Which LVAD to Use for a Patient with Cardiogenic Shock?

After excluding any mechanical complications from AMI, the treatment for patients with cardiogenic shock is to restore the coronary blood flow as soon as possible by the support of an intra-aortic balloon pump (IABP), TANDEM HEART (Cardiac Assist Inc. Pittsburgh, PA), or IMPALLA (ABIOMED, Inc. Danvers, MA) ventricular assist device. The safety and efficacy of a percutaneous left ventricular assist device versus intra-aortic balloon pumping for treatment of cardiogenic shock caused by MI follow. ***LVAD in Cardiogenic Shock Methodology:*** This is a prospective, randomized study with 26 patients with cardiogenic shock. The primary endpoint was the change of the cardiac index (CI) from baseline to 30 min after implantation. Secondary endpoints included lactic acidosis, hemolysis, and mortality after 30 days. ***Results:*** The CI after 30 minutes of support was significantly increased in patients with the Impella LP2.5 compared with patients with IABP (Impella: delta CI = 0.49 +/− 0.46 L/min/m²; IABP: delta CI = 0.11 +/− 0.31 L/min/m²; P = 0.02). Overall 30-day mortality was 46% in both groups. ***Practical Applications:*** The use of the Impella device is safe and feasible and provides superior hemodynamic support compared with standard treatment using an IABP. Therefore, this may be a valuable tool for acute PCI in patients presenting with cardiogenic shock caused by AMI.[27]

Is IABP Beneficial in Cardiogenic Shock?

This is a systematic review and meta-analysis of intra-aortic balloon pump therapy in STEMI patients with cardiogenic shock. The first meta-analysis included seven randomized trials (n = 1009) of STEMI. IABP showed neither a 30-day survival benefit nor improved left ventricular ejection fraction while being associated with significantly higher stroke and bleeding rates. The second meta-analysis included nine cohorts of STEMI patients with cardiogenic shock (n = 10,529). In patients treated with thrombolysis, IABP was associated with an 18% (95% CI, 16-20%; P < 0.0001) decrease in 30-day mortality, although with significantly higher revascularization rates compared to patients without support. In contrast, in patients treated with PCI, IABP was associated with a 6% (95% CI, 3-10%; P < 0.0008) increase in 30-day mortality. *Mechanism of Difference:* The pooled randomized data do not support IABP in patients with high-risk STEMI. The meta-analysis of cohort studies in the setting of STEMI complicated by cardiogenic shock supported IABP therapy adjunctive to thrombolysis. In contrast, the observational data did not support IABP therapy adjunctive to primary PCI.[28]

How to Perform PCI in Patients with STEMI, Complex Bleeding, and Thrombotic Problems

Bleeding or intra-arterial thrombosis before, during, or after PCI of STEMI could be a major (or possibly fatal) problem triggering a small to full-scale crisis situation. Different problems and solutions with bleeding or thrombosis mainly from anecdotal reports are discussed here. Because of the small number of patients, there are no evidence-based guidelines for how to manage these patients. If the benefits outweigh the risks, then the patient should have PCI, provided that there is a strong indication. The family and the patient need to understand the benefits and the risks clearly and agree with the proposed treatment.

STEMI in >400-Pound Patients

The weight limit for a table in the cardiac catheterization laboratories is usually 400 lb. The difficulty is femoral access; usually this kind of patient requires a transradial approach. While using FT, there are no guidelines for dosage because in the RCTs, all overweight patients were excluded.[16]

STEMI in Patients with Bleeding

In general, if the bleeding can be stopped by a mechanical mean (compressing or ligating the artery), then the patient can tolerate four hours of anticoagulant during PCI. The favorite anticoagulant is UFH because of its short half-life and because it can be reversed by protamine.[16]

AMI Patients with Gastric Bleeding

If the patient has gastric bleeding and is hemodynamically stable, a gastroenterologist could do a gastroscopy and stop the bleeding by stapling the culprit artery. After that, the patient should be treated with an H2 antagonist and could tolerate short-term anticoagulant and oral antiplatelet (clopidogrel and ASA) for stenting of the IRA. GP 2b3a inhibitors should be avoided.[16]

AMI Patients with Very Recent Noncardiac Surgery

In a case report, a patient developed STEMI after removal of the right kidney. He underwent balloon angioplasty of the IRA with a standard dose of UFH to keep an ACT of 250 to 300. No stent was used and no UFH was given after the procedure. If the patient had a clean surgery, then he or she could have the stent placed because the bleeding problem with long-term ASA and clopidogrel therapy is quite low.[16]

AMI Patients with Concurrent Stroke

If the AMI patient has ischemic stroke, after getting the agreement from the neurologist to give a short-term anticoagulant (UFH or DTI) and a long-term oral antiplatelet drug, then the patient may undergo PCI and stenting. The following are two major concerns: (1) the risk of hemorrhagic conversion of the ischemic stroke with anticoagulant therapy, and (2) the risk of cerebral emboli from the protruding plaque in the aortic arch if they were the cause of stroke in the first place. If the benefits outweigh the risks, then the patient should have PCI provided that a strong indication is present. The family and the patient need to understand clearly the benefits and the risks, as the PCI procedure may convert a stable stroke into an unstable one. The mortality of a patient with AMI complicated by a stroke is also very high.[16]

AMI Patients Right After CABG

Sometimes, shortly after returning from the operating room (OR) after CABG, the patient is found to have ST segment elevation in one of the areas just bypassed. The patient should be brought back to the OR or the cardiac catheterization laboratory to recheck the patency of the bypass grafts. If there is a need for PCI, a full dose of UFH should be given, as the prior anticoagulation during CABG is reversed by protamine. The patient can tolerate DES stenting and subsequent clopidogrel therapy without a problem. The risk of returning to the OR is higher because of bleeding caused by clopidogrel; however, the full therapeutic effect of clopidogrel is not complete (>80% of platelets inhibited) until 24 hours later.

AMI Patients with AF on Coumadin, INR>2

Because coumadin does not have any effect on platelets, patients with therapeutic levels of INR can still develop STEMI. During PCI, the patient can be given oral loading and maintenance doses of antiplatelet drugs as usual. If the patient has a high INR, no UFH is needed. If the INR is less than 2, then the patient can be given UFH (as in the treatment of pulmonary embolism). Again, a transradial approach is preferred because of fewer bleeding complications at the vascular access site.

AMI Patients with Heparin-Induced Thrombocytopenia

Heparin-induced thrombocytopenia (HIT) is an immune-mediated complication of UFH. It involves a decrease in circulating platelets (thrombocytopenia) and an increased tendency to form blood clots, which can have devastating clinical consequences, such as limb ischemia requiring amputation (10–20%), MI, stroke, pulmonary embolism, and even death (20–30%). In patients with HIT, LMWH cannot be used because it has cross-reactivity. Either bivalirudin or argatroban can be used during PCI.[16]

AMI Patients with Hemophilia

Hemophilia B is a severe, inherited coagulopathy caused by mutations in the gene that encodes factor IX. Surgical and invasive procedures in patients suffering from this congenital disease are considered at high risk for hemorrhage. Regularly, the patient with hemophilia has been administered recombinant factor VIII pre- and postprocedure to maintain activity levels between 60 and 80% in order to prevent bleeding. Bivalirudin can be safely used in patients with a very high risk of bleeding (hemophilia) undergoing PCI.[16]

TAKE-HOME MESSAGE

Data Collecting Collect focused data about the patient's history (chest pain, history of HTN, DM, high cholesterol level), family history (of early sudden death due to heart disease, history of early CAD), and from a focused physical examination (signs of prior stroke, CAD, PAD, carotid murmur, weak peripheral pulses), all of which add weight to the clinical decision-making process.

Data Mining Recommend safe, appropriate, and efficacious investigation (including urgent ECG, fasting blood glucose, BUN, and creatinine levels, weight, PT, PTT).

Management Recommend safe, appropriate, and efficacious therapy. Based on worldwide availability of facilities, logistics, and resource affordability, especially in developing countries, the benchmark reperfusion strategy remains fibrinolytic therapy (FT). It is important to use those agents that the practitioner knows best. The earliest administration of any agent is better than the delayed administration of the best agent. If experienced operators are available and if the interval between door and balloon is less than 90 minutes, it is highly suggested that patients undergo primary intervention. Pay special attention to early acute stent thrombosis, especially in patients with initial TIMI-0 to TIMI-1 flow. Adjunctive therapies, especially ACEIs, beta blockers, and statins, should be given to improve short- and long-term outcomes.

References

1. Gibson, C. M.: The time dependent open vascular hypothesis. Cardiol Rounds. 2000;4:10.

2. Antman, E. M., Anbe, D. T., Armstrong, P. W., et al.: ACC/AHA guidelines for the management of patients with ST-elevation myocardial infarction: A report of the American College of Cardiology/American Heart Association Task Force on Practice Guidelines (Committee to Revise the 1999 Guidelines for the Management of Patients with Acute Myocardial Infarction). J Am Coll Cardiol. 2004;44:E1–E211.
3. Indications for fibrinolytic therapy in suspected acute myocardial infarction: collaborative overview of early mortality and major morbidity results from all randomised trials of more than 1000 patients. Fibrinolytic Therapy Trialists' (FTT) Collaborative Group. Lancet. 1994 Feb 5;343(8893):311-322-3.
4. Antman, E. M., Morrow, D. A., McCabe, C. H., et al.: Enoxaparin versus unfractionated heparin with fibrinolysis for ST-elevation myocardial infarction. N Engl J Med. 2006;354:1477–1488.
5. Keeley, E. C., Boura, J. A., Grines, C. L.: Primary angioplasty versus intravenous thrombolytic therapy for acute myocardial infarction: a quantitative review of 23 randomised trials. Lancet. 2003; Jan 4;361 (9351):13–20.
6. Stone, G. W., Witzenbichler, B., Guagliumi, G., and the HORIZONS-AMI Trial Investigators.: Bivalirudin during primary PCI in acute myocardial infarction. N Engl J Med. 2008; May 22;358(21):2218–2230.
7. Stone, G. W., Witzenbichler, B., Guagliumi, G., et al.: Bivalirudin during primary PCI in acute myocardial infarction. N Engl J Med. 2008; 358:2218–2230.
8. Dangas, G.: Stent thrombosis in the HORIZON AMI trial presented at the late Breaking Clinical Trial Session during the i2 Summit at the American College of Cardiology 2009 Scientific Sessions, Orlando FL, March 2009.
9. Smith, S. S., et al.: ACC/AHA/SCAI 2005 Guideline update for percutaneous coronary intervention. Cath Cardiovasc Intervent. 2006; 67:87–112.
10. Mehta, S.R.: The results of the CURRENT-OASIS 7 presented at the European Society of Cardiology Congress 2009 Barcelona September 2009.
11. Sabatine, M., Morrow, D., Montalescot, G., et al.: Clopidogrel as Adjunctive Reperfusion Therapy (CLARITY) TIMI 28 trial. Circulation. 2005;112:3846–3854.
12. Chen, Z. M., Pan, H. C., Chen, Y. P., for the COMMIT (Clopidogrel and Metoprolol in Myocardial Infarction Trial) collaborative group: Early intravenous then oral metoprolol in 45,852 patients with acute myocardial infarction: randomised placebo-controlled trial. Lancet 2005;366(9497):1587–1589.
13. ACE Inhibitor Myocardial Infarction Collaborative Group: Indications for ACE inhibitors in the early treatment of acute myocardial infarction: systematic overview of individual data from 100,000 patients in randomised trials. Circulation. 1998;97:2202–2212.
14. White, H. D., Aylward, P. E., Huang, Z., et al. for the VALIANT Investigators: Heart Failure Mortality and Morbidity Remain High Despite Captopril and/or Valsartan Therapy in Elderly Patients With Left Ventricular Systolic Dysfunction, Heart Failure, or Both After Acute

Myocardial Infarction: Results From the Valsartan in Acute Myocardial Infarction Trial (VALIANT). Circulation. 2005;112: 3391–3399.

15. Bavry, A. A., Mood, G. R., Kumbhani, D. J., et al.: Long-term benefit of statin therapy initiated during hospitalization for an acute coronary syndrome: a systematic review of randomized trials. Am J Cardiovasc Drugs. 2007;7(2):135–141.

16. Nguyen, T., ed: ST Segment Elevation Myocardial Infarction, in Management of Complex Cardiovascular Problems. Philadephia, PA.: Blackwell Futura, 2007, pp 19–50.

17. http://www.wikidoc.org/index.php/Plasmapheresis (accessed 7/2009).

18. Lawal, L., Lange, R., Schulman, S.: Acute myocardial infarction in two young women without significant risk factors. J Invasive Cardiol. 2009, 21:e3–e5.

19. Al-Aqeedi, R. F., Al-Nabti, A. D.: Drug-eluting stent implantation for acute myocardial infarction during pregnancy with use of glycoprotein IIb/IIIa inhibitor, aspirin and clopidogrel. J Invasive Cardiol. 2008;20(5):E146–E149.

20. Davies, J. O., Hunt, B. J.: Myocardial infarction in young patients without coronary atherosclerosis: assume primary antiphospholipid syndrome until proved otherwise. Int J Clin Pract. 2007;61(3): 379–384.

21. Mukherjee, D.: Management of Cocaine-Associated Chest Pain and Myocardial Infarction: A Scientific Statement From the American Heart Association Acute Cardiac Care Committee of the Council on Clinical Cardiology. http://www.medscape.com/viewarticle/572723 (accessed 6/9/2009).

22. Herzog, C., Ma, J., Collins, A.: Poor long-term survival after acute myocardial infarction among patients on long-term dialysis. N Engl J Med. 1998;339:799–805.

23. Herzog, C.: Acute MI in dialysis patients: How can we improve the outlook? J Crit Illness. 1999;14:613–621.

24. Simonson, J. S., Schiller, N. B.: Sonorespirometry: A new method for non-invasive estimation of mean right atrial pressure based on 2-D echocardiographic measurements of the inferior vena cava during measured inspiration. J Am Coll Cardiol. 1988;11:557–564.

25. Hochman, J. S., Lamas, G. A., Buller, C. E., et al.: Coronary intervention for persistent occlusion after myocardial infarction. N Engl J Med. 2006;355(23):2395–407.

26. Mehilli, J., et al. The results of the BRAVE-3: Bavarian Reperfusion Alternatives Evaluation-3 Trial, presented at the ACC/SCAI late Breaking Clinical Trials results, at the ACC Annual Scientifc Sessions Chicago, March 2008.

27. Seyfarth, M., Sibbing, D., Bauer, I., et al.: A randomized clinical trial to evaluate the safety and efficacy of a percutaneous left ventricular assist device versus intra-aortic balloon pumping for treatment of cardiogenic shock caused by myocardial infarction. J Am Coll Cardiol. 2008;52(19):1584–1588.

28. Thiele, H., and Schuler, G.: A systematic review and meta-analysis of intra-aortic balloon pump therapy in ST-elevation myocardial infarction: should we change the guidelines? Eur Heart J. 2009;30:389–390.

Peripheral Arterial Disease

John Reilly, Ho Thuong Dung, Ainol Sahar, and Vijay Dave

Chapter Outline

DEFINITION

Peripheral arterial disease (PAD) conventionally refers to vascular diseases of the lower extremities, although it actually encompasses noncoronary vascular diseases in aggregate. Renovascular and carotid disease are typically each considered separately due to specific pathophysiology of these vascular beds.

Patient Population in Focus

An important determinant of the reported incidence and prevalence of disease is the definition used for the presence of disease. Some studies of the prevalence of PAD rely on patient-reported symptoms, while others rely on noninvasive imaging as a sensitive measure of disease. Many, in fact, most people with PAD are ignorant of their disease and remain asymptomatic, and therefore those studies that rely on patient-reported symptoms underestimate the true prevalence of the disease. The World Health Organization (WHO) Rose questionnaire is a standardized questionnaire developed to elicit and characterize claudication symptoms. The Framingham Heart Study employed this Rose questionnaire to identify those among its cohort of 5209 men and women aged 28 to 62 who had intermittent claudication.[1] The questionnaire was administered every two years, beginning in 1948. Among those 30 to 44 years old, the annual incidence of PAD, as defined by claudication by the Rose questionnaire, was 0.06% of the men and 0.03% of the women. This increased to 0.6% and 0.5% among men and women, respectively, between the ages of 65 and 74 years.

Strategic Programming

The first step is to identify patients with PAD through data collecting with a comprehensive history of claudication and physical examination (especially an examination of the pulses in the lower extremities). The next step is to perform data processing in order to formulate a preliminary diagnosis and a short list of differential diagnoses (e.g., aortic dissection). Then, using the method of data mining, tests could be ordered (ankle-brachial index [ABI], magnetic resonance angiography [MRA]) in order to confirm (data converting) the main diagnosis of PAD and to rule out (data filtering) the differential diagnoses.

Risk Factors

The most common cause of PAD is atherosclerosis; thus, the risk factors for coronary artery disease (CAD) are shared with those of PAD. Hypertension, hypercholesterolemia, diabetes mellitus, and tobacco use all increase the risk of developing PAD, as do unconventional risk factors such as hyperhomocysteinemia or elevated levels of C-reactive protein. A history of tobacco use is the dominant risk for the development of PAD. Those with a history of smoking are at such high risk that approximately 80% of patients with PAD are current or former smokers.[2,3] Tobacco use is a greater risk for the development of PAD than it is for the development of CAD; it is two to three times as likely to cause PAD as CAD.[4] Smoking increases the risk of PAD and claudication between two to ten times when compared with those who have never smoked.[3,5,6]

Diabetes mellitus increases the risk of PAD to nearly the same degree as a history of tobacco use. The incidence of PAD is increased from two- to four-fold in patients with diabetes. Nearly one in five people with PAD have diabetes.[7] Diabetes particularly affects the smaller, more distal vessels of the coronary tree. Similarly, among patients with diabetes and PAD, the smaller infrapopliteal vessels are more likely to be significantly involved. These smaller caliber, infrapopliteal vessels become diffusely diseased, which is why patients with diabetes are at increased risk for developing critical limb ischemia and for requiring limb amputation.[8-10] Some reports estimate that diabetics are at a 15-fold increased risk for lower extremity amputation.[11]

Each of the lipid abnormalities that is associated with an increase in atherosclerotic heart disease has been shown to increase the risk of PAD. Increasing levels of cholesterol are correlated with increasing incidence of PAD.[12, 13] Lower levels of high-density lipoprotein (HDL) and higher levels of low-density lipoprotein are found in patients with PAD as compared to matched controls without PAD.[12,13,14] Although a causal relationship between hyperhomocysteinemia, elevated C-reactive protein, and atherosclerosis is less well established, both are associated with increased risk of PAD. Hyperhomocysteinemia carries a two- to three-fold risk for PAD as compared to those with normal levels of homocysteine.[15, 16] The Physicians' Health Study revealed that those with the highest levels of C-reactive protein were at twice the risk of developing PAD.[17]

DATA COLLECTING

Investigation Master Plan

When a physician sees a patient suspected of having PAD, there are seven main areas of interest for data collecting (history and physical examination).

The main area of interest: The arterial system of the legs. In general, the patient with PAD is asymptomatic. There are subjective symptoms or physical findings related directly to PAD. This is a hardware problem with tight linear interaction and loose coupling with the pulmonary or renovascular system (zone A).

The **upstream area for** PAD is the arterial segment proximal to the index lesion (zone B).

The **downstream area is** the leg or lower leg (zone C).

The **system configuration:** There is no problem with the configuration of the vascular system. However, the index lesion obstructs the blood flow to the distal segment (zone E).

The **work-around configuration:** There are collaterals (zone D).

The **cardiovascular system:** There is direct interaction between the arterial system of the leg with the cardiovascular system.

The **network (the whole body):** Long-standing, uncontrolled PAD can cause ischemic neuropathy, damaging the electrical system. However, PAD has no effect on the pulmonary, cerebral, or renal system (zone F). A person can live without a leg.

History

The majority of patients with PAD are asymptomatic. This absence of symptoms is the underlying fact that has pushed researchers to employ objective noninvasive studies, such as the ABI, to define the presence of disease.

Claudication

The classic symptom of PAD due to lower extremity ischemia is claudication. At rest, the individual does not experience any discomfort because there is sufficient blood flow. With the increased demand of movement or exercise, the individual with claudication experiences discomfort, pain, weakness, or fatigue in specific muscle groups. Most commonly, the calf muscles are the first to become involved, although these symptoms may then extend proximally. The muscle groups involved are determined by the level of occlusive disease.

Stenosis of the common or superficial femoral artery produces claudication of the calf. More proximal stenoses, such as terminal aorta or iliac disease, result in symptoms of the hips, buttocks, and thighs as well as the calf muscles.

Those with infrapopliteal disease may experience pain or numbness of the feet. However, since there are three vessels below the knee, this disease must be extensive to produce claudication on the basis of isolated infrapopliteal disease. Importantly, the symptoms of exertional claudication are reproducible with similar levels of exertion and are promptly relieved with rest. Two classification systems qualify the severity of ischemia, those of Fontaine and Rutherford, and create a standardized language in which clinicians can communicate to one another (Table 18-1). Changes of body position have no effect on vascular causes of claudication. If the individual must sit down or bend over to relieve symptoms, claudication is not the cause of the discomfort.

TABLE 18-1: Classification of Clinical Status of Patients with PAD

Fontaine		Rutherford		
Stage	Characteristics	Grade	Category	Characteristics
I	Asymptomatic	0	0	Asymptomatic
IIa	Mild Claudication	I	1	Mild Claudication
IIb	Moderate-Severe Claudication	I	2	Moderate Claudication
		I	3	Severe Claudication
IIII	Ischemic Rest Pain	II	4	Ischemic Rest Pain
		III	5	Minor tissue loss
IV	Ulceration or Gangrene	IV	6	Ulceration or Gangrene

Critical Limb Ischemia

As opposed to the patient with claudication, the patient with critical limb ischemia (CLI) has insufficient perfusion to maintain the limb at rest. Untreated, such ischemia would require limb amputation within six months. Patients with CLI experience pain at rest, ulcers, and ischemic gangrene. Resting pain in CLI is often exacerbated when the patient is supine and may improve by dangling the foot over the edge of the bed. Narcotics are often required for relief of pain.

However, patients who have developed neuropathy secondary to diabetes or ischemia may not report pain at rest even when presenting with CLI. Patients presenting with CLI and their physicians may be ignorant of underlying PAD because it is often the initial presentation of PAD. Atherosclerotic arterial disease is the most common cause of CLI, and this disease is frequently diffuse and affects more than one anatomic level. The infrapopliteal vessels are almost uniformly involved. Thromboagiitis obliterans (Buerger disease), vasculitis, thromboembolic or atheroembolic events, trauma, and popliteal entrapment may also critically impair circulation and produce CLI. Vasospastic disease, severely low cardiac output states, and diabetes may all impair microvascular blood flow, thereby exacerbating CLI.

Acute Limb Ischemia

The presentation of CLI may be of acute or chronic onset. CLI typically refers to the latter; those patients with acute critical limb ischemia are managed significantly differently from those who present chronically and therefore should be specifically distinguished as having acute limb ischemia.

DATA DECODING TIPS (CLINICAL PEARLS)
Differentiating Chronic and Acute Limb Ischemia

When obtaining the history from the patient with CLI, the duration and onset of symptoms are the most important elements of the history. There is an extensive potential for collateral development to the lower leg through the internal iliac and profunda femoris arteries; this collateral bed allows obstructive disease to develop on multiple levels with limited symptoms. The balance is finally tipped in the patient with CLI in that the collateral flow is insufficient to counterbalance the obstruction in the major vessels of the limb, and enough ischemia is present to threaten the limb's viability. Patients with acute limb ischemia, in contrast, have not had sufficient time to develop this collateral circulation when a sudden, new obstruction creates limb-threatening ischemia. The distinction between acute limb ischemia and CLI is important because the acutely ischemic limb must be recognized and urgently revascularized. Pain, paralysis, parasthesia, pulselessness, and pallor are the classic five "Ps" that aid in identifying patients with acutely ischemic limbs. The ischemic limb is also subjectively and objectively cool (poikilothermia) to the patient and clinician.

Atheroembolic or thromboembolic disease is often a cause of the acutely ischemic limb, as these phenomena produce a sudden obstruction to flow that may cause acute limb ischemia. Branching points in the arterial system produce a sudden reduction in the caliber of the vessel as opposed to more gradual tapering in nonbranching segments. Emboli are commonly found in these bi- or trifurcations, and the experienced clinician pays particular attention to these segments of the anatomy. Aneurysms more proximal in the arterial tree and the atria or ventricles of the heart are possible sources of these emboli. Another mechanism for the sudden development of an ischemia-producing lesion is in-situ thrombotic occlusion superimposed on preexisting plaque.

Physical Examination
Examination of the Pulses of the Lower Extremities

The pulses of each lower extremity are checked in four locations. The femoral pulse is palpated just below the inguinal ligament, two finger-breadths lateral to the public tubercle. In obese patients, external rotation of the hip may facilitate palpation of the artery. The popliteal pulse is more difficult to feel, as it lies in the popliteal space. With the patient supine and the knee slightly flexed, the examiner should hook the fingertips of the hands around the medial and lateral knee tendons and press the fingertips into the popliteal space. The pulse usually lies slightly lateral to the midline. The dorsalis pedis is a terminal branch of the anterior tibial artery and is found in the mid-dorsum of the foot between the first and second metatarsals. The posterior tibial is found behind the medial malleolus, while the peroneal artery terminates at the ankle and is not palpable on physical exam.[18]

Grading of the Pulses of the Lower Extremities

Grading of pulses is subjective, and a simple method is to describe the pulses as normal, diminished, or absent and symmetric versus asymmetric in relation to the other side. Numbered grading systems can also be used, although these may vary among institutions. An example of a pulse grading system is 0, absent; 1+, diminished; 2+, normal; 3+, prominent, the last suggesting local aneurysm. If a pulse is not palpable, further assessment with a continuous-wave Doppler test should be pursued. Doppler signals should be qualified as triphasic, biphasic, or monophasic, with the triphasic signal considered normal. In the absence of a palpable pulse, biphasic and monophasic signals correlate with moderate and severe arterial occlusive disease, respectively. In severe cases of acute lower-extremity ischemia or chronic critical ischemia, the only Doppler signal in the foot may be a soft continuous venous signal.[18]

Inspection of the Leg and Foot

This process may reveal important signs of acute and chronic arterial insufficiency. Acute insufficiency will produce definite changes of pallor followed by cyanosis or skin mottling. In addition, muscle weakness or paralysis, especially of the foot dorsiflexors (anterior compartment), may become obvious. After 24 hours of acute ischemia, the leg often becomes swollen, and the skin may blister.

Chronic claudication may have no findings on inspection other than mild muscle atrophy and/or hair loss on the leg or foot. Critical lower-extremity ischemia, however, is associated with elevation pallor and dependent rubor of the forefoot. Additionally, skin breakdown in the toes or forefoot tissue may occur, and nonhealing ulcers or gangrene will appear. Neuropathic ulcers are difficult to distinguish from those that are primarily ischemic by inspection alone, as they both occur in the same distribution. Dry gangrene with black tissue or wet gangrene with draining purulence and foul odor may be present in the setting of neuropathic and ischemic ulcers, and often there is a mixed component.[18]

Palpation

This technique is also helpful in the assessment of acute extremity ischemia. Skin coldness and the level of temperature demarcation can be detected by palpation with the back of the examiner's hand and fingers. Acute ischemia also may be associated with tenderness and tenseness of the calf muscles, especially the anterior compartment. In addition, acute ischemia may cause sensory nerve damage, detectable by pinprick sensory examination or testing of proprioception in the toes.[18]

Auscultation

This examination of lower-extremity arteries is most useful in the femoral area, where bruits indicate local femoral artery disease or more proximal aortoiliac disease with bruits transmitted to the groin. If there is a question about the presence of a femoral bruit, walking the patient for 25 to 50 steps at the bedside often will increase lower-extremity flow enough to increase the severity of the bruit. Auscultation is also important when an arteriovenous fistula is suspected, which generally has a characteristic continuous to-and-fro bruit.[18]

DATA DECODING TIPS (CLINICAL PEARLS)
Examination of Patients with Critical Limb Ischemia (CLI)

Careful examination of pulses is imperative during examination of limbs with critical ischemia in order to determine the likely level of stenosis or occlusion. When dependent, the extremity develops rubor that quickly blanches upon elevation and sluggish capillary filling is present. Livido reticularis suggests atheroembolic disease as a cause of CLI. Ulcers should be carefully examined; arterial ulcers are painful and tender to the touch unless neuropathy clouds the scenario. The surrounding tissue often has concomitant cellulitis. Venous ulcers are typically located over the malleoli as opposed to ulcers of arterial origin.

DATA FILTERING (DIFFERENTIAL DIAGNOSIS)

There are many causes of lower extremity pain or weakness that may be confused with claudication or "pseudoclaudication." Nerve root compression, spinal stenosis, arthritis, chronic compartment syndrome, venous claudication, and symptomatic Baker cyst may each manifest with symptoms that mimic true claudication. The astute clinician must be wary of elements of the patient's history that suggest that the discomfort does not arise from insufficient circulation. Spinal stenosis typically requires a change in position, such as sitting down, leaning over at the waist, or bending over a shopping cart to relieve discomfort. Symptoms that are not promptly relieved by rest suggest arthritis, spinal stenosis, or radicular pain. Radicular and arthritic pains as well as symptomatic Baker cysts may be causes of pain at rest. Intermittent claudication occurs at the same level of exertion consistently; radicular pain often occurs nearly immediately after onset of exertion; the pain of spinal stenosis may begin after prolonged standing; the onset of arthritic pain is variably related to exertion.

DATA MINING (WORK-UP)
Ankle Brachial Index

The ankle brachial index (ABI) is the single most valuable diagnostic tool for the evaluation of PAD. It is simple to perform, noninvasive, and risk-free. The results of the ABI are both diagnostic of and prognostic for PAD. The ABI is an ideal test for these reasons; therefore the cardiovascular specialist must understand the ABI and how it is performed.

An ABI ≤ 0.9 is abnormal and diagnostic of obstructive peripheral arterial disease; therefore, an abnormal ABI has been used in epidemiologic studies as the definition for the presence of PAD and as pathognomonic. The ABI is inversely proportional to the degree of stenosis or total "burden" of stenosis and correlates with the severity of symptoms. An ABI that is ≤ 0.9 is consistent with symptoms of intermittent claudication, ABI measurements between 0.71 and 0.9 suggest mild obstruction, and those with measurements between 0.41 and 0.7 have moderate obstruction. Those patients with ABIs ≤ 0.4 have severe obstructive disease consistent with critical limb ischemia in the proper clinical presentation. Although the ABI is proportional to the degree of obstruction, by itself it is not sufficient to make the diagnosis of claudication. The presence of symptoms in patients with obstructive disease is determined by the extent of collateral circulation and the time course over which these obstructions develop.

 JOB DESCRIPTION:

How to Measure the Ankle Brachial Index

The ABI can be readily performed in a physician's office with a manual blood pressure cuff and hand-held Doppler probe. The ankle brachial index indexes the lower extremity blood pressure against the upper extremity blood pressure as the reference point. The ABI is calculated as the lower extremity pressure over the upper extremity pressure. The systolic blood pressure is measured manually in each arm; the higher value of these two measurents is then used as the denominator. Patients who have PAD may have obstructive disease of the subclavian artery, reducing the measured pressure, which is why the higher pressure is used to calculate the ABI for both lower extremities. For example, the right arm may serve as the denominator to determine the ABI for both lower extremities. The cuff is then placed above the ankle, and systolic pressures of the dorsalis pedis and posterior tibialis arteries are measured using the Doppler probe to obtain the systolic pressure. The higher value measured at the ankle is then used as the numerator to calculate the ABI for the respective lower extremities (Figure 18-1). Performing the ABI can be done even more simply with an automated blood pressure cuff.

Right ABI = <u>Higher Right Ankle Pressure</u>   Right ABI = <u>Higher Left Ankle Pressure</u>
            Higher Arm Pressure   **Higher Arm Pressure**

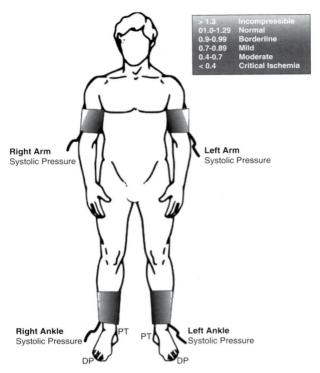

> 1.3	Incompressible
01.0-1.29	Normal
0.9-0.99	Borderline
0.7-0.89	Mild
0.4-0.7	Moderate
< 0.4	Critical Ischemia

Right Arm Systolic Pressure

Left Arm Systolic Pressure

Right Ankle Systolic Pressure   PT   PT   **Left Ankle** Systolic Pressure

DP   DP

Figure 18-1 Ankle-brachial Index. The higher arm pressure is the denominator for the ABI of both lower extremity ABIs. The higher pressure measured in the DP or PT is the denominator for the respective extremity. DP = Dorsalis pedis artery, PT = Posterior tibial artery.

⚬ DATA DECODING TIPS (CLINICAL PEARLS)
False Positives and Negatives of ABI

If sufficient collaterals have developed to compensate for stenosis, the resting ABI may be normal. Those patients with symptoms strongly suggestive of claudication whose ABI is normal should undergo ABI measurement after exercise. The arteriolar dilatory response to exercise reduces vascular resistance, reducing the systolic pressure in the lower extremity, thereby lowering the ABI. In other patients, particularly those with diabetes or renal failure, the infrapopliteal vessels may become calcified and incompressible, artificially increasing the ABI. Thus, an ABI ≥ 1.3 does not exclude PAD. In these cases, a toe-brachial index (TBI) should be employed. Small cuffs are used to compress the digital arteries, which are spared the calcification of the infrapopliteal vessels, and the TBI is calculated in the same manner as the ABI.

As an extension of the ABI, the vascular laboratory may be asked to perform segmental pressure measurements. Plethysmographic cuffs are placed on the upper and lower thighs and the upper and lower portions of the lower legs. Analogous to those of the ABI, these lower extremity pressures may be indexed against the brachial artery. Segmental pressure measurements provide the additional information of localizing the stenosis; a pressure gradient between the brachial artery pressure and the upper thigh suggests aortic or iliac stenosis. When the gradient is between the upper and lower thighs, the lesion will be found in the superficial femoral artery (SFA). A 20-mm difference in pressures is generally accepted as significant.

Vascular Ultrasound

The cardiovascular specialist is well acquainted with the merits and potential for ultrasound evaluation through familiarity with echocardiography. Ultrasonography displays anatomic vascular details in gray-scale images (Figure 18-2). In addition to displaying vessel lumen narrowing, plaque can be visualized, allowing the assessment of the degree of calcification. Ultrasound also displays aneurysm, arterial dissection, lymphatic disease, soft-tissue impingement, and popliteal entrapment. Although the imaging capability of ultrasound is enticing, combining this anatomic imaging with the physiologic information derived from Doppler measurements of blood velocity is what strengthens the role of duplex ultrasonography. Duplex ultrasound is widely available, relatively inexpensive, noninvasive, and risk-free. When needed, it can be performed at the bedside for hospitalized patients. Imaging quality and interpretability are dependent upon the skill and effort of the ultrasonographer performing the exam and therefore may be variable.

Peak systolic velocities are measured at identified stenoses and in the segment immediately proximal to the stenosis. If the velocity within the stenosis is twice that of the proximal segment, the lesion is interpreted to be at least 50% stenotic[19, 20] (Figure 18-3). Some investigators have attempted to use velocity measurements to distinguish lesions between 50 and 75% and those between 75 and 99%.[21, 22] Totally occluded vessels have no flow and therefore the Doppler measured velocity for 100% lesions is zero. The sensitivity and specificity for the detection of a ≥50% stenosis from the iliac to the popliteal artery are 90% to 95%. The diagnostic accuracy of duplex imaging is impaired when the vessel is difficult to image, such as when there is excessive bowel gas in pelvic vessels or dense calcification causing shadowing of acoustic waves. If

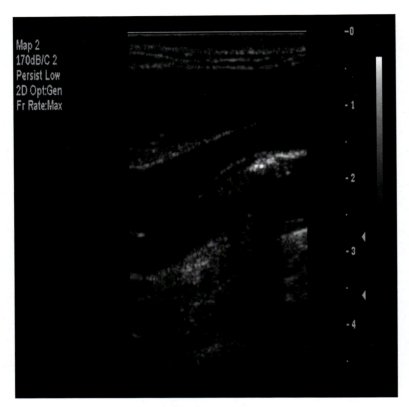

Figure 18-2 Vascular ultrasound demonstrating gray-scale image of vessel as well as plaque present within the wall, although the lumen is preserved.

significant tortuosity of the vessel causes the sonographer to obtain an inadequate Doppler signal, the accuracy of the study will be negatively affected (Figures 18-4 and 18-5).

In most cases, the diagnosis of obstructive PAD can be made without duplex ultrasound, since history, physical exam, and an abnormal ABI should establish the diagnosis. Duplex ultrasound should be employed in those patients who may benefit from revascularization. From the ultrasound exam the location and degree of stenosis can be determined and can predict suitability for endovascular repair in 84 to 92% of cases.[23, 24] Duplex ultrasonography has also been used to select the appropriate infrapopliteal vessel for distal anastomosis of surgical bypass grafts.[25, 26] Patients who have had surgical revascularization with conduits routinely undergo surveillance duplex ultrasonography in an

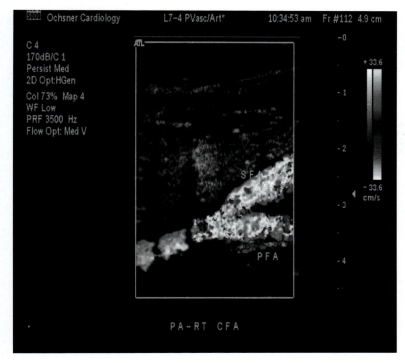

Figure 18-3 Duplex ultrasound of the bifurcation of the right common femoral artery (CFA) into the superficial femoral artery (SFA) and the profunda femoris (PFA). When using instrument equipped with color flow, color coding of Doppler-derived flow velocities demonstrates turbulent flow at the bifurcation, resulting in a mosaic of red and blue. This turbulent flow suggests stenosis at the bifurcation.

effort to improve graft patency. This surveillance is more sensitive for the development of graft-threatening lesions than history, physical exam, or ABI.[27-31] In one report, grafts with abnormal duplex exams that were revised had a 90% patency rate at one year that was similar to the rate in patients with normal duplex exams at surveillance. In contrast, those with abnormal duplex exams that were not revised had a patency rate of 66%.[29] Although it is not widely adapted or studied, a similar policy of surveillance following endovascular intervention may improve long-term patency.

Magnetic Resonance Angiography

Magnetic resonance angiography (MRA) can be used to evaluate the location and degree of stenosis. Unlike CT angiography, MRA depicts

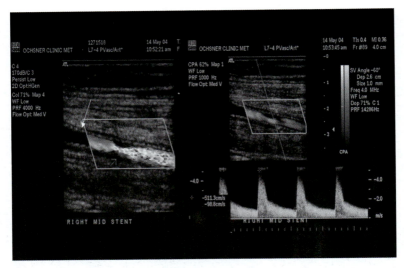

Figure18-4 In instrument equipped with color, color duplex ultrasound on the left demonstrates a stent (white arrow) with focal in stent restenosis demonstrated by the turbulent flow (thin arrow). Right panel demonstrates increased velocity through the restenotic segment.

the lumina of vessels, more comparable to conventional angiography. Several techniques may be employed to perform MRA, including two-dimensional time of flight, three-dimensional imaging, bolus chase, and contrast-enhanced imaging with gadolinium. Recently, gadolinium has been implicated as the cause of nephrogenic systemic fibrosis (NSF), which is a debilitating disease that affects the skin, muscles, and internal organs. While gadolinium had once been considered a less nephrotoxic option for digital subtraction angiography, patients with acute or chronic renal insufficiency with a glomerular filtration rate less than 30 mL/min should not receive gadolinium. Thus a noncontrasted technique or another imaging modality should be employed whenever possible.

Comparison of MRA and conventional angiography reveals a high degree of correlation. The sensitivity and specificity of MRA to detect lesions more than 50% obstructed were between 90 and 100% using conventional angiography as the control.[32] Some reports suggest that MRA may be a better test to demonstrate the patency of infrapopliteal vessels in patients with CLI. In 24 patients with diabetes and CLI, nearly 40% had pedal vessels that had escaped detection by conventional angiography.[33] Other reports dispute this claim, and it is logical that its basis is dependent upon the quality of each exam.[34-36]

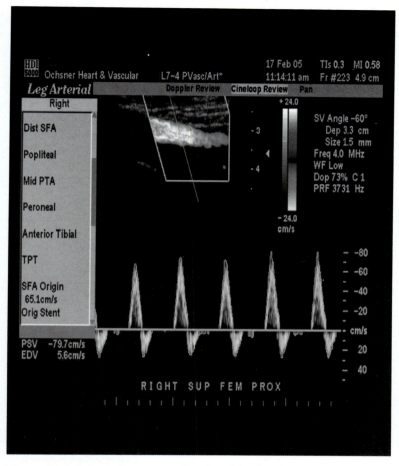

Figure 18-5 Pulse volume recording (PVR) in the above normal superficial femoral artery (SFA) demonstrates a velocity pattern that is similar to an invasive arterial tracing. With obstruction, this pattern becomes blunted distal to the stenosis.

MRA does not require exposure to the ionizing radiation that CT and conventional angiography require. Also, iodinated contrast medium must be used for all conventional and CT angiograms. While the safety of gadolinium for contrast enhancement is now in doubt, by employing other techniques, MRA can be accomplished without the injection of an intravenous contrast agent. Patients with permanent pacemakers, implanted defibrillators, preclude performing an MR exam. Metal clips and stents may cause sufficient artifact to significantly reduce accuracy. Turbulent flow in a stenosis may cause overestimation of stenosis. Retrograde collateral flow may create significant artifact at the time of flight studies.

MRA and CT angiography provide the same information—the location and degree of stenosis—with the caveats mentioned above. The degree of accuracy when compared to conventional angiography is similar. A comparison of MRA with gadolinium with CT angiography with a 16-slice scanner reveals greater interobserver agreement for MRA.[37,38] Heavy clacification can cause disagreement among observers, particularly in infrapopliteal vessels (Table 18-2).

TABLE 18-2: Relative Merits and Limitations of Noninvasive Vascular Imaging Studies

	Benefits	Limitations
ABI	Can be office-based Diagnoses presence of PAD when <0.9	Medical calcinosis may produce non-compressible vessels (diabetics, renal failure patients, elderly)
ABI with exercise	Increased sensitivity for Iliac disease Correlates symptoms with ABI	Requires treadmill
Duplex USG	Diagnoses and images PAD Useful for revascularization patients Surgical graft surveillance	Pelvic vessels may be difficult to image due to bowel gas Dense calcium deposits may cause shadowing
CTA	Assesses lesion anatomic characteristics Assesses eligibility for revascularization Quick and reproducible Imaging of stents and clips	Ionizing radiation Iodinated contrast may cause contrast induced nephropathy (CIN)
MRA	Assesses anatomic characteristics of lesion Assesses lesion eligibility for revascularization Stents produce artifact Implants preclude MRA (i.e., PPM, ICD)	May overestimate stenosis Stents produce artifact Implants preclude MRA (i.e., PPM, ICD)

ABI: ankle brachial index, PAD: peripheral artery disease, USG: ultrasound, CTA: computed tomographic angiography, MRA: magnetic resonance angiogram, PPM: pacemaker, ICD: implantable cardioverter defibrillator.

Computed Tomographic Angiography

With the development of the multidetector computed tomography (CT) scanner and other technologic advances, the ability to perform angiography noninvasively has been achieved. The ability of the CT scanner to cover larger territories more quickly has improved as these scanners can follow a bolus of intravenous contrast dye as it flows through the aorta to the lower extremities. This test is minimally invasive, requiring the insertion of an intravenous catheter in a superficial vein, typically in the antecubital fossa. As opposed to invasive angiography, there is no requirement for observed recovery after the procedure and no risk of significant bleeding. Patients are still exposed to ionizing radiation and intravenous contrast dye and the attendant risks of these exposures. Careful consideration should be paid prior to subjecting younger patients to radiation, as they are more likely to develop a radiation-associated cancer in their lifetime when compared to older subjects. Patients with previous contrast dye allergies must be premedicated with antihistamines and steroids prior to undergoing CT angiography. A prior history of renal insufficiency, diabetes mellitus, contrast-induced nephropathy, heart failure, or dehydration increases the potential for contrast-induced nephropathy.[39-41] One report would suggest that intravenous contrast agent may be less deleterious to renal function than the intra-arterial injection required for traditional angiography.[42]

Unlike imaging with magnetic resonance (MR), the presence of implants, such as permanent pacemakers and implantable cardiac defibrillators, pose no contraindication for CT angiography. The presence of surgical clips or prosthetic joint implants may cause some artifacts; however, this usually is limited to the immediate adjacent structures and does not prevent interpretation of the study.

CT angiography produces images that correlate well with conventional invasive angiography, corroborated by studies prior to the development of multidetector CT.[43,44] Rubin and coworkers compared CT angiography performed with a four detector CT scanner with DSA and found 100% concordance between the two modalities among the 24 patients studied. In addition, CT angiography successfully imaged 26 vessels that were not seen on DSA due to tight upstream stenoses producing slow flow.[45] Similarly Martin and colleagues. examined 41 patients with both modalities and found an 87% sensitivity and 98% specificity for stenoses, while the sensitivity and specificity for occlusion were 92% and 97%, respectively. An additional 110 segments were visualized on MDCT that were not seen by DSA.[46] Contrast injection for CT angiography occurs over 15 to 20 seconds, such that collateralized vessels and vessels that fill slowly owing to stenoses have a greater opportunity to be visualized compared to short duration contrast injections performed immediately before DSA acquisition. The interpretation of CT angiograms is bolstered by the ability to manipulate the acquired images to evaluate the angiogram in an infinite number of angles. Even rotational digital subtraction angiograms have a finite number of angles that may be reviewed. In addition to the lumen of the angiogram, CT angiography allows evaluation of the vessel wall and surrounding parenchymal structures.

When performed properly, CT angiography can replace traditional invasive angiography, and therefore it is an excellent tool to define which patients are potential candidates for revascularization. CT angiography can identify the location and degree of stenosis. It provides excellent characterization of the lesion: length, diameter, side branches, and plaque composition. Runoff vessels distal to the stenosis to be revascularized are also well visualized. In patients with an indication for revascularization, CT angiography should be considered prior to referring the patient for revascularization. CT angiography should also be considered when one of the vasculidities is in the differential diagnosis in order to evaluate the vessel wall, which cannot be performed by conventional angiography. Obstruction secondary to extrinsic compression, such as a Baker's cyst compressing the popliteal artery, can be readily evaluated by CT imaging, which is not restricted to looking at the lumen of the vessels.

Risk Stratification

The natural history of atheroslerotic limbs has not been extensively studied. The limbs of patients who present with claudication generally indicate a good prognosis. Patients with claudication in isolation are not at increased risk of limb loss through ten years of follow-up.[47] The addition of an abnormal ABI or a history of diabetes mellitus are predictors of the development of ischemic ulcers or pain at rest in these patients. By definition, patients with CLI are at greatly increased risk of limb loss. The number and extent of stenotic lesions, as well as the potential for successful revascularization, determine the likelihood of limb salvage. Patients with acute limb ischemia must be promptly evaluated for evidence of a threatened limb, such as paralysis or anesthesia, and referred for rapid revascularization as appropriate. Among patients who present with CLI, 25% will undergo major limb amputation within the following year.[48]

There is considerable overlap among populations of people with coronary artery disease, cerebrovascular disease, and peripheral arterial disease. Atherosclerosis is a systemic disease that affects the entire vascular system. Approximately one out of four people with coronary artery disease have vascular disease in multiple vascular territories.[49, 50] Sixty percent of people with PAD also have evident atherosclerosis in coronary or cerebrovascular arteries. Patients with PAD are at increased risk for myocardial infarction (MI) and cerebrovascular accident (CVA).[48] The

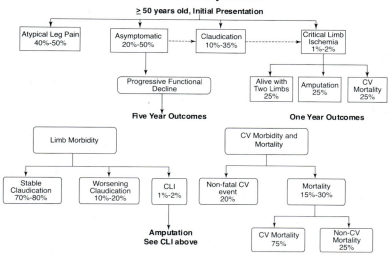

Figure 18-6 This algorithm demonstrates the natural history of PAD. The upper half describes the initial presentation with PAD. The lower half demonstrates the outcomes five years after initial presentation. Adapted from Hirsch et al., Circulation. 113(11);e463-e654[68]

severity of PAD has been shown to directly correlate with the severity of carotid artery disease; therefore the 40% increased incidence of ischemic neurologic events among those with PAD is not surprising.[51] The Edinburgh Artery Study confirms this relationship between increasing severity of PAD and increased incidence of transient ischemic attacks (TIA) and stroke; PAD patients were at a four-to-fivefold increased risk of TIA or stroke compared to those without PAD.[52] The risk of MI is increased 20 to 60%, and there is a two- to sixfold increase in coronary death.[51-56] Vascular patients with CLI are the sickest of all of these groups. They are arguably among the sickest patients across all specialties and subgroups. During the first year after presentation with CLI, the mortality rate is 25% and increases to as high as 45% in those patients with CLI who undergo limb amputation[56-59] (Figure 18-6).

PROGRAMMED MANAGEMENT

Strategic Programming

Atherosclerosis is the dominant cause of PAD and a systemic disease and therefore must be treated systemically. Treatment of their underlying cardiovascular risk factors is of paramount importance in reducing the morbidity and mortality among patients with PAD. Patients with PAD have an increased risk of cardiovascular events, such as death, MI, and stroke.[48-55] This treatment should include therapy for lipid abnormalities, hypertension, and diabetes. Lifestyle modification should include daily aerobic exercise and elimination of cigarette smoking. These treatments should be instituted for all patients with PAD, regardless of clinical scenario, including those who are asymptomatic and those with chronic claudication and acute limb ischemia.

Unlike the ischemia discovered by an abnormal stress test, an abnormal ABI or other noninvasive vascular study does not demand revascularization. Aside from the lifestyle and risk factor modifications discussed in the preceding section, there is no therapy indicated for the patient without symptoms or signs of lower extremity PAD (Table 18-3).

Statins

Patients with PAD are regarded as "high risk" for future cardiovascular events when considering the National Cholesterol Education Program Adult Treatment Panel III guidelines for lipid therapy. The goal of treatment is to achieve an LDL of 100 mg/dL or less, although if PAD is associated with other risk factors for atherosclerosis, that goal should be less than 70 mg/dL. Statin therapy reduces the likelihood of MI and death from cardiovascular causes by approximately 30%.[60] Retrospective analysis of the Scandanavian Simvastatin Survival Study found that the development or worsening of claudication was reduced with simvastatin, a result that was supported in a prospective trial of atorvastatin, which found that the walking distance to onset of claudication was longer on statin therapy.[61, 62]

Antihypertensive Therapy

This strategy reduces the risk of stroke, heart failure, and death and should be used when treating patients with PAD. There is no evidence that beta blockers adversely affect claudicants, and as they have been

TABLE 18-3: Management Master Plan	
Data management	Keep BP below 140/90 or 120/80 mm Hg
	Low-sodium diet
	Preventive measures with statin
	Pharmacologic therapy
Root-cause correction	Angioplasty and stenting
Work-around management	Bypass surgery
System replacement	None available

shown to reduce the risk of MI and death, they should be prescribed as indicated. Angiotensin-converting enzyme inhibitors were studied in the Heart Outcomes Prevention Evaluation study, including more than 4000 patients with PAD. Ramipril reduced the risk of major adverse cardiovascular events among these patients by 25%, as it did in the overall population.[63] Caution is advised when treating patients with critical limb ischemia, as distal perfusion may be dependent upon blood pressure. Those patients with PAD who quit smoking have a lower risk of death, MI, and amputation than those who continue to smoke. Treating physicians must educate their patients regarding the risks of tobacco use and identify strategies to improve success at smoking cessation.[64]

Antiplatelet Therapy

This is a cornerstone treatment for atherosclerotic diseases. Antiplatelet therapy produces a 22% reduction in odds of MI, stroke, or vascular death among patients with PAD.[77] This benefit is equally shared among those with claudication and those with endovascular or surgical revascularization. An analysis of a spectrum of aspirin doses revealed that although higher doses of aspirin resulted in greater reductions in vascular events, this was at the expense of increased intracranial or gastrointestinal bleeding.[65] Doses smaller than 75 mg did not afford significant protection against vascular events, and doses higher than 325 mg significantly increased bleeding risk; therefore 75 mg to 325 mg should be prescribed for patients with lower extremity PAD. One prospective trial compared aspirin to clopidogrel in patients with a history of vascular disease. The event rate for cardiovascular events was reduced by 8.7%; among PAD patients, clopidogrel reduced this risk by 24% more than aspirin.[66] This additional benefit was achieved without increased bleeding risk. Patients with PAD should receive antiplatelet therapy, aspirin, or clopidogrel to reduce their risk of MI stroke and vascular death.

Antcoagulation Therapy

Anticoagulation with warfarin or its derivatives has not been shown to be beneficial on balance. There are a paucity of data specifically addressing anticoagulation therapy for PAD. Drawing inferences from data on the use of warfarin in patients with CAD, the risk reduction for vascular events is coupled with increased risk of bleeding. Treatment with the goal International Normalized Ratio (INR) of 2.8 to 4.8 was associated with a 4.5-fold increase in major bleeding, although a significant reduction in death and MI was achieved. With goal INR between 2 and 3, no significant reduction was achieved for stroke or death or for MI, but bleeding increased nearly eightfold.[67] One trial specifically examining the benefit of aspirin versus warfarin for infrainguinal graft patency showed no significant difference.

Exercise Training

Among patients with claudication or discomfort in the legs when walking, the initial treatment is more walking. In the most recent ACC/AHA guidelines for the treatment of PAD, exercise training receives a Class I indication as the initial treatment modality for patients with claudication.[68, 69] The mechanisms for the benefit derived from exercise training are not completely understood, are likely multifactorial, and include improvement in muscle metabolism, endothelial function, muscular strength, and alteration in gait. Exercise training results in improvement in pain-free walking time and maximal walking time.[70] In order to be of benefit, exercise must be performed for at least 30 minutes and occur at least three times a week. Benefit has been reported to occur as early as one month after initiating training and to continue to improve for six months. Treadmill exercise is the best form of exercise to relieve lower extremity claudication; treadmill speed and resistance should initially be set to provoke claudication at three to five minutes. When they develop moderate claudication, patients are allowed to rest until symptoms resolve and then exercise again. As the population with claudication frequently has concomitant CAD, an exercise stress test should be performed prior to initiating exercise training. Those patients who develop cardiac ischemia prior to exertion limitation by claudication should undergo appropriate further evaluation for obstructive CAD. Supervised exercise programs are considered to be superior to patients walking independently, and this can be accommodated in most cardiac rehabilitation programs.

Pharmacologic Therapy

Cilostazol

Cilostazol has been shown to have beneficial effects on HDL and triglycerides. It is a phosphodiesterase inhibitor, and it inhibits platelets and vasodilates. Cilostazol has also been shown to improve walking distance by 40 to 60%.[71] Patients are typically started on 50 mg twice daily and increased to 100 mg twice a day as tolerated. The side effects may include headache, diarrhea, palpitations, and dizziness. Cilostazol should not be used in patients with heart failure, as there is a potential for excess mortality; the FDA has a black-box warning for patients with heart failure.

Pentoxyfylline

This derivative of methylxanthine acts as a hemorheologic agent. It has been shown to have a statistically significant improvement in pain-free and maximal walking distances.[72, 73] The magnitude of its benefit is not as great as that of cilostazol, and therefore it is considered a second-line agent to cilostazol. Pentoxyfylline is administered as 400 mg three times a day and has no black-box warning. It is generally well tolerated, although dyspepsia, nausea, diarrhea, and sore throat have been reported.

ADVANCED MANAGEMENT

Revascularization therapy may be considered for patients with intermittent claudication that limits their vocation or prevents them from enjoying activities that are important to their lifestyle. Fontaine IIb claudication describes symptoms that are significantly limiting and may merit revascularization. As discussed earlier, ACC/AHA guidelines recommend a trial of exercise training and pharmacologic therapy as the initial therapy for claudication. Individuals with Fontaine IIb claudication who are considered for revasclarization will undergo further diagnostic testing to determine if their anatomy is amenable to revascularization and for which type of revascularization they may be eligible.

Surgical Revascularization

If surgical revascularization is being considered, then identification of the level of stenosis, an appropriate target for distal anastomosis, and the patency of the vessels distal to the point of distal anastomosis, is sufficient information. The exact length, degree, and morphology of the stenosis are less important considerations for patients undergoing surgical revascularization. Identification of healthy segments for anastamosis and good runoff of the infrapopliteal vessels are important determinants of short- and long-term success. Duplex ultrasound and segmental pressures will localize the level and degree of stenosis but to fully evaluate the patient for revascularization, an angiogram is required.

Surgical revascularization is associated with greater morbidity and mortality than percutaneous endovascular procedures.[74, 75] The threshold to operate on an individual for claudication, then, is higher as compared to PTA/stent. An appropriate preoperative evaluation should be performed given the high prevalence of coronary and cerebrovascular disease in this population.[49, 50] Surgical therapy for iliac disease has a higher likelihood of long-term success than bypass for femoral artery disease, particularly when compared with below the knee bypass for femoral artery disease. The conduit material is also an important determinant of success for femoral artery bypass, autologous veins having better durability then polytetrafluoroethylene (PTFE) synthetic grafts. The five-year patency rate for venous bypass grafts is 80%, for PTFE with distal anastomosis above the knee 75%, and for PTFE with a distal anastomosis below the knee 65%.[76]

Given these midterm results for surgical revascularization and the morbidity and mortality of the procedure, a strategy of endovascular revascularization as a first option should be employed. The experienced interventionalist should assess the probability of procedural success based on angiographic characteristics. These angiograms may be invasive or noninvasive angiograms. When considering endovascular revascularization, the exact location, length, degree, and morphology of the stenosis are important predictors of technical success. In addition, tortuosity of vessels proximal to the lesion, the angulation of the aortic bifurcation, and having an appropriate vessel to obtain vascular access all contribute to the technical difficulty for endovascular revascularization. Angiography will provide these details to decipher the likelihood of success for endovascular therapy. A noninvasive angiogram with CTA or MRA provides this road map to identify which patients should not be offered endovascular therapy before performing an invasive angiogram. The relative merits and deficiencies of these two techniques are discussed earlier in the chapter, but the experience and expertise with each technique at the practitioner's institution are important determinants of which modality to use.

Endovascular Treatment

Endovascular treatment of PAD employs balloons and stents most commonly, although mechanical and laser atherectomy, cutting balloons, cryoangioplasty, and thrombectomy are used as adjunctive therapies. Technology for endovascular therapy continues to improve and evolve. The common iliac artery has the most durable results after endovascular therapy. The response and durability of endovascular therapy are poorer the more distal in the vascular tree the intervention is performed. Lesion-specific characteristics such as longer lesions, serial stenoses, and poor runoff vessels distal to the point of intervention predict poor long-term success. Smoking, renal failure, and diabetes are patient characteristics that also bode poorly for durability of intervention. The TransAtlantic Society Consensus (TASC) Working Group created a scheme to classify lesions, categorizing them as to those that may be most appropriate for endovascular therapy and those that may be most appropriate for surgical revascularization. These categories are meant to reflect the relative likelihood for success and of risk. Although this scheme provides a frame of reference, the expertise of the operator may increase or decrease the likelihood of success, thus affecting the decision for surgical versus endovascular therapy. As endovascular technology improves, the likelihood of procedural success will continue to increase. Although the TASC document classification set out to define which patients should be treated endovascularly and which should be treated surgically, advances in endovascular technology will challenge these classifications.

Patients who present with CLI frequently have critical stenoses at more than one level of the vascular tree, iliac and femoral or femoral and tibial. Due to the extensive nature of disease, both revascularization methods face a greater challenge to restore flow. Although collateral blood flow may be sufficient to sustain tissue, patients with tissue loss require the reestablishment of pulsatile in-line flow to the foot, particularly in the area of tissue loss. CLI progresses to tissue necrosis; thus evaluation and treatment for CLI must be rapid. Patients who present with acute limb-threatening ischemia must be evaluated and treated on an emergent basis, with efforts to achieve complete revascularization to the foot promptly. Patients who present with subacute or chronic CLI should be treated promptly but may not require emergent revascularization. These patients may initially be treated for upstream or inflow stenosis and subsequently undergo revascularization of outflow stenosis. For all patients with CLI, the arterial anatomy, clinical presentation, and comorbid conditions will determine whether surgical or endovascular therapy is initiated in efforts to salvage the limb.

TAKE-HOME MESSAGE

Peripheral arterial disease is a significant cause of morbidity. Because of the prevalence of coexisting coronary and cerebrovascular disease, patients with PAD are at increased risk for mortality. The cardiovascular specialist must be cognizant of PAD and its presentations and remain vigilant for evidence of its presence. The physician who is well versed in PAD and the techniques for the evaluation thereof will gain insight into the patient's overall vascular health.

References

1. Kannel, W. B., Skinner, J. J. J., Schwartz, M. J.: Intermittent claudication: incidence in the Framingham Study. Circulation. 1970;41: 875–883.
2. Meijer, W. T., Hoes, A. W., Rutgers, D., et al.: Peripheral arterial disease in the elderly: the Rotterda Study. Arterioscler Thromb Vasc Biol. 1998; 18:185–192.
3. Smith, G. D., Shipley, M. J., Rose, G.: Intermittent claudication, heart disease risk factors, and mortality. The Whitehall Study. Circulation. 1990;82:1925–1931.
4. Price, J. F., Mowbray, P. I., Lee, A. J., et al.: Relationship between smoking and cardiovascular risk factors in the development of peripheral arterial disease and coronary artery disease: Edinburgh Artery Study. Eur Heart J. 1999;20:344–353.
5. Bowlin, S. J., Medalie, J. H., Flocke, S. A., et al.: Epidemiology of intermittent claudication in middle-aged men. Am J Epidemiol. 1994; 140: 418–430.
6. Kannel, W. B., McGee, D. L.: Update on some epidemiologic features of intermittent claudication: the Framingham Study. J Am Geriatr Soc. Jan 1985;33(1):13–18.
7. Hiatt, W. R., Hoag, S., Hamman, R. F.: Effect of diagnostic criteria on the prevalence of peripheral arterial disease. The San Luis Valley Diabetes Study. Circulation. 1995;91:1472–1479.
8. Dormandy, J. A., Murray, G. D.: The fate of the claudicant—a prospective study of 1969 claudicants. Eur J Vasc Surg. Apr 1991;5(2):131–133.

9. McDaniel, M. D., Cronenwett, J. L.: Basic data related to the natural history of intermittent claudication. Ann Vasc Surg. Jul 1989;3(3): 273–277.

10. Most, R. S., Sinnock, P.: The epidemiology of lower extremity amputations in diabetic individuals. Diabetes Care. Jan-Feb 1983;6(1):87–91.

11. Bild, D. E., Selby, J. V., Sinnock, P., et al.: Lower-extremity amputation in people with diabetes. Epidemiology and prevention. Diabetes Care. Jan 1989;12(1):24–31.

12. Ingolfsson, I. O., Sigurdsson, G., Sigvaldason, H., et al.: A marked decline in the prevalence and incidence of intermittent claudication in Icelandic men 1968-1986: a strong relationship to smoking and serum cholesterol—the Reykjavik Study. J Clin Epidemiol. Nov 1994;47(11): 1237–1243.

13. Murabito, J. M., D'Agostino, R. B., Silbershatz, H., et al.: Intermittent claudication. A risk profile from The Framingham Heart Study. Circulation. 1997;96:44–49.

14. Horby, J., Grande, P. A. V., et al.: High density lipoprotein cholesterol and arteriography in intermittent claudication. Eur J Vasc Surg. 1989; 3:333–337.

15. Boushey, C. J., Beresford, S. A., Omenn, G. S., et al.: A quantitative assessment of plasma homocysteine as a risk factor for vascular disease. Probable benefits of increasing folic acid intakes. JAMA. Oct 4 1995; 274(13):1049–1057.

16. Graham, I. M., Daly, L. E., Refsum, H. M., et al.: Plasma homocysteine as a risk factor for vascular disease. The European Concerted Action Project. JAMA. Jun 11 1997;277(22):1775–1781.

17. Ridker, P., Cushman, M., Stampfer, M., et al.: Plasma concentration of C-reactive protein and risk of developing peripheral vascular disease. Circulation. 1998;97:425–428.

18. Rasmussen, T. E., Clouse, W. D., Tonnessen, B. H.: Handbook of Patient Care in Vascular Diseases, 5th ed, Philadelphia, PA: Lippincott Williams & Wilkins, 2008.

19. Moneta, G. L., Yeager, R. A., Lee, R. W., et al.: Noninvasive localization of arterial occlusive disease: a comparison of segmental Doppler pressures and arterial duplex mapping. J Vasc Surg. Mar 1993;17(3): 578–582.

20. Pinto, F., Lencioni, R., Napoli, V.: Peripheral ischemic occlusive arterial disease: comparison of color Doppler pressure and arterial duplex mapping. J Vasc Surg. 1996;17:578–582.

21. Sacks, D., Robinson, M. L., Marinelli, D. L., et al.: Peripheral arterial Doppler ultrasonography: diagnostic criteria. J Ultrasound Med. Mar 1992;11(3):95–103.

22. Whelan, J. F., Barry, M. H., Moir, J. D.: Color flow Doppler ultrasonography: comparison with peripheral arteriography for the investigation of peripheral vascular disease. J Clin Ultrasound. Jul-Aug 1992;20(6):369–374.

23. Edwards, J. M., Coldwell, D. M., Goldman, M. L., et al.: The role of duplex scanning in the selection of patients for transluminal angioplasty. J Vasc Surg. Jan 1991;13(1):69–74.

24. Van der Heijden, F., Legemate. D., Van Leeuwen, M.: Value of duplex scanning in the selection of patients for percutaneous transluminal angioplasty. Eur J Vasc Surg. 1993;7:71–76.

25. Ascher, E., Mazzariol, F., Hingorani, A., et al.: The use of duplex ultrasound arterial mapping as an alternative to conventional arteriography for primary and secondary infrapopliteal bypasses. Am J Surg. Aug 1999;178(2):162–165.
26. Proia, R. R., Walsh, D. B., Nelson, P. R., et al.: Early results of infragenicular revascularization based solely on duplex arteriography. J Vasc Surg. Jun 2001;33(6):1165–1170.
27. Bandyk, D. F., Schmitt, D. D., Seabrook, G. R., et al.: Monitoring functional patency of in situ saphenous vein bypasses: the impact of a surveillance protocol and elective revision. J Vasc Surg. Feb 1989;9(2):286–296.
28. Laborde, A. L., Synn, A. Y., Worsey, M. J., et al.: A prospective comparison of ankle/brachial indices and color duplex imaging in surveillance of the in situ saphenous vein bypass. J Cardiovasc Surg (Torino). Jul-Aug 1992;33(4):420–425.
29. Mattos, M. A., van Bemmelen, P. S., Hodgson, K. J., et al.: Does correction of stenoses identified with color duplex scanning improve infrainguinal graft patency? J Vasc Surg. Jan 1993;17(1):54–64; discussion 64–66.
30. Mills, J. L., Harris, E. J., Taylor, L. M., Jr., et al.: The importance of routine surveillance of distal bypass grafts with duplex scanning: a study of 379 reversed vein grafts. J Vasc Surg. Oct 1990;12(4):379–386; discussion 387–389.
31. Taylor, P. R., Tyrrell, M. R., Crofton, M., et al.: Colour flow imaging in the detection of femoro-distal graft and native artery stenosis: improved criteria. Eur J Vasc Surg. May 1992;6(3):232–236.
32. Nelemans, P. J., Leiner, T., de Vet, H. C., et al.: Peripheral arterial disease: a meta-analysis of the diagnostic performance of MR angiography. Radiology. 2000;217:105–114.
33. Kreitner, K. F., Kalden, P., Neufang, A., et al.: Diabetes and peripheral arterial occlusive disease: prospective comparison of contrast enhanced three dimensional MR angiography with conventional digital subtraction angiography. Am J Roentgenol. 2000;174:171–179.
34. Leyendecker, J. R., Elsass, K. D., Johnson, S. P., et al.: The role of infrapopliteal MR angiography in patients undergoing optimal contrast angiography for chronic limb-threatening ischemia. J Vasc Interv Radiol. 1998;9:545–551.
35. Oser, R. F., Picus, D., Hicks, M. E., et al.: Accuracy of DSA in the evaluation of patency of infrapopiteal vessels. J Vasc Interv Radiol. 1995;6:589–594.
36. Hartnell, G.: MR angiography compared with digital subtraction angiography. Am J Roentgenol. 2000;175:1188–1189.
37. Ouwendijk, R., de Vries, M., Pattynama, P. M., et al.: Imaging peripheral arterial disease: a randomized controlled trial comparing contrast-enhanced MR angiography and multi-detector row CT angiography. Radiology. Sep 2005;236(3):1094–1103.
38. Ouwendijk, R., Kock, M. C., Visser, K., et al.: Interobserver agreement for the interpretation of contrast-enhanced 3D MR angiography and MDCT angiography in peripheral arterial disease. AJR Am J Roentgenol. Nov 2005;185(5):1261–1267.

39. Mehran, R., Aymong, E. D., Nikolsky, E., et al.: A simple risk score for prediction of contrast-induced nephropathy after percutaneous coronary intervention: development and initial validation. J Am Coll Cardiol. Oct 6 2004;44(7):1393–1399.

40. Mehran, R., Nikolsky, E.: Contrast-induced nephropathy: definition, epidemiology, and patients at risk. Kidney Int Suppl. Apr 2006(100): S11–S15.

41. Nikolsky, E., Aymong, E. D., Dangas, G., et al.: Radiocontrast nephropathy: identifying the high-risk patient and the implications of exacerbating renal function. Rev Cardiovasc Med. 2003;4 Suppl 1:S7–S14.

42. Lufft, V., Hoogestraat-Lufft, L., Fels, L. M., et al.: Contrast media nephropathy: intravenous CT angiography versus intraarterial digital subtraction angiography in renal artery stenosis: a prospective randomized trial. Am J Kidney Dis. Aug 2002;40(2):236–242.

43. Lawrence, J. A., Kim, D., Kent, K. C., et al.: Lower extremity spiral CT angiography versus catheter angiography. Radiology. Mar 1995;194(3): 903–908.

44. Riecker, O., Duber, C., Schmiedt, W.: Prospective comparison of CT angiography of the legs with intrarterial digital subtraction angiography. Am J Roentgenol. 1996;182:269–276.

45. Rubin, G. D., Schmidt, A. J., Logan, L. J., et al.: Multi-detector row CT angiography of lower extremity arterial inflow and runoff: initial experience. Radiology. Oct 2001;221(1):146–158.

46. Martin, M. L., Tay, K. H., Flak, B., et al.: Multidetector CT angiography of the aortoiliac system and lower extremities: a prospective comparison with digital subtraction angiography. Am J Roentgenol. 2003;180:1085–1091.

47. Muluk, S. C., Muluk, V. S., Kelley, M. E., et al.: Outcome events in patients with claudication: a 15-year study in 2777 patients. J Vasc Surg. Feb 2001;33(2):251–257; discussion 257–258.

48. Weitz, J. I., Byrne, J., Clagett, G. P., et al.: Diagnosis and treatment of chronic arterial insufficiency of the lower extremities: a critical review. Circulation. Dec 1 1996;94(11):3026–3049.

49. Bhatt, D. L., Steg, P. G., Ohman, E. M., et al.: International prevalence, recognition, and treatment of cardiovascular risk factors in outpatients with atherothrombosis. JAMA. Jan 11 2006;295(2):180–189.

50. Ohman, E. M., Bhatt, D. L., Steg, P. G., et al.: The REduction of Atherothrombosis for Continued Health (REACH) Registry: an international, prospective, observational investigation in subjects at risk for atherothrombotic events-study design. Am Heart J. Apr 2006;151(4): 786;781–790.

51. Zheng, Z. J., Sharrett, A. R., Chambless, L. E., et al.: Associations of ankle-brachial index with clinical coronary heart disease, stroke and preclinical carotid and popliteal atherosclerosis: the Atherosclerosis Risk in Communities (ARIC) Study. Atherosclerosis. 1997(131): 115–125.

52. Leng, G. C., Lee, A. J., Fowkes, F. G., et al.: Incidence, natural history and cardiovascular events in the general population. Int J Epidemiol. 1996(25):1172–1181.

53. Smith, G. D., Shipley, M. J., Rose, G.: Intermittent claudication, heart disease risk factors, and mortality. The Whitehall Study. Circulation. 1990(82):1925–1931.
54. Kornitzer, M., Dramaix, M., Sobolski, J., et al.: Ankle/arm pressure index in asymptomatic middle-aged males: an independent predictor of ten-year coronary heart disease mortality. Angiology. Mar 1995;46(3): 211–219.
55. Vogt, M. T., Cauley, J. A., Newman, A. B., et al.: Decreased ankle/arm blood pressure index and mortality in elderly women. JAMA. Jul 28 1993;270(4):465–469.
56. Criqui, M. H., Langer, R. D., Fronek, A., et al.: Mortality over a period of 10 years in patients with peripheral arterial disease. N Engl J Med. Feb 6 1992;326(6):381–386.
57. Luther, M.: The influence of arterial reconstructive surgery on the outcome of critical limb ischaemia. Eur J Vasc Surg. 1994(8):682–689.
58. Kazmers, A., Perkins, A. J., Jacobs, L. A.: Major lower extremity amputation in Veteran Affairs medical centers. Ann Vasc Surg. 2000(14): 216–222.
59. Dormandy, J. A., Heeck, L., Vig, S.: The fate of patients with critical leg ischemia. Semin Vasc Surg. 1999;12:142–147.
60. Sacks, F. M., Pfeffer, M. A., Moye, L. A., et al.: The effect of pravastatin on coronary events after myocardial infarction in patients with average cholesterol levels. Cholesterol and Recurrent Events Trial investigators. N Engl J Med. Oct 3 1996;335(14):1001–1009.
61. Mohler, E. R., 3rd, Hiatt, W. R., Creager, M. A.: Cholesterol reduction with atorvastatin improves walking distance in patients with peripheral arterial disease. Circulation. Sep 23 2003;108(12):1481–1486.
62. Pedersen, T. R., Kjekshus, J., Pyorala, K., et al.: Effect of simvastatin on ischemic signs and symptoms in the Scandinavian simvastatin survival study (4S). Am J Cardiol. Feb 1 1998;81(3):333–335.
63. Yusuf, S., Sleight, P., Pogue, J., et al.: Effects of an angiotensin-converting-enzyme inhibitor, ramipril, on cardiovascular events in high-risk patients. The Heart Outcomes Prevention Evaluation Study Investigators. N Engl J Med. Jan 20 2000;342(3):145–153.
64. Jonason, T., Bergstrom, R.: Cessation of smoking in patients with intermittent claudication. Effects on the risk of peripheral vascular complications, myocardial infarction and mortality. Acta Med Scand. 1987;221(3):253–260.
65. Collaborative meta-analysis of randomised trials of antiplatelet therapy for prevention of death, myocardial infarction, and stroke in high risk patients. BMJ. Jan 12 2002;324(7329):71–86.
66. A randomised, blinded, trial of clopidogrel versus aspirin in patients at risk of ischaemic events (CAPRIE). CAPRIE Steering Committee. Lancet. 1996;348:1329–1339.
67. Anand, S. S., Yusuf, S.: Oral anticoagulants in patients with coronary artery disease. J Am Coll Cardiol. Feb 19 2003;41(4 Suppl S):62S–69S.
68. Hirsch, A. T., Haskal, Z. J., Hertzer, N. R., et al.: ACC/AHA 2005 Practice Guidelines for the management of patients with peripheral arterial disease (lower extremity, renal, mesenteric, and abdominal aortic): a

collaborative report from the American Association for Vascular Surgery/Society for Vascular Surgery, Society for Cardiovascular Angiography and Interventions, Society for Vascular Medicine and Biology, Society of Interventional Radiology, and the ACC/AHA Task Force on Practice Guidelines (Writing Committee to Develop Guidelines for the Management of Patients With Peripheral Arterial Disease): endorsed by the American Association of Cardiovascular and Pulmonary Rehabilitation; National Heart, Lung, and Blood Institute; Society for Vascular Nursing; TransAtlantic Inter-Society Consensus; and Vascular Disease Foundation. Circulation. Mar 21 2006;113(11):e463–e654.

69. Hirsch, A. T., Haskal, Z. J., Hertzer, N. R., et al.: ACC/AHA 2005 guidelines for the management of patients with peripheral arterial disease (lower extremity, renal, mesenteric, and abdominal aortic): executive summary, a collaborative report from the American Association for Vascular Surgery/Society for Vascular Surgery, Society for Cardiovascular Angiography and Interventions, Society for Vascular Medicine and Biology, Society of Interventional Radiology, and the ACC/AHA Task Force on Practice Guidelines (Writing Committee to Develop Guidelines for the Management of Patients With Peripheral Arterial Disease) endorsed by the American Association of Cardiovascular and Pulmonary Rehabilitation; National Heart, Lung, and Blood Institute; Society for Vascular Nursing; TransAtlantic Inter-Society Consensus; and Vascular Disease Foundation. J Am Coll Cardiol. Mar 21 2006; 47(6):1239–1312.

70. Tsuchikane, E., Fukuhara, A., Kobayashi, T., et al.: Impact of cilostazol on restenosis after percutaneous coronary balloon angioplasty. Circulation. Jul 6 1999;100(1):21–26.

71. Money, S. R., Herd, J. A., Isaacsohn, J. L., et al.: Effect of cilostazol on walking distances in patients with intermittent claudication caused by peripheral vascular disease. J Vasc Surg. Feb 1998;27(2):267–274; discussion 274–275.

72. Lindgarde, F., Jelnes, R., Bjorkman, H., et al.: Conservative drug treatment in patients with moderately severe chronic occlusive peripheral arterial disease. Scandinavian Study Group. Circulation. Dec 1989; 80(6):1549–1556.

73. Porter, J. M., Cutler, B. S., Lee, B. Y., et al.: Pentoxifylline efficacy in the treatment of intermittent claudication: multicenter controlled double-blind trial with objective assessment of chronic occlusive arterial disease patients. Am Heart J. Jul 1982;104(1):66–72.

74. Franco, C. D., Goldsmith, J., Veith, F. J., et al.: Management of arterial injuries produced by percutaneous femoral procedures. Surgery. Apr 1993;113(4):419–425.

75. Lumsden, A. B., Miller, J. M., Kosinski, A. S., et al.: A prospective evaluation of surgically treated groin complications following percutaneous cardiac procedures. Am Surg. Feb 1994;60(2):132–137.

76. Hunink, M. G., Wong, J. B., Donaldson, M. C., et al.: Patency results of percutaneous and surgical revascularization for femoropopliteal arterial disease. Med Decis Making. Jan-Mar 1994;14(1):71–81.

Carotid Arterial Disease

Gianluca Rigatelli, Paolo Cardaioli, Yidong Wei, and Nguyen Thuong Nghia

CHAPTER

19

Chapter Outline

DEFINITION

Carotid artery occlusive disease is defined as obstruction of the blood flow from atherosclerosis in a carotid artery lumen, which includes the internal carotid artery (ICA) and occasionally the common carotid artery (CCA).

Patient Population in Focus

ICA occlusive disease (ICAD) includes asymptomatic and symptomatic patients with proven lesions. The prevalence of asymptomatic ICAD in persons >65 years is estimated to be 5–10% for ≥50% stenosis and ≃1% for >80% stenosis. In asymptomatic patients with >50% stenosis, the annual risk of stroke is 1–4.3%, being more relevant proportionally to stenosis severity.[1]

Strategic Programming

The first step is to identify the patients with carotid artery disease through data collecting with a comprehensive history and physical examination. The next step is to perform data processing in order to formulate a preliminary diagnosis and a short list of differential diagnoses (e.g., carotid artery dissection, vertebral artery disease). Then, using the method of data mining, tests may be ordered (e.g., carotid ultrasound and Doppler studies) in order to confirm (data converting) the main diagnosis of carotid artery disease and to rule out (data filtering) the differential diagnoses.

DATA COLLECTING

Investigation Master Plan

When a physician sees a patient suspected of having carotid artery disease, there are seven main areas of interest for data collecting (history and physical examination).

The main area of interest: Carotid Artery Disease (zone A). In general, the patient with ICAD is asymptomatic. There are no subjective symptoms unless the disease is in a late state. The physical finding related directly to ICAD is the carotid artery murmur. Obstruction of the blood flow to the central nervous system is a hardware problem.

The upstream area for carotid artery disease is the heart (zone B). However, there are no signs or symptoms from the heart when there is early stenosis of the carotid artery.

The downstream area of the carotid artery is the brain (zone C). There are no signs or symptoms from the brain when there is early stenosis of the carotid artery.

The system configuration: The lesion is in the carotid artery (zone E). There is no abnormality of the configuration.

The work-around configuration: When there is a significant lesion in the index carotid artery, there is increased flow to the contralateral carotid artery and more collaterals to the index side of the brain. However, there are no signs or symptoms from the collaterals (zone D).

The cardiovascular system: The heart is the organ upstream from the carotid artery. There are no symptoms and signs.

The network (the whole body): It seems that there is no relation between a carotid lesion and other systems of the body. However, when a patient has a large stroke, the mortality is very high even though the patient might have a perfect cardiovascular, pulmonary, or renal system (zone F).

History

Typical Symptoms

Typical symptoms include a variety of cerebral syndromes, ranging from contralateral transient ischemic attack (TIA) to ischemic stroke. Usually the first manifestation is loss of strength that can progress to complete paralysis (hemiplegia) of an arm or a leg or both, associated with asymmetry of the labial rims as well as ptosis of a palpebral rim. Often slurred speech anticipates other symptoms. Partial vision loss (hemianopsis) or sensory deficit (paresthesia) may present less frequently.

Atypical Symptoms

Atypical symptoms may present as lipotimia or even loss of consciousness (syncope) by (1) conditions of low cardiac output in the setting of severe stenosis of the ICA, or (2) stimulation of carotid glomus in the presence of a tight stenosis of the ICA.

DATA DECODING TIPS (CLINICAL PEARLS)
Vertebral-Subclavian Steal

Vertebral-subclavian steal is suspected when a patient develops symptoms during or immediately after manual work or even after brushing his or her hair. It is associated with signs of reduced cerebral flow, such as vertigo, lipotimia, or even syncope with fatigue or paralysis of the arm. This clinical picture is usually caused by obstruction of the subclavian artery before the origin of the vertebral artery. There is stealing of blood flow from the posterior vertebral circulation to the distal subclavian artery. It is usually diagnostic when a blood pressure difference of 30 mm Hg between the arms is detected.[2]

DATA DECODING TIPS (CLINICAL PEARLS)
Noncarotid Conditions Mimicking Cerebral Ischemia

Anxiety attacks in anxious-depressive syndrome may mimic transient ischemic attack. Normally, signs such as loss of strength or paralysis are diffuse (both arms, both legs).

Physical Examination

There are no typical findings in the physical examination. Sometimes a bruit at the neck auscultation in the absence of aortic valve stenosis may be heard. Classic signs of cardiovascular risk factors, including hypertension, smoking, hypercholesterolemia, and diabetes, should be detected.

DATA FILTERING (DIFFERENTIAL DIAGNOSES)
Spontaneous Cervical Dissection

Spontaneous dissection is a nontraumatic tear in the wall of the ICA or the vertebral arteries, a common event in young people of both genders (25% of strokes in patients < 45 years of age). In 90% of cases, it causes carotid territory ischemia with local signs and symptoms on the side of dissection, but in 10% of patients it is asymptomatic. Head, facial, and neck pain or pulsatile tinnitus are the most frequent symptoms. Urgent magnetic resonance imaging (MRI) or computed tomography angiography (CTA) is warranted to define the diagnosis when an ischemic stroke is preceded by these symptoms and signs.[3]

DATA DECODING TIPS (CLINICAL PEARLS)
Clinical Clues for Spontaneous Carotid Dissection

When treating a patient with a suspected spontaneous carotid artery dissection, the physician should check for a history of minor trauma preceding a new onset of headache or neck pain. Neuroimaging should be performed early; it is not uncommon for a spontaneous carotid artery dissection to seal itself hours or days after symptoms, leaving physicians without a certain diagnosis.

Cardiac Embolism

Atrial fibrillation (AF) is the most common cause of cardiac embolism and cardiac–related stroke; its diagnosis should always be ascertained by electrocardiogram or 24-hour Holter electrocardiogram, even in the presence of a significant carotid disease. Transthoracic (TTE) and transesophageal echocardiography (TEE) should evaluate the function, volume, and diameter of the left atrium and possibly the presence of left atrial thrombi.

Embolism from an aortic plaque is a frequent event; patients with stroke but without carotid disease should be accurately evaluated by TEE in order to detect possible aortic plaques and assess their severity (Montgomery classification). The treatment includes antiplatelet drugs. In selected cases, heparin as well as statins should be started promptly to prevent further embolization.

Paradoxical embolism through a patent foramen ovale (PFO) may lead to stroke and represents another condition that warrants accurate cardiac evaluation, especially in patients under 50 to 55 years of age. Transcranial Doppler is the most sensitive test to detect a suspected right-to-left shunt. If this test is positive, a TEE with contrast or normal saline injection should be performed in order to define the diagnosis, shunt severity, and anatomical indications for eventual transcatheter PFO closure.

Other sources of cardiac emboli include infected cardiac valves or thrombosed aortic and mitral valvular prostheses. A new cerebral ischemic event in a patient with a known valvular prosthesis or systemic signs of infection or sepsis warrants a careful evaluation of valvular function rather than looking for an unlikely etiology such as carotid artery disease.[4]

DATA DECODING TIPS (CLINICAL PEARLS)
Clinical Clues for Paradoxical Embolism

Young age (<50-55 years), absence of classic cardiovascular risk factors, and history of migraine with aura should be the high suspicion markers for paradoxical embolism through a PFO rather than carotid artery disease.

Acute Aortic Dissection

Acute aortic dissection usually causes a sudden onset of excruciating, ripping pain. The ascending aortic dissections tend to manifest with pain in the midline of the anterior chest, while descending aortic dissections manifest with pain in the back. Aortic dissections usually occur in the presence of risk factors, including hypertension, pregnancy, atherosclerosis, and other conditions that lead to degeneration of the aortic media, such as Marfan syndrome or EHI Danlos syndrome.

DATA DECODING TIPS (CLINICAL PEARLS)
When Aortic Dissection Needs Emergency Surgery

When a patient with an ischemic cerebral syndrome is suspected of having dissection of the aorta, look for the transient diastolic murmur of aortic regurgitation. Check for any differences in timing and strength of the pulses in the carotid, radial, and femoral arteries. In cases of retrograde extension of the dissection flap to the common carotid arteries, these signs precede the cerebral ischemic syndrome. In a known case of aortic dissection, new cerebral ischemic events indicate extension of the dissection, which should require surgical intervention.

DATA MINING (WORK-UP)

In symptomatic patients, once a cerebral ischemic event (stroke or TIA) occurs and potential cerebral lesions are ruled out by brain CT or MRI, the suspected diagnosis of ICAD should be confirmed by Doppler ultrasound, MRI, or CTA of the supra-aortic vessels. In asymptomatic patients, ICAD is usually suspected as a part of screening in patients with multiple risk factors or in patients scheduled for major surgical procedures such as major general surgery or cardiac surgery. Initial evaluation with Doppler ultrasonography should be implemented with MRI or CT.[5]

Doppler Ultrasound

Duplex ultrasound is a well-validated screening tool for carotid artery stenosis; however, it is operator- and patient-dependent. The results need to be confirmed by additional testing such as color Doppler, spectral Doppler waveform analysis, power Doppler (a technique that displays the total amplitude of the returning Doppler signal without distinguishing direction), and Doppler velocity—which is the main tool used to evaluate the stenosis severity (Table 19-1). The criteria distinguishing between normal and diseased ICA have a specificity of 84% and a sensitivity of 99% when compared to digital subtraction angiography. The accuracy for detecting 50% to 99% diameter stenosis is 93%. Duplex

TABLE 19-1: Criteria for Classification of Internal Carotid Artery Disease by Duplex Scanning with Spectral Waveform Analysis

Degree of Stenosis %	ICA Peak Systolic Velocity cm/s
Normal	<125
<50	<125
50-69	125-230
>70	>230
Subtotal occlusion	>300
Occlusion	0

ultrasound can distinguish between soft (unstable) and hard calcified (stable) plaques, giving crucial information for clinical decision making.[6]

SMART THINKING:

Do We Need to Screen for ICAD in Asymptomatic Patients?

Methodology: The recent U.S. Preventive Services Task Force reviews the evidence on the natural history of ICAD and the accuracy of screening tests in asymptomatic patients. *Results:* The most feasible screening for ICAD is duplex ultrasound. Despite a good sensitivity (86-90%) and specificity (87-94%), the test has many false-positive results after confirmation by digital subtraction angiography. Confirmatory test suchs as MRI are expensive and have some inaccuracies. *Mechanism of Difference:* The net benefit from reduction in stroke rates with endarterectomy of asymptomatic patients is approximately 5% over 5 to 6 years. If ultrasound screenings were followed by MRI confirmation, about 23 strokes would be prevented over 5 years by screening 100,000 people with a prevalence of ICAD of about 1%. *Practical Applications:* The adult general population should not be screened with ultrasound or other tests because the harms of inappropriate imaging and surgeries outweigh the benefits.[7]

Magnetic Resonance Imaging (MRI)

The MRI techniques used in carotid and intracranial arteries include both multislice (two-dimensional) and volumetric (three-dimensional) time-of-flight techniques. However carotid MRI is currently performed with gadolinium-enhanced sequences to improve the examination speed, anatomic coverage, and small-vessel resolution. Initial confirmatory study for ICAD is performed with an unenhanced time-of-flight MRI and subsequently with gadolinium-enhanced MRI. Gadolinium-enhanced MRI was found to have a sensitivity of 95% and a specificity of 93% for stenosis >70% when compared with standard MRI and CT. MRA of the carotid artery can be coupled with cerebral perfusion imaging to create a map of cerebral blood volume and cerebral blood flow. It can detect the ischemic changes much better than noncontrast study within minutes of stroke onset.[8]

Computed Tomographic Angiography

Computed tomographic angiography (CTA) is an emerging technique in the evaluation of the carotid arteries. The sixty-four-row scanner allows acquisition of high-resolution volumetric data sets that can be viewed in multiple planes. With these techniques, the sensitivity and specificity of CTA are 89% and 84%, respectively, and for >70% stenosis lesion, the sensitivity is 100%, despite the fact that it may slightly overestimate the degree of stenosis (Table 19-2).

Carotid Angiography

Carotid artery angiography with digital subtraction carries a risk of 1.3% of stroke but is still considered the diagnostic standard on which carotid interventions should be based. At this present time, it is not indicated to confirm the initial diagnosis, except in the case of suspected cervical artery dissection.

 TECHNOLOGY ASSESSMENT AND ECONOMIC ANALYSIS:

MRA Versus Doppler Ultrasound and DSA in Symptomatic Patients

Methodology: From 1997 to 2000, 350 patients were included in a blinded, consecutive cohort study. The sensitivities and specificities of

TABLE 19-2: Advantages and Disadvantages of Carotid MRA and CTA		
	Advantages	**Disadvantages**
MRA	No radiation exposure Combination with cerebral perfusion scan	Gadolinium still has nephrotoxic effects Long acquisition time
CTA	Speed of examination Comfort Ability to evaluate stented vessel	Long interpretation time\ Interference from calcium Potentially nephrotoxic contrast Radiation exposure Artifacts from dental implants and swallowing

CTA: computed tomographic angiography, MRA: magnetic resonance angiography.

US and MRA were estimated by using DSA as the reference standard; the actual costs of performing imaging and endarterectomy were estimated. *Results:* The US had 88% sensitivity and 76% specificity. MRA had 92% sensitivity and 76% specificity. Combined concordant US and MRA had 96% sensitivity and 80% specificity. *Cost-Effectiveness Analysis:* The US alone was the most efficient strategy. Adding MRA led to a marginal increase in quality-adjusted life-years (QALY) gained but at prohibitive cost (cost-effectiveness ratio > 1.500.000 euro per QUALY gained). Performing DSA for discordant US and MRA led to extra costs and QALY loss owing to complications. *Practical Applications:* US without additional imaging is cost-effective in symptomatic patients who are suitable for endarterectomy.[9]

PROGRAMMED MANAGEMENT

Strategic Programming

In general, the goals of the management of patients with ICAD are (1) secondary prevention of previous cerebral ischemic events, and (2) primary prevention of new cerebral ischemic events. The current standard treatment includes inhibition of platelets by ASA, lowering cholesterol level with statins, and pharmacologic treatment of hypertension and diabetes if present. Variation in this standard treatment includes the additional use of ticlopidin, clopidogrel, or warfarin. Carotid stenting or surgical endarterectomy is performed if indicated (Table 19-3A).

Management for Asymptomatic Patients

Aspirin

Aspirin (ASA) is a weak platelet inhibitor; it irreversibly inhibits the acetylating cyclooxygenase. ASA suppresses the production of the

TABLE 19-3A: Management Master Plan	
Data management	Control blood pressure
	Low-sodium diet
	Preventive measures
	with antiplatelet medications or
	anticoagulant or cholesterol-
	lowering drug
Root-cause treatment	Stenting of the carotid artery
	Carotid artery endarterectomy
Work-around management	Bypass graft surgery
System replacement	None available

pro-aggregatory arachidonic-acid–mediated effect of thromboxane A_2. ASA is indicated in all patients with significant (>50% stenosis) ICAD. Low dose ASA, 75-150 mg/day, is best. Higher-dose ASA (75 mg or more) is no more effective than lower-dose ASA at preventing cardiovascular events.[10]

Ticlodipine

Ticlopidine hydrochloride is a thienopyridine that inhibits adenosine disphosphate–induced fibrinogen binding to platelets. It has been shown to be effective for the prevention of vascular outcomes in patients with cerebrovascular disease in several randomized studies. Ticlopidine is associated with 1% of incidence of neutropenia, and >60 cases of associated thrombotic thrombocytopenia purpura have been reported.[10]

Optimal Medical Therapy in Symptomatic Patients

Clopidogrel

Clopidogrel is a thienopyridine derivative that inhibits the binding of adenosine diphosphate to its platelet receptors. It has been shown to be more effective than ASA in reducing the combined risk of ischemic stroke at 75 mg per day. There are no major differences between ASA and clopidogrel in terms of safety; serious hemorrhages occurred at a slightly higher rate among patients taking ASA.[10]

BENEFITS, HARMS, AND COST-EFFECTIVENESS ANALYSIS:

Clopidogrel +ASA versus Clopidogrel in the MATCH Trial

Methodology: 7599 patients with a recent stroke or TIA were randomized to receive clopidogrel (75 mg per day) versus clopidogrel (75 mg per day) plus low dose aspirin (75 mg per day). *Results:* During 18 months of follow-up, there was no statistically significant difference in the rate of ischemic events between the treatment groups. *Harms:* In the patients treated with the combination of clopidogrel plus ASA, there was a statistically significant increase in life-threatening bleeding (2.6% versus 1.3%). Intracranial hemorrhage occurred in 25 patients in the clopidogrel group versus 40 in the combination therapy group. *Practical Applications:* Administration of clopidogrel is as effective as clopidogrel plus ASA in reducing the rate of ischemic events. Moreover, it is safer than combination therapy.[11]

SMART THINKING:

Aspirin and Extended-Release Dipyridamole Versus Clopidogrel for Recurrent Stroke The PRoFESS Study

Methodology: 20,332 patients with a recent stroke or TIA were randomized to receive clopidogrel (75 mg per day) versus ASA (25 mg daily) plus extended-release dipyridamole (200 mg per day). *Benefits:* During 2.5 years of follow-up there was no statistically significant difference in the rate of ischemic events between the treatment groups: 13.1% in both groups. The net risk of recurrent stroke was similar in both groups (11.4 versus 11.7%). *Harms:* There were more major hemorrhagic events including intracranial hemorrhage among combined therapy recipients than among monotherapy patients. *Practical Applications:* Clopidogrel is as safe and effective as the combination of dipyridamole plus ASA, without any evidence of superiority between these two protocols.[12]

BENEFITS, HARMS, AND COST-EFFECTIVENESS ANALYSIS:

Clopidogrel +Dipyridamole versus Clopidogrel Versus ASA

Methodology: Data sets of ESP-2 trial were used to create a health economic model that estimates the incremental cost and cost-effectiveness of ASA/extended release dipyridamole or clopidogrel versus ASA. *Benefits:* ASA/extended release dipyridamole was cost-effective when compared with ASA (US$ 28,472). Clopidogrel was not cost-effective when compared with ASA (cost for stroke averted, US$161,316) *Practical Applications:* The combination of ASA/extended release dipyridamole is a cost-effective alternative to ASA for the prevention of recurrent stroke.[13]

Warfarin

Despite a number of randomized trials comparing ASA with warfarin in the secondary prevention of noncardioembolic stroke, there is no evidence of superiority of warfarin over ASA. There are, however, consistent data about an increase of major bleeding with warfarin therapy. Nevertheless, some case series and nonrandomized studies have shown a benefit concerning the risk of recurrent noncardioembolic stroke with warfarin, including patients with cervical artery dissection or severe carotid disease prior to revascularization.

ADVANCED MANAGEMENT

DECISION POINT:

When Does a Patient with ICAD Need to Be Revascularized?

Revascularizations (endarterectomy or percutaneous carotid stenting) are not recommended in symptomatic and asymptomatic patients with low-grade carotid stenosis (stenosis <50% in symptomatic and <60% in asymptomatic patients) in whom optimal medical therapy should be administered. In patients with moderate to severe carotid stenosis, judgment about revascularization should be distinguished in symptomatic and asymptomatic patients.[1] Although the questions about revascularization in asymptomatic and symptomatic patients appear to be quite sufficiently answered, there are still many unanswered issues about which revascularization techniques should be used (CEA versus CAS) and which clinical settings (symptomatic high-risk versus asymptomatic patients) are preferable. This is mainly due to (1) a lack of a combined endpoint of stroke death and acute myocardial infarction in surgical trials, (2) lack of sufficient endovascular experiences of surgical teams participating in endovascular trials, (3) differences in preprocedural classification of patients and inclusion criteria among surgical and endovascular trials.

Carotid Endarterectomy (CEA)

Carotid endarterectomy (CEA) is the current standard of care to prevent stroke in asymptomatic and symptomatic patients.

Symptomatic Patients

Among symptomatic NASCET patients with stenosis of 50 to 69%, the five-year rate of any ipsilateral stroke has been reduced from 22.2 to 15.7% by endarterectomy.[14] In patients with stenosis of 70 to 99%, the risk of ispilateral stroke has been reduced from 26 to 9%. Results from the ECST trial had similar findings supporting surgical revascularization in symptomatic for hemispheric stroke patients with stenosis 50 to 99%[15] (Table 19-3B).

Asymptomatic Patients

The Veterans Affairs Cooperative Study (stenosis >50%), the Asymptomatic Carotid Atherosclerotic Study (stenosis >60%), and the Asymptomatic Carotid Surgery Trial (stenosis >60%) included 5223

TABLE 19-3B: Surgical Clinical Trials (Included Surgical Harms of CAS Versus CEA Trials) of Symptomatic Patients.

Trial Name	No. of Patients	30-day DS, %	30-day D/MS, %	1-year D/S, %
VACS[16]	91	7.7	4.7	—
NASCET[14]	1415	6.5	—	15.8 (2 years)
ECTS[15]	1742	7.5	3.6	—
CAVATA[17]	253	9.9	5.9	—
EVA-3S[18]	259	3.9	1.5	6.1 (6 months)
SPACE[19]	584	6.5	3.8	—

D/S: death and stroke, D/MS: death and all major stroke

TABLE 19-4: Surgical Clinical Trials of Asymptomatic Patients

Trial Name	No. of Patients	30-day D/S/MI,%	30-day D/S,%	30-day D/SM,%	1-year D/S	5-year D/S
VACS[16]	211	6.5	4.7	4.7	10.3	—
ACAS[20]	825	—	2.7	—	6.5	31.9
ACST[21]	1560	—	3.1	—	—	28.9

D/S: death and stroke, D/MS: death and all major stroke, D/S/MI: death/stroke/myocardial infarction

patients with moderate to severe carotid stenosis.[16, 20-21] The incidence of perioperative stroke or death was 2.8%, with patients in surgical groups faring better than patients in medical therapy.

In asymptomatic patients with moderate to severe carotid stenosis (≥60%), carotid endarterectomy plus medical management should be recommended as long as the perioperative risk is low. There are no strong recommendations for CAS in asymptomatic patients at this time (Table 19-4).

Carotid Artery Stenting (CAS)

CAS is an emerging alternative revascularization technique to prevent stroke. This is a technique in evolution that recently included different embolic protection devices (neuroprotection) and a variety of open and closed cell stents. Many reports exist about the supposed benefits and harms of CAS in both symptomatic (Table 19-5) and asymptomatic patients (Table 19-6).

Although data have been produced by different groups, it is still difficult to compare each study or to compare different endovascular trials against surgical trials. There are too many confounding factors such as differences in definition of endpoints, lack of medications

TABLE 19-5: Endovascular Clinical Trials of Symptomatic Patients

Trial Name	No. of Patients	30-day D/S, %	30-day D/MS, %	1-year D/S
WALLSTENT[22]	107	12.1	—	12.1
CAVATAS[17]	251	10	6.4	—
CREST[23]	1246	5.6	—	—
EVA-3S[18]	261	9.6	3.4	11.7 (6 months)
SPACE[19]	605	6.8	4.7	—

D/S: death and stroke, D/MS: death and all major stroke

TABLE 19-6: Endovascular Clinical Trials of Asymptomatic Patients

Trial Name	No. of Patients	30-day D/S/MI, %	30-day D/S, %	30-day D/SM, %	1-year D/S/MI, %	1-year D/S, %
BEACH[24]	557	5	4.3	2.7	8	13.6
CASES-PMS[25]	1158	4.7	—	—	—	—
CREST[23]	1246	—	3.4	—	—	—
CAPTURE[26]	3017	5.4	—	—	—	—
CaRESS[27]	99	2.1	2.1	2.1	10.9	10
SAPPHIRE[28]	117	5.8	4.5	2.6	10.3	6.8

D/S: death and stroke, D/MS: death and all major stroke, D/S/MI: death/stroke/myocardial infarction

against risk factors in surgical trials, differences in baseline cardiovascular risk factors, inexperience of the endovascular team (e.g., WALL-STENT,[22] SPACE[19] and EVA-3S,[18] and particularly differences in devices (no neuroprotection devices in CAVATAS[17]) and technology used (open versus closed cell stent).

SMART THINKING:

When to Suggest CAS and CEA for Asymptomatic Patients?

From the body of literature produced until now, CEA remains the procedure of choice for asymptomatic patients with significant carotid stenosis (60 to 99%) if performed with ≤3% perioperative risk of stroke and death. It reduces the ipsilateral stroke rate but not the midterm mortality rate. CAS appears to have a perioperative risk of stroke and death within or very near to the "3% rule" in asymptomatic patients at average risk. It can be an option when treating asymptomatic patients at increased surgical risk, especially with stenosis ≥80%.[29]

TECHNOLOGY ASSESSMENT AND ECONOMIC ANALYSIS:

CAS Versus CEA

Methodology: A group of 94 asymptomatic patients, with 46 patients in the CAS group and 48 patients in the CEA group, were enrolled. Clinical outcomes such as perioperative mortality, adverse events (death, stroke, MI, length of stay, incidence of hemodynamic instability) were analyzed. Total costs, indirect costs, and direct procedural costs associated with hospitalizations were evaluated. *Benefits and Harms:* CAS was associated with a shorter length of stay (1.2 versus 2.1 days) compared with CEA. Differences in perioperative mortality (0 versus 2%), major adverse events (2 versus 10%), strokes (2 versus 4%), and myocardial infarction (0 versus 4%) were not statistically significant between the CAS and CEA groups. *Cost Analysis:* CAS was associated with higher total procedural costs (US$17,402 versus US$12,112) and direct costs (US$10,522 versus US$7227). The differences in indirect costs were not significant. *Practical Applications:* CAS with neuroprotection was associated with similar outcomes when compared with CEA but with higher hospital costs. Utilization of CAS over CEA should be based upon patient's surgical risk and economic resources.[30]

SMART THINKING:

CAS Versus CEA in High-Risk Patients

Although CEA reduces the incidence of cerebral infarction in symptomatic and asymptomatic patients, its benefits should be balanced with perioperative risks associated with the procedure. Even in today's technology, many patients cannot safely undergo CEA for different unfavorable anatomic and clinical reasons (Table 19-7). Usually, patients enrolled in surgical trials were carefully selected at low risk of periprocedural complications: for example, age >75 years has not always been included in the randomized trials, and indeed the benefits of CEA in patients > 75 years of age has not yet been established.

TABLE 19-7: Criteria for Increased Surgical Risk

Anatomic Characteristics

Surgically inaccessible lesions (≥C2 level, or below clavicle)
Previous neck or head radiation therapy or surgery
Spinal immobility
Restenosis after carotid endarterectomy
Controlateral laryngeal palsy
Tracheal stoma
Controlateral carotid occlusion

Comorbidities

Age>75 years
New York Heart Association class III-IV
Canadian Cardiovascular Society Classification III-IV
Left main ≥2 vessel coronary disease
Acute myocardial infarction < 30 days before
Left ventricle ejection fraction ≤30%
Heart surgery scheduled within 1 month
Severe lung and renal diseases

TABLE 19-8: Endovascular Clinical Trials of High-Risk Patients

Trial Name	No. of Patients	30-day D/S/MI, %	30-day D/S, %	1-year D/S, %
ARCHeR[31]	581	8.3	6.9	9.6
BEACH[26]	480	5.8	—	9.1
CABERNET[32]	454	3.8	—	4.5
CAPTURE[26]	3500	6.3	5.7	—
CREATE[33]	419	6.2	5.2	—
MAVERIC[34]	399	—	5.3	—
SECURITY[35]	305	8.5	—	—

D/S: death and stroke, D/MS: death and all major stroke, D/S/MI: death/stroke/ myocardial infarction

CAS has been investigated extensively in high-risk patients because it is less invasive than CEA (Table 19-8). From the body of evidence produced, it is clear that CAS is not inferior to CEA in high-risk populations, and despite the rate of complications it is still better than CEA in average risk patients. However, from a long-term perspective, the data suggest that CAS is the treatment of choice for patients with ICAD. After following up patients for a decade, the investigators from the CAVATAS study reported more stroke and severe restenosis in patients receiving CEA. The results of the study appeared in the October issue of *Lancet Neurology* but were published on line August 29 2009.

 EVIDENCE-BASED MEDICINE:

Lesson from the SAPPHIRE Trial

Methodology: This was a multicenter, prospective, randomized trial enrolling 747 patients (>70% of asymptomatic patients) at high risk for CEA. The endpoint was the 1-year incidence of major adverse events, including stroke, death, MI within 30 days plus death and ipsilateral stroke between 31 days and 1 year. Of the 747 patients, 334 were randomized (167 CEA and 167 CAS); 413 patients refused CEA because of excessive risk and entered a CAS registry; 7 patients refused CAS and entered a CEA registry. *Results:* The rates of major events were almost the same for CAS (2.6%) and CEA (2.5%). The one-year primary composite endpoint demonstrated statistically significant noninferiority for CAS (12.2%) compared with CEA (20.1%). In the asymptomatic high risk patients, CAS did better than CEA (adverse major effect rate 10.5% for CAS and 20.3% for CEA) owing to a large difference in non-Q wave MI. In symptomatic high-risk patients there was no statistically significant difference between

CAS and CEA in terms of 30-day rate of stroke, death, and MI (2.1% versus 9.3%) or one-year primary endpoint (16.8% versus 16.5%). *Practical Application:* Although not conclusively, the trial suggests that high surgical risk patients may benefit from the CAS over the CEA approach, even though the rate of adverse events is still high.[28]

ICAD Management in Patients Scheduled for Cardiac Surgery

Carotid artery stenosis is often associated with advanced coronary artery disease. The coexistence of carotid and coronary artery disease adds complexity to the medical decision-making process and brings increasing challenge to the perioperative management of coronary artery bypass graft (CABG) surgery. Postoperative stroke remains one of the most devastating complications of CABG, thereby contributing to the increased risk of mortality following CABG. Carotid artery disease causes approximately one-third of post-CABG stroke and thus needs to be addressed while preparing a patient for CABG. While CEA has been the gold standard for carotid artery revascularization, carotid artery stenting may not be inferior to CEA in patients with increased surgical risks. Thus, a consensus as how to best revascularize patients with carotid artery stenosis before CABG is yet to emerge. Current guidelines state that carotid endarterectomy is probably recommended before or concomitant with coronary artery bypass grafting, but the best management strategy for patients with concomitant surgical coronary artery disease in need of CABG and significant carotid artery stenosis should be still based on individual patient characteristics, urgency of revascularization, prioritization based on the symptomatic vascular territory, and local expertise with an integrated team approach by interventionalists, neurologists, and cardiothoracic surgeons, preferably in high-volume cardiac centers.[36-37]

TAKE-HOME MESSAGE

Data Collecting Collect all the data about the patient's history (of smoking, high-sodium, high-cholesterol diet, alcohol abuse, lack of exercise, HTN, DM, high cholesterol level), family history (of early sudden death due to heart disease, history of early stroke, CAD), social history (work and behaviors) and from a complete physical examination (signs of prior stroke, TIA, CAD, PAD, carotid murmur, weak peripheral pulses), all of which add weight to the clinical decision-making process.

Data Mining Recommend safe, appropriate, and efficacious investigation including carotid ultrasound and Doppler studies. Fasting lipid profile, fasting blood glucose, BUN and creatinine levels, weight, BMI, and waist circumference would help to control risk factors.

Management Recommend safe, appropriate, and efficacious therapy to maintain the stable health status of the patient over time (ASA, dipyridamole, and in selected cases warfarin). No clear recommendations can be made about preferred medical therapy in asymptomatic patients. CAS still carries some additive risk and high costs in non–high-risk patients when compared to CEA with current technology.

Patient-Centered Education and Care Get the patients involved in their own lifestyle modification to increase compliance with diet, exercise, medication, office visits, and testing in order to provide continuity of care.

References

1. Hobson, R. W. 2nd, Mackey, W. C., Ascher, E., et al.: Society for Vascular Surgery. Management of atherosclerotic carotid artery disease: clinical practice guidelines of the Society for Vascular Surgery. J Vasc Surg. 2008 Aug;48(2):480–486.
2. Rigatelli, G., Zanchetta, M.: Endovascular therapies for noncoronary atherosclerosis in the elderly: supra-aortic vessels and thoracoabdominal aorta lesions. Am J Geriatr Cardiol. 2005. May-Jun;14(3):142–147.
3. Caplan, L. R.: Dissections of brain-supplying arteries. Nat Clin Pract Neurol. 2008 Jan;4(1):34–42.
4. Rigatelli, G.: Patent foramen ovale: the evident paradox between the apparently simple treatment and the really complex pathophysiology. J Cardiovasc Med. 2007 Apr;8(4):300–304.
5. Josephs, S. C., Rowley, H. A., Rubin, G. D.: American Heart Association Writing Group 3. Atherosclerotic Peripheral Vascular Disease Symposium II: vascular magnetic resonance and computed tomographic imaging. Circulation. 2008; Dec 16;118(25):2837–2844.
6. Gerhard-Herman, M., Gardin, J. M., Jaff, M., et al.: American Society of Echocardiography; Society for Vascular Medicine and Biology. Guidelines for noninvasive vascular laboratory testing: a report from the American Society of Echocardiography and the Society for Vascular Medicine and Biology. Vasc Med. 2006 Nov;11(3):183–200.
7. U.S. Preventive Services Task Force. Screening for carotid artery stenosis: U.S. Preventive Services Task Force recommendation statement. Ann Intern Med. Dec 18, 2007;147(12):854–859.
8. Debrey, S. M., Yu, H., Lynch, J. K., et al.: Diagnostic accuracy of magnetic resonance angiography for internal carotid artery disease: a systematic review and meta-analysis. Stroke. Aug 2008;39(8):2237–2248.
9. Buskens, E., Nederkoorn, P. J., Buijs-Van Der Woude, T., et al.: Imaging of carotid arteries in symptomatic patients: cost-effectiveness of diagnostic strategies. Radiology. Oct 2004;233(1):101–112.
10. Albers, G. W., Amarenco, P., Easton, J. D., et al.: Antithrombotic and thrombolytic therapy for ischemic stroke: the Seventh ACCP Conference on Antithrombotic and Thrombolytic Therapy. Chest. Sept. 2004; 126(3 Suppl):483S–512S.

11. Diener, H.C., Bogousslavsky, J., Brass, L.M., et al.: MATCH investigators. Aspirin and clopidogrel compared with clopidogrel alone after recent ischaemic stroke or transient ischaemic attack in high-risk patients (MATCH): randomised, double-blind, placebo-controlled trial. Lancet. 2004;364:331–7.

12. Sacco, R. L., Diener, H. C., Yusuf, S., et al. and the PRoFESS Study Group: Aspirin and extended-release dipyridamole versus clopidogrel for recurrent stroke. N Engl J Med. 2008;359:1238–1251.

13. Shah, H., Gondek, K.: Aspirin plus extended-release dipyridamole or clopidogrel compared with aspirin monotherapy for the prevention of recurrent ischemic stroke: a cost-effectiveness analysis. Clin Ther. Mar. 2000;22(3):362–370.

14. North American Symptomatic Carotid Endarterectomy Trial Collaborators (NASCET). Beneficial effect of carotid endarterectomy in symptomatic patients with high-grade carotid stenosis. N Engl J Med. 1991;325:445–453.

15. European Carotid Surgery Triallists'Collaborative Group. Randomized trial of endarterectomy for recently symptomatic carotid stenosis: final results of the MRC European Carotid Surgery Trial (ECST). Lancet 1998; 339:1379–87.

16. Hobson, R. W. II, Weiss, D. G., Fields, W. S., et al.: Veterans Affairs Cooperative Study (VACS) Group. Efficacy of carotid endarterectomy for asymptomatic carotid stenosis. N Engl J Med. 1993;328:221–227.

17. Endovascular versus surgical treatment in patients with carotid stenosis in the Carotid and Vertebral Artery Transluminal Angioplasty Study (CAVATAS): a randomised trial. Lancet. 2001;357:1729–1737.

18. Mas, J. L., Chatellier, G., Beyssen, B., and the EVA-3S Investigators: Endarterectomy versus stenting in patients with symptomatic severe carotid stenosis. N Engl J Med. 2006;355:1660–1671.

19. SPACE Collaborative Group, Ringleb, P. A., Allenberg, J., Bruckmann, H., et al.: 30 Day results from the SPACE trial of stent-protected angioplasty versus carotid endarterectomy in symptomatic patients: a randomised non-inferiority trial. Lancet. 2006;368:1239–1247.

20. Executive Committee for the Asymptomatic Carotid Atherosclerosis Study (ACAS). Endarterectomy for asymptomatic carotid artery stenosis. JAMA. 1995;273:1421–1428.

21. Halliday, A., Mansfield, A., Marro, J., et al.: MRC Asymptomatic Carotid Surgery Trial (ACST) Collaborative Group. Prevention of disabling and fatal strokes by successful carotid endarterectomy in patients without recent neurological symptoms: randomised controlled trial [published correction appears in Lancet. 2004;364:416]. Lancet. 2004; 363:1491–1502.

22. lberts MJ. Results of a multicenter prospective randomized trial of carotid artery stenting versus carotid endarterectomy. Stroke 2001:32: 325 d-abstract.

23. Hobson, R. W. 2nd, Howard, V. J., Roubin, G. S., et al.: CREST Investigators. Carotid artery stenting is associated with increased complications in octogenarians: 30-day stroke and death rates in the CREST lead-in phase. J Vasc Surg. 2004;40:1106–1111.

24. White, C. J., Iyer, S. S., Hopkins, L. N., et al.: BEACH Trial Investigators. Carotid stenting with distal protection in high surgical risk patients: the BEACH trial 30 day results. Catheter Cardiovasc Interv. 2006;67:503–512.
25. Yadav, J. S., Criado, F., Schrieber, T., The CASES-PMS carotid stenting surveillance study: final 30-day results. Abstract presented at Transcatheter Cardiovascular Therapeutics 2006; October 22–27, 2006; Washington, DC.
26. Gray, W. A., Yadav, J. S., Verta, P., et al.: The CAPTURE registry: results of carotid stenting with embolic protection in the post approval setting. Catheter Cardiovasc Interv. 2007;69:341–348.
27. CaRESS Steering Committee. Carotid Revascularization Using Endarterectomy or Stenting Systems (CaRESS) phase I clinical trial: 1-year results. J Vasc Surg. 2005;42:213–219.
28. Yadav, J.S., Wholey, M.H., Kuntz, R.E., et al.: Stenting and angioplasty with protection in patients at high risk for endarterectomy investigators. Protected carotid-artery stenting versus endarterectomy in high-risk patients. N Engl J Med. 2004; Oct 7;351(15):1493–501.
29. Bates, E. R., Babb, J. D., Casey, D. E. Jr., et al. ACCF/SCAI/SVMB/SIR/ASITN 2007 clinical expert consensus document on carotid stenting: a report of the American College of Cardiology Foundation Task Force on Clinical Expert Consensus Documents (ACCF/SCAI/SVMB/SIR/ASITN Clinical Expert Consensus Document Committee on Carotid Stenting) [published correction appears in J Am Coll Cardiol. 2007;49: 924]. J Am Coll Cardiol. 2007;49:126–170.
30. Park, B., Mavanur, A., Dahn, M., et al.: Clinical outcomes and cost comparison of carotid artery angioplasty with stenting versus carotid endarterectomy. J Vasc Surg. 2006; Aug;44(2):270–276.
31. Gray, W. A., Hopkins, L. N., Yadav, S., et al.: ARCHeR Trial Collaborators. Protected carotid stenting in high-surgical-risk patients: the ARCHeR results. J Vasc Surg. 2006;44:258–268.
32. Hopkins, L. N., Myla, S., Grube, E., et al.: Carotid artery revascularization in high surgical risk patients with the NexStent and the Filterwire EX/EZ: 1-year results in the CABERNET trial. Catheter Cardiovasc Interv. 2008;71:950–960.
33. Safian, R.D., Bresnahan, J.F., Jaff, M.R., et al.: CREATE Pivotal Trial Investigators.Protected carotid stenting in high-risk patients with severe carotid artery stenosis. J Am Coll Cardiol. 2006; Jun 20;47(12): 2384–2389.
34. Ramee, S., Higashida, R.: Evaluation of the Medtronic self-expanding carotid stent system with distal protection in the treatment of carotid artery stenosis. Am J Cardiol. 2004;94:61E.
35. SECURITY Investigators. U.S. Food and Drug Administration, Center for Devices and Radiological Health. Xact® Carotid Stent System - P040038. Summary of safety and effectiveness.
36. Das, P., Clavijo, L. C., Nanjundappa, A., et al.: Revascularization of carotid stenosis before cardiac surgery. Expert Rev Cardiovasc Ther. 2008; Nov;6(10):1393-1396.

37. Guzman, L. A., Costa, M. A., Angiolillo, D. J., et al.: A systematic review of outcomes in patients with staged carotid artery stenting and coronary artery bypass graft surgery. Stroke. 2008; Feb;39(2):361–365.
38. Reimers, B., Sievert, H., Schuler, G. C., et al.: Proximal endovascular flow blockage for cerebral protection during carotid artery stenting: results from a prospective multicenter registry. J Endovasc Ther. 2005;12: 156–165.
39. Coppi, G., Moratto, R., Silingardi, R., et al.: PRIAMUS–proximal flow blockage cerebral protection during carotid stenting: results from a multicenter Italian registry. J Cardiovasc Surg (Torino). 2005;46:219–227.
40. Yadav, J. S., Wholey, M. H., Kuntz, R. E., et al. Stenting and Angioplasty with Protection in Patients at High Risk for Endarterectomy Investigators. Protected carotid-artery stenting versus endarterectomy in high-risk patients. N Engl J Med. 2004;351:1493–1501.

Section V

Arrhythmias

Atrial Fibrillation

*Chansheng Ma, Dayi Hu,
Pham Nhu Hung, and Thach Nguyen*

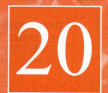

Chapter Outline

DEFINITION

Atrial fibrillation (AF) is the most common persistent tachyarrhythmia characterized by disorganized atrial depolarization without effective atrial contraction. There are four kinds of AF.

- Lone AF is AF in patients younger than 60 years without evidence of structural heart disease.
- Persistent AF is AF lasting more than seven days and requires intervention for termination.
- Permanent AF is AF that has existed for many years and cannot be consistently terminated with cardioversion.
- Paroxysmal AF is AF that terminates spontaneously within seven days.

Secondary AF is caused by an acute and possibly reversible cause, such as hyperthyroidism, acute alcohol intoxication, or after thoracic surgery.

Patient Population in Focus

AF is found in 0.1% of adults younger than 55 but in more than 9% of those aged 80 or older.[1]

Strategic Programming

The first step is to identify patients with AF through data collecting with a comprehensive history and physical examination. The next step is to perform data processing in order to formulate a preliminary diagnosis and a short list of differential diagnoses (e.g., AF, supraventricular tachycardia, ventricular arrhythmia causing palpitation). Then, using the method of data mining, tests may be ordered (electrocardiogram [ECG], echocardiography, thyroid function, 24-hour Holter monitoring, stress testing, coronary angiography if needed) in order to confirm (data converting) the main diagnosis of AF and to rule out (data filtering) the differential diagnoses. The therapeutic goal is to reduce and prevent the thromboembolic events, relieve related symptoms with ventricular rate control, or restore sinus rhythm.

DATA COLLECTING

Investigation Master Plan

When a physician sees a patient suspected of having AF, there are seven main areas of interest for data collecting (history and physical examination).

The main area of interest: The right atrium (zone A).

There are no upstream areas for AF identified (zone B).

The downstream area for AF is the ventricular response (zone C).

The system configuration: There is nothing wrong with the configuration of the system (zone E).

The work-around configuration: (not identified yet) (zone D).

The cardiovascular system: If there is long-standing uncontrolled AF, the heart can become dilated. The symptoms and signs are of the end-organ damage or failure and not due to AF per se.

The network (the whole body): Long-standing AF can cause stroke, transient ischemic attack (TIA), thromboemboli to the peripheral arteries causing critical limb ischemia, and kidney and splenic infarction (zone F).

History

The symptoms of AF are highly variable and depend on several factors, including ventricular rate, cardiac function, concomitant medical problems, and individual patient perception. The rapid and irregular rhythm and the loss of synchronized atrial activity contribute to impaired cardiac performance and symptoms. The complaints associated with AF include palpitations, chest pain, shortness of breath on exertion, fatigue, dizziness, and, rarely, syncope.[2]

However, many patients who present with palpitations, are asymptomatic. AF may be felt as palpitations during exercise or at rest. However, palpitation is worse when there is concomitant structural heart disease. Because of possible reversion of sinus rhythm with ablation intervention, the term "permanent AF" is not appropriate in the context of patients undergoing catheter and/or surgical ablation of AF[3] (Table 20-1).

Physical Examination

The classic physical exam findings are as follows: a slight reduction in intensity of the first heart sound, absence of the *a* wave in the jugular venous pulse, and an irregularly irregular ventricular rhythm. The other

TABLE 20-1: Information Needed During History Interview

Pattern of Arrhythmia
Paroxysmal, permanent, persistent
Symptoms
Concomitant cardiovascular diseases or etiologies of AF
History
Onset of first episode of AF and of current episode
Frequency, duration, precipitating factors, severity of symptoms, and mode of termination of AF
History of prior evaluation and response to prior management
History of stroke and risk factors for stroke
Family history of arrhythmia and sudden cardiac death

findings are from the causes of AF, including structural heart disease (including valvular disease), coronary artery disease, or hyperthyroidism.

DATA FILTERING (DIFFERENTIAL DIAGNOSIS)

For patients with AF, if the ventricular rhythm becomes regular, the following conditions should be suspected: conversion to sinus rhythm, atrial tachycardia, and atrial flutter with a constant ratio of conducted beats. AF needs to be distinguished from atrial flutter when the typical flutter waves are not prominent or have a varying ventricular conduction ratio. The absolutely irregular ventricular rhythm and disordering of AF waves in some leads may help to differentiate AF from atrial flutter.

DATA MINING (WORK-UP)

Electrocardiogram

The typical characteristics of AF in the electrocardiogram (ECG) are as follows: disappearance of the P wave; fine and irregular baseline undulations, i.e., f waves; the fast frequency of the f wave at a rate of 350 to 600 beats/min; and irregularly irregular ventricular response (VR). In patients with Wolff-Parkinson-White syndrome, the VR during AF can at times exceed 300 beats/min and lead to ventricular fibrillation (Table 20-2).

2-D Echocardiography

Echocardiography can help to find the possible causes of AF (rheumatic mitral valve disease, hypertrophic cardiomyopathy, and other organic

TABLE 20-2: Information Needed from Tests	
Laboratory Tests	
Blood electrolytes, glucose levels Liver and renal function tests Thyroid function	
12-Lead ECG	
Chest XR	Evidence of left ventricular (LV) hypertrophy, heart size, and evidence of cardiac diseases such as mitral stenosis; pulmonary diseases
Echocardiogram	To diagnose underlying structural heart diseases, such as valvular diseases, LV hypertrophy, and cardiomyopathies; to assess left atrial size, LV size, and function
Holter Monitoring	To diagnose paroxysmal AF, to assess ambulatory ventricular rate during AF
Exercise Stress Test	To diagnose CAD and exercise-induced AF

cardiac diseases) and may provide information that is useful in stratifying thromboembolic risk. Among high-risk AF patients, impaired left ventricle systolic function, the presence of thrombi, dense spontaneous echo contrast (SEC), or reduced velocity of blood flow in the left atrium appendage have been associated with thromboembolism events.

Transesophageal Echocardiography (TEE)

TEE is the most sensitive and specific technique to detect cardiogenic thrombi.[4] TEE has been used to stratify stroke risk in patients with AF and to guide cardioversion. For patients with AF of greater than 48-hours' duration, a TEE-guided strategy or the traditional strategy of anticoagulation for three weeks before and four weeks after elective cardioversion resulted in similar rates of thromboembolism.[1]

Holter Monitoring

Asymptomatic AF is more common in patients with PAF. Ambulatory monitoring can provide more detailed information on the duration and frequency of AF onset and also help to detect the long pause during AF or at AF conversion. This has important implications for deciding whether a patient needs chronic anticoagulation therapy and for evaluating the potential risks of antiarrhythmic agents. Repeated episodes of premature atrial beats triggering AF warrant an electrophysiologic study (EPS) and catheter ablation.

Stress Testing

AF may be triggered or may worsen during exercise. During a stress test, the patient exercises on a treadmill or stationary bicycle for information on heart rate increase with activities. The stress test can also be used to detect coronary artery disease.

Exercise testing should be performed if myocardial ischemia is suspected and should be done prior to initiating type IC antiarrhythmic drug therapy. Another reason for exercise testing is to study the adequacy of rate control across a full spectrum of activity (not only at rest) in patients with persistent or permanent AF.

PROGRAMMED MANAGEMENT

The goals of management include (1) to control the heart rate, (2) to convert to sinus rhythm, (3) to prevent recurrence of AF (or maintain sinus rhythm), and (4) to prevent thromboembolism.

Strategic Planning

A hemodynamically unstable patient should undergo emergency direct current cardioversion. For hemodynamically stable patients, the goal of therapy is to control the VR with a target heart rate of <100 beats/min. Oral or intravenous calcium channel blockers or beta blockers are the first-line agents. Diltiazem is generally preferable to verapamil because it is associated with fewer negative inotropic effects and less peripheral vasodilation. Beta blockers are more effective for patients with higher adrenergic tones, such as those with postoperative AF. Some patients with infrequent but highly symptomatic acute episodes of AF can be managed without regular dosing of flecainide or propafenone. This so-called pill-in-the pocket is taken by the patient at the first sign of AF. This therapy should be initiated in a monitored setting so that the risk of proarrhythmia can be assessed. Any patients, especially young patients, with paroxysmal AF and rapid ventricular rates who are still symptomatic with rate control should have a rhythm control approach by cardioversion[5] (Table 20-3).

🔴 DATA MANAGEMENT TIPS (CLINICAL PEARLS)
Treatment of AF and Mortality

No current findings suggest that treating the AF contributes to a reduction in any potentially enhanced mortality rate. Therefore, patients cannot be counseled to undergo any form of rhythm control with the expectation of improving their chances of survival. The reasons for the

TABLE 20-3: Management Master Plan

Data management	Keep HR below 80 bpm
	Low-sodium diet
	Preventive measures
	Pharmacologic therapy
Enhanced intrinsic correction	Rate control with drug, AV node ablation
Index problem	Pulmonary vein ablation, pharmacologic or electrical cardioversion
System configuration correction	None
Work-around management	None
System replacement	None

absence of such findings may be that mortality rates associated with AF are not enhanced to begin with or that the proarrhythmic potential of antiarrhythmic agents is offset by the procedural risks associated with invasive therapies.[5]

Rhythm or Rate Control

Besides prevention of the risk of thromboembolism, another goal of management of the patient with AF is symptom control. The actual clinical consideration is mainly focused on the selection of strategy, rhythm control, or rate control.

 EVIDENCE-BASED MEDICINE:

A Comparison of Rate Control and Rhythm Control in Patients with Atrial Fibrillation. The AFFIRM Study.[6]

Methodology: The AFFIRM study was a randomized, multicenter clinical trial to compare two treatment strategies (rate control vs. rhythm control) in patients with AF and a high risk of stroke or death. The primary endpoint was overall mortality. ***Results:*** A total of 4060 patients (69.7+/−9.0 years) were enrolled. At the five-year follow up, the mortality of the rhythm-control group was similar to that of the rate-control group (23.8% vs. 21.3%, HR 1.15; 95% CI, 0.99−1.34; P = 0.08). More patients in the rhythm-control group than in the rate-control group were hospitalized, and there were more adverse drug effects in the rhythm-control group as well. ***Evidence-Based Applications:*** The results indicate that management of AF with the rhythm-control strategy offers no survival advantage over the rate-control strategy.

In theory, rhythm control should have advantages over rate control; however, in the AFFIRM trial, there was no difference in outcomes between the two strategies. One reasonable interpretation is that the hazards of proarrhythmic effects with antiarrhythmic drugs (AAD) may outweigh the benefits of sinus rhythm restored with antiarrhythmic drugs. This study might suggest that attempts to restore sinus rhythm with presently available antiarrhythmic drugs are not beneficial. Future medications with fewer side effects may show the benefits of restoring RSR. The AFFIRM study also did not address AF in younger, symptomatic patients with little underlying heart disease in whom restoration of sinus rhythm by cardioversion, antiarrhythmic drugs, or nonpharmacologic interventions still must be considered.

Rate Control

In many patients, especially elderly patients with minimal symptoms related to AF, rate control is a reasonable strategy. The goal is to achieve a resting ventricular rate of 70 to 80 beats per minute and a maximal exercise rate of less than 120 beats per minute.

Beta Blockers

Beta blockers effectively decrease the ventricular rate when AF recurs and relieve or abolish its associated symptoms. When given intravenously, the short-acting beta blocker (esmolol) may have modest efficacy for pharmacologic cardioversion of new-onset AF, but it is not useful in patients with persistent AF. Beta blockers have moderate but consistent efficacy to prevent AF recurrence or reduce the frequency of paroxysmal AF. They may cause lack of awareness of recurrent AF and potentially aggravate vagally mediated AF.

⊙ DATA MANAGEMENT TIPS (CLINICAL PEARLS)
Rationale for the Selection of Rate-Control Medications

In patients with heart failure and AF, relief of pulmonary congestion by diuretics and vasodilators may aid in decreasing the heart rate. Digoxin has both negative chronotropic and positive inotropic effects and therefore is an appropriate first-line drug in such patients. Since the effect of digoxin on ventricular rate is mediated by its vagotonic effect on the AV node, the onset of action may take several hours; furthermore, digoxin is usually ineffective in acute settings, as the parasympathetic tone is low.[7, 8] Therefore, in many situations, especially in post-thoracotomy patients, a beta blocker or calcium channel blockers are the preferred agents for slowing the ventricular rate. These drugs should be used with caution in patients with hypotension or heart failure and should be started at low doses and administered slowly. In most of these patients, hypotension or heart failure is the result of rapid heart rate and may improve when rate control is achieved. After rate control has been achieved, possible underlying causes for AF should be investigated and cardioversion of AF should be considered.[2]

Digitalis

Compared with placebo, digoxin is generally not more effective for conversion of new-onset AF to sinus rhythm. Digoxin was less effective in suppressing recurrent AF. When given intravenously, digoxin slows the rapid VR and improves LV function in patients with acute MI or severe LV dysfunction. Digoxin is not recommended as the only medicine to control the VR in patients with paroxysmal AF. For patients with AF and a preexcitation syndrome, digoxin may paradoxically accelerate the VR and is contraindicated.

Rhythm Control

Cardioversion

Within the first 24 hours, up to 70 to 80% of patients with new-onset AF convert back to sinus rhythm.[7] If a patient does not convert spontaneously, pharmacologic or electrical cardioversion should be attempted. In general, in patients with nonvalvular AF of less than 48 hours, cardioversion can be safely performed with a low risk of thromboembolism after anticoagulation with heparin. However, in patients with an AF longer than 48 hours or in those with a higher risk of thromboembolism due to underlying valvular heart disease, three weeks of oral anticoagulation prior to cardioversion are recommended. Alternatively, transesophageal echocardiography to exclude atrial thrombi allows immediate cardioversion with intravenous heparin coverage, even with a patient history of a prior embolic event.[10] When the left atrial appendage cannot be adequately visualized, cardioversion should be performed after three weeks of oral anticoagulation.[8]

DATA MANAGEMENT TIPS (CLINICAL PEARLS)
Tips for Drugs That Maintain Sinus Rhythm

Because of the limited efficacy of all forms of drug therapy, a drug that maintains sinus rhythm for months or years should probably be given at least one more trial after a repeat cardioversion. Practically, for patients with idiopathic AF, flecainide and propafenone are recommended as front-line drugs of choice because they have low toxicity and low incidence of proarrhythmia. For patients with hypertension and LV hypertrophy, propafenone is the first drug of choice because it does not prolong the QT interval and there is less chance of the occurrence of torsades de pointes. For post-MI patients, sotalol and amiodarone are the first choices because they have neutral effects on the survival of these patients.[9,10] For patients with congestive heart failure, the best drug is amiodarone.[11,12] Caution should be applied for potential adverse effects when using AADs for suppression of AF in patients with structural heart disease.[8,13,14] The risk of drug-induced torsades de pointes is enhanced by metabolic disturbances, LV dysfunction, a history of ventricular tachycardia, prolongation of the QT interval, and relative bradycardia. Amiodarone appears to have a lower risk of proarrhythmia as compared to other AADs. Whether patients with recurrent sustained AF should undergo repeated cardioversion remains unclear. However, repeated cardioversion should be performed in patients who have significant symptoms despite adequate rate control and for those who maintain sinus rhythm for a significant period of time after a previous cardioversion.

DATA MANAGEMENT TIPS (CLINICAL PEARLS)
Side Effects of AADs

Flecainide should not be used for patients with coexisting heart disease. Although amiodarone is associated with a lower risk of proarrhythmia than flecainide, its use is limited by serious extracardiac organ toxicity. Dofetilide can be administered to patients with systolic dysfunction, but its use requires inpatient observation, careful dose initiation and titration, and monitoring of the QT interval. Neither dofetilide nor sotalol can be administered to patients with serious renal dysfunction. For patients with LV hypertrophy, dofetilide and sotalol are relatively contraindicated, and amiodarone is preferred. Dofetilide is less useful for patients with paroxysmal AF.[5]

Prevention of Recurrence

While treatment with AADs may successfully reduce the frequency of paroxysms, a significant number of treated patients will continue to have symptomatic arrhythmias. Furthermore, suppression of the patients' symptomatic AF episodes may not abolish the arrhythmia. Many of these patients still have asymptomatic episodes that are associated with an increased risk of thromboembolism. In a subset of patients with vagally triggered AF, digoxin and beta blockers may aggravate the arrhythmia but disopyramide or flecainide may be particularly effective. In those patients with adrenergic-triggered AF, beta blocker, propafenone, or sotalol may be useful. Class Ia and Class Ic agents can be given to patients who have no clear-cut pattern of arrhythmia and no structural heart disease. Because of the unfavorable long-term side-effect profile, amiodarone should only be administered to patients with significant heart disease and used as a last resort after failure with other drugs.[20]

Because AF usually combines with some organic cardiac disease, such as hypertension, coronary artery disease, or rheumatoid valvular disease, effective control of primary conditions will decrease the development of AF.

Some clinical trials suggest that ACE inhibitors, angiotensin receptor blockers, and statins may reduce the occurrence and recurrence of AF.[11,13-14] There is no sufficient evidence to recommend any medication for primary prevention of AF. Do amiodarone or beta blockers prevent recurrence of AF after successful cardioversion? How frequently should amiodarone be given? The answers depend on the results of the trial that follows.

SMART THINKING:

Effects of Amiodarone in the Prevention of AF

This trial was conducted to compare major events in patients randomized to receive episodic amiodarone treatment with those who received continuous amiodarone treatment while still aiming to prevent AF. *Methodology:* This is a randomized trial of 209 ambulatory patients with recurrent symptomatic persistent AF. Patients were randomly assigned to receive either episodic or continuous amiodarone treatment after electrical cardioversion following amiodarone loading. Episodic amiodarone treatment was discontinued after a month of sinus rhythm and reinitiated if AF relapsed. In the continuous treatment group, amiodarone was maintained throughout. The primary endpoint was a composite of amiodarone and underlying heart disease–related major events. The secondary endpoints were all-cause mortality and cardiovascular hospitalizations. *Results:* After a median follow-up of 2.1 years (range, 0.4-2.5 years), 51 (48%) of those receiving episodic treatment versus 64 (62%) receiving continuous treatment had sinus rhythm (P = 0.05). There were 85 AF recurrences (80%) among the episodic treatment group versus 56 (54%) in the continuous treatment group (P < 0.001). All-cause mortality and cardiovascular hospitalizations were higher among those receiving episodic treatment (56 [53%] vs. 35 [34%], P = 0.02). *Practical Applications:* In this study population, there was no difference in the composite of amiodarone and cardiac major adverse events between groups. However, patients receiving episodic treatment had a significantly increased rate of AF recurrence and a significantly higher rate of all-cause mortality and cardiovascular hospitalizations.[15]

SMART THINKING:

Use of Metoprolol CR/XL to Maintain Sinus Rhythm After Conversion from Persistent AF

This was a randomized, double-blind, placebo-controlled study.[10] *Methodology:* After successful conversion to sinus rhythm, 394 patients with persistent AF were randomly assigned to treatment with metoprolol CR/XL or placebo. The two treatment groups were similar with respect to all pretreatment characteristics. The symptomatic relapses or adverse events were followed up during the six months after cardioversion. *Results:* In the metoprolol CR/XL group, 96 patients (48.7%) had a relapse to AF compared with 118 patients (59.9%) in the placebo group (P = 0.005). Heart rate in patients after a relapse into AF was significantly lower in the metoprolol group (98 +/− 23 bpm) than in the placebo group (107 +/− 27 bpm). The rate of adverse events reported was similar in both groups. *Practical Applications:* Beta blockers are effective in preventing early recurrence after cardioversion of AF compared with placebo and will slower VR as well.[16]

Prevention of Embolic Stroke

Indications for Antithrombotic Therapy

Based on serial clinical trials results, the guideline of the ACC/AHA/ESC[1] recommended antithrombotic therapy to prevent thromboembolism for all patients with AF except those with lone AF or contraindications. Anticoagulation with warfarin is recommended for patients with more than one moderate risk factor. Such factors include age of 75 years or more, hypertension, HF, impaired LV systolic function (ejection fraction 35% or less or fractional shortening less than 25%), and diabetes mellitus. Aspirin is recommended as an alternative to vitamin K antagonists in low-risk patients or in those with contraindications to oral anticoagulation. In patients with AF for whom anticoagulation therapy was unsuitable, a recent trial indicates that the combination of aspirin and clopidogrel can reduce the risk of major vascular events, especially stroke.[18]

EVIDENCE-BASED MEDICINE:

The CHADS2 Index

In order to assess the predictive value of classification schemes that estimate stroke risk in patients with AF, two existing classification schemes were combined into a new stroke-risk scheme, the CHADS2 index, and all three classification schemes were validated. *Methodology:* The CHADS2 was formed by assigning one point each for the presence of CHF, HTN, age 75 years or older, and diabetes mellitus and by assigning two points for history of stroke or transient ischemic attack. Data from the National Registry of AF (NRAF) consist of 1733 Medicare beneficiaries aged 65–95 years who had nonrheumatic AF and were not prescribed warfarin at hospital discharge. The main outcome measure is hospitalization for ischemic stroke. *Results:* During 2121 patient-years of follow-up, 94 patients were readmitted to the hospital for ischemic stroke (stroke rate, 4.4 per 100 patient-years). As indicated by a *c* statistic greater than 0.5, the two existing classification schemes predicted stroke better than chance: *c* of 0.68 (95% CI, 0.65–0.71) for the scheme developed by the Atrial Fibrillation Investigators (AFI) and *c* of 0.74 (95% CI, 0.71–0.76) for the Stroke Prevention in Atrial Fibrillation (SPAF) III scheme. However, with a *c* statistic of 0.82 (95% CI, 0.80–0.84), the CHADS2 index was the most accurate predictor of stroke. The stroke rate per 100 patient-years without antithrombotic therapy increased by a factor of 1.5 (95% CI, 1.3–1.7) for each one-point increase in the CHADS2 score:

1.9 (95% CI, 1.2–3.0) for a score of 0

2.8 (95% CI, 2.0–3.8) for 1

4.0 (95% CI, 3.1–5.1) for 2

5.9 (95% CI, 4.6–7.3) for 3

8.5 (95% CI, 6.3–11.1) for 4

12.5 (95% CI, 8.2–17.5) for 5

18.2 (95% CI, 10.5–27.4) for 6

The two existing classification schemes and especially the new stroke risk index, CHADS2, can quantify the risk of stroke for patients who have AF and may aid in the selection of antithrombotic therapy.[17]

The schemes for stratification of stroke risk identifying patients who benefit most and least from anticoagulation are controversial. Referring to the AHA/ACC/ESC 2006 guideline[1] for the management of patients with AF, the risk factors include female gender, coronary artery disease, hypertension, heart failure, advanced age, previous stroke, or embolism. The recommended anticoagulation therapy was performed according to the risk category (Table 20-4).

Aspirin and Clopidogrel

Aspirin is used to prevent the thromboembolism (TE) events in patients with AF but concomitant with low risk of TE or contradictory to warfarin. Aspirin can only offer modest protection against stroke for patients with AF[18] but may be more efficacious for AF patients with hypertension or diabetes.[7]

TABLE 20-4: Antithrombotic Therapy for Patients with AF

Risk Category	Recommended Therapy
No risk factors	Aspirin, 81 to 325 mg daily
One moderate-risk factor	Aspirin, 81 to 325 mg daily, or warfarin(INR 2.0 to 3.0, target 2.5)
Any high-risk factor or more than 1 moderate-risk factor	Warfarin (INR 2.0 to 3.0, target 2.5)

Less Validated or Weaker Risk Factors	Moderate-Risk Factors	High-Risk Factors
Female gender	Age ≥ 75y	Previous stroke, TIA or embolism
Age 65 to 74	Hypertension	
Coronary artery disease	Heart failure	Mitral stenosis
Thyrotoxicosis	LV ejection fraction 35% or less	Prosthetic heart valve*
	Diabetes mellitus	

*If mechanical valve, target international normalized ratio (INR) greater than 2.5.

INR: international normalized ratio; LV: left ventricle; TIA: transient ischemic attack.

EVIDENCE-BASED MEDICINE:

Effect of Clopidogrel Added to Aspirin in Patients with Atrial Fibrillation (The ACTIVE Trial)[18]

Methodology: A total of 7554 patients with AF who had an increased risk of stroke but were unsuitable for Coumadin therapy were randomly assigned to receive clopidogrel (75 mg) plus aspirin (group A) or aspirin plus placebo (group B). The primary outcome was the composite of stroke, myocardial infarction, non–central nervous system systemic embolism, or death from vascular causes. *Results:* At 3.6 years of follow-up, major vascular events had occurred in 832 patients from group A (6.8% per year) and in 924 patients, from group B (7.6% per year) (P = 0.01). The difference was primarily due to a reduction in the rate of stroke with clopidogrel. Stroke occurred in 296 patients from group A (2.4% per year) and 408 patients from group B (3.3% per year) (P < 0.001). *Harms:* Major bleeding occurred in 251 patients in group A (2.0% per year) and in 162 patients from group B (1.3% per year) (P < 0.001). *Evidence-Based Applications:* The combination of clopidogrel and aspirin, as compared with aspirin alone, can minimally reduce the rate of major TE among patients with AF who were at increased risk for stroke and for whom therapy with a vitamin K antagonist was considered unsuitable. This reduction was primarily due to a reduction in the risk of stroke. There was a significant increase in the risk of major hemorrhage.[18]

Coumadin (Warfarin)

Patients with AF who had rheumatic heart disease or prosthetic heart valves had a higher risk of ischemic stroke and systemic embolism. In addition, the risk of stroke in patients with nonvalvular AF is 5~7 times greater than that in controls without AF.[19, 20] Anticoagulation (warfarin) therapy is approximately 33% more effective than aspirin therapy for the prevention of ischemic stroke in patients with AF.[7] Several clinical guidelines[1, 3] suggested that any patient with AF who has risk factors for stroke should be treated with warfarin with an international normalized ratio (INR) range of 2.0 to 3.0. Warfarin is also applied for the periprocedure stroke prevention of cardioversion to sinus rhythm. Patients who have AF longer than two days should receive warfarin to achieve an INR of 2.0 to 3.0 for three weeks before cardioversion and for four weeks after reversion to sinus rhythm.[1] But for elderly (> 75 years) patients with AF, warfarin should be used with caution and carefully monitored because of the potentially increased risk of intracranial hemorrhage.

DATA MANAGEMENT TIPS (CLINICAL PEARLS)
CAVEATS in Antithrombotic Therapy

Atrial flutter should be treated with antithrombotic therapy, as in patients with AF. All patients with paroxysmal, persistent, or permanent AF should receive antithrombotic treatment unless contraindicated. AADs do not reduce the need for long-term antithrombotic therapy aimed at preventing stroke. Most of the ischemic strokes in the rhythm control arm of AFFIRM occurred after warfarin was discontinued. Strokes are not unexpected among patients with seemingly successful restoration of sinus rhythm, given the fact that asymptomatic AF is common. Long-term antithrombotic therapy should still be strongly considered after successful ablation. The combination of aspirin and clopidogrel should not be considered an adequate substitute for warfarin-based anticoagulation for patients with AF. The risk of stroke is 1.72-fold higher for patients taking aspirin plus clopidogrel than for those taking adjusted-dose warfarin. Antithrombotic therapy for patients with a drug-eluting coronary stent and AF should be individualized, with consideration given to the use of adjusted-dose warfarin plus clopidogrel without aspirin.[3, 5]

ADVANCED MANAGEMENT
Catheter Ablation

For those patients who were refractory to antiarrhythmic drugs, catheter ablation approaches have been applied successfully. Radiofrequency ablation aimed at electrical isolation of the pulmonary veins is 70 to 85%

effective in patients with paroxysmal AF and 50 to 70% effective in patients with persistent AF.[1,3,21] With the advance of ablative techniques and strategy, the clinical application of catheter ablation on AF has expanded to wider indications. But little information is available about the late success and prognosis of ablation in patients with AF.

SMART THINKING:

Catheter Ablation Versus Antiarrhythmic Drugs for AF: The A4 Clinical Trial

Methodology The A4 trial enrolled 112 patients with symptomatic paroxysmal AF and randomized to an ablation group (n = 53) or antiarrhythmic drugs group (n = 59). The primary endpoint was absence of recurrent AF between months 3 and 12, absence of recurrent AF after up to three ablation procedures, or changes in antiarrhythmic drugs during the first three months. *Results:* Crossover from the anti-arrhythmic drugs and ablation groups occurred in 37 (63%) and 5 patients (9%), respectively (P = 0.0001). At the one-year follow-up, 13 of 55 patients (23%) and 46 of 52 patients (89%) had no recurrence of AF in the antiarrhythmic drug and ablation groups, respectively (P < 0.0001). Symptom score, exercise capacity, and quality of life were significantly higher in the ablation group. *Practical Applications:* Catheter ablation is superior to antiarrhythmic drugs in patients with symptomatic AF with regard to maintenance of sinus rhythm and improvement in symptoms, exercise capacity, and quality of life.[22]

SMART THINKING:

Pulmonary Vein Isolation for AF in Patients with Heart Failure: The PABA-CHF Trial[23]

Methodology: The PABA-CHF trial randomly assigned patients (n = 81) with symptomatic, drug-resistant AF, an ejection fraction of 40% or less, and New York Heart Association Class II or III heart failure to undergo either pulmonary vein isolation (n = 41) or atrioventricular node ablation with biventricular pacing (n = 40). Over a six-month period, all patients completed the Minnesota Living with Heart Failure questionnaire, underwent echocardiography and a 6-minute walk test, and were monitored for both symptomatic and asymptomatic episodes of AF. *Results:* The composite primary endpoint favored the group that underwent pulmonary vein isolation, with an improved questionnaire score at six months (60 vs. 82 in the group that underwent atrioventricular node ablation with biventricular pacing; P < 0.001), a longer 6-minute-walk distance (340 m vs.

297 m, P < 0.001), and a higher ejection fraction (35% vs. 28%, P < 0.001). In the group that underwent pulmonary vein isolation, 88% of patients receiving antiarrhythmic drugs and 71% of those not receiving such drugs were free of AF at six months. *Practical Applications:* Pulmonary vein isolation was superior to atrioventricular node ablation with biventricular pacing in patients with heart failure who had drug-refractory AF for symptom relief and prognosis improvement.

Indications for Catheter Ablation of AF.

The ACC/AHA/ESC 2006 Guidelines[1] for the Management of Patients with AF suggested that "catheter ablation is a reasonable alternative to pharmacologic therapy to prevent recurrent AF in symptomatic patients with little or no LA enlargement" (Class 2A recommendation, level of evidence C. The HRS/EHRA/ECAS Expert Consensus Statement on Catheter and Surgical Ablation of AF[3] stated that "the primary indication for catheter AF ablation is the presence of symptomatic AF refractory or intolerant to at least one Class 1 or 3 anti-arrhythmic medications." In rare clinical situations, catheter ablation of AF is also appreciated in patients with heart failure, cardiomyopathy, or other organic cardiac diseases. We should recognize that catheter ablation of AF is a demanding technical procedure that may result in complications. Patients should only undergo AF ablation after carefully weighing the risks and benefits of the procedure.

Dronedarone

Dronedarone is a new antiarrhythmic drug that is being developed for the treatment of patients with atrial fibrillation. *Methodology:* This is a multicenter trial to evaluate the use of dronedarone in 4628 patients with atrial fibrillation who had additional risk factors for death. Patients were randomly assigned to receive dronedarone, 400 mg twice a day, or placebo. The primary outcome was the first hospitalization due to cardiovascular events or death. Secondary outcomes were death from any cause, death from cardiovascular causes, and hospitalization due to cardiovascular events. *Results:* The mean follow-up period was 21 ± 5 months, with the study drug discontinued prematurely in 696 of the 2301 patients (30.2%) receiving dronedarone and in 716 of the 2327 patients (30.8%) receiving placebo, mostly because of adverse events. The primary outcome occurred in 734 patients (31.9%) in the dronedarone group and in 917 patients (39.4%) in the placebo group, with a hazard ratio for dronedarone of 0.76 (95% CI, 0.69 to 0.84; P<0.001). There were 116 deaths (5.0%) in the dronedarone group and 139 (6.0%) in the placebo group (hazard ratio, 0.84; 95% CI, 0.66 to 1.08; P = 0.18). There were 63 deaths from cardiovascular causes (2.7%) in the dronedarone group and 90 (3.9%) in the placebo group (hazard ratio, 0.71; 95% CI, 0.51 to 0.98; P = 0.03), largely due to a reduction in the rate of death from arrhythmia with dronedarone. The dronedarone group had higher rates of bradycardia, QT-interval prolongation, nausea, diarrhea, rash, and an increased serum creatinine level as compared to the placebo group. Rates of thyroid- and pulmonary-related adverse events were not significantly different between the two groups. *Practical Applications:* Dronedarone reduced the incidence of hospitalizations due to cardiovascular events or death in patients with atrial fibrillation.[24]

TROUBLE-SHOOTING AND DEBUGGING

Is Warfarin Safe for the Elderly (>80 Years Old)?

Although age older than 75 years is a moderate risk factor of thromboembolism for patients with AF, the potential risk of hemorrhage with anticoagulation in elderly patients should not be underevaluated. Major hemorrhage and tolerability of warfarin are major problems among elderly patients with AF.[17] *Methodology:* From 2001 to 2003, 472 patients (≧65 years) who accepted warfarin therapy and their outcomes were investigated including major hemorrhage, time to termination of warfarin, and reason for discontinuation during the first year. *Results:* The cumulative incidence of major hemorrhage for patients ≧80 years of age was 13.1 per 100 person-years and 4.7 for those < 80 years of age (P = 0.009). Within the first year, 26% of patients ≧80 years of age stopped taking warfarin. Perceived safety issues accounted for 81% of them. *Practical Applications:* Anticoagulation therapy among elderly patients with AF remains a challenging and pressing health concern, and efficacy and security of treatment should be weighed simultaneously.[25] However, a new drug, dabigatran, given at a dose of 110 mg, was associated with rates of stroke and systemic embolism that were similar to those associated with warfarin as well as lower rates of major hemorrhage. Dabigatran administered at a dose of 150 mg, as compared with warfarin, was associated with lower rates of stroke and systemic embolism but similar rates of major hemorrhage. Hopefully, the patient with AF, especially elderly patients, would benefit from the lower complication profile of dagibatran.[26]

How to Treat AF in Patients with Hyperthyroidism

The action of thyroid hormone affects cardiac performance. It is related to heart rate, myocardial contractility, and LV muscle mass and its predisposition to arrhythmia. Hyperthyroidism can worsen preexisting heart diseases or cause cardiovascular complications in patients with structurally normal hearts. AF is the most common cardiac complication in patients with hyperthyroidism. The incidence is increased with advancing age, and it occurs more in men than women.

Treatment of AF in hyperthyroidism includes controlling ventricular rate and anticoagulation. Cardioversion is not recommended until the euthyroid state is restored and maintained. Beta blockers and calcium channel blockers are used to control ventricular rate. IV calcium channel blockers causing hypotension due to a further fall in SVR should be avoided. The restoration of sinus rhythm depends on the duration of AF, left atrial size, age, and underlying heart disease.

TAKE-HOME MESSAGE

AF is a common and growing problem due to the aging of the population. It is associated with substantial morbidity, mortality, and resource consumption. The optimal treatment strategies for AF include controlling the ventricular rate and maintaining sinus rhythm with AADs and chronic anticoagulation. Restoration and maintenance of sinus rhythm should reduce symptoms and improve hemodynamic status and potentially decrease the risk of thromboembolic complications and mortality. Furthermore, if AF is successfully suppressed, the need for and risk of long-term anticoagulation can be eliminated. Decisions for immediate or delayed cardioversion, pharmacologically or electrically, and anticoagulation have to be made based on the clinical presentation and the individual patient's need for restoration and maintenance of sinus rhythm. The chance of maintaining sinus rhythm and the risk of adverse side-effects should be considered when long-term AAD therapy is used to suppress AF. In some patients, ventricular rate control by drugs or catheter ablation with pacemakers and antithrombotic prophylaxis may be preferable to cardioversion and long-term AAD therapy. The limited efficacy and risk of pharmacologic therapy for preventing AF have stimulated interest in nonpharmacologic approaches to maintain sinus rhythm, such as the use of surgery, atrial pacing, AADs, and catheter ablation.

References

1. Zipes, D. P., Camm, A. J., Borggrefe, M., et al.: ACC/AHA/ESC 2006 Guidelines for Management of Patients With Ventricular Arrhythmias and the Prevention of Sudden Cardiac Death: a report of the American College of Cardiology/American Heart Association Task Force and the European Society of Cardiology Committee for Practice Guidelines (writing committee to develop Guidelines for Management of Patients With Ventricular Arrhythmias and the Prevention of Sudden Cardiac Death): developed in collaboration with the European Heart Rhythm Association and the Heart Rhythm Society. Circulation. 2006;114: e385–e484.

2. Tse, H. F., Lau, C. P. Atrial fibrillation. In Nguyen T., Hu D., et al., eds. Management of Complex Cardiovacular problems, Blackwell Futura, Boston MA, 2007, pp 287–318.

3. Calkins, H., Brugada, J., Packer, D. L., et al.: HRS/EHRA/ECAS expert Consensus Statement on catheter and surgical ablation of atrial fibrillation: recommendations for personnel, policy, procedures and follow-up. A report of the Heart Rhythm Society (HRS) Task Force on catheter and surgical ablation of atrial fibrillation. Heart Rhythm. 2007;4: 816–861.

4. Pearson, A. C., Labovitz, A. J., Tatineni, S., et al.: Superiority of trans-esophageal echocardiography in detecting a cardiac source of embolism in patients with cerebral ischemia of uncertain etiology. J Am Coll Cardiol. 1991; 17:66–72.

5. Mark, A., Crandall David, J., Bradley Douglas, L., et al.: Contemporary Management of Atrial Fibrillation: Update on Anticoagulation and Invasive Management Strategies. Mayo Clin Proc. 2009;84:643–662.

6. Wyse, D. G., Waldo, A. L., DiMarco, J. P., et al.: A comparison of rate control and rhythm control in patients with atrial fibrillation. N Engl J Med. 2002;347:1825–1833.

7. The efficacy of aspirin in patients with atrial fibrillation. Analysis of pooled data from 3 randomized trials. The Atrial Fibrillation Investigators. Arch Intern Med. 1997; 157:1237–1240.

8. Effect of clopidogrel added to aspirin in patients with atrial fibrillation. N Engl J Med. 2009;360:2066–2078.

9. Khan, M. N., Jais, P., Cummings, J., et al.: Pulmonary-vein isolation for atrial fibrillation in patients with heart failure. N Engl J Med. 2008; 359:1778–1785.

10. Hylek, E. M., Evans-Molina, C., Shea, C., et al.: Major hemorrhage and tolerability of warfarin in the first year of therapy among elderly patients with atrial fibrillation. Circulation. 2007;115:2689–2696.

11. Ueng, K. C., Tsai, T. P., Yu, W. C., et al.: Use of enalapril to facilitate sinus rhythm maintenance after external cardioversion of long-standing persistent atrial fibrillation. Results of a prospective and controlled study. Eur Heart J. 2003;24:2090–2098.

12. Hsu, L. F., Jais, P., Sanders, P., et al.: Catheter ablation for atrial fibrillation in congestive heart failure. N Engl J Med. 2004; 351:2373–2383.

13. Pedersen, O. D., Bagger, H., Kober, L., et al.: Trandolapril reduces the incidence of atrial fibrillation after acute myocardial infarction in patients with left ventricular dysfunction. Circulation. 1999;100: 376–380.

14. Siu, C. W., Lau, C. P., Tse, H. F.: Prevention of atrial fibrillation recurrence by statin therapy in patients with lone atrial fibrillation after successful cardioversion. Am J Cardiol. 2003;92:1343–1345.

15. Singh, B., Singh, S., Reda, D., et al.: for the Sotalol Amiodarone Atrial Fibrillation Efficacy Trial (SAFE-T) Investigators Amiodarone versus Sotalol for Atrial Fibrillation N Engl J Med. 2005;352:1861–1872.

16. Kuhlkamp, V., Schirdewan, A., Stangl, K., et al.: Use of metoprolol CR/XL to maintain sinus rhythm after conversion from persistent atrial fib-

rillation: a randomized, double-blind, placebo-controlled study. J Am Coll Cardiol. 2000;36:139–146.

17. Gage, B. F., Waterman, A. D., Shannon, W., et al.: Validation of clinical classification schemes for predicting stroke: Results From the National Registry of Atrial Fibrillation. JAMA. 2001;285:2864–2870.

18. Hart, R. G., Benavente, O., McBride, R., et al.: Antithrombotic therapy to prevent stroke in patients with atrial fibrillation: a meta-analysis. Ann Intern Med. 1999; 131:492–501.

19. Flegel, K. M., Shipley, M. J., Rose, G.: Risk of stroke in non-rheumatic atrial fibrillation. Lancet. 1987;1:526–529.

20. Wolf, P. A., Abbott, R. D., Kannel, W. B.: Atrial fibrillation as an independent risk factor for stroke: the Framingham Study. Stroke. 1991; 22:983–988.

21. Cappato, R., Calkins, H., Chen, S. A., et al.: Worldwide survey on the methods, efficacy, and safety of catheter ablation for human atrial fibrillation. Circulation. 2005;111:1100–1105.

22. Jais, P., Cauchemez, B., Macle, L., et al.: Catheter ablation versus antiarrhythmic drugs for atrial fibrillation: the A4 study. Circulation. 2008;118:2498–2505.

23. Khan, M. N., Jais, P., Cummings, J., et al.: Pulmonary-vein isolation for atrial fibrillation in patients with heart failure. N Engl J Med. 2008,359:1778–1785.

24. Hohnloser, S. H., Crijns, H. J. G. M., van Eickels, M., et al.: Effect of dronedarone on cardiovascular events in atrial fibrillation. N Engl J Med. 2009;360:668–678.

25. Hylek, E. M., Evans-Molina, C., Shea, C., et al.: Major hemorrhage and tolerability of warfarin in the first year of therapy among elderly patients with atrial fibrillation. Circulation. 2007;115:2684–6.

26. Connolly, S. J., Ezekowitz, M. D., Yusuf, S., et al.: Dabigatran versus warfarin in patients with atrial fibrillation. N Engl J Med. 2009; Published at www.nejm.org August 30, 2009.

Ventricular Tachycardia

*Thomas Bump, Pham Quoc Khanh,
Phan Nam Hung, Pham Nhu Hung,
Ta Tien Phuoc, and Huynh Van Minh*

Chapter Outline

DEFINITION

Ventricular tachycardia (VT) is a rapid cardiac rhythm that originates in the ventricles and presents with wide QRS complexes and a heart rate greater than 120 beats per minute (bpm). The rhythm may be regular or irregular. The QRS complexes during tachycardia are identical to each other in the case of *monomorphic* VT and vary in the case of *polymorphic* VT. Episodes of VT that terminate spontaneously within 30 seconds of their onset are said to be *nonsustained*, and the term "sustained" is applied to episodes that last longer than 30 seconds or require therapy for termination. Ventricular fibrillation (VF) is an arrhythmia in which distinct beats are not discernible in the surface electrocardiogram (ECG).

Etiologies

VTs are caused by a variety of mechanisms. Monomorphic VT in a patient with a healed myocardial infarction (MI) is usually due to reentry.[1] The VT arising in the setting of digitalis toxicity is probably due to triggered automaticity arising from late afterdepolarizations.[2] Patients with dilated cardiomyopathy are subject to a type of monomorphic VT, usually with a left bundle branch block morphology that is due to macroreentry with a wavefront that travels antegradely down the right bundle branch, across the interventricular septum, retrogradely up the left bundle branch, and into the bundle of His before starting another circuit.[3] Torsades de pointes (TdP), a polymorphic VT that arises in various settings, may be initiated by triggered automaticity due to early afterdepolarizations.[4] The early afterdepolarizations are in turn caused by disorders of potassium or sodium channels. A catecholamine-dependent VT that typically originates from the right ventricular outflow tract of patients with structurally normal hearts may be due to cyclic adenosine monophosphate (cAMP)–mediated triggered activity.[5] The same mechanism may underlie repetitive monomorphic VT, which occurs at rest and usually originates from the right or left ventricular outflow tract.[6] A verapamil-sensitive VT that typically originates in the region of the left posterior fascicle in patients with structurally normal hearts may be caused by reentry in which one link of the circuit is calcium-dependent.[7] A catecholamine-induced polymorphic VT that occurs in young people with structurally normal hearts is likely due to delayed after-depolarizations that arise as a result of disordered intracellular calcium handling due to a mutation in either the cardiac ryanodine receptor 2 or calsequestrin 2.[8] VF is probably caused by multiple simultaneous reentrant wavefronts that migrate through the ventricles.

DATA COLLECTING
History

In obtaining the medical history, special attention is paid to eliciting information about the severity of symptoms. For example, patients with syncope from VT should be treated more aggressively than certain patients who are asymptomatic from their VT. It is important to determine how often VT occurs in a particular patient because implantable cardioverter defibrillator (ICD) therapy might not be indicated as solo therapy for a patient with frequent episodes of VT, since frequent shocks are poorly tolerated.

Other important historical information includes any clues as to the possible presence of any causative factors, such as electrolyte disturbance, drug use (illicit or prescribed), elevated catecholamines, previous MI, ongoing ischemia, left ventricular dysfunction, valvular abnormalities, and family history of VT, syncope, or premature sudden cardiac death. The physician must identify what therapies might have already been used for the patient and with what degree of success they were met.

Physical Examination

The physical examination during an episode of wide complex tachycardia (WCT) must immediately focus on vital signs and other indicators of the adequacy of perfusion. The patient's blood pressure, respiratory rate, and presence or absence of diaphoresis, mental status changes, and peripheral hypoperfusion must immediately be assessed, because the findings will determine how aggressively the rhythm should be treated or cardioverted or defibrillated. The presence of intermittent cannon a-waves in the jugular venous pulse is evidence of atrioventricular dissociation, which would support the diagnosis of VT rather than SVT with aberrant conduction.

DATA FILTERING (DIFFERENTIAL DIAGNOSES)

Supraventricular tachycardia (SVT) can mimic VT whenever either bundle branch block or ventricular preexcitation is also present. It is important for the physician to differentiate SVT from VT because SVT usually carries a more benign prognosis than VT and because therapeutic options are different for SVT and VT. Electrocardiographic artifact and rapid ventricular pacing can also mimic VT but should not cause any diagnostic challenges.

DATA MINING (WORK-UP)

Depending on the type of presentation of VT or VF, the patient might be evaluated for an acute MI by serial cardiac enzymes and ECGs. Also, the patient with VT might be evaluated through other laboratory tests for electrolyte disturbances such as hyperkalemia, hypokalemia, or hypomagnesemia; or for drug toxicity.

Electrocardiogram

The 12-lead ECG during tachycardia is invaluable. It heightens the ability of the physician to differentiate between VT and SVT with aberrant conduction (Table 21-1). It also aids the physician in determining if the patient has a VT, which could be particularly amenable to ablation, such as idiopathic VT arising from the right or left ventricular outflow tracts; idiopathic VT arising from the inferoseptal left ventricle; or bundle branch reentry. Furthermore, the 12-lead ECG obtained during clinical VT can eventually be compared with ECGs obtained during subsequent electrophysiologic (EP) studies to determine if the VT that is induced during the study is the same as that which the patient had outside the laboratory.

Rhythm Strips

Other types of electrocardiography are also useful in selected patients. Rhythm strips, in the hospital or in the outpatient setting, often provide the first evidence that WCT has occured in a particular patient. Furthermore, monitor strips can provide information that might not be available from the 12-lead ECG, such as the nature of the onset, duration, and termination of the WCT. Although it is not as powerful as a 12-lead ECG, a one- or two-channel rhythm strip can be used to determine whether a WCT is a VT or whether it is one of the conditions

TABLE 21-1: Electrocardiographic Criteria Suggestive of Ventricular Tachycardia

Atrioventricular dissociation
Absence of RS complex in any precordial lead
If there is an RS complex in at least one precordial lead, the interval from the onset of the R wave to the nadir of the S wave is at least 100 msec
If bundle branch block is present during sinus rhythm, the QRS morphology during tachycardia is different from the QRS morphology during sinus rhythm

that mimics VT—namely, SVT, electrocardiographic artifact, or a burst of rapid ventricular pacing. Rhythm strips are produced by a variety of techniques, including bedside monitoring, Holter recording, event monitoring, and storage of electrograms within implanted devices, including pacemakers and implantable cardioverter defibrillators. Therefore if a patient with a pacemaker or defibrillator experiences palpitations or syncope, the device can be examined to see if it has stored signals that correspond with the episode. And during routine surveillance of device function, a patient might be found to have had episodes of VT.

Signal-Averaged Electrocardiography and T-Wave Alternans

Two other types of electrocardiography have been advanced as being helpful for risk stratification of cardiac patients: signal-averaged electrocardiography and T-wave alternans testing. Signal averaging and filtering reduce signals that are produced by noise and permit detection of low amplitude signals not seen in traditional ECGs, such as activation of the sinus node, AV node, His bundle, and bundle branches. In addition, delayed activation ("late potentials") in ventricular myocardium can be detected in some patients, indicating slow conduction, which is one of the prerequisites for reentry. The finding of late potentials is a sensitive but not specific marker for risk of VT, and its use for risk stratification is limited to testing for slow conduction in the right ventricle as a marker for the presence of arrhythmogenic right ventricular dysplasia (ARVD). Another specialized electrocardiographic procedure, testing for T-wave alternans, has been found to help discriminate between patients who are at high or low risk for developing VT. Alternating T-wave morphology and amplitude have been found in patients who are susceptible to VT but also are found in other people; therefore a positive T-wave alternans result is a nonspecific finding. On the other hand, a negative test for T-wave alternans accurately predicts freedom from VT, at least over a short follow-up period. Therefore testing for T-wave alternans can be used to determine if a particular cardiac patient might reasonably be followed without an implantable defibrillator for primary prevention against sudden cardiac death.

Cardiac Imaging

This helps to identify patients who are at risk of developing VT, and in patients with known VT, it can be used to identify the cause. Echocardiography permits analysis of left ventricular function, which is an important codeterminant of prognosis in patients with VT. In patients with chronic ischemic heart disease, the risk of developing fatal VT rises as the left ventricular ejection fraction falls.[9] In addition, the echocardiogram can provide evidence of other conditions that are associated with

VT, including hypertrophic cardiomyopathy (HCM) and arrhythmogenic right ventricular dysplasia (ARVD). Magnetic resonance imaging also is used in the evaluation of patients with suspected ARVD. Stress testing is an important diagnostic tool in patients with known or suspected VT because it screens for ischemia and also because it screens for exercise-induced VT. Coronary arteriography is a reasonable diagnostic option in any patient with VT who is suspected of having coronary insufficiency.

Genetic Testing

This is available for use in highly selected patients to screen for the presence of any of the mutations that cause hereditable VT or VF, such as the long QT syndrome, Brugada syndrome, catecholaminergic polymorphic VT, arrhythmogenic right ventricular dysplasia, and high-risk hypertrophic cardiomyopathy. Patients who might benefit from genetic testing include family members of patients with identified hereditable VT or VF, family members of subjects who died from unexplained sudden cardiac death, and patients with syncope and an ECG that raises suspicions of one of the heritable syndromes of VT or VF.

Electrophysiologic (EP) Testing

This is performed in specialized cardiac catheterization laboratories that are equipped with a programmable stimulator, EP amplifiers, and recording equipment. These devices are connected to multipolar electrode catheters that are advanced to various intracardiac positions such as the high right atrium, the His bundle position, and the right ventricular apex. The timing of local activation during different cardiac rhythms can be measured from bipolar recordings that are made through closely spaced electrodes on the catheters.

Different rhythms may be induced in susceptible patients by provocative stimulation protocols that are delivered through the catheters from the programmable stimulator. The electrophysiologist can compare the rate and electrocardiographic appearance of the induced rhythm with that of previously documented tachycardias in order to determine if the induced rhythm reproduces a previously documented "clinical" rhythm. The electrophysiologist can then analyze the intracardiac recordings of activation of multiple cardiac sites during the induced rhythm and determine if a particular rhythm is VT or if it is SVT with aberrant conduction.

EP testing can also be used for risk stratification. In certain situations, the presence of inducible VT indicates that the patient has an increased risk of developing spontaneous VT, and the absence of inducible VT implies a more benign prognosis. The predictive accuracy of EP testing varies greatly according to the type of VT that is being investigated and the nature of the heart disease that is present. For example, polymorphic VT can be induced by aggressive provocative stimulation protocols, even in patients who are known to be at minimal risk for developing spontaneous VT or VF. Thus, induced polymorphic VT is a nonspecific finding of EP studies, particularly when closely spaced triple premature beats are required for induction. The induction of monomorphic VT is usually taken to be a meaningful finding, but induction of very rapid monomorphic VT (in the range of 300 or more bpm) has less specificity than induction of slower monomorphic VTs. The sensitivity of EP for detecting susceptibility to VT is high in patients with left ventricular dysfunction due to coronary disease and relatively low in patients with nonischemic cardiomyopathy.

EP studies can be helpful in defining the level of risk for lethal ventricular tachycardia in patients, especially when there might be uncertainty concerning whether an implantable defibrillator might be helpful. In a patient with persistent severe left ventricular dysfunction with an ejection fraction of less than 35%, an EP study is not necessary to determine if an ICD is indicated. However, in patients with a history of myocardial infarction, nonsustained ventricular tachycardia, and an ejection fraction of less than 40%, those with inducible VT have improved survival with ICDs. This suggests that EP testing should be considered in patients with nonsustained VT, a history of myocardial infarction, and an ejection fraction of 35 to 40%. On the other hand, EP studies have such a low sensitivity in the presence of nonischemic cardiomyopathy that they are generally not performed in these patients unless syncope, near syncope, or a sustained wide complex tachycardia has occurred.

EP Drug Testing

In the past, patients with inducible VT in the baseline state were repeatedly brought back to the EP laboratory in order to perform serial EP studies to try to identify a drug or drugs that might render the VT noninducible, based on the premise that noninducibility in the laboratory should predict a favorable long-term clinical response to the drug. This approach was abandoned after serial EP drug testing was found not to provide better outcomes for patients than those provided by selection of drug therapy according to which drug produced the greatest suppression of ventricular ectopy on Holter monitoring.[10]

Another indication for EP testing is to evaluate the patient for possible cure of the arrhythmia by catheter ablation (discussed below). Candidates for catheter ablation first undergo EP evaluation to determine if VT can be induced in the laboratory and to see if the induced VT is similar or identical to the VT that the patient has had in the past. The hemodynamic status of the patient during the induced VT is evaluated to determine if the patient is stable enough during VT to undergo possibly prolonged efforts to locate the site in the ventricles where a small lesion might eradicate the VT. Testing is performed to see if the patient has multiple forms of VT, which, if present, might render attempts at catheter ablation futile.

EP testing is relatively safe. The chief risks are vessel damage, thrombophlebitis, and perforation of a vessel or the heart. The patient may require electrical defibrillation during the study. The risk of death as a complication of an EP study is approximately 1 in 10,000. If the EP study leads to catheter ablation, then other risks may be encountered. These risks are discussed in the sections that follow.

PROGRAMMED MANAGEMENT

A variety of therapies are available for patients with VT or with an increased risk of developing VT. These include correction of predisposing factors such as electrolyte abnormalities, drug toxicity, and myocardial ischemia; antiarrhythmic drugs (AADs); electrical therapies including antitachycardia pacing, external cardioversion and implantable cardioverter-defibrillator therapy (ICD); and catheter ablation.

Strategic Programming

VT can be lethal in one patient and benign in another. The physician must seek to prevent the death of patients with lethal forms of VT without over treating patients who have relatively benign forms of ventricular arrhythmias. To this end, the physician must assess the present and likely future impact of VT on the patient at hand and weigh the therapeutic options with their risks and potential benefits. VTs do not respond uniformly well to a single kind of therapy. Therefore, the physician must be acquainted with different therapies, including antiarrhythmic drugs, antitachycardia pacing, electrical cardioversion and defibrillation, catheter ablation.

Pharmacologic Treatment

The 2005 Advanced Cardiac Life Support guidelines include amiodarone, lidocaine, and procainamide as potentially useful drugs in the acute management of VT and VF. In the setting of out-of-hospital cardiac arrest from refractory VF or pulseless VT (unresponsive to at least three precordial shocks), paramedic administration of amiodarone has been found to increase survival compared to placebo and lidocaine.[11, 12]

Amiodarone

This drug has a broad spectrum of activity against VT (see farther on). Lidocaine is ineffective against reentrant VT but may be effective against

VT resulting from acute ischemia, digitalis toxicity, or mutation of the sodium channel (torsades in the LQT3 variant of the long QT syndrome).

Procainamide
This drug is occasionally effective against reentrant VT but must be avoided in all patients with long QT syndrome.

Verapamil
This drug can be effective against a particular form of idiopathic VT that arises from the inferoseptal wall of the left ventricle but should be avoided in all other forms of VT.

Flecainide and Propafenone
These drugs have not been shown to improve survival in any group of patients but can be used to improve the quality of life of patients with symptomatic ventricular ectopy in the absence of coronary artery disease or structural heart disease.

Beta Blocking Drugs
A variety of drugs, including sotalol and amiodarone, are the most important drugs for the management of VT and VF and deserve further comment. Beta blocking drugs are invaluable in managing patients who have VT or are at risk for developing VT. They have repeatedly been shown to reduce mortality rates in patients with ischemic heart disease and those with left ventricular dysfunction.[13] They are also a mainstay in the treatment of patients with hypertrophic cardiomyopathy and patients with the most common form of the long QT syndrome, LQT1. Beta blockers directly attenuate the proarrhythmic effects of sympathetic hyperactivity, which include shortening of ventricular refractoriness and increase of ventricular automaticity; and beta blockers indirectly reduce morbidity and mortality from VT by reducing ischemia and preventing infarction. Potential adverse effects of beta blockers include excessive bradycardia or hypotension, bronchospasm, exacerbation of left ventricular systolic dysfunction (in rare cases), easy fatigability, impaired sexual function, and increased risk of hypoglycemia in diabetic patients. The family of beta blockers is large and heterogeneous (Table 21-2).

DATA MANAGEMENT TIPS (CLINICAL PEARLS)
Selection of Beta Blockers

Characteristics of the patient and goals of therapy should determine which beta blocker is selected for each patient. For example, if the patient has a history of episodes of bronchospasm, a beta-1 selective drug such as nebivolol, bisoprolol, metoprolol, or atenolol should be chosen.

TABLE 21-2: Selective Characteristics of Some Commonly Used Beta Blockers

Drug	β-1 Selectivity	Lipid Solubility	Ancillary Properties	Half-Life (h)	Elimination	Pregnancy Cat. (US)
Acebutolol	+	Moderate	ISA, MSA	3-4	R, H	B
Atenolol	++	Weak		6-8	R	D
Bisoprolol	++	Weak		9-12	R, H	C
Carvedilol	+	High	α-Blockade	7-10	H	C
Esmolol	++	Weak		9 min	B	C
Labetalol	0	Weak	α-Blockade	3-4	H	C
Metoprolol	++	Moderate		3-4	H	C
Nadolol	0	Weak		14-24	R	C
Nebivolol	+++	Weak		12-19	H, R	C
Pindolol	0	Moderate	ISA	3-4	R	C
Propranolol	0	High		3-4	H	C
Sotalol	0	Weak	Class III	9-10	R	B
Timolol	0	Weak		4-5	R	C

Pregnancy Class: A — controlled studies show no fetal risk; B — no controlled studies but no evidence of fetal risk; fetal harm unlikely; C — fetal risk cannot be excluded; drug should be used only if potential benefits outweigh potential risks D — definite fetal risk; drug should be avoided unless in a life-threatening situation or safer alternatives do not exist; X — contraindicated in pregnancy.

ISA: intrinsic sympathomimetic activity, MSA: membrane stabilizing action.

If the patient has severe renal insufficiency, a drug that is cleared by the liver should be chosen, such as metoprolol or propranolol. If the patient has hepatic insufficiency, then a drug that is cleared by the kidneys should be chosen, such as nadolol or atenolol. If a long half-life is desired, then nadolol is a good choice. If bradycardia needs to be avoided, then a drug with intrinsic sympathomimetic activity (ISA), such as acebutolol or pindolol, should be chosen. If a patient has symptomatic arrhythmia while taking a beta blocker, then switching to sotalol could be a reasonable option. If a pregnant woman in the United States needs a beta blocker, then acebutolol would be given preference because its risk of harming the fetus is ranked Category B in the United States; atenolol would be avoided because it is ranked Category D. These considerations don't apply to pregnant women in Australia, where all beta blockers are ranked as having a Category C risk for injuring the fetus.

Sotalol

This is an interesting drug in that its levo-enantiomer has beta blocking effects while both of its enantiomers have Class III antiarrhythmic effects that are mediated by blockade of I_{Kr}. In the Electrophysiologic Study Versus Electrocardiographic Monitoring trial, racemic sotalol was found to have a significantly more favorable effect on survival than mexiletine, pirmenol, quinidine, procainamide, or propafenone. Sotalol has been reported to have a beneficial effect on patients with arrhythmogenic right ventricular dysplasia.[10] It can be very helpful as adjunct therapy in patients who have an implantable cardioverter-defibrillator (ICD), in whom it has been found to reduce the occurrence of defibrillator shocks for VT and VF.[14]

Unfortunately, sotalol, like other drugs that block potassium channels, can cause proarrhythmia: specifically, a drug-induced long QT syndrome with torsades de pointes (TdP). In fact, d-sotalol caused increased mortality compared to placebo in SWORD, a study of patients with left ventricular dysfunction following myocardial infarction. Therefore, sotalol is not generally relied upon as solo therapy to prevent arrhythmic morbidity in patients at high risk for VT. Also, initiation or up-titration of sotalol should be performed in an inpatient setting for the first five doses, watching for excessive prolongation of the QT interval or the appearance of TdP.[15]

Amiodarone

This is a popular drug for treatment of VT. It blocks the sodium channel, calcium channel, and multiple repolarizing currents: I_{to}, I_{Kr}, I_{Ks}, $I_{K, Na}$, and $I_{K, Ach}$. It causes sinus bradycardia, slowing of AV nodal conduction, and marked prolongation of the QT interval. Amiodarone is also a potent and noncompetitive α- and β-adrenergic antagonist; and it affects the relationship between thyroid hormone and the heart by decreasing the peripheral conversion of thyroxine (T_4) to triiodothyronine

(T_3), inhibiting entry of T_3 into cardiac myocytes and inhibiting binding of T_3 to its nuclear receptors.

Compared to other antiarrhythmic drugs, amiodarone is notable for a long half-life that is conductive to once-daily dosing, relative efficacy, freedom from causing proarrhythmias, and lack of negative inotropic effect that enable its use in patients with left ventricular systolic dysfunction. It was found to be more effective than conventional antiarrhythmic drugs at secondary prevention of sudden cardiac death in the Cardiac Arrest in Seattle Conventional Versus Amiodarone Drug Evaluation in which patients who had been resuscitated from VF were randomly assigned to amiodarone or conventional antiarrhythmic drug therapy.[16] In the European Myocardial Infarction Amiodarone Trial and the Canadian Myocardial Infarction Amiodarone Trial, amiodarone significantly reduced cardiac mortality and episodes of VF but did not reduce all-cause mortality compared to placebo in these patients with recent acute myocardial infarction.[17,18] In the Sudden Cardiac Death in Heart Failure Trial, amiodarone was no better than placebo and was significantly worse than ICD at improving survival in patients with left ventricular systolic dysfunction and NYHA class II or III heart failure.[19] But in the Optimal Pharmacological Therapy in Cardioverter Defibrillator Patients study, patients with ICD therapy were less likely to receive shocks if they were taking amiodarone rather than sotalol.[20]

Two other studies compared amiodarone with placebo in patients with left ventricular dysfunction. The Grupo de Estudio de la Sobrevida en la Insuficincia Cardiaca en Argentina trial reported a 28% reduction in mortality in patients with heart failure who were treated with low-dose amiodarone compared with patients who were treated with placebo.[21] However, the Congestive Heart Failure-Survival Trial of Antiarrhythmic Therapy did not show any difference in survival between patients treated with amiodarone and patients treated with placebo.[22] It is thought that the discrepancy in these findings may be related to the fact that there were more patients with ischemic cardiomyopathy in CHF-STAT than there were in GESICA. Subgroup analysis in CHF-STAT revealed that amiodarone was no better than placebo in patients with ischemic cardiomyopathy. In contrast, amiodarone therapy was associated with a reduction of mortality in patients with nonischemic cardiomyopathy in CHF-STAT, just as had been the case in GESICA.

Amiodarone is metabolized by the cytochrome P-450 sub-family of enzymes to N-desethylamiodarone, which has antiarrhythmic activity. Amiodarone inhibits the P-450 enzymes, causing increased levels of digoxin, quinidine, procainamide, warfarin, dextromethorphan, cyclosporine, simvastatin, and many other drugs. When amiodarone is administered intravenously, hypotension is the most common side effect, occurring in about 16% of patients. Fatal hepatocellular necrosis has occurred in two patients who received high doses of intravenous amiodarone. Oral amiodarone can cause pulmonary fibrosis, cirrhosis, hypothyroidism or hyperthyroidism, skin discoloration, visual disturbances, peripheral neuropathy, and ataxia.

In summary, AADs are an important therapeutic option in patients with ventricular arrhythmias (Tables 21-3 and 21-4). However, these drugs have not been found to improve survival in patients with VT or other forms of ventricular ectopy in the setting of ischemic or nonischemic cardiomyopathy compared to the best medical therapy without antiarrhythmic drugs. In patients with a history of cardiac arrest or with left ventricular systolic dysfunction, ICD therapy has been found to help survival more than antiarrhythmic drug therapy. The main roles for antiarrhythmic drug therapy are in the acute management of VT in a monitored setting, the reduction in frequency of episodes of VT in patients who have ICDs, and improvement of quality of life in patients with symptomatic ventricular arrhythmias in certain specific situations.

Nonpharmacologic Therapy

Nonpharmacologic therapies are important options in the management of VT. Either antitachycardia pacing (ATP) or direct current shock can terminate episodes of tachycardia, and in some cases pacing can prevent recurrences of tachycardia. These therapies can be delivered either by external devices or by ICDs. Other treatments that are potentially curative include catheter ablation and cardiac surgery.

Antitachycardia Pacing

Reentrant tachycardias are vulnerable to termination by antitachycardia pacing when the reentry circuit is anatomically defined and there is an excitable gap between a circulating wavefront and its wake of refractoriness. Given these conditions, it is possible for a stimulated impulse to invade the circuit and create a bidirectional block. The latter will occur if the invading impulse proceeds in both directions in the circuit, clockwise and counterclockwise. In one direction, the invading impulse collides with and extinguishes the reentering wavefront; in the other direction, it is itself extinguished when it runs into the wake of refractoriness of the reentering impulse. ATP cannot terminate VF or polymorphic VT.

The usual technique of ATP is to deliver a train of stimuli at a somewhat faster rate than that of the tachycardia. A train of stimuli is more likely than a single stimulus to produce an impulse that penetrates the reentrant circuit. With trains of stimuli, however, there is a risk that one stimulus will terminate a tachycardia and a subsequent one will restart the tachycardia. It may be necessary to literally deliver dozens of trains of stimuli of different rates and durations until a train is finally delivered that fortuitously ends with a pulse that extinguishes the tachycardia

TABLE 21-3: Clinical Usage Information for Oral Antiarrhythmic Drugs

Drug	Oral Loading Dose (mg)	Oral Maintenance Dose	Time to Peak Plasma Concentration	Effective Serum or Plasma Concentration (μ/mL)	Elimination Half-Life (h)	Major Route of Elimination	Pregnancy Class
Quinidine	800 to 1000	300 to 600 q6h	1.5 to 3.0	3 to 6	5 to 9	Liver	C
Procainamide	500 to 1000	250 to 1000 q4h to q6h	1	4 to 10	3 to 5	Kidneys	C
Disopyramide	200 to 300	100 to 300 q6h to q8h	1 to 2	2 to 5	8 to 9	Kidneys	C
Mexiletine	400-600	150 to 300 q8h to q12h	2 to 4	0.75 to 2	10 to 17	Liver	C
Flecainide	200 to 300	100 to 200 q12h	3 to 4	0.2 to 1	20	Liver, Kidneys	C
Propafenone	600 to 900	150 to 300 q8h to q12h	1 to 3	0.2 to 3	5 to 8	Liver	C
Amiodarone	800 to 1600 qd for 7-14 days	100 to 400 qd	3 to 7	0.5 to 1.5	56 days	Liver	D
Sotalol	Not to be loaded	80 to 320 q12h	2.5 to 4	2.5 to 4	12	Kidneys	B
Dofetilide	Not to be loaded	0.125 to 0.5 q12h			7 to 13	Kidneys	C

Pregnancy Class: A — controlled studies show no fetal risk; B — no controlled studies but no evidence of fetal risk; fetal harm unlikely; C — fetal risk cannot be excluded; drug should be used only if potential benefits outweigh potential risk; D — definite fetal risk; drug should be avoided unless in a life-threatening situation or safer alternatives or safer alternatives do not exist; X — contraindicated in pregnancy.

TABLE 21-4: Risks of Antiarrhythmic Drugs

Drug	Proarrhythmia	Effect on Contractility	Extracardiac Side Effects	Drug Interactions	Pregnancy Class
Quinidine	Torsades de pointes		Hypotension (alpha-adrenergic blockade), diarrhea, thrombocytopenia	Digoxin, inhibits CYP450	C
Procainamide	Torsades de pointes		Lupus-like syndrome, agranulocytosis		C
Disopyramide	Torsades de pointes	Decrease	Urinary outflow obstruction, exacerbation of glaucoma		C
Lidocaine			Central neurologic (seizure, depressed consciousness); nausea		B
Mexiletine			Central neurologic (seizure, depressed consciousness); nausea		C
Phenytoin			Central neurologic (ataxia, nystagmus, seizure, stupor, coma), nausea, hyperglycemia, pseudolymphoma, gingival hyperplasia, megaloblastic anemia)		D
Flecainide	Incessant monomorphic VT	Decrease	Blurred vision, headache, confusion		C
Propafenone	Incessant monomorphic VT	Decrease	Blurred vision, headache, confusion		C
Moricizine			Central neurologic, nausea		B

(continued)

TABLE 21-4: Risks of Antiarrhythmic Drugs *(continued)*

Drug	Proarrhythmia	Effect on Contractility	Extracardiac Side Effects	Drug Interactions	Pregnancy Class
Amiodarone	Sinus bradycardia		Pneumonia, hepatitis, hyperthyroidism, hypothyroidism, corneal microdeposits, skin discoloration, neuropathy, gait disturbance	Digoxin, warfarin	D
Bretylium			Transient hypertension, hypotension, nausea		C
Sotalol	Torsades de pointes, sinus bradycardia				B
Dofetilide	Torsades de pointes				C
Ibutilide	Torsades de pointes				C
Verapamil	AV block	Decrease	Hypotension, constipation	Digoxin	C

rather than reinducing it. As this process may take several minutes, ATP is usually used for VTs that do not cause immediate hemodynamic compromise. Also, ATP often causes VT to accelerate or even degenerate into VF. For this reason, ATP must be used only when back-up electrical defibrillation is available. The typical indication for ATP is for treatment of a recurrent reentrant sustained VT that is refractory to drugs and does not cause immediate hemodynamic compromise. ATP would be used in preference to electrical cardioversion, since patients tolerate the former much better. Most ICDs have the capacity to deliver ATP as first-line therapy for VT, with direct-current shock to be automatically delivered subsequently if necessary.

Direct-Current Cardioversion

This technique can be delivered by either an external or an implanted device and has the broadest spectrum of antiarrhythmic activity of any therapy. Properly applied, it is nearly always effective against those arrhythmias that are thought to result from reentry. In addition, high doses of electricity can defibrillate the heart, which is not surprising, since VF probably often arises from a reentrant mechanism. Finally, direct-current cardioversion can terminate TdP, even though it may result from a nonreentrant mechanism—namely, triggered activity.

DATA MANAGEMENT TIPS (CLINICAL PEARLS)
VT Refractory to Direct Cardioversion

Some forms of VT are refractory to direct current cardioversion. For example, direct current cardioversion is ineffective against tachycardias that arise from enhanced automaticity. Arrhythmias in this category include sinus tachycardia, some forms of ectopic atrial tachycardia, multifocal atrial tachycardia, accelerated junctional rhythm, and even some cases of VT. Also, arrhythmias that occur in the setting of digitalis intoxication can be exacerbated by direct-current shock, probably because shocks depolarize sympathetic nerve terminals in the heart, causing them to release norepinephrine, which then accelerates the tachycardia or even causes a more malignant arrhythmia to appear. Finally, electrical shock can fail to terminate incessant VT that is caused by Class IC antiarrhythmic drugs (i.e., flecainide, encainide, and possibly propafenone), even though this rhythm is probably caused by reentry.[23] Arrhythmias that cannot be terminated by cardioversion are often referred to as incessant.

In order to terminate fibrillation, a shock must produce a sufficient voltage gradient throughout the fibrillating chamber to bring all myocardial cells to the same electrical state. When all of the cells within a reentrant circuit are depolarized, a condition of electrical homogeneity is established that is inimical to reentry. This is because ongoing reentry requires that at all times some part of the chamber not be depolarized, so that this part can be next in line to be activated. In order to be successful, a shock must produce a period of electrical homogeneity that persists for a sufficient period of time. In an elegant series of animal experiments, fibrillation was demonstrated to reappear immediately if the period of homogeneity lasted for less than 130 milliseconds.[24] Reentrant arrhythmias that are more organized, such as atrial flutter or VT, may require depolarization of only the excitable portion of the reentry circuit. This may explain the clinical observation that less energy and current are necessary to terminate these arrhythmias than is the case with atrial or ventricular fibrillation.

The minimum amount of energy required to defibrillate the heart is called the defibrillation threshold. Even in a single individual, the defibrillation threshold is not a single value but rather is described by a sigmoidal dose-response relationship: the greater the energy in a shock, the more likely it is to defibrillate a given heart.[25] Typical energy thresholds for external defibrillation of the atria or ventricles are between 50 and 100 J. Defibrillation thresholds for intracardiac electrodes, such as are used in ICD systems, are in the neighborhood of 10 J. Biphasic shocks have lower thresholds than monophasic shocks.

DATA MANAGEMENT TIPS (CLINICAL PEARLS)
Variabilities in Transthoracic Impedance

There is marked variability from patient to patient in the energy threshold for external defibrillation, mainly because of interpatient differences in transthoracic impedance. The latter has several determinants: interelectrode distance (chest size), electrode size, electrode–chest wall contact pressure, couplant ("electrode paste"), and respiratory phase. Increases in transthoracic impedance during lung expansion have implications for patients receiving mechanical ventilation and positive end-expiratory pressure. Impedance declines after repeated shocks, partly because of hyperemia and edema in the current pathway.[26] Because current, not energy, is the determinant of successful defibrillation, an external defibrillator has been developed that automatically delivers more energy when the impedance has been found to be high.[27]

Other factors besides transthoracic impedance can influence the defibrillation threshold. Lidocaine, flecainide, and amiodarone have been found to raise defibrillation thresholds significantly.[28-32] Sotalol lowers defibrillation thresholds.[32] Most other antiarrhythmic drugs have neutral or else very mild effects on defibrillation thresholds. Beta agonists and aminophylline lower defibrillation thresholds.[33, 34] The duration of VF prior to attempted defibrillation affects defibrillation threshold in a biphasic manner. The energy requirement may actually decrease after two minutes of VF perhaps because of a favorable increase in extracellular potassium.[35] When VF has persisted for more than 10 minutes, it becomes increasingly difficult and ultimately impossible to defibrillate the heart.

Implantable Cardiac Defibrillators

ICDs are invaluable for treating patients with VT. These devices can be programmed to deliver different types of therapy for different types of VT, such as antitachycardia pacing or direct current shocks ranging from 1 J to 40 J. When a milder treatment fails to convert a tachycardia, the device can proceed to deliver a stronger therapy; this is called "tiered therapy." ICD systems include an ICD pulse generator plus one, two, or three leads that have electrodes for sensing cardiac rhythm and for delivery of pacing stimuli or shocks of up to 40 J to the heart. The usual current pathway for an ICD shock is between an electrode coil in the right ventricular apex and the can of the pulse generator. Other electrodes may also be employed in the high voltage shocking circuit, such as a proximal electrode coil situated in the superior vena cava and less frequently electrodes that are located either on the epicardium or subcutaneously. ICDs can deliver antitachycardia pacing even while charging internal capacitors in preparation for automatically shocking the heart. After charging and before shocking, the ICD reexamines the heart rate to see if VT is still present. If VT is reconfirmed, a shock is delivered to the heart. Even ICDs with single leads have algorithms that are able to differentiate supraventricular tachycardia (SVT) from VT based on the morphology of the intracardiac signal, the suddenness of onset, and the regularity of the ventricular rhythm. Other ICDs have both an atrial lead and a ventricular lead(s), which greatly enhances their capacity to distinguish VT from other rhythms such as atrial fibrillation with rapid response, sinus tachycardia, and other forms of SVT. This greatly diminishes the incidence of inappropriate shocks or therapies that could be delivered when the heart rate increases because of SVT rather than VT. Some ICDs offer atrial therapies for treating SVT, atrial flutter, and atrial fibrillation in addition to shocking and pacing therapies for VT. Some ICD systems incorporate both right and left ventricular pacing leads, enabling biventricular pacing (also known as cardiac resynchronization) that produces greater synchrony than right ventricular pacing alone. Biventricular pacing ICD systems improve the survival of patients with left bundle branch block and congestive heart failure.[36]

ICDs have been found to reduce total mortality when used in patients who are at high risk of developing lethal VT or VF (Table 21-5, Table 21-6, and Table 21-7). For example, patients with a history of cardiac arrest or syncope from VT in the absence of transient or correctible factors are at high risk for a lethal recurrence. In these patients, ICD therapy serves as secondary prevention. In addition, patients who have never had a cardiac arrest or syncope from VT might still be at high risk if they have characteristics such as severe left ventricular systolic dysfunction, hypertrophic cardiomyopathy with complications

(text continues on page 597)

TABLE 21-5: Trials of the Efficacy of ICD Therapy for Primary Prevention of Death in Patients with Left Ventricular Dysfunction

Trial (Year)	N	Inclusion Criteria	Comparison	Primary Endpoint	Annual Mortality Rate in Controls (%)	Main Findings
Multicenter Automatic Defibrillator Implantation Trial (MADIT) (1996)	196	Age 25-80 yr, NYHA I-III, EF<0.35, nonrecent MI (>3 wk) or CABG (>3 mo), spontaneous NSVT, and inducible VT	ICD vs. best medical therapy that could include amiodarone	All-cause mortality	17	56% risk reduction in primary endpoint (P = 0.009) with ICD 22.8% absolute risk reduction
Multicenter Unsustained Tachycardia Trial (MUSTT) (1999)	704	Age < 80 yr, NYHA I, II, or III, EF <0.40, nonrecent MI (>4 days), spontaneous NSVT, and inducible VT	ICD vs. antiarrhythmic therapy (amiodarone and class I agents)	All-cause mortality	13	76% relative reduction in primary endpoint (P<0.001) with ICD 23% absolute risk reduction
Second Multicenter Automatic Defibrillator Implantation Trial (MADIT-II) (2002)	1232	NYHA I-III, EF <0.30, remote MI (>1 mo)	ICD vs. best medical therapy	All-cause mortality	10	31% relative reduction in primary endpoint (P = .02) with ICD 5.4% absolute risk reduction

CABG: coronary artery bypass graft surgery, EF: ejectionf raction, ICD: implantable cardioverter defibrillator, MI: myocardial infarction, NSVT: non-sustained ventricular tachycardia, NYHA: New York Heart Association, PVC: premature ventricular contraction, VT: ventricular tachycardia.

Amiodarone Versus Implantable Cardioverter-Defibrillator Trial (AMIOVERT) (2003)	103	NYHA I-IV, EF <0.35, dilated cardiomyopathy, nonsustained VT	ICD vs. best medical therapy	All-cause mortality	4	No significant alteration (P = .8) with ICD 1.7% absolute risk reduction
Cardiomyopathy Trial (CAT) (2002)	104	NYHA II-III, EF <0.30, dilated cardiomyopathy, recent onset heart failure (<9 mo)	ICD vs. best medical therapy	All-cause mortality	4	No significant alteration (P = .6) with ICD 5.4% absolute risk reduction
Comparison of Medical Therapy, Pacing, and Defibrillation in Heart Failure (COMPANION) (2004)	903 1676 458	NYHA III-IV, EF <0.35, nonrecent MI or CABG (>60 days), QRS >120 msec, PR >150 msec, recent heart failure hospitalization (<12 mo), and nonrecent onset of heart failure (>6 mo)	Resynchronization ICD vs. best medical therapy	All-cause death or hospitalization	19	20% relative reduction in primary endpoint (P = .01) with resynchronization ICD 7.3% absolute risk reduction

(continued)

TABLE 21-5: Trials of the Efficacy of ICD Therapy for Primary Prevention of Death in Patients with Left Ventricular Dysfunction *(continued)*

Trial (Year)	N	Inclusion Criteria	Comparison	Primary Endpoint	Annual Mortality Rate in Controls (%)	Main Findings
Sudden Cardiac Death Heart Failure Trial (SCD-HeFT) (2005)	1676	NYHA II-III, EF <0.35, nonrecent MI or revascularization (>30 days), nonrecent heart failure onset (>3 mo)	ICD vs. placebo	All-cause mortality	7	23% relative reduction in primary endpoint ($P < .01$) with ICD 6.8% absolute risk reduction
Defibrillators in Non-Ischemic Cardiomyopathy Treatment Evaluation (DEFINITE) (2005)	458	NYHA I-III, EF <0.35, dilated cardiomyopathy, nonsustained VT or >10 PVCs/hr	ICD vs. best medical therapy	All-cause mortality	7	35% relative reduction in primary endpoint ($P = .08$) with ICD 5.2% absolute risk reduction

From Exner DV. Clinical trials of defibrillator therapy. In Ellenbogen KA, Kay GN, Lau C-P, Wilkoff BL. Clinical Cardiac Pacing, Defibrillation, and Resynchronization Therapy. Philadelphia, PA. WB Saunders, 2007.

TABLE 21-6: Trials of the Efficacy of ICD Therapy for Secondary Prevention of Death in Patients with a History of Sustained or Symptomatic VT or VF

Trial (Year)	N	Inclusion Criteria	Comparison	Primary Endpoint	Annual Mortality Rate in Controls (%)	Main Findings
Antiarrhythmics vs. Implantable Defibrillators (1999)	1016	Resuscitated VF, sustained VT and syncope, or sustained VT with EF <0.40 and severe symptoms; no reversible cause	ICD vs. antiarrhythmic drugs (amiodarone)	All-cause mortality	12	31% relative reduction in primary endpoint (P<0.02) with ICD 8.2% absolute risk reduction
Canadian Implantable Defibrillator Study (CIDS) (2000)	659	Resuscitated VF, sustained VT and EF< 0.35, or unmonitored syncope with subsequent spontaneous or inducible VT, no reversible cause	ICD vs. amiodarone	All-cause mortality	10	20% relative reduction in primary endpoint (P = 0.1) with ICD 4.3% absolute risk reduction
Cardiac Arrest Study (CASH) (2000)	228	Cardiac arrest secondary to VT or VF not related to a reversible cause	ICD vs. drug therapy (amiodarone, metoprolol, propafenone)	All-cause mortality	9	23% relative reduction in primary endpoint (P = 0.2) with ICD 8.1% absolute risk reduction

From Exner, D. V.: Clinical trials of defibrillator therapy. In Ellenbogen, K. A., Kay, G. N., Lau, C-P, Wilkoff, B L.: Clinical Cardiac Pacing, Defibrillation, and Resynchronization Therapy. Philadelphia, PA.: WB Saunders, 2007.

TABLE 21-7: Trials of the Efficacy of ICD Therapy for Primary Prevention of Death in Patients with Recent Myocardial Infarction or Undergoing Coronary Artery Bypass Surgery

Trial (Year)	N	Inclusion Criteria	Comparison	Primary Endpoint	Annual Mortality Rate in Controls (%)	Main Findings
CABG-Patch Trial (1996)	900	EF <0.35, undergoing CABG, abnormal signal-averaged ECG	ICD vs. best medical therapy	All-cause mortality	8	No significant alteration (P = 0.6) with ICD 1.7% absolute increase in risk with ICD
Defibrillators in Acute Myocardial Infarction Trial	674	NYHA I-III, EF <0.35%, recent MI (6-40 days), depressed heart rate variability or elevated average 24-hr heart rate	ICD vs. best medical therapy	All-cause mortality	7	No significant alteration (P = 0.7) with ICD 1.7% absolute increase in risk with ICD
Beta Blocker Strategy plus ICD (BEST-ICD) (2005)	148	EF <0.3 *and* one or more of the following: >10 PVCs/hr, reduced heart rate variability, abnormal signal-averaged ECG; Recent MI (<1 mo)	Invasive strategy (ICD if inducible VT, otherwise medical therapy) vs. conservative therapy (medical therapy)	All-cause therapy	14	No significant alteration (P = 0.4) with an invasive vs. a conservative strategy 2.4% absolute increase in the primary endpoint with an invasive strategy

(e.g., extreme septal hypertrophy, history of syncope, nonsustained VT, or family history of sudden cardiac death), or familial sudden cardiac death syndromes, such as certain forms of the long QT syndrome, Brugada syndromes, catecholaminergic polymorphic ventricular tachycardia, or arrhythmogenic right ventricular dysplasia. ICD therapy in these patients serves as primary prevention.

ICDs have drawbacks, however. They are expensive and require surgery for implantation. The surgical technique is similar to that employed during pacemaker implantation. Surgical risks include bleeding complications, infection, lead dislodgement, and pneumothorax. ICDs do not always prevent syncope because it can take 10 to 20 seconds for the device to complete a cycle of arrhythmia detection, capacitor charging, and shock delivery. Also, shocks delivered to conscious patients are not well tolerated. Defibrillators, unfortunately, may deliver inappropriate shocks when the patient is not in VT. For example, a rapid ventricular rate during atrial fibrillation or sinus tachycardia can cause the rate threshold for detection of VT to be exceeded, triggering a shock. In fact, the first shock or two may cause the patient enough distress to cause the heart rate during atrial fibrillation or sinus tachycardia to remain elevated so that multiple shocks are triggered.

ICD therapy has been associated with increased hospitalizations for congestive heart failure.[37] This has been attributed to right ventricular pacing, which activates the ventricles in an asynchronous pattern similar to that produced by left bundle branch block. Taking care to minimize ventricular pacing from the defibrillator can mitigate this problem.[38]

ICDs can malfunction as a result of lead dislodgement, poor connection between the lead and the pulse generator, lead fracture, or breakdown of insulation of the lead. Rarely, the ICD pulse generator may malfunction because of a flaw in manufacturing. Occasionally, manufacturers have issued recalls or technical warnings, causing physicians and their patients to have to weigh whether to remove and replace a possibly defective device.

Catheter Ablation

This is an excellent nonpharmacologic option for some types of VT. The goal of catheter ablation is to destroy the substrate of the tachycardia with as small a lesion as possible. The first step in catheter ablation is to position an electrode catheter so that its ablating electrode is adjacent to the arrhythmogenic substrate, through a process called mapping. The ablating electrode is almost always at the distal end of the catheter and is usually larger than the other electrodes on the catheter. For example, the ablating electrode is usually 4 to 10 mm in length instead of the 1 or 2 mm length of pacing or stimulating electrodes.

Once it is determined that the ablating electrode is in a suitable location, adjacent either to the focus of a tachycardia or to a vulnerable point of a reentrant circuit, up to 100 Watts of radiofrequency electrical energy (150 kHz to 1 MHz) is then delivered through the electrode to a reference electrode patch on the patient's chest wall. The purpose is to heat the myocardium adjacent to the ablating electrode and to destroy the arrhythmogenic substrate. Radiofrequency catheter ablation (RFCA) creates injury by heating myocardium at the electrode tissue interface to a temperature of up to 70° C. The residuum of RFCA is a well-demarcated spherical or oval zone of coagulation necrosis.

Ablation can also be performed by removing heat from cardiac tissues, through a process known as cryotherapy. However, cryotherapy catheters are presently too stiff to permit mapping and ablation of VT. Other catheter-based approaches are undergoing evaluation, including microwave energy and ultrasound.

Different mapping techniques are used for different types of VT. For VTs that arise from a small focus, such as the idiopathic VT that arises from the right ventricular outflow tract, the electrophysiologist uses activation-mapping and pace-mapping. In activation-mapping the ablating electrode is positioned at the site in the ventricle that is activated earliest during each beat of tachycardia. This is the site from which the VT arises. Local activation of this site is usually 20 to 40 milliseconds earlier than the onset of the QRS in the 12-lead surface ECG during VT. In pace-mapping, the concept is that pacing at the exact focus where the VT originates should duplicate the QRS morphology of the clinical VT. The chance for a successful ablation at such a site will be high.[39] Success rates of at least 90% have been reported for ablation of these VTs.[39]

In the case of idiopathic VTs arising from the inferoseptal wall of the left ventricle, the ablating catheter is also positioned at the site of earliest activation during VT. The electrical signal at this site usually has a distinct high-frequency potential, similar to a His bundle potential, which appears before the onset of the QRS on the surface ECG. This has led to speculation that this VT may be caused by reentry involving the left posterior fascicle. Again, success rates of 90% can be expected for ablation of this kind of VT.

In the case of bundle branch reentrant VT, the ablating electrode is positioned near the distal right bundle branch, which can easily be found by first locating the His bundle and then moving the tip of the catheter more distally until the distal electrode records the electrical signal of the distal right bundle branch. This potential looks like a His bundle potential, but its timing is much closer to the onset of the surface QRS during sinus rhythm than is the His bundle potential. The reentry circuit of bundle branch reentrant VT is vulnerable at this point, and often this VT can be eliminated by an application of energy here without producing complete heart block (although permanent right bundle branch block will be produced).[40] Success rates of close to 100% may be expected for this kind of VT. Unfortunately, many patients with bundle branch reentrant VT have severe left ventricular dysfunction and are subject to other forms of VT that are not eliminated by ablation of the right bundle branch.

Mapping techniques are different in the case of VTs that originate from the region of a previous infarction. These VTs are usually caused by reentry circuits that include a zone of slow conduction that passes through the scar. During VT this zone produces an activation signal that occurs after one surface QRS complex and before the next (that is, when the bulk of normal ventricular myocardium is in diastole—therefore, this signal is called a "diastolic potential"). Usually there are other areas in the scar that also conduct slowly and exhibit diastolic potentials during VT, even though they do not participate in the reentry circuit. Therefore, diastolic potentials are not a specific finding. In order to determine if a site with diastolic potentials is part of the reentry circuit, pacing stimuli are delivered through the mapping/ablating catheter at a rate slightly faster than the tachycardia. If the site is within the reentry circuit, the pacing stimuli should produce paced QRS complexes with morphology similar to the QRS complexes during VT; and during pacing the interval from the stimulus to the onset of the paced QRS should be identical to the interval from the diastolic potential to the QRS during VT. If the site is in a zone of slow conduction that is not part of the reentry circuit, then the interval of pacing stimulus to the onset of paced QRS is much longer than the interval of diastolic potential to the onset of QRS during VT.[41, 42] The success rate of ablation for treatment of postinfarction VT is highly dependent on patient selection. Higher success rates (perhaps 80 to 90%) are achieved in patients who have one slow, hemodynamically stable VT. Lower success rates are achieved in patients with multiple different types of VT (that is, a history of VTs with different rates and morphologies), severe left ventricular dysfunction, and rapid, hemodynamically unstable VT.

Catheter ablation carries a small risk. Complete heart block can be produced by inadvertent destruction of the normal AV conduction system. Other complications can include vascular damage (hematoma, arteriovenous fistula, or pseudoaneurysm), cardiac perforation with tamponade, thromboembolism, valvular damage (particularly when mapping or ablating catheters are advanced retrogradely across the aortic valve), infection, and adverse reactions to drugs used during the procedure. The risk of a serious complication is less than 5%. Catheter ablation procedures can last many hours unless an arbitrary limit is placed on the permissible duration of the procedure. Exposure to fluoroscopic radiation can be considerable and is a concern for both patient and staff.

Cardiac Surgery

This technique can be used to treat VT. The site from which the VT emerges can be identified through EP mapping. Once it is localized, it can be surgically excised, ablated with radiofrequency energy, or frozen by cryosurgery.[43] An alternative approach is to use visual guidance and remove scarred endocardium, for the reentrant loop seems to pass through endocardial scar in most cases.[44] With either approach the efficacy rate is approximately 75%, with a perioperative mortality rate of 10 to 15%. This is a reasonable therapeutic option for patients with discrete anterior or apical aneurysms, especially if the patient might benefit hemodynamically from aneurysmectomy or if the patient needs concomitant coronary bypass surgery. Inferior wall aneurysms are not as accessible to the surgeon, and inferior wall surgery is more likely to compromise the papillary muscles and mitral apparatus. Other therapeutic options, such as the implantable defibrillator, are more attractive than endocardial resection for patients with inferior aneurysms.

Emergent Management of VT

Patients who present with wide complex tachycardia (WCT) must undergo scrutiny into whether they have VT or one of the conditions that mimics VT: supraventricular tachycardia with aberrant conduction, rapid ventricular pacing, or electrocardiographic artifact. The ECGs obtained during sinus rhythm and during tachycardia should be inspected and compared. The diagnosis of VT is made with certainty if atrioventricular dissociation is present during tachycardia, but this finding is apparent in only 21% of ECGs obtained during VT. Other electrocardiographic criteria have also been found to be very helpful (see Table 21-1). When a diagnosis cannot be reached with certainty using the ECGs, EP testing can be definitive, as long as the clinical tachycardia can be induced in the laboratory.

At the same time, and with the highest priority, the hemodynamic status of the patient must be evaluated. Cardiac arrest from VT or VF must be managed with cardiopulmonary resuscitation, including airway management, mechanical ventilation, chest compressions, and immediate electrical defibrillation with 120 to 200 J biphasic shock or 360 J monophasic shock. In general, successful defibrillation is closely correlated to the time to delivery of countershock.[45] If the patient remains in pulseless VT despite these measures, 1.0 mg of 1:10,000 epinephrine or 40 units of vasopressin should be given intravenously, followed by another attempt at electrical defibrillation. This dose of epinephrine should be repeated every five minutes while the patient remains in pulseless VT or VF. When VT persists, either intravenous amiodarone (a bolus of 300 mg followed if necessary by an additional 150 mg) or lidocaine (an initial intravenous bolus of 1 mg/kg followed by repeated boluses of 0.5 mg/kg every eight minutes to a total of 3 mg/kg) may be given. Throughout this process, the utmost attention must be paid to recognizing and correcting metabolic abnormalities. Once an adequate rhythm is restored, evidence for underlying myocardial ischemia or infarction should be sought; this may dictate the need for specific interventions such as intra-aortic balloon pumping or emergent coronary revascularization. Mild hypothermia (cooling to 32° to 34° C) can increase the likelihood of the patient's making a good neurologic recovery.

Many episodes of VT do not cause cardiovascular collapse. If the patient is hemodynamically stable, a 12-lead ECG and rhythm strip should be obtained and the diagnosis of VT confirmed from among the other causes of wide QRS complex tachycardia. The conscious patient with VT does not need to be electrically cardioverted on an emergent basis, but preparations can be made for elective synchronized cardioversion. In the meantime, intravenous amiodarone, lidocaine, or procainamide can be administered in the hope of a pharmacologic conversion. Rarely, the consultant may have the option of pace-terminating the episode of VT (in patients who have an implanted pacing device or temporary ventricular pacing lead).

Certain types of VT are refractory to electrical shock and to the usual antiarrhythmic drugs. These include VT arising from hyperkalemia, proarrhythmia due to flecainide or propafenone, or digitalis intoxication. Extreme hyperkalemia (with serum potassium concentration >8 mEq/L) can cause an incessant VT with a sinusoidal morphology. It should be treated with intravenous calcium (10 to 30 mL of 10% calcium gluconate given over one to five minutes), hypertonic glucose plus insulin, and sodium bicarbonate (44 to 132 mEq, or 1 to 3 ampules). Flecainide and propafenone cause a similar VT that occasionally responds to lidocaine but can be highly refractory. Theoretically, this arrhythmia might respond best to hypertonic sodium, which would counteract the sodium channel blocking effects of the flecainide or propafenone.[46, 47] Another VT that is refractory to direct-current shock and to most AAD is a rare form of verapamil-responsive VT, that occurs in young patients with no identifiable heart disease.[48] The QRS morphology of this VT resembles right bundle branch block with left axis deviation. This VT provides an exception to the rule that verapamil has no role in the management of VT. Finally, refractory VT or VF can be the terminal event in patients with truly end-stage heart disease in which mechanical cardiac function is so severely diminished that the patient would not survive even if the VT could be terminated. In this situation the arrhythmia is called secondary VF or VT.

VT from digitalis intoxication may require management with antidigoxin antigen binding fragments (Fab). The dose of antidigoxin Fab to be delivered can be calculated by calculating the total body load of digoxin as the serum concentration of digoxin (in ng/L) multiplied by the volume of distribution (equal to the patient's weight in kilograms multiplied by 5.6 L/kg). The total body load of digoxin is then divided by 600 (the number of nanograms of digoxin bound by each vial) to determine the number of vials that should be administered to the patient. Antidigoxin Fab also binds digitoxin, and the same calculations can be used to determine the number of vials to be given, except that the volume of distribution of digitoxin is 0.56 L/kg. Patients usually respond clinically to the antibody fragments within 30 minutes of administration.[49] The serum concentration of digoxin climbs after administration of the antibody fragments because they remove digoxin from extravascular binding sites. The Fab-digitalis complexes are excreted by the kidneys and have a half-life of 16 to 20 hours in patients with normal renal function. It is not clear how the complexes are eliminated in patients with renal insufficiency; however, such patients have responded well to antidigoxin Fab.

Once the presenting episode of VT or VF has been terminated, the next step is to prevent recurrence. Success depends on accurate identification of the specific type of VT that is being treated. The patient must be screened for transient or reversible causes such as infarction, ischemia, electrolyte abnormalities, and drug toxicity. Acute myocardial infarction (AMI) is associated with different types of VT, including a rapid polymorphic VT associated with normal QT interval that occurs during the first few minutes of AMI and sometimes when the patient has severe left ventricular systolic dysfunction or ongoing ischemia. There may be recurrences of this VT in the short term, which can respond to lidocaine, amiodarone, beta-blocking drugs, and intra-aortic balloon pumping. In the long run, this VT is not likely to recur when severe left ventricular systolic dysfunction is not present, especially if reperfusion can be provided. A slow monomorphic VT or accelerated idioventricular rhythm typically occurs in the subacute phase of AMI (4 to 36 hours after the onset of the AMI). It carries a benign prognosis and doesn't require acute or chronic therapy. In the posthospitalization phase of AMI, lethal postinfarction VT is less likely to occur if patients are treated with beta blocking drugs. The prognosis of these patients is also improved if their coronary risk factors are controlled.

It is important to recognize when acute ischemia has been the cause of VT or VF. A typical presentation would be the occurrence of VT or VF during exercise in a patient who is then identified as having coronary insufficiency. If revascularization can be performed and left ventricular systolic function is preserved, then ICD therapy may not be necessary. The same can be true when VT has been secondary to drug toxicity. And if electrolyte abnormalities appear to be contributing to the VT, they must be identified and corrected. However, the physician should not expect that the correction of electrolytes is sufficient to prevent recurrence of VT. In the registry of the Antiarrhythmics vs. Implantable Defibrillators (AVID) study, a high mortality rate was found in patients whose physicians believed that their VT was caused by a reversible electrolyte imbalance and who therefore were not given an ICD.[50]

Many patients with VT do not have an identifiable correctable cause of their arrhythmia. Effective antiarrhythmic therapy for each patient must be identified prior to discharge from a monitored setting. The physician should not be falsely encouraged by an absence of VT during monitoring after conversion of an episode of sustained VT; it is the nature of some cases of sustained VT to recur after long periods of remission. As described previously in this chapter, EP testing is often used at this point to confirm that the patient is susceptible to VT and not SVT with aberrant conduction. EP testing is more useful for patients who have had VT or a sustained wide complex tachycardia than it is for patients who have had VF.[51] In the former group of patients, EP testing can identify which patients are suitable candidates for catheter ablation. These include patients with bundle branch reentry and patients with a single inducible VT that is hemodynamically stable enough to permit careful mapping. Patients with structurally normal hearts and idiopathic monomorphic VT (such as tachycardia arising from the right or left ventricular outflow tract or tachycardia arising from the inferoseptal left ventricle) are especially good candidates for catheter ablation.

Patients with a history of sustained VT in the setting of severe left ventricular systolic dysfunction are best treated with ICD therapy, since ICDs have been shown to improve survival in patients with ejection fractions less than 35%, even when no VT has ever been previously documented.[19] Rarely, a temporary exception might be made if the VT is curable by catheter ablation and the left ventricular systolic dysfunction is highly likely to be reversible, such as in cases in which the patient might have tachycardia-mediated tachycardia or when the patient has left ventricular systolic dysfunction secondary to a large territory of ischemic but viable myocardium that can be addressed by revascularization. If such a patient is not treated with an ICD, there must be follow-up to determine if left ventricular function has returned to normal. In general, though, ICD therapy is the first line of therapy for patients who have had sustained VT in the setting of severe left ventricular dysfunction. If VT recurs, then an AAD can be used to reduce the frequency of VT and thereby reduce the frequency of shocks from the ICD.

Polymorphic VT arises in different clinical settings. It appears in various genetic syndromes such as the long QT syndrome, the Brugada syndrome, the catecholaminergic polymorphic VT syndrome, and the short QT syndrome. It can appear in patients with acquired long QT syndromes such as are caused by Class IA and Class III drugs, neurologic disorders (subarachnoid hemorrhage, stroke, or encephalitis), hypomagnesemia, and hypokalemia. It also can appear in acute ischemia; therefore patients with polymorphic VT should be screened for coronary insufficiency unless another cause is apparent.

Torsades de Pointes (TdP)

This process receives its name, which translates as "twisting of the points," from the manner in which the QRS complexes appear to rotate around the isoelectric baseline, with variability in axis and morphology. It often occurs in the setting of a prolonged QT interval. Other features of TdP include episodes that are often nonsustained. Some forms of TdP are catecholamine-dependent, while others are pause-dependent. Often there is T-wave alternans prior to episodes, and occasionally the episodes degenerate into VF.

The acute management of TdP includes electrical cardioversion to terminate sustained VT, prevention of recurrences by beta blockade, correction of electrolyte abnormalities, withdrawal of offending drugs, pharmacologic doses of magnesium sulfate,[53] and temporary pacing. Lidocaine can be effective in the treatment of the LQT3 form of TdP. Procainamide, quinidine, disopyramide, sotalol, dofetilide, and ibutilide should be avoided because they can further prolong the QT interval and exacerbate the VT. As a last resort in a patient with a storm of polymorphic VT, amiodarone can be tried. In such a desperate case, the patient should be screened for ischemia, and consideration should be given to emergency revascularization or intra-aortic balloon pumping.

Congenital TdP and Long QT Syndrome

The chronic management of patients with congenital TdP and long QT syndrome begins with beta blockade. If VT or syncope recurs despite beta blockade, then ICD therapy should be recommended. Beta blockers are more likely to be effective in the LQT1 form of TdP than in other forms. The LQT2 variant is especially dangerous, especially in female patients. Pause-dependent TdP (including most of the commonly acquired forms) can be treated by pacing with or without concomitant beta blockade, although if a pacemaker is to be implanted it would be reasonable to use an ICD rather than a pacemaker.

Brugada Syndrome

Brugada syndrome and the catecholaminergic polymorphic VT syndrome also produce episodes of polymorphic VT. Since neither has been found to reliably respond to antiarrhythmic drugs, symptomatic patients and high-risk asymptomatic patients are best treated with implantation of an ICD. Asymptomatic patients are considered to be high risk if they have documented VT or otherwise unexplained syncope.

Hypertrophic Cardiomyopathy

Patients with hypertrophic cardiomyopathy can be at increased risk for lethal VT. High-risk characteristics include a family history of sudden cardiac death, a very thick interventricular septum, the presence of nonsustained VT, and otherwise unexplained syncope. ICD therapy is warranted in high-risk patients.

High-Risk Patients without Documented VT

Patients with unexplained palpitations, near-syncope or syncope should be evaluated to find out if VT is the cause of any of their symptoms. Evaluation of these patients includes electrocardiographic monitoring and provocative testing. Monitoring can be performed in the hospital or on an outpatient basis with ambulatory electrocardiographic recording, transtelephonic arrhythmia monitoring, implantable event recording, or continuous outpatient telemetry. Provocative testing might include exercise stress testing, epinephrine infusion to test for long QT syndrome, procainamide infusion to test for the Brugada syndrome, and electrophysiologic (EP) testing. Patients with syncope should also be screened for structural heart disease and left ventricular systolic dysfunction since, for example, ICD therapy would be offered to patients who have otherwise unexplained syncope in the context of severe left ventricular dysfunction or hypertrophic cardiomyopathy.

All patients with heart disease should be evaluated for the presence of characteristics that reveal a significant risk for lethal ventricular arrhythmias (Table 21-8). Measurement of left ventricular function is particularly important. Good left ventricular function is associated with a good prognosis even in patients with nonsustained VT as long as there are no other markers of high risk. The presence of severe left ventricular dysfunction alone is evidence of high risk for developing lethal VT and can be an indication for placement of an implantable cardioverter-defibrillator (ICD). The MADIT-2 and SCD-HeFT studies showed that ICDs improve the chances for survival in patients with persistent severe

---

TABLE 21-8: Characteristics That Indicate Increased Risk of Lethal Ventricular Tachyarrhythmias

LV dysfunction (EF −30 or 35%)
Symptomatic congestive heart failure
Unrevascularized CAD with myocardial ischemia
Hypertrophic cardiomyopathy with any of the following:
   History of syncope
   History of nonsustained or sustained VT
   Markedly thickened septum, greater than 25 mm
   Genetic markers of mutations that are high risk for VT
   Family history of SCD
Familial disorders of VT
   Long QT syndrome
   Arrhythmogenic RV dysplasia
   Brugada syndrome

CAD: coronary artery disease; EF: ejection fraction; LV: left ventricular; RV: right ventricular; SCD: sudden cardiac death; VT: ventricular tachycardia

left ventricular dysfunction (left ventricular ejection fraction less than 0.30 or 0.35, respectively). The COMPANION trial revealed that biventricular pacing defibrillators improve the chances for survival in patients with persistent severe left ventricular dysfunction and left bundle branch block.

ICDs have not been found to improve the survival of patients with left ventricular dysfunction in certain specific conditions. In CABG-Patch, patients with left ventricular dysfunction who were undergoing coronary artery bypass were randomized to receive or not to receive an ICD at the time of surgery. In DINAMIT, patients who had left ventricular dysfunction in the setting of recent (less than one month) acute myocardial infarction were randomized to receive or not to receive an ICD. ICDs did not improve survival in either of these studies. It is thought that left ventricular function improved sufficiently in enough subjects in these trials to reduce the overall risk of death from VT or VF so that the potential benefit of ICD therapy was reduced relative to the risk of ICD therapy.

TAKE-HOME MESSAGE

A few generalizations about the management of VT are possible. Reversible causes of VT should be identified and corrected. These include ischemia, drug toxicity, and electrolyte abnormalities. Patients with left ventricular dysfunction should be treated with an angiotensin converting enzyme inhibitor or angiotensin receptor blocker, and metoprolol or carvedilol. Reversible forms of left ventricular dysfunction should be identified and treated, including alcoholic cardiomyopathy and tachycardia-mediated cardiomyopathy. Antiarrhythmic drugs, catheter or surgical ablation, and ICDs may be used, alone and in combination, depending on the patient's condition.

The selection of optimal therapy for a particular patient can be a challenge. Paradoxes abound. For example, ICDs are valuable in treating patients with persistent left ventricular systolic dysfunction but no better than placebo in treating patients with left ventricular systolic dysfunction in the setting of a recent myocardial infarction or patients with left ventricular systolic dysfunction who are undergoing bypass surgery. Similarly, beta blockers are very effective treatment for patients with the LQT1 variant of the long QT syndrome but are relatively ineffective in patients with the LQT2 and LQT3 variants. Not every one with a history of sustained VT should receive an ICD; catheter ablation is a better option for patients with idiopathic VT arising from the right or left ventricular outflow tracts or inferoseptal left ventricle. The risks and potential benefits of available therapies fluctuate over time. Technologic progress usually is beneficial but occasionally is unexpectedly detrimental, such as when a newly designed ICD lead turns out to be unreliable.

The algorithms for managing patients who have VT or who are at risk of developing VT are therefore complex and continuously evolving.

References

1. Harris, L., Downar, E., Mickleborough, L., et al.: Activation sequence of ventricular tachycardia: Endocardial and epicardial mapping studies in the human ventricle. J Am Coll Cardiol. 1987;10:1040–1047.
2. Wieland, J. M., Marchlinski, F. E.: Electrocardiographic response of digoxin-toxic fascicular tachycardia to Fab fragments: Implications for tachycardia mechanism. PACE. 1986;9:727–738.
3. Caceres, J., Jazayeri, M., McKinnic, J., et al.: Sustained bundle branch reentry as a mechanism of clinical tachycardia. Circulation. 1989; 79:256–270.
4. Benson, D. W., MacRae, C. A., Vesely, M. R., et al.: Missense mutation in the pore region of HERG causes familial long QT syndrome. Circulation. 1996;93:1791–1795.
5. Lerman, B. B.: Response of nonreentrant catecholamine-mediated ventricular tachycardia to endogenous adenosine and acetylcholine: Evidence for myocardial receptor-mediated effects. Circulation. 1993; 87:382–390.
6. Lerman, B. B., Stein, K., Engelstein, E. D., et al.: Mechanism of repetitive monomorphic ventricular tachycardia. Circulation. 1995;92:421–429.
7. Okumura, K., Matsuyama, K., Miyagi, H., et al.: Entrainment of idiopathic ventricular tachycardia of left ventricular origin with evidence for reentry with an area of slow conduction and effect of verapamil. Am J Cardiol. 1988;62:727–732.
8. Nam, G. B., Burashnikov, A., Antzelevitch, C.: Cellular mechanisms underlying the development of catecholaminergic ventricular tachycardia. Circulation. 2005;111:2727–2733.
9. Stecker, E. C., Vickers, C., Waltz, J., et al.: Population-based analysis of sudden cardiac death with and without left ventricular systolic dysfunction: two-year findings from the Oregon Sudden Unexpected Death Study. J Am Coll Cardiol. 2006;47:1161-1166.
10. Mason, J. W. for the Electrophysiologic Study Versus Electrocardiographic Monitoring Investigators: A comparison of electrophysiologic testing with Holter monitoring to predict antiarrhythmic-drug efficacy for ventricular tachyarrhythmias. N Engl J Med. 1993;329:445–451.
11. Kudenchuk, P. J., Cobb, L. A., Copass, M. K., et al.: Amiodarone for resuscitation after out-of-hospital cardiac arrest due to ventricular fibrillation. N Engl J Med. 1999;341:871–878.
12. Dorian, P., Cass, D., Schwartz, B., et al.: Amiodarone as compared with lidocaine for shock-resistant ventricular fibrillation. N Engl J Med. 2002;346:884–890.
13. Freemantle, N., Cleland, J., Young, P., et al.: Beta blockade after myocardial infarction: Systematic review and meta regression analysis. BMJ. 1999;318:1730–1737.
14. Pacifico, A., Hohnloser, S. H., Williams, J. H., et al.: Prevention of implantable-defibrillator shocks by treatment with sotalol. N Engl J Med. 1999;340:1855–1862.

15. Waldo, A.L., Camm, A.J., de Ruyter, H., et al.: Effects of d-sotalol on mortality in patients with left ventricular dysfunction after recent and remote myocardial infarction. Lancet. 1996;348:7-12.

16. The CASCADE Investigators. Randomized antiarrhythmic drug therapy in survivors of sudden cardiac death (the CASCADE study). Am J Cardiol. 1993;72:280–287.

17. Julian, D. G., Camm, A. J., Frangin, G., et al.: Randomized trial of the effect of amiodarone on mortality in patients with left ventricular dysfunction after recent myocardial infarction: EMIAT. Lancet. 1997; 349:667–674.

18. Cairns, J., Connolly, S., Roberts, R., et al.: Randomized trial of outcome after myocardial infarction in patients with frequent or repetitive ventricular premature depolarizations: CAMIAT. Lancet. 1997; 349:675–682.

19. Klein, H., Auricchio, A., Reek, S., et al.: New primary prevention trials of sudden cardiac death in patients with left ventricular dysfunction: SCD-HeFT and MADIT-II. Am J Cardiol. 1999;83:91D–97D.

20. Connolly, S. J., Dorian, P., Roberts, R. S., et al.: Comparison of beta blockers, amiodarone plus beta blockers, or sotalol for prevention of shocks from implantable cardioverter defibrillators. The OPTIC Study: a randomized trial. JAMA. 2006;295:165–171.

21. Doval, H.C., Nul, D.R., Grancelli, H.O., et al.: Randomised trial of low-dose amiodarone in severe congestive heart failure. Grupo de Estudio de la Sobrevida en la Insuficiencia Cardiaca en Argentina (GESICA). Lancet. 1994;344:493-498.

22. Singh, S.N., Fletcher, R.D., Fisher, S.G., et al.: Amiodarone in patients with congestive heart failure and asymptomatic ventricular arrhythmia. Survival trial of antiarrhythmic therapy in congestive heart failure. N Engl J Med. 1995;333:77-82.

23. Winkle, R. A., Mason, J., Griffin, J. C., et al.: Malignant ventricular tachyarrhythmias associated with the use of encainide. Am Heart J. 1981;102:857–864.

24. Chen, P. S., Shibata, N., Dixon, E. G., et al.: Activation during ventricular defibrillation in open-chest dogs. Evidence of complete cessation and regeneration of ventricular fibrillation after unsuccessful shocks. J Clin Invest. 1986;77:810–823.

25. Davy, J. M., Fain, E. S., Dorian, P., et al.: The relationship between successful defibrillation and delivered energy in open-chest dogs: Reappraisal of the "defibrillation threshold" concept. Am Heart J. 1987;113:77–84.

26. Sima, S. J., Kieso, R. A., Fox-Eastham, K. J., et al.: Mechanisms responsible for the decline in thoracic impedance after direct current shock. Am J Physiol. 1989;257:H180.

27. Kerber, R. E., Martins, J. B., Kienzle, M. G., et al.: Energy, current, and success in defibrillation and cardioversion: Clinical studies using an automated impedance-based method of energy adjustment. Circulation. 1988;77:1038–1046.

28. Ujhelyi, M. R., Schur, M., Frede, T., et al.: Differential effects of lidocaine on defibrillation threshold with monophasic versus biphasic shock waveforms. Circulation. 1995;92:1644–1650.

29. Hernandez, R., Mann, D. E., Breckinridge, S., et al.: Effects of flecainide on defibrillation thresholds in the anesthetized dog. J Am Coll Cardiol. 1989;14:777–781.
30. Guarnieri, T., Levine, J. H., Veltri, E. P., et al.: Success of chronic defibrillation and the role of antiarrhythmic drugs with the automatic implantable cardioverter/defibrillator. Am J Cardiol. 1987;60:1061–1064.
31. Jung, W., Manz, M., Pizzulli, L., et al.: Effects of chronic amiodarone therapy on defibrillation threshold. Am J Cardiol. 1992;70:1023–1027.
32. Wang, M., Dorian, P.: DL and D sotalol decrease defibrillation energy requirements. PACE. 1989;12:1522–1529.
33. Ruffy, R., Schechtman, K., Monje, E., et al.: Adrenergically mediated variations in the energy required to defibrillate the heart: Observations in closed-chest, nonanesthetized dogs. Circulation. 1986;73:374–380.
34. Ruffy, R., Monje, E., Schechtman, K.: Facilitation of cardiac defibrillation by aminophylline in the conscious, closed-chest dog. J Electrophysiol. 1988;2:450–454.
35. Babbs, C. F., Whistler, S. J., Kim, G. K. W., et al.: Dependence of defibrillation threshold upon extracellular/intracellular K+ concentrations. J Electrocardiol. 1980;13:73–78.
36. Bristow, M. R., Saxon, L. A., Boehmer, J., et al.: The Comparison of Medical Therapy P, Defibrillation in Heart Failure (COMPANION) Investigators. Cardiac-resynchronization therapy with or without an implantable defibrillator in advanced chronic heart failure. N Engl J Med. 2004;350:2140–2150.
37. Bloomfield, D.M., Steinman, R.C., Namerow, P.B., et al.: Microvolt T-wave alternans distinguishes between patients likely and patients not likely to benefit from implanted cardiac defibrillator therapy: A solution to the Multicenter Automatic Defibrillator Implantation Trial (MADIT) II Conundrum. Circulation. 2004:110:1885–1889.
38. Olshansky, B., Day, J.D., Moore, S., et al.: Is dual-chamber programming inferior to single-chamber programming in an implantable cardioverter-defibrillator? Results of the INTRINSIC RV (Inhibition of Unnecessary RV Pacing With AVSH in ICDs) study. Circulation. 115: 2007; 9–16.
39. Klein, L. S., Shih, H. T., Hackett, F. K., et al.: Radiofrequency catheter ablation of ventricular tachycardia in patients without structural heart disease. Circulation. 1992;85:1666–1674.
40. Tchou, P., Jazayeri, M., Denker, S., et al.: Transcatheter electrical ablation of right bundle branch. A method of treating macroreentrant ventricular tachycardia attributed to bundle branch reentry. Circulation. 1988;78:246–257.
41. Stevenson, W. G., Weiss, J. N., Weiner, I., et al.: Resetting of ventricular tachycardia: Implications for localizing the area of slow conduction. J Am Coll Cardiol. 1988;11:522–529.
42. Fitzgerald, D. M., Friday, K. J., Wah, J., et al.: Electrogram patterns predicting successful catheter ablation of ventricular tachycardia. Circulation. 1988;77:806–814.
43. Horowitz, L. N., Harken, A. H., Kastor, et al.: Ventricular resection guided by epicardial and endocardial mapping for treatment of recurrent ventricular tachycardia. N Engl J Med. 1980;302:589–593.

44. Kehoe, R., Zheutlin, T., Finkelmeler, B., et al.: Visually directed endocardial resection for ventricular arrhythmia: Long term outcome and functional status. J Am Coll Cardiol. 1985;5(suppl 2):497.
45. Kerber, R. E., Samat, W. : Factors influencing the success of ventricular defibrillation in man. Circulation. 1979;60:226–230.
46. Winkelmann, B. R., Leinberger, H.: Life-threatening flecainide toxicity. Ann Intern Med. 1987;106:807–814.
47. Pentel, P. R., Goldsmith, S. R., Salerno, D. M., et al.: Effect of hypertonic sodium bicarbonate on encainide overdose. Am J Cardiol. 1986; 57:878–880.
48. German, L. D., Packer, D. L., Bardy, G. H., et al.: Ventricular tachycardia induced by atrial stimulation in patients without symptomatic cardiac disease. Am J Cardiol. 1983;52:1202–1507.
49. Wenger, T. L., Butler, V. P. Jr, Haber, E., et al.: Treatment of 63 severely digitalis-toxic patients with digoxin-specific antibody fragments. J Am Coll Cardiol. 1985;5:118A.
50. Anderson, J. L., Hallstrom, A. P., Epstein, A. E., et al.: Design and results of the antiarrhythmics vs implantable defibrillators (AVID) registry. Circulation. 1999;99:1692–1699.
51. Poole, J. E., Mathisen, T. L., Kudenchuk, P. J., et al. : Long-term outcome in patients who survive out of hospital ventricular fibrillation and undergo electrophysiologic studies: Evaluation by electrophysiologic subgroups. J Am Coll Cardiol. 1990;16:657–665.

INDEX